Ruppel's
Manual of Pulmonary Function Testing

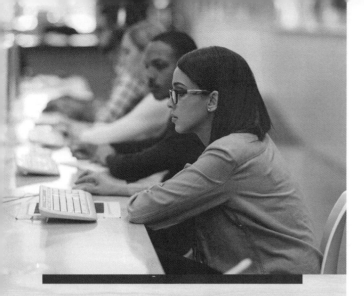

Set a course for success with individualized quizzing

Elsevier Adaptive Quizzing (EAQ) offers a bank of high-quality practice questions that allows students to advance at their own pace — based on their performance — through multiple mastery levels for each chapter, topic, or concept. EAQ integrates seamlessly into the curriculum to help students of all skill levels focus their study time and effectively prepare for class, course exams, and summative exams.

- **Elsevier's trusted, market-leading content** serves as the foundation for all questions, which are written, reviewed, and leveled by experienced educators, item writers, and authors.

- **Detailed rationales for each question and essential test-taking tips and strategies** help students learn how to successfully dissect and tackle different question types and improve test-taking skills for both course exams and summative exams.

- **A robust performance dashboard** highlights usage and performance summaries and areas of strength and weakness tied to topics.

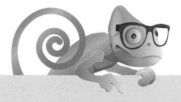

Find out how EAQ can help improve learning and program outcomes!

VISIT
myevolve.us/EAQ

ELSEVIER

Ruppel's
Manual of Pulmonary Function Testing

TWELFTH EDITION

Carl D. Mottram, RRT, RPFT, FAARC
Associate Professor of Medicine
President – PFWConsulting LLC

ELSEVIER

Elsevier
3251 Riverport Lane
St. Louis, Missouri 63043

RUPPEL'S MANUAL OF PULMONARY FUNCTION TESTING,
TWELFTH EDITION

ISBN: 978-0-323-76261-8

Notice

Previous editions copyrighted 2017, 2013, 2009, 2003, 1998, 1994, 1991, 1986, 1982, 1979, 1975.

Senior Content Strategist: Yvonne Alexopoulos
Content Development Specialist: Andrae Akeh
Publishing Services Manager: Shereen Jameel
Senior Project Manager: Manikandan Chandrasekaran
Design Direction: Julia Dummitt

Printed in India

Last digit is the print number: 9   8   7   6   5   4   3   2

Working together
to grow libraries in
developing countries

www.elsevier.com • www.bookaid.org

List of Contributors

The editor(s) would like to acknowledge and offer grateful thanks for the input of all previous editions' contributors, without whom this new edition would not have been possible.

Susan Blonshine, BS, RRT, RPFT, FAARC, AE-C
CEO and President
Management
TechEd Consultants, INC.
Mason, MI

Jeffrey M. Haynes, RRT, RPFT, FAARC
Clinical Coordinator
Pulmonary Function Laboratory
Elliot Health System
Manchester, NH

Katrina M. Hynes, MHA, RRT, RPFT
Sr. Manager, Customer Education
People and Culture
Vyaire Medical Inc.
Mettawa, IL

David A. Kaminsky, MD
Professor of Medicine
Pulmonary and Critical Care Medicine
University of Vermont;
Attending Physician
Pulmonary and Critical Care Medicine
University of Vermont Medical Center
Burlington, VT

Preface

The primary functions of the lung are oxygenation of mixed venous blood and removal of carbon dioxide. Gas exchange depends on the integrity of the entire cardiopulmonary system, including airways, pulmonary blood vessels, alveoli, respiratory muscles, and respiratory control mechanisms. A few pulmonary function tests assess individual parts of the cardiopulmonary system. However, most lung function tests measure the status of the lungs' components in an overlapping way.

This twelfth edition describes the most common pulmonary function tests, their techniques, and the pathophysiology that may be evaluated by each test. Topics covered include the following:

- Basic tests of lung function, including spirometry, lung volume measurements (i.e., body plethysmography, nitrogen washout, and helium dilution), diffusing capacity, and blood gas analysis
- Ventilation and ventilatory control, cardiopulmonary exercise tests, and pediatric and infant pulmonary function testing
- Specialized test regimens that focus on exhaled nitric oxide measurements, forced oscillation techniques, metabolic studies, disability determination, and preoperative evaluation
- Bronchial challenge tests that assist the clinician in characterizing the hyperreactivity of the airways
- Pulmonary function testing equipment, quality assurance, and reference values and interpretation

DISTINCTIVE FEATURES

The twelfth edition includes many of the features from the previous editions:

- Learning objectives for entry-level and advanced practitioners are again included at the beginning of each chapter.

- Each test section includes criteria for acceptability and repeatability, as well as interpretive strategies with criteria that are organized to help those who perform pulmonary function tests adhere to recognized standards.
- Most of the testing criteria are based on the American Thoracic Society and European Respiratory Society (ATS-ERS) statements, with a few based on the clinical practice guidelines of the American Association for Respiratory Care.
- The interpretive strategies are presented as a series of questions that can be used as a starting point for test interpretation. In this edition, we include a flowchart process for systematically interpreting the basic lung function tests.
- Case Studies with real-life patient scenarios, questions, and discussion topics are included at the end of the chapters.
- How To boxes populate specific testing chapters. These are step-by-step guides for performing function tests. When possible, we provide illustrations. These procedures take the guesswork out of performing an accurate test.
- The Evolve Learning Resources feature updated Case Studies in PowerPoint format so that instructors can utilize them during class discussions. Clinical Scenario slides, organized by disease process, provide an in-depth case analysis, with figures and charts noting lab values and treatment options. Instructors and student study groups can use these to supplement their own clinical experiences.

TEXT UPDATES

- Chapter 1 includes updates related to the 2019 ATS-ERS technical standard.

- Chapter 2 is updated per the 2019 ATS-ERS Technical Standard published in 2019.
- Chapter 3 is now aligned with the 2017 ATS-ERS technical standard for the Global Lung Initiative (GLI).
- The ERS published their methacholine technical standard in late 2017 and their indirect testing (e.g., mannitol, exercise, hyperventilation, cold air) technical standard in 2018. Both have been incorporated into Chapter 9.
- Updates to several sections are included in Chapter 10:
  - Respiratory muscle strength testing—Respiratory Muscle Strength testing section has been updated to include the 2019 ERS Testing Standard and the 2017 reference set for children
  - Exhaled nitric oxide—Exhaled nitirc oxide testing has been updated to include the 2017 ERS Technical Standard on Exhaled Biomarkers and the 2021 ATS Clinical Practice Guideline on the Use of FENO to Guide Treatment
  - Spirometry sections modified based on new 2019 ATS-ERS technical standard
- Chapter 11 has been updated to reflect new equipment and vendors.
- Chapter 12 covers the new version of QMS01, the quality management system document. The components of the ATS Pulmonary Function Laboratory (PFL) Accreditation Program are included.
- Chapter 13 includes the new GLI diffusion of lung capacity for carbon monoxide reference, published in 2019 and the 2020 GLI Lung Volume reference set.

As in previous editions, each chapter includes self-assessment questions. The questions in this edition are divided into entry-level and advanced categories. The answers may be found in Appendix A. A selected bibliography at the end of each chapter is arranged according to topics within the chapter, including standards and guidelines.

USING THIS BOOK

This manual is intended to serve as a text for students of pulmonary function testing and as a reference for technologists and physicians. Because of the wide variety of methods and equipment used in pulmonary function evaluation, some tests are discussed in general terms. For this reason, readers are encouraged to use the selected bibliographies provided. The presentation of indications, pathophysiology, and the clinical significance of various tests presumes a basic understanding of cardiopulmonary anatomy and physiology. Again, readers are urged to refer to the General References included in the selected bibliographies to refresh their background knowledge of lung function. The terminology used is that of the American College of Chest Physicians (ACCP)-ATS Joint Committee on Pulmonary Nomenclature. In some instances, test names reflect common usage that does not follow the ACCP-ATS recommendations.

EVOLVE ANCILLARIES

- Evolve is an interactive learning environment designed to work in coordination with *Ruppel's Manual of Pulmonary Function Testing*, twelfth edition.

For the student, our Evolve Learning Resources include:
- Practice tests to help students apply the knowledge learned within the text
- Conversion and correction factors
- Helpful equations
- Reference tables
- Sample calculations
- Electronic image collection consisting of images from the textbook

For the instructor, our Evolve Learning Resources include:
- PowerPoint presentations of Case Studies and Clinical Scenarios
- Test Bank containing approximately 600 questions
- Electronic image collection consisting of images from the textbook

Instructors may use Evolve to provide an Internet-based course component that reinforces and expands the concepts presented in class. Evolve may be used to publish the class syllabus, outlines, and lecture notes; set up virtual office hours and e-mail communication; share important dates and information through the online class calendar; and encourage student participation through chat rooms and discussion boards. Evolve allows instructors to post examinations and manage their grade books online. For more information, visit http://evolve.elsevier.com or contact an Elsevier sales representative.

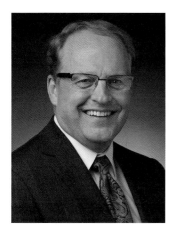

I would like to acknowledge a few key colleagues and friends who have contributed to my professional success. First, I had the honor of being educated and mentored by Drs. Fred Helmholtz and Robert (Bob) Hyatt, both giants in their field. Dr. Helmholtz, along with colleagues, assisted in the development of the G-suit during World War II and the nitrogen washout test. After his retirement, he continued to have a significant impact on the field through his contributions to the National Board for Respiratory Care's credentialing system and specifically the initiation of the pulmonary function credentialing exam. Dr. Hyatt was the first to describe the flow-volume curve and tests for evaluating respiratory muscle strength. I had the privilege of sharing an office with Dr. Hyatt in the later stages of his career, and I learned so much about his passion for pulmonary physiology testing. Drs. Paul Scanlon, David Driscoll, Bruce Staats, and Ken Beck treated me as they would a pulmonary fellow in training and later as a colleague. These individuals were tremendously instrumental in my understanding of pulmonary physiology and my professional development. Jeff Ward, MEd, RRT, FAARC, Mayo Clinic's former respiratory therapy program director, started me on my professional journey with the mindset of inquiry and yearning for knowledge. I would not be the professional I am today without all of their guidance and tutelage.

I would personally like to thank the contributors to this edition, Susan Blonshine, Dr. David Kaminsky, Jeffrey Haynes, and Katrina Hynes, for their excellent subject review. I would also like to thank the staff members and leadership of the Mayo Clinic Pulmonary Function Laboratories, especially Drs. Alex Niven and Kaiser Lim. They continue to carry forward the incredible work the laboratory has been renown for since its inception by championing Mayo's primary value of "the needs of the patient come first."

Carl D. Mottram, RRT, RPFT, FAARC

Contents

Chapter 1

Indications for Pulmonary Function Testing

CHAPTER OUTLINE

LEARNING OBJECTIVES

After studying the chapter and reviewing the figures, tables, and case studies, you should be able to do the following:

Entry-level

1. Categorize pulmonary function tests according to specific purposes.
2. List indications for spirometry, lung volumes, and diffusing capacity.
3. Identify at least one obstructive and one restrictive pulmonary disorder.
4. Relate pulmonary history to indications for performing pulmonary function tests.

Advanced

1. Identify three indications for exercise testing.
2. Name at least two diseases in which air trapping may occur.
3. Describe which services are available during Level I and Level II of a pandemic.
4. Describe the use of an operator-adapted protocol for pulmonary function studies.

KEY TERMS

β_2 agonist
body plethysmograph
bronchial challenge
capnography
diffusing capacity (D_{LCO})
edema
forced vital capacity (FVC)
hypercapnia

hyperventilation
hypoventilation
maximal expiratory flow volume (MEFV)
maximal midexpiratory flow rate (MMFR)
maximal voluntary ventilation (MVV)

oximetry
pulse oximetry
personal protective equipment (PPE)
resting energy expenditure (REE)
spirometry
vital capacity (VC)

The chapter provides an overview of pulmonary function testing. Common pulmonary function tests are introduced, and the indications for each test are discussed. Diseases that commonly require pulmonary function tests are described, and guidelines regarding patient preparation and assessment are presented. Adequate patient preparation, physical assessment, and pulmonary history help the tests provide answers to clinical questions. The importance of patient instruction in obtaining valid data is discussed. These topics are developed more fully in subsequent chapters.

PULMONARY FUNCTION TESTS

Many different tests are used to evaluate lung function. These tests can be divided into categories based on the aspect of lung function they measure (Box 1.1). Although the tests can be performed individually, they are often performed in combination. Fig. 1.1 shows a sample pulmonary function test (PFT) report that includes spirometry, lung volumes, diffusing capacity, and respiratory muscle strength measurements in a commonly used format. Determining which tests to do depends on the *clinical question* to be answered. This question may be explicit, such as "Does the patient have *asthma*?" or less obvious, such as "Does this patient who needs thoracic surgery have any pulmonary diseases that might complicate the procedure?" In either case, indications for specific tests are useful (see Boxes 1.2–1.6).

Airway Function Tests

The most basic test of pulmonary function is the measurement of **vital capacity (VC).** This test simply measures the largest volume of air that can be moved into or out of the lungs. In the mid-1800s,

a surgeon named Hutchinson developed a simple water-sealed *spirometer* that allowed measurement of what he named *vital capacity,* or "vital breath," as he noted its relationship to survival. Hutchinson popularized the concept of using VC to assess lung function and named several other lung compartments with terms that are still used today. He observed that VC was related to the standing height of the patient. He also developed tables to estimate the expected VC for a healthy patient. The VC was usually graphed on chart paper, which allowed subdivisions of the VC to be identified (see Chapter 2).

PF TIP 1.1

Pulmonary function data are usually grouped into categories (see Fig. 1.1). The patient's demographic data (age, height, gender, race, weight) are usually at the top of the report. The PFT data are presented in several columns. These columns show the predicted (expected) values, the lower limit of normal (LLN) or upper limit of normal (ULN), measured values obtained during testing, and the percentage of predicted values for each test (actual/predicted × 100). Be sure to identify which column is actual and which is predicted.

Forced vital capacity (FVC) is an enhancement of the simple VC test. During the 1930s, Barach observed that patients with asthma or emphysema exhaled more slowly than healthy patients. He noted that airflow out of the lungs was important in detecting obstruction of the airways. Barach used a rotating chart drum *(kymograph)* to display VC changes as a *spirogram.* He even evaluated the effects of bronchodilator medications using the FVC traced as a spirogram.

BOX 1.1	CATEGORIES OF PULMONARY FUNCTION TESTS

A. Airway function
  1. Simple spirometry
    a. Vital capacity (VC), expiratory reserve volume (ERV), inspiratory capacity (IC)
  2. Forced vital capacity (FVC) maneuver
    a. FVC, forced expired volume in the first second (FEV_1), forced expiratory flow (FEF), peak expiratory flow (PEF)
      (1) Prebronchodilator and postbronchodilator
      (2) Prebronchochallenge and postbronchochallenge
    b. Maximal expiratory flow-volume (MEFV) curves
      (1) Prebronchodilator and postbronchodilator
      (2) Prebronchochallenge and postbronchochallenge
  3. Maximal voluntary ventilation (MVV)
  4. Airway resistance (Raw) and compliance (C_L)
B. Lung volumes and ventilation
  1. Functional residual capacity (FRC)
    a. Open-circuit (N_2 washout)
    b. Closed-circuit/rebreathing (He dilution)
    c. Thoracic gas volume (V_{TG})
  2. Total lung capacity (TLC), residual volume (RV), RV/TLC ratio
  3. Minute ventilation, alveolar ventilation, and dead space
  4. Distribution of ventilation
    a. Multiple-breath N_2
    b. He equilibration
    c. Single-breath techniques
C. Diffusing capacity (D_{LCO}) tests
  1. Single-breath (breath holding)
  2. Steady state
  3. Other techniques
D. Blood gases and gas exchange tests
  1. Blood gas analysis and blood oximetry
    a. Shunt studies
  2. Pulse oximetry
  3. Capnography
E. Cardiopulmonary exercise tests
  1. Simple, noninvasive tests
  2. Tests with exhaled gas analyses
  3. Tests with blood gas analyses
  4. Tests with flow-volume loops
  5. Tests with direct laryngoscopy
F. Specialized tests
  1. Respiratory muscle strength testing
    a. Maximal respiratory pressures (maximal inspiratory pressure [MIP]/maximal expiratory pressure [MEP])
    b. Cough peak flow (CPF)
    c. Sniff nasal inspiratory pressures (SNIPs)
  2. Exhaled nitric oxide
  3. Forced oscillatory technique
G. Metabolic measurements
  1. Resting energy expenditure (REE)

In 1947, Tiffeneau described measuring the volume expired in the first second of a maximal exhalation in proportion to the maximal volume that could be inspired (FEV_1/IVC [inspiratory vital capacity]) as an index of airflow obstruction (i.e., the Tiffeneau index). Around 1950, Gaensler began using a microswitch in conjunction with a water-sealed spirometer to time FVC. He observed that healthy patients consistently exhaled approximately 80% of their FVC in 1 second and almost all of the FVC in 3 seconds. He used the forced expired volume in the first second (FEV_1) to assess airway obstruction. In 1955, Leuallen and Fowler demonstrated a graphic method used to assess airflow. They measured airflow between the 25% and 75% points on a forced expiratory spirogram. This measure was described as the **maximal midexpiratory flow rate (MMFR).** This and similar measurements have been used to describe airflow from both healthy and airflow-obstructed patients. To stan-

dardize terminology, the MMFR is now referred to as the *forced expiratory flow 25% to 75%* ($FEF_{25\%-75\%}$).

In addition to displaying FVC as a volume–time spirogram, it can be represented by plotting airflow against volume. In the late 1950s, Hyatt and others began using the flow-volume display to assess airway function. The tracing was termed the **maximal expiratory flow-volume (MEFV)** curve. By combining the forced expiration with an inspiratory maneuver, a closed loop can be displayed. This figure is called the *flow-volume loop* (see Chapter 2).

Peak expiratory flow (PEF) is measured using either a flow-sensing spirometer or a *peak flow meter*. In the 1960s, Wright and McKerrow popularized the use of peak flow to monitor patients with asthma. Peak flow can be readily assessed from the flow-volume loop as well. Recently, portable peak flow meters that allow monitoring at home, as well as in the hospital or clinic, have been developed.

Pulmonary Function Report

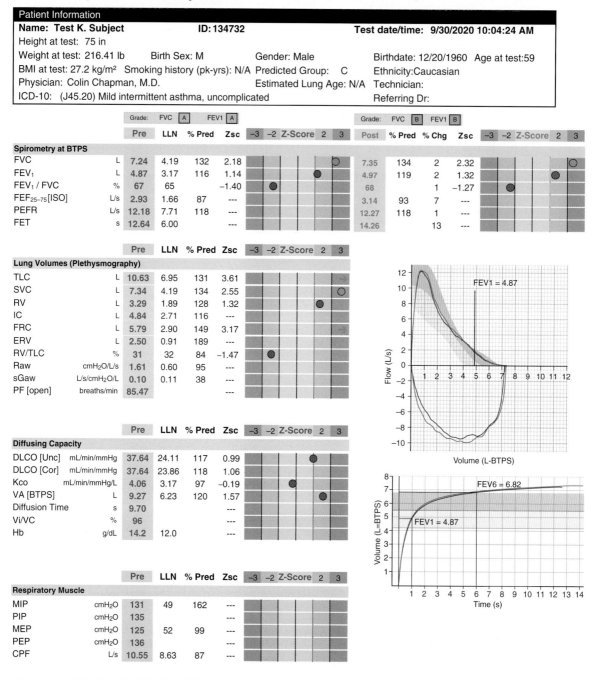

Patient Information			
Name: Test K. Subject	ID: 134732		Test date/time: 9/30/2020 10:04:24 AM
Height at test: 75 in			
Weight at test: 216.41 lb	Birth Sex: M	Gender: Male	Birthdate: 12/20/1960 Age at test:59
BMI at test: 27.2 kg/m²	Smoking history (pk-yrs): N/A	Predicted Group: C	Ethnicity:Caucasian
Physician: Colin Chapman, M.D.		Estimated Lung Age: N/A	Technician:
ICD-10: (J45.20) Mild intermittent asthma, uncomplicated			Referring Dr:

Grade: FVC [A]   FEV1 [A]   Grade: FVC [B] FEV1 [B]

Spirometry at BTPS		Pre	LLN	% Pred	Zsc	-3 -2 Z-Score 2 3	Post	% Pred	% Chg	Zsc	-3 -2 Z-Score 2 3
FVC	L	7.24	4.19	132	2.18		7.35	134	2	2.32	
FEV₁	L	4.87	3.17	116	1.14		4.97	119	2	1.32	
FEV₁ / FVC	%	67	65		-1.40		68		1	-1.27	
FEF₂₅₋₇₅[ISO]	L/s	2.93	1.66	87	---		3.14	93	7	---	
PEFR	L/s	12.18	7.71	118	---		12.27	118	1	---	
FET	s	12.64	6.00		---		14.26		13	---	

Lung Volumes (Plethysmography)		Pre	LLN	% Pred	Zsc	-3 -2 Z-Score 2 3
TLC	L	10.63	6.95	131	3.61	
SVC	L	7.34	4.19	134	2.55	
RV	L	3.29	1.89	128	1.32	
IC	L	4.84	2.71	116	---	
FRC	L	5.79	2.90	149	3.17	
ERV	L	2.50	0.91	189	---	
RV/TLC	%	31	32	84	-1.47	
Raw	cmH₂O/L/s	1.61	0.60	95	---	
sGaw	L/s/cmH₂O/L	0.10	0.11	38	---	
PF [open]	breaths/min	85.47			---	

Diffusing Capacity		Pre	LLN	% Pred	Zsc	-3 -2 Z-Score 2 3
DLCO [Unc]	mL/min/mmHg	37.64	24.11	117	0.99	
DLCO [Cor]	mL/min/mmHg	37.64	23.86	118	1.06	
Kco	mL/min/mmHg/L	4.06	3.17	97	-0.19	
VA [BTPS]	L	9.27	6.23	120	1.57	
Diffusion Time	s	9.70			---	
Vi/VC	%	96			---	
Hb	g/dL	14.2	12.0		---	

Respiratory Muscle		Pre	LLN	% Pred	Zsc	-3 -2 Z-Score 2 3
MIP	cmH₂O	131	49	162	---	
PIP	cmH₂O	135			---	
MEP	cmH₂O	125	52	99	---	
PEP	cmH₂O	136			---	
CPF	L/s	10.55	8.63	87	---	

FIG. 1.1 Sample pulmonary function test report. Lung function tests are grouped by category. The post-bronchodilator data also include the percent (%) change. Both the lower limit of normal (LLN) and Z scores are displayed, the latter with an associated graph, along with the flow–volume loop and volume–time graphs.

Past Pulmonary Function Results for this Patient

Parameter	Today				Previous Test Results - Most Recent to Past									
	FVC	FEV1	FVC	FEV1		FVC	FEV1			FVC	FEV1			
Spirometry Grading	A	A	B	A		E	E			B	B			
	9/30/2020		8/25/2020	% Diff	Abs	8/17/2020	% Diff	Abs		7/6/2020	% Diff	Abs		
FVC			7.02	4	0.22	7.06	3	0.18		7.22	1	0.02		
FEV₁			4.86	1	0.01	4.89	<1	-0.02		4.80	2	0.07		
TLC			----	----	----	10.57	1	0.06		----	----	----		
DLCO [Unc]			----	----	----	----	----	----		----	----	----		

(continued columns)

	FVC	FEV1			
Spirometry Grading	A	B			
	6/2/2020	% Diff	Abs		
FVC	7.43	-2	-0.19		
FEV₁	5.29	-8	-0.42		
TLC	10.76	-1	-0.13		
DLCO [Unc]	31.69	16	5.95		

Six Minute Walk Study

		Resting	1 min	2 min	3 min	4 min	5 min	6 min	Recovery		
									Min 1	Min 2	Min 3
SpO₂	(%)	98.1	98.0	97.8	97.6	97.1	96.8	96.2	96.0	97.2	97.8
HR	(bpm)	66	67	69	71	73	80	86	97	90	74
BP	(mmHg)	122 / 80						134 / 82			
Dyspnea	(1 - 10)							3			

Total distance walked in 6 minutes: 733 meters
Predicted distance: 656 meters
Percent of predicted: 112 %

Supplemental oxygen during the test: O2 Label Units
Previous Test:
Last Test Date: 9/30/2020   Last Test Distance:

Technologist Comments:

Good test subject effort and cooperation. Albuterol delivered with a 12-min waiting period.

Computer Impression:

Normal spirometric values indicate the absence of any significant degree of obstructive pulmonary impairment and/or restrictive ventilatory defect.

Bronchodilator therapy was administered followed by repeat spirometric testing. Post-bronchodilator testing failed to demonstrate a significant change in FVC, FEV1, or FEF 25-75. This indicates that this patient may not benefit from continued bronchodilator therapy.
The total lung capacity is increased indicating hyperinflation. The carbon monoxide diffusing capacity is normal indicating normal alveolar-capillary surface area for gas exchange. Maximal respiratory muscle pressures are normal.

Oxygen saturation by pulse oximetry is satisfactory. The MVV is consistent with the level of FEV1.

FIG. 1.1, CONT'D

The FVC, FEV_1, and other flows, along with flow-volume loops, are all used to measure the patient's response to bronchodilator medications (see Chapter 2). Tests are performed before and after inhalation of a bronchodilator, and the percentage of change is calculated. The same tests may be used to assess airway response after a challenge to the airways. These tests are referred to as **bronchial challenge** or *bronchial provocation* tests. The challenge may be in the form of a nonspecific inhaled agent (e.g., *methacholine*) or a physical agent (e.g., exercise). In either case, airflow is assessed before and after the challenge. The percent change (normally a decrease) after the challenge is calculated (see Chapter 9).

Maximal voluntary ventilation (MVV) was described as early as 1941. Cournand and Richards originally called it the *maximal breathing capacity* (MBC). In the MVV test, the patient breathes rapidly and deeply for 12 to 15 seconds. The volume of air exchanged is expressed in liters per minute. The MVV gives an estimate of the peak ventilation available to meet physiologic demands.

Measurement of respiratory muscle strength is accomplished by assessing maximal inspiratory pressure (MIP) and maximal expiratory pressure (MEP). This is done using either a pressure *transducer* or a simple aneroid *manometer*. MIP and MEP are important adjuncts to spirometry for monitoring respiratory muscle function in a variety of pulmonary and nonpulmonary diseases. Black and Hyatt developed the first device to assess these parameters and called the device a "bugle" because the expiratory maneuver and the device used to measure the pressure were like blowing into a bugle.

Raw measurements date back to the development of the **body plethysmograph** in the early 1950s. Comroe, DuBois, and others perfected a technique that provided estimates of alveolar pressure. The patient sits in an airtight box called a *plethysmograph* (see Chapter 11). The plethysmographic method allows the calculation of the pressure drop across the airways related to flow at the mouth (see Chapter 4). This technique originally required complicated monitoring and recording devices. Microprocessors have simplified the measurement of the required signals so that plethys-

mography is now widely used. The same equipment can also be used to measure thoracic gas volume (V_{TG}) rapidly and accurately.

Lung compliance is measured by passing a small balloon into the esophagus to measure pleural pressure. Intrapleural pressure can then be related to volume changes to estimate the distensibility of the lung (see Chapter 4). Other less invasive techniques are available but not widely used.

Lung Volume and Ventilation Tests

Measurement of lung volume dates to the early 1800s, well before Hutchinson's development of spirometry. Various techniques have been used to estimate the volume of gas remaining in the lung after a complete exhalation. Davy used a hydrogen-dilution technique to estimate residual air. This technique was later improved by Meneely and Kaltreider using helium (He) instead of hydrogen. Around the same time, Darling, Cournand, and Richards began using oxygen breathing to wash nitrogen (N_2) out of the lungs. The collection and analysis of the volume of exhaled N_2 allowed the functional residual capacity (FRC) to be estimated. Using simple spirometry combined with FRC determinations allows total lung capacity (TLC) and residual volume (RV) to be calculated. The other commonly used method for measuring lung volumes uses the body plethysmograph to measure V_{TG} or FRC. Estimation of lung volumes from chest radiographs is possible but is not widely used. Lung volume can also be estimated from computed tomography (CT) scans, but such measurements are seldom performed just for the purpose of measuring lung volume.

Closed-circuit (He-dilution) and open-circuit (N_2-washout) techniques are both widely used to measure FRC. Besides determining lung volumes, each technique provides some limited information about the distribution of ventilation within the lungs. The pattern of N_2 washout can be displayed graphically. The time required for He to equilibrate during rebreathing provides a similar index of the evenness of ventilation. In the early 1950s and 1960s, Fowler developed a single-breath N_2-washout technique. This method plots the N_2 concentration in expired gas after a single breath of 100% oxygen. The single-breath N_2 washout also provides limited information about gas distribution in the lungs and allows estimates of the lung volume at which airway closure occurs when the patient exhales completely (see Chapter 4).

Measurement of resting ventilation requires only a simple gas-metering device and a means of collecting expired air. Portable computerized spirometers allow minute ventilation, tidal volume (V_T), and breathing rate to be readily measured in almost any setting. Determination of alveolar ventilation or dead space (wasted ventilation) requires measurement of the arterial partial pressure of carbon dioxide ($Paco_2$) in addition to total ventilation. Alternately, the partial pressure of carbon dioxide (Pco_2) can be estimated from expired CO_2. The availability of blood gas analyzers and exhaled CO_2 analyzers makes these measurements routine.

Diffusing Capacity Tests

The basis for the modern single-breath **diffusing capacity (D_{LCO})** test was described by August and Marie Krogh in 1911. They showed that small but measurable differences existed between inspired and expired gas containing carbon monoxide (CO). This change could be related to the uptake of gas across the lung. Although they used the method to test a series of patients, they did not use the single-breath technique for clinical purposes. Around 1950, Forrester and others revisited the method. They developed it as a tool to measure the gas exchange capacity of the lung. At about the same time, Filley and others were promoting other techniques using CO to measure D_{LCO}. Most of these techniques allowed patients to breathe normally rather than hold their breath. These methods are called *steady-state techniques*. Each method has certain limitations. However, the single-breath technique is the most widely used and standardized in the United States and Europe (see Chapter 3).

Blood Gases and Gas Exchange Tests

Measurement of gases (O_2 and CO_2) in the blood began with volumetric methods used since the early 1900s. In 1957, Sanz introduced the glass electrode to measure the *pH* of fluids potentiometrically. In 1958, Severinghaus added an outer jacket containing a bicarbonate buffer to the glass electrode. The electrode buffer was separated from the blood being analyzed by a membrane permeable to CO_2. This allowed the pressure of CO_2 in the blood to be measured as a pH change in the electrode. In 1956, Leland Clark covered a platinum electrode with a polypropylene membrane. When a voltage was applied to the electrode, O_2 was reduced at the platinum *cathode* in proportion to its partial pressure. These three electrodes (pH, Pco_2, and partial pressure of oxygen [Po_2]) were the basic measurement devices in blood gas analyzers for many years. Miniature electrodes gradually replaced the traditional electrodes. Today, blood gas analyzers use a variety of electrochemical techniques (see Blood Gas Analyzers, Chapter 11) to measure not only pH, Pco_2, and Po_2 but also the various fractions of Hb, such as oxyhemoglobin (O_2Hb) and carboxyhemoglobin (COHb). Similar methods to measure electrolytes (K^{++}, Na^{++}, Cl^-) are also included in many blood gas analyzer systems. Transcutaneous electrodes using techniques like the classical blood gas electrodes are available for the measurement of O_2 and CO_2 tensions ($tcpO_2$ and $tcpCO_2$).

Blood **oximetry** was developed during World War II to monitor the effects of exposure to high-altitude flight. During the 1960s, spectrophotometric analyzers that could measure the total Hb, along with O_2Hb and COHb levels, were perfected. Blood oximetry testing is commonly combined with blood gas analysis so that both can be accomplished with a single instrument. **Pulse oximetry** was developed in the 1970s because of efforts to monitor cardiac rate by using a light beam to sense pulsatile blood flow. It was quickly discovered that the pulse could be sensed, and changes in light absorption could also be used to estimate arterial oxygen saturation. Modern microprocessors have allowed pulse oximeters that are small and portable, with some devices capable of measuring COHb in addition to O_2 saturation.

Capnography, or monitoring of exhaled carbon dioxide, was developed in conjunction with the infrared gas analyzer (see Chapter 11). This sensitive and rapidly responding analyzer allows exhaled CO_2 to be monitored continuously. Most critical care units, operating rooms, and emergency departments use some combination of blood gas analysis, pulse oximetry, and capnography for patient monitoring. Blood gas analysis is an integral part of routine pulmonary function testing because it is the definitive test of the basic functions of the lung.

Exhaled nitric oxide (eNO), although not a measure of blood gas or gas exchange, has emerged as an important parameter for assessing inflammatory changes in the lungs. Asthma, chronic obstructive pulmonary disease (COPD), and other pathologies characterized by inflammation of the airways or lung tissue can be monitored by analyzing trace amounts of nitric oxide (NO) in exhaled gas.

Cardiopulmonary Exercise Tests

Exercise tests commonly use a treadmill or cycle ergometer to impose an external workload that stresses the cardiovascular and musculoskeletal systems. The simplest types of exercise tests are those in which the patient performs work and only noninvasive measurements are made. Such measurements include heart rate and rhythm monitoring using an electrocardiogram (ECG). Other simple, noninvasive measurements are blood pressure and respiratory rate monitoring. Analysis of exhaled gas is noninvasive, but the patient does have to breathe through a mouthpiece or mask. Ventilation and V_T can be estimated by collecting the exhaled air. Analysis of expired gases permits oxygen consumption and CO_2 production to be measured. When invasive measures (blood gas analysis, arterial catheters, pulmonary artery catheters) are used, the entire range of physiologic variables that affect exercise can be monitored. Computerized exhaled gas analysis allows sophisticated measurements to be made rapidly while the patient continues to exercise (breath-by-breath gas analysis). Simple exercise field tests, such as the 6-Minute Walk Test (6MWT), have become popular because the distance walked correlates well with more sophisticated exercise measurements and with clinical outcomes in a variety of diseases.

Metabolic Measurements

Measurement of energy expenditure and caloric requirements dates to the early 1900s. The *basal metabolic rate* (BMR) was measured by allowing subjects to rebreathe from a volume spirometer containing added oxygen. Plotting the rate at which oxygen was consumed derived an estimate of energy expenditure. Similar techniques are used today, except that oxygen consumption and carbon dioxide production are monitored using exhaled gas analysis. **Resting energy expenditure (REE)** has replaced BMR as the primary variable related to metabolic needs. Although BMR was used to detect disorders that affected metabolism, REE is used to manage critically ill patients whose caloric requirements may be difficult to estimate.

INDICATIONS FOR PULMONARY FUNCTION TESTING

Each category of pulmonary function testing includes specific reasons that the test may be necessary. These reasons for testing are called *indications*. Some PFTs have well-defined indications. The same indications that apply to one type of test (e.g., spirometry) may also apply to other categories.

Spirometry

Spirometry is the PFT performed most often because it is indicated in many situations (see Box 1.2). Spirometry is often performed as a screening procedure. It may be the first test to indicate the presence of pulmonary disease. Spirometry is either recommended or required for the diagnosis of obstructive lung disease by the Global Initiative for Chronic Obstructive Lung Disease (GOLD), the Global Initiative for Asthma (GINA), and numerous other organizations concerned with the diagnosis of lung diseases. However, spirometry alone may not be sufficient to completely define the extent of disease, response to therapy, preoperative risk, or level of impairment. Spirometry must be performed correctly because of the serious impact its results can have on the patient's life. It is one of the few tests that yield a false-positive response if performed poorly because low values are the result. These low results may lead to further testing, inappropriate diagnosis and treatment, and increased costs for the patient and the health care delivery system.

BOX 1.2   INDICATIONS FOR SPIROMETRY

Diagnosis

1. To evaluate symptoms, signs, or abnormal laboratory results
   a. Dyspnea, cough, chest discomfort, phlegm production
   b. Decreased breath sounds, chest wall abnormalities
   c. Abnormal chest x-ray or computed tomography, abnormal arterial blood gases or pulse oximetry
2. To measure the physiologic effect of the disease or disorder
3. To screen individuals at risk of having pulmonary disease
   a. Smokers > 45 with symptoms
   b. Working in a hazardous or dusty environment
4. To assess preoperative risk
   a. Lung resection (lobectomy, pneumonectomy)
   b. Upper abdominal procedures
5. To assess prognosis

Monitoring

1. To assess response to therapeutic intervention
2. To monitor disease progression
3. To monitor patients for exacerbations of disease and recovery from exacerbations
4. To monitor people for adverse effects of exposure to injurious agents
   a. Employees participating in a respiratory protection program
5. To watch for adverse reactions to drugs with known pulmonary toxicity
   a. For example, bleomycin, amiodarone

Disability/Impairment Evaluations

1. To assess patients as part of a rehabilitation program
2. To assess risks as part of an insurance evaluation
3. To assess individuals for legal reasons

Other

1. Research or clinical trials
2. Epidemiologic surveys
3. Derivation of reference equations
4. Preemployment and lung health monitoring for at-risk conditions
5. To assess health status before beginning at-risk physical activities

---

Lung Volumes

The determination of lung volume usually includes the VC and its subdivisions, along with the FRC. From these two basic measurements, TLC and other lung volumes can be calculated (see Chapter 4). Lung volumes are almost always measured in conjunction with spirometry, although the indications for them are distinct (see Box 1.3). The most common reason for measuring lung volumes is to identify restrictive lung disease. A reduced VC (or FVC) measured with spirometry may suggest restriction, particularly if airflow is normal. Measurement of FRC and determination of TLC are necessary to confirm restriction because a low FVC can be caused by either restriction or obstruction. If TLC is reduced below the 5th percentile of the predicted value, restriction is present. The severity of the restrictive process is determined by the extent of reduction of the TLC. TLC and its components can be determined by several methods. For patients with obstructive lung diseases (COPD, asthma), lung volumes measured by body plethysmography may be indicated (see Chapter 4) because multiple-breath or single-breath dilution techniques may underestimate TLC. In obstructive lung disease, lung volumes are necessary to determine whether air trapping or hyperinflation is present. The degree of hyperinflation, measured by indices

---

BOX 1.3   INDICATIONS FOR LUNG VOLUME DETERMINATION

A. Lung volume determinations may be indicated to diagnose or assess the severity of restrictive lung disease (reduced total lung capacity [TLC])
B. Differentiate between obstructive and restrictive disease patterns
C. Assess response to therapeutic interventions
   1. Bronchodilators, steroids
   2. Lung transplantation, resection, reduction
   3. Radiation or chemotherapy
D. Make preoperative assessments of patients with compromised lung function
E. Determine the extent of hyperinflation
F. Assess gas trapping by comparison of plethysmographic lung volumes with gas-dilution lung volumes
G. Standardize other lung function measures (e.g., specific conductance)

such as the IC/TLC ratio, correlates with increased mortality in patients who have COPD.

Diffusing Capacity

Diffusing capacity is measured by having the patient inhale a low concentration of CO and a *tracer* gas to determine gas exchange within the lungs (DLco). Several methods of evaluating the uptake of CO from the lungs are available, but the single-breath technique (DLcosb) is most used. This method is also called the *breath-hold technique* because CO transfer is measured during 8 to 12 seconds of breath holding. DLco is usually measured in conjunction with spirometry and lung volumes. Although many pulmonary and cardiovascular diseases reduce DLco (see Box 1.4), it may be abnormally increased in some cases (see Chapter 3). DLco testing is commonly used to monitor diseases caused by dust (pneumoconiosis). These are conditions in which lung tissue is infiltrated by substances such as silica or asbestos that disrupt the normal structure of the gas exchange units. DLco testing is also used to evaluate pulmonary involvement in systemic diseases such as rheumatoid arthritis. DLco measurements are often included in the evaluation of patients with obstructive lung disease, particularly in emphysema. DLco tests may be indicated to monitor changes in lung function (i.e., gas exchange) induced by drugs used to treat cardiac arrhythmias, as well as changes caused by chemotherapy and radiation therapy for lung cancer.

Blood Gases

Blood gas analysis is often done in conjunction with pulmonary function studies. Blood is drawn from a peripheral artery without being exposed to air (i.e., anaerobically). The radial artery is often used for a single arterial puncture or indwelling catheter. Blood gas analysis includes the measurement of pH, along with Pco_2 and Po_2. Other calculated parameters (HCO_3^-, base excess, etc.) are often included in the standard blood gas report. The same specimen may be used for blood oximetry to measure total Hb, O_2Hb saturation, COHb, and *methemoglobin* (MetHb).

Blood gas analysis is the ideal measure of pulmonary function because it assesses the two primary functions of the lung (oxygenation and CO_2 removal). Evaluation of many pulmonary disorders may include blood gas analysis. Specific indications for blood gas analysis are listed in Box 1.5. Blood gas analysis is most often used to determine the need for supplemental oxygen and to manage patients who require ventilatory support. Some pulmonary function measurements require blood gas analysis as an integral part of the test (i.e., shunt or dead-space studies). Blood gas analysis is invasive; noninvasive measurements of oxygenation or gas exchange are often preferred because they are safer

---

BOX 1.4   INDICATIONS FOR DLco

A. Diffusing capacity (DLco) measurements may be indicated to evaluate or follow the progress of parenchymal lung diseases
   1. Dusts (asbestos, silica, metals)
   2. Organic agents (allergic alveolitis)
   3. Drugs (amiodarone, bleomycin)
B. Evaluate pulmonary involvement in systemic diseases
   1. Rheumatoid arthritis
   2. Sarcoidosis
   3. Systemic lupus erythematosus
   4. Systemic sclerosis
   5. Mixed connective tissue disease
C. Evaluate obstructive lung disease
   1. Follow the progression of disease
      a. Emphysema
      b. Cystic fibrosis

   2. Differentiate types of obstructions
      a. Emphysema
      b. Chronic bronchitis
      c. Asthma
   3. Predict arterial desaturation during exercise in chronic obstructive pulmonary disease
D. Evaluate cardiovascular diseases
   1. Primary pulmonary hypertension
   2. Acute or recurrent pulmonary thromboembolism
   3. Pulmonary edema and congestive heart failure
E. Quantify disability associated with interstitial lung disease
F. Evaluate pulmonary hemorrhage, polycythemia, or left-to-right shunts (increased DLco)

BOX 1.5 INDICATIONS FOR BLOOD GAS ANALYSIS

A. Blood gas analysis and/or blood oximetry may be indicated to evaluate adequacy of lung function
  1. Ventilation (Pa_{CO_2})
  2. Acid–base status
    a. pH
    b. Pa_{CO_2}
  3. Oxygenation and oxygen-carrying capacity
    a. Pa_{O_2}
    b. Total Hb, O_2Hb, COHb, MetHb
  4. Intrapulmonary shunt
  5. V_D/V_T ratio
B. Determine need for supplemental oxygen (for clinical or reimbursement purposes)
  1. Presence or severity of resting hypoxemia
  2. Exercise desaturation
  3. Nocturnal desaturation
  4. Adequacy of oxygen prescription
C. Monitor ventilatory support
  1. Assess or follow respiratory failure
  2. Adjust therapy to improve oxygenation (positive end-expiratory pressure [PEEP], continuous positive airway pressure [CPAP], pressure support)
D. Document the severity or progression of known pulmonary disease
E. Provide data to correct or corroborate other pulmonary function measurements
  1. Correct D_{LCO} measurements (Hb and COHb)
  2. Determine accuracy of pulse oximetry, transcutaneous monitors, or indwelling blood gas devices

---

or less costly. Many noninvasive techniques (e.g., pulse oximetry, transcutaneous monitoring, and capnography) rely on a blood gas analysis to verify their validity (see Chapter 6).

Exercise Tests

Physical exercise stresses the heart, the lungs, and the pulmonary and peripheral circulatory systems. Exercise testing allows simultaneous evaluation of the cellular, cardiovascular, and ventilatory systems. Cardiopulmonary exercise tests can be used to determine the level of fitness or extent of dysfunction. Appropriately designed tests can determine the role of cardiac or pulmonary involvement. COPD, interstitial lung disease, pulmonary vascular disease, and exercise-induced bronchospasm are respiratory disorders that often require exercise evaluation. Understanding the physiologic basis for the patient's inability to exercise is an important aspect in prescribing effective therapy (i.e., cardiac or pulmonary rehabilitation). Exercise testing may also be required for the determination of disability. Box 1.6 lists specific indications for exercise tests.

Equipment used to measure oxygen consumption and CO_2 production during exercise can also measure resting metabolic rates. This allows estimates of caloric needs in patients who are critically ill. Indications for performing studies of REE are detailed in Chapter 10.

BOX 1.6 INDICATIONS FOR EXERCISE TESTING

A. Exercise testing may be indicated to evaluate exercise intolerance or level of fitness
B. Document or diagnose exercise limitation because of fatigue, dyspnea, or pain
  1. Cardiovascular diseases
    a. Myocardial ischemia or dyskinesis
    b. Cardiomyopathy
    c. Congestive heart failure
    d. Peripheral vascular disease
    e. Selection for heart transplantation
  2. Pulmonary diseases
    a. Airway obstruction (including cystic fibrosis) or hyperreactivity
    b. Interstitial lung disease
    c. Pulmonary vascular disease
  3. Mixed cardiovascular and pulmonary etiologies
  4. Unexplained dyspnea
    a. Deconditioning
    b. Upper airway abnormalities (e.g., vocal cord dysfunction)
C. Exercise evaluation for cardiac or pulmonary rehabilitation
  1. Exercise desaturation/hypoxemia
  2. Oxygen prescription
D. Assess preoperative risk, particularly lung resection or reduction
E. Assess disability, particularly related to occupational lung disease
F. Evaluate therapeutic interventions such as heart or lung transplantation

PATTERNS OF IMPAIRED PULMONARY FUNCTION

Patients are usually referred to the pulmonary function laboratory to evaluate signs or symptoms of lung disease. In some instances, the clinician may wish to exclude a specific diagnosis, such as asthma. Indications for different categories of PFTs have been described previously. Sometimes, patients display patterns during testing that are consistent with a specific diagnosis. This section presents an overview of some commonly encountered forms of impaired pulmonary function.

Obstructive Airway Diseases

An obstructive airway disease is one in which airflow into or out of the lungs is reduced. This simple definition includes a variety of pathologic conditions. Some of these conditions are closely related in how they cause airway obstruction. For example, mucus hypersecretion is a component of *chronic bronchitis,* asthma, and *cystic fibrosis* (CF), although their causes are distinct.

Chronic Obstructive Pulmonary Disease

The term *COPD* is often used to describe long-standing airway obstruction caused by emphysema, chronic bronchitis, or sometimes asthma, which is not fully reversible. These three conditions may be present alone or in combination (Fig. 1.2). *Bronchiectasis* is sometimes considered a component of COPD. COPD is characterized by dyspnea at rest or with exertion, often accompanied by a productive cough. Delineation of the type of obstruction depends on the history, physical examination, and pulmonary function studies. Unfortunately, the term *COPD* is used to describe the clinical findings of dyspnea or cough without attention to the actual cause. This may lead to inappropriate therapy. Other similar terms include *chronic obstructive lung disease* (COLD) and *chronic airway obstruction* (CAO).

Emphysema

Emphysema means "air trapping" and is defined morphologically. The air spaces distal to the terminal bronchioles are abnormally increased in

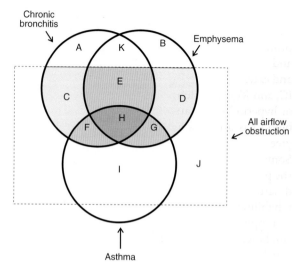

FIG. 1.2 Nonproportional diagram depicting the relationship between various components of chronic obstructive pulmonary disease (COPD). Emphysema, chronic bronchitis, and asthma overlap to varying degrees *(shaded areas).* Chronic obstruction in small airways and all airway obstructive diseases *(large dashed square)* also overlap. (A) Patients with chronic bronchitis but no airflow obstruction. (B) Patients with anatomic changes related to emphysema but no obstruction. (C) Patients with chronic cough and airflow obstruction. (D) Patients with emphysema and obstruction, as demonstrated by spirometry. (E) Combined chronic bronchitis and emphysema, commonly occurring in the same patient, because of cigarette smoking. (F) Combined chronic bronchitis and asthma. (G) Combined emphysema and asthma. (H) Combined asthma, chronic bronchitis, and emphysema. (I) Patients with asthma manifested by reversible obstruction (spirometry or peak flow). (J) Other forms of airway obstruction, including cystic fibrosis, bronchiolitis obliterans, or upper airway abnormalities (e.g., vocal cord dysfunction), are not considered part of COPD. (K) Patients with cough and morphologic evidence of emphysema but no obstruction. (Modified from American Thoracic Society. [1995]. Standards for the diagnosis and care of patients with chronic obstructive pulmonary disease. *American Journal of Respiratory and Critical Care Medicine, 152,* S77–S120.)

size. The walls of the alveoli undergo destructive changes. This destruction results in the overinflation of lung units. If the process mainly involves the respiratory bronchioles, the emphysema is termed *centrilobular.* If the alveoli are also involved, the term *panlobular emphysema* is used to describe the pattern. These distinctions require the examination of lung tissue either by biopsy or at postmortem. Because this is often impractical, emphysema is suspected when there is airway obstruction with air trapping. Physical assessment, chest x-ray or CT studies, and pulmonary function studies are the primary diagnostic tools. Spirometry (FVC, FEV_1, and FEV_1/FVC) is used to determine the presence and extent of obstruction. Lung volumes (TLC, RV, IC, and RV/TLC) define the pattern of air trapping or hyperinflation caused by emphysema. D_{LCO} and blood gas analyses are useful in tracking the degree of gas exchange abnormality in emphysema. Some form of exercise testing may be necessary if the patient with emphysema is suspected of oxygen desaturation with exertion or to plan pulmonary rehabilitation.

Emphysema is caused primarily by cigarette smoking. Repeated inflammation of the respiratory bronchioles results in tissue destruction. As the disease advances, more and more alveolar walls are destroyed. Loss of elastic tissue results in airway collapse, air trapping, and hyperinflation. Some emphysema is caused by the absence of a protective enzyme, α_1-antitrypsin. The lack of this enzyme is caused by a genetic defect. The enzyme α_1-antitrypsin inhibits proteases in the blood from attacking healthy tissue. Deficiency of α_1-antitrypsin causes the gradual destruction of alveolar walls, resulting in panlobular emphysema. Chronic exposure to environmental pollutants can also contribute to the development of emphysema. The natural aging of the lung also causes some changes that resemble the disease entity. The natural decline of elastic recoil in the lung reduces maximal airflow and increases lung volume as people age. Surgical removal of lung tissue sometimes causes the remaining lung to overinflate.

The main symptom of emphysema is breathlessness, either at rest or with exertion. Hypoxemia may contribute to this dyspnea, particularly in advanced emphysema. However, the destruction of alveolar walls also causes loss of the capillary bed. Ventilation-perfusion matching may be relatively well preserved in patients with emphysema. As a result, oxygen levels may be only slightly decreased, particularly at rest. This type of patient is sometimes called the "pink puffer." As the disease advances, the loss of alveolar surface causes a decreased ability to oxygenate mixed venous blood. D_{LCO} is reduced. The patient becomes increasingly breathless, particularly with exertion. Muscle

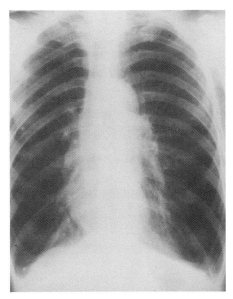

FIG. 1.3 Chronic obstructive pulmonary disease (COPD) radiograph with hyperinflation.

wasting seems to be common in emphysema, and patients are often below their ideal body weight. As noted, symptoms of chronic bronchitis and asthma may be present as well.

The chest x-ray film of a patient with emphysema shows flattened diaphragms and increased air spaces. The lung fields appear hyperlucent (dark), with little vascularity. The heart appears to be hanging from the great vessels (Fig. 1.3). CT scans, especially spiral CT scans, show a three-dimensional picture of enlarged air spaces and loss of supporting tissue. CT scans also delineate whether the emphysematous changes are localized or spread throughout the lungs.

The physical appearance of the chest confirms what is shown radiographically. The chest wall is immobile with the shoulders elevated. The diameter of the chest is increased in the anterior-posterior aspect (so-called *barrel chest*). There is little diaphragmatic excursion during inspiration. Intercostal retractions may be prominent. Accessory muscles (neck and shoulders) are used to lift the chest wall. Breath sounds are distant or absent. Patients may need to support the arms and shoulders to catch their breath. Breathing is often done through pursed lips to alleviate the sensation of dyspnea (Fig. 1.4).

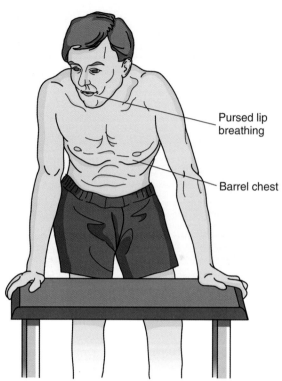

Pursed lip breathing

Barrel chest

FIG. 1.4 Chronic obstructive pulmonary disease (COPD) signs. Note pursed lips, intercostal retractions, and need to use arms and shoulder for support to catch breath.(From Henry, M., & Stapleton, E. [2010]. *EMT prehospital care* [4th ed.]. St. Louis, MO: Mosby JEMS.)

Chronic Bronchitis

Chronic bronchitis is diagnosed by clinical findings. It is present when there is excessive mucus production with a productive cough on most days for at least 3 months for 2 years or more. The diagnosis is made by excluding other diseases that also result in excess mucus production. These include CF, tuberculosis, abscess, tumors, and bronchiectasis.

Chronic bronchitis, like emphysema, is caused primarily by cigarette smoking. It may also result from chronic exposure to environmental pollutants and second hand smoke. Chronic bronchitis causes the mucous glands that line the airways to hypertrophy and increase in number. There is also chronic inflammation of the bronchial wall with infiltration of leukocytes and lymphocytes. The

number of ciliated epithelial cells decreases. This causes impairment of mucus flow in the airways. Similar changes occur in respiratory bronchioles. Excessive mucus and poor clearance make the patient susceptible to repeated infections. Some patients who have chronic bronchitis caused by cigarette smoking experience a decrease in cough and mucus production after smoking cessation. Some airway changes, however, usually persist. Spirometry is useful in evaluating the extent of airway obstruction caused by bronchitic changes. D_{LCO} may be helpful in distinguishing emphysema and chronic bronchitis; patients with bronchitis may have preserved D_{LCO}, whereas patients with emphysema tend to have reduced D_{LCO}. However, D_{LCO} is usually not normal in chronic bronchitis because of the mismatching of ventilation and perfusion caused by bronchial obstruction.

Chronic cough is the defining symptom of chronic bronchitis. Some patients do not consider cough abnormal and refer to it as "smoker's cough" or "morning cough." In addition to cough, chronic bronchitis may produce dyspnea, particularly with exertion. Blood gas abnormalities usually accompany chronic bronchitis. Ventilation-perfusion mismatching causes hypoxemia. If hypoxemia is significant and persists, the patient may develop secondary polycythemia. *Cyanosis* may be present because of the combination of arterial desaturation and increased Hb levels. Chronic hypoxemia may also lead to right-sided heart failure *(cor pulmonale)* with peripheral edema, particularly in the feet and ankles. Advanced chronic bronchitis is also often accompanied by CO_2 retention (**hypercapnia**).

Unlike the patient with emphysema, the patient with chronic bronchitis may show few clinical signs of underlying disease. Body weight may be normal or increased, with minimal changes to the chest wall. Patients with bronchitis may appear normal except for cough and dyspnea. The chest x-ray film in chronic bronchitis differs markedly from that in emphysema. The congested airways are easily visible. The heart may appear enlarged, with the pulmonary vessels prominent. The diaphragms may appear normal or flattened, depending on the degree of air trapping present. If there is right-sided heart failure, swelling (**edema**) of the lower extremities is often present.

Pulmonary infections can seriously aggravate chronic bronchitis, and patients who have chronic bronchitis tend to have an increased number of chest infections. The appearance of the sputum produced can help predict worsening function. If it is normally white, a change to discolored sputum indicates the beginning of an infection. This may be accompanied by worsened hypoxemia and shortness of breath. Early treatment can potentially reverse an otherwise serious complication. Failure to manage the chest infection can result in severe hypoxemia and hypercapnia with exacerbation of right-sided heart failure. Acute respiratory failure superimposed on chronic failure is a common cause of death in patients with COPD.

Bronchiectasis

Bronchiectasis is pathologic dilatation of the bronchi. It usually results from the destruction of the bronchial walls by severe repeated infections, but some individuals are born with it (congenital bronchiectasis). The terms *saccular, cystic,* and *tubular* are used to describe the appearance of the bronchi. Most bronchiectasis involves prolonged episodes of infection. Bronchiectasis is common in CF and after bronchial obstruction by a tumor or foreign body. When the entire bronchial tree is involved, it is assumed that the disease is inherited or caused by developmental abnormalities.

The main clinical feature of bronchiectasis is a very productive cough. The sputum is usually purulent and foul-smelling. *Hemoptysis* is also common. Frequent bronchopulmonary infections lead to gas exchange abnormalities like those of chronic bronchitis. Right-sided heart failure follows the advancement of the disease. Chest x-ray studies, bronchograms, and CT scans are used to identify the type and extent of the disease. As in chronic bronchitis, spirometry may be useful for assessing the degree of obstruction and response to therapy.

Treatment of bronchiectasis includes vigorous bronchial hygiene. Regular antibiotic therapy is used to manage the repeated infections. Bronchoscopy and surgical resection are sometimes required to manage localized areas of infection. Patients with recurrent hemoptysis may require a resection of the offending lobe.

Management of Chronic Obstructive Pulmonary Disease

GOLD, a World Health Organization (WHO) program, works with health care professionals to raise awareness and improve the prevention and treatment of COPD. COPD is the third-leading cause of morbidity and mortality throughout the world. COPD often includes components of emphysema and chronic bronchitis (see Fig. 1.2). This association most likely is due to the common risk factor of cigarette smoking. *Hyperreactive* airways disease (asthma) may also be present. Reversibility of obstruction, however, is usually less than in uncomplicated asthma. Bronchiectasis and bronchiolitis are also commonly found in patients with COPD.

An essential ingredient in COPD management is early diagnosis. GOLD requires spirometry as the primary tool in the diagnosis of COPD. It also classifies airflow limitation into four grades (GOLD 1, mild; GOLD 2, moderate; GOLD 3, severe; and GOLD 4, very severe). Spirometry is recommended for all smokers with ≥ 20 years of smoking and chronic cough, dyspnea on exertion, mucus hypersecretion, or wheezing.

Treatment of COPD begins with smoking cessation and avoiding irritants that inflame the airways. The rate of decline in lung function (FEV_1) in smokers is approximately twice that of nonsmokers. Smoking cessation decreases the accelerated decline in most, but not all, smokers. Other measures aimed at keeping the airways open are also important. Inhaled bronchodilators, especially β_2 **agonists,** are commonly used. Combinations of β_2 agonists and anticholinergic bronchodilators, together with inhaled corticosteroids (ICSs), provide relief for many patients with COPD. This is often the case even when there is little improvement in airflow assessed by spirometry. Some patients require oral steroids (e.g., prednisone) to manage chronic inflammation. Antibiotics are commonly used at the first sign of respiratory infections, and vaccination against viral and bacterial (pneumococcus) infection is recommended. Digitalis and *diuretics* are most often prescribed for the management of cor pulmonale.

Breathing retraining, bronchial hygiene measures, and physical reconditioning are important therapeutic modalities in addition to pharmacologic management. Breathing retraining is especially important for the patient with advanced COPD. Grossly altered pulmonary mechanics favor hyperinflation and the use of accessory muscles. Training in the use of the diaphragm for slow, relaxed breathing can significantly improve gas exchange. Pulmonary rehabilitation, particularly physical reconditioning, permits many patients with otherwise debilitating disease to maintain their quality of life (Fig. 1.5).

Supplemental O_2 therapy is indicated in COPD when the patient's oxygen tension at rest or during exercise is less than 55 mm Hg. Oxygen may also be prescribed when signs of cor pulmonale are present. Many patients desaturate with exertion only. Exercise testing is the only reliable method of detecting exertional desaturation. Low-flow O_2 therapy can be implemented by several methods,

including portable systems. Chronic O_2 supplementation has been shown to improve survival in patients with COPD.

Single-lung transplantation has been used for patients with end-stage COPD who meet the inclusion criteria. Although lung transplantation causes an immediate improvement in pulmonary function, there are factors that need to be considered. The cost of hospitalization and follow-up care is extensive, and the lack of donor organs means that many patients with COPD die while awaiting transplantation. The prognosis for those receiving lung transplants is generally good. In some transplant recipients, a severe form of airway obstruction *(bronchiolitis obliterans)* has been found to occur in the transplanted lung. The reason for this obstructive process is unclear, but the progression is rapid. Spirometry is used to monitor transplant recipients to detect early changes associated with bronchiolitis obliterans (Fig. 1.6).

Lung volume reduction surgery (LVRS) has also been used to treat end-stage COPD. In this procedure, poorly perfused lung tissue is surgically removed. This allows the remaining lung units to expand with improved ventilation-perfusion matching. This technique works particularly well when there are well-defined areas of trapped gas with little perfusion (bullae). The procedure can be performed by sternotomy or by using a flexible thoracoscope. With both methods, lung volumes (TLC and RV) are reduced, and spirometry and gas exchange improve. Spirometry, lung volume measurement, and blood gas analysis are used to monitor changes in these patients. Lung volume reduction is expensive, carries significant risk, and does not appear to benefit all patients who have air trapping.

Hyperreactive Airway Disease: Asthma

Asthma is characterized by reversible airway obstruction. Obstruction is caused by inflammation of the mucosal lining of the airways, bronchospasm, and increased airway secretions. Bronchospasm is usually reversed by the inhalation of bronchodilators but may be persistent and severe in some patients. Inflammation is the essential element in the asthmatic response. Increased airway

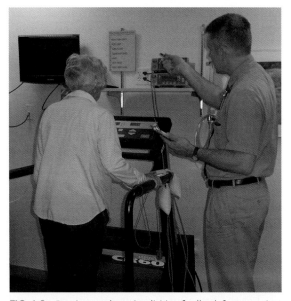

FIG. 1.5 Respiratory therapist eliciting feedback from a patient during a pulmonary rehabilitation exercise session.

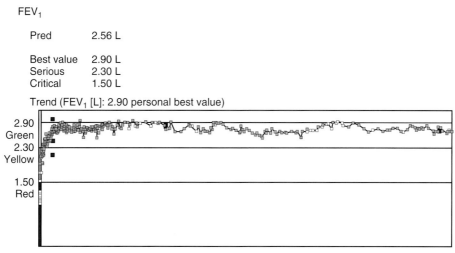

FEV$_1$

Pred	2.56 L
Best value	2.90 L
Serious	2.30 L
Critical	1.50 L

Trend (FEV$_1$ [L]: 2.90 personal best value)

FIG. 1.6   Home spirometry trend in a patient following lung transplant.

responsiveness is related to the inhalation of antigens, viral infections, air pollution, occupational exposure, cold air, and exercise. Spirometry is the most useful tool for detecting reversible airway obstruction. Improvement in the FEV$_1$ or FVC (see Chapter 2) is the hallmark of reversibility. Raw and specific airway conductance (sGaw) are also useful in the evaluation of reversible obstruction. PEF, measured using portable peak flow meters, can provide immediate information for a clinician or patient to modify therapy. Analysis of eNO can detect inflammatory changes in the airways even in the absence of spirometric or peak flow abnormalities.

Asthma can occur at any age but often begins during childhood. Even infants can have hyperreactive airways (see Chapter 8). Some children with asthma outgrow the disease, but in others, the disease continues into adulthood. In some individuals, asthma begins in adulthood, usually after age 40. There appears to be a hereditary component to asthma; many cases occur in patients who have a family history of asthma or allergic disorders.

Agents or events that cause an asthmatic episode are called *triggers* (Box 1.7). Antigens such as animal dander, pollens, and dusts are the most common triggers. Other common triggers include exposure to air pollutants, exercise in cold or dry air, occupational exposure to dusts or fumes, and viral upper respiratory infections. Aspirin or other drugs can

---

BOX 1.7   ASTHMA TRIGGERS

A. Allergic agents
   1. Pollens
   2. Animal dander (proteins)
   3. House dust mites
   4. Molds
B. Nonallergic agents
   1. Viral infections
   2. Exercise
   3. Cold air
   4. Air pollutants (sulfur, nitrogen dioxides)
   5. Cigarette smoke
   6. Drugs (aspirin, beta-blockers)
   7. Food additives
   8. Emotional upset
C. Occupational exposure
   1. Toluene 2,4-diisocyanate (TDI)
   2. Cotton, wood dusts
   3. Grain
   4. Metal salts
   5. Insecticides

---

also trigger asthma, as can food additives (e.g., metabisulfites) or emotional upset (e.g., crying, laughing). All these triggers act on the hyperresponsive airway to produce the symptoms of asthma.

The most common presentation of asthma includes wheezing, cough, and shortness of breath. The severity of asthmatic episodes varies, even in the same individual at different times. In many patients, airway function is relatively normal between intermittent episodes or attacks. Some patients have only cough or chest tightness that subsides spontaneously. However, severe episodes may be life-threatening. In its worst presentation, asthma causes continuous chest tightness and wheezing that may not respond to the usual therapy. Dyspnea and cough can both be extreme, and if unresolved, they can progress to respiratory failure.

During an attack, there is usually wheezing, noisy breathing, and prolonged expiratory times. If the attack is severe, there may be significant air trapping with decreased breath sounds, similar to the pattern seen in patients with emphysema. Accessory muscles of ventilation are used, and breathing may be labored. Spirometry or peak flows provide a simple means of tracking response to bronchodilators. Arterial blood gas testing may be necessary during severe asthmatic episodes. Hypoxemia is commonly present because of ventilation-perfusion mismatching. This usually results in acute alveolar hyperventilation that presents itself as respiratory alkalosis or metabolic alkalosis in chronic patients and deteriorates into respiratory acidosis, which suggests impending respiratory failure.

Bronchial provocation tests using methacholine, histamine, mannitol, exercise, or hyperventilation are often used to make the diagnosis of hyperreactive airways in patients who appear normal but have episodic symptoms. Skin testing is also used to demonstrate sensitivity to inhaled antigens. Elevated eNO levels are also predictive of the airway inflammation common in the patient with asthma and usually correlate with hyperresponsiveness measured by conventional bronchial challenge tests (see Chapter 9).

Management of Asthma

GINA, a WHO-sponsored program, and the National Asthma Education Prevention Program (NAEPP) are two resources that provide guidance on asthma management.

The first step in asthma management is avoiding known triggers. In some instances, this is easily accomplished. However, in the case of air pollution or occupational exposure, avoiding the offending substance may be expensive or impossible. Asthma education usually focuses on helping affected individuals identify and avoid triggers, monitoring their peak flows daily, and instructing them on the proper use of medications.

Pharmacologic management of asthma is usually based on a combination of bronchodilator, steroid, and antiinflammatory therapy. For some patients with mild asthma, a β_2 agonist bronchodilator from a metered-dose inhaler (MDI) may be the only treatment required. Various β_2 agonists are available, and these drugs are typically used as rescue medications. In moderate or severe asthma, long-acting β_2 agonist bronchodilators (e.g., salmeterol) are usually inhaled on a dosing schedule. Anticholinergic bronchodilators (e.g., ipratropium or tiotropium) have become widely prescribed for use in conjunction with β_2 agonists. Anticholinergic bronchodilators may be preferred in patients who experience tachycardia or tremor caused by adrenergic drugs. Although most β_2 agonists have a rapid onset of action (5–15 minutes), anticholinergic bronchodilators typically take 30 to 60 minutes for peak effect to occur but with much longer-lasting effects.

ICSs (e.g., beclomethasone, fluticasone, budesonide, and mometasone) are the most effective treatment for mild, moderate, and severe asthma. Steroids act primarily as antiinflammatory agents in the airways and may allow bronchodilators to work more effectively. Several different preparations are available in MDIs or dry-powder inhalers. Combinations of inhaled steroids and long-acting β_2 agonist bronchodilators seem to be highly effective at preventing asthma symptoms. Children and adolescents may not respond to inhaled steroids. Corticosteroids, in general, have several adverse side effects, including a reduction in bone density and adrenal suppression. Inhaled steroids have relatively fewer side effects; fungal infection of the oral cavity is a common problem. Inhaled steroids decrease bone density, and their effect on growth in children is not completely understood.

Cromolyn sodium or *nedocromil* is used to prophylactically prevent bronchoconstriction by blocking the release of mediators from mast cells in the airways. They cannot be used for acute episodes but may decrease the amount of corticosteroids or bronchodilators necessary. Cromolyn derivatives are available as a nebulized solution, inhaled powder, or MDI.

Leukotriene receptor antagonists are also used to reduce airway inflammation in asthma. They block the release of leukotrienes, which potentiate inflammatory mediators. These drugs may be effective in cases in which inhaled steroids are not and have been successfully used in conjunction with steroids. Some patients may better accept oral preparations of leukotriene inhibitors.

Some patients who have severe asthma caused by allergies may benefit from drugs that block immunoglobulin E (IgE)-mediated responses. Omalizumab blocks IgE from binding to mast cells and prevents activation that can lead to inflammation.

A significant tool in the management of asthma is the portable peak flow meter (see Chapters 2 and 11). This device allows simple monitoring of airway function by the patient at home, as well as by caregivers in a variety of settings. Measuring peak flow provides objective data to guide both the patient and physician in modifying bronchodilator therapy or seeking early treatment. Computerized peak flow meters that include symptom history (i.e., an electronic diary) allow asthma management to be tailored to the individual patient's asthmatic needs.

Cystic Fibrosis

CF is a disease that primarily affects the mucus-producing apparatus of the lungs and pancreas. CF is an inherited disorder, transmitted as an autosomal-recessive trait. In whites, it occurs in approximately 1 in 2500 to 3000 live births; in African Americans, CF is much less common, occurring in only 1 of 17,000 live births. There are approximately 70,000 to 100,000 people living worldwide with CF. A simple test, the sweat test, measures the chloride level in sweat, which is elevated in CF. Some states require a screening blood test for CF in newborns. CF was once considered a pediatric disease because affected individuals rarely lived to adulthood. Improved detection and aggressive treatment have increased the median survival age well into adulthood.

CF is characterized by the malabsorption of food because of pancreatic insufficiency and progressive suppurative pulmonary disease. In infancy and early childhood, gastrointestinal manifestations seem to predominate. As the child gets older, respiratory complications related to the tenacious mucus production take over. Other organ systems may be involved as well. Children with CF tend to remain chronically infected with respiratory *pathogens,* such as *Staphylococcus aureus, Pseudomonas aeruginosa,* or *Burkholderia cepacia.*

Clinical manifestations of CF include chronic cough and sinusitis, bronchiectasis, and atelectasis. Hemoptysis and pneumothorax are common. Pulmonary function studies may be used to follow the progression of the disease. Spirometry (FEV_1) is frequently measured as an index of the need for lung transplantation. Chest x-ray studies show changes consistent with bronchiectasis and honeycombing. Atelectasis commonly affects entire lobes because of mucus impaction. Other complications center on gastrointestinal manifestations (e.g., bowel obstruction and vitamin deficiencies). Most individuals with CF are diagnosed in infancy or early childhood, based on elevated sweat chloride levels. Occasionally, some young adults are not diagnosed until after age 15. In many instances, adolescents or even adults are misdiagnosed as having asthma or related pulmonary diseases. Misdiagnosis usually occurs in individuals who have mild CF with few complications.

Management of Cystic Fibrosis

Removal of the excess mucus produced in CF is the primary focus of management. This usually requires bronchial hygiene measures and pharmacologic intervention. Bronchodilators are used to reverse the bronchospasm that commonly accompanies chronic inflammation. A genetically engineered enzyme is now used to reduce mucus viscosity in patients with CF. This enzyme (rhDNase) is administered via an aerosol. This reduces the viscosity of secretions and improves airflow. Corticosteroids are used to combat both pulmonary inflammation and bronchial hyperreactivity. Continuous or intermittent antibiotics are also a mainstay of care in the patient with CF. Proper nutrition is similarly important in managing CF. Pancreatic insufficiency increases the patient's metabolic rate, even though nutrients are poorly absorbed in the intestine. Pancreatic enzyme supplements and vitamins are required, particularly in children with CF. For individuals with severe CF, lung transplantation has become a life-saving treatment. Pulmonary function studies are routinely used to assess lung function following transplantation.

Upper or Large Airway Obstruction

Many obstructive diseases involve the medium or small airways. Sometimes, airway obstruction occurs in the upper airways (nose, mouth, or pharynx) or in the large thoracic airways (trachea, main-stem bronchi). Obstruction can also occur where the upper and lower airways meet at the vocal cords. When obstruction occurs below the vocal cords, the degree of obstruction may vary with changes in thoracic pressure. This occurs because the airways themselves change size as thoracic pressure rises or falls. Obstructive processes above the vocal cords are not influenced by thoracic pressures but may still vary with airflow, depending on the type of lesion involved. Regardless of the location of the problem, large airway obstruction results in increased work of breathing. Extrathoracic or intrathoracic airway obstruction is frequently diagnosed using the flow-volume loop or measurements of Raw (see Chapters 2 and 4).

Vocal cord dysfunction (VCD) or damage can result in significant airway obstruction. The vocal cords are normally held open or abducted during inspiration. When damaged, the vocal cords move toward the midline, narrowing the airway opening. This type of obstruction limits flow primarily during inspiration. In some cases, expiratory flow may be reduced as well, but inspiratory flow is typically lower. Common causes of VCD include laryngeal muscle weakness or mechanical damage, as sometimes occurs during intubation of the trachea. Severe infections involving the larynx can leave scar tissue on the vocal cords or supporting structures. VCD often mimics asthma. It may become noticeably worse when ventilation is increased, such as during exercise. Neuromuscular disorders can cause paralysis of the vocal cords, also resulting in variable extrathoracic airway obstruction (see Chapter 2).

Tumors are a common cause of large airway obstruction. Lesions that invade the trachea or main-stem bronchi can significantly diminish airflow. The decrease in flow is related to the decrease in the cross-sectional area of the airway. If the airway lumen (i.e., the part not obstructed) varies in cross-sectional area with inspiration and expiration, the obstruction is described as *variable*. During inspiration, thoracic pressure decreases, and large airways increase their cross-sectional area. During expiration, the opposite occurs. If the airway is partially obstructed by a tumor, airflow will be decreased during inspiration and expiration but more so during expiration. If the tumor reduces the cross-sectional area of the airway but does not cause it to change with the phase of breathing, the obstruction is fixed. In this instance, both inspiratory and expiratory flows are reduced approximately equally (see Chapter 2). Tumors involving the upper airway may cause variable or fixed obstruction. If an extrathoracic tumor causes the airway cross section to vary with breathing, inspiratory flow is usually reduced. An easy way to remember the cause and effect is to use the mnemonic, "What's in is out, what's out is in." In other words, if the obstruction is within the thoracic cage, it will affect the expiratory flow-volume curve. In contrast, if the obstruction is outside of the thoracic cage (i.e., VCD), it will affect the inspiratory portion of the flow-volume loop.

Neuromuscular disorders that affect the muscles of the upper airway can also affect airway patency. When the muscles of the pharynx or larynx are relaxed (reduced muscle tone), airway collapse may occur during the inspiratory phase of breathing. Any disorder that affects the innervation of the pharyngeal muscles can cause similar obstructive patterns. Abnormal airflow patterns are sometimes seen in patients who have obstructive sleep apnea, although flow measurements cannot predict sleep apnea. Myasthenia gravis affects the muscles of respiration, including the muscles of the upper airway. Generalized weakness of these muscles can result in variable extrathoracic obstruction.

Both extrathoracic and intrathoracic large airway obstructions commonly result from trauma to the airways. This can occur as a result of motor vehicle accidents or falls. Scarring or stenosis of the trachea may also occur after prolonged endotracheal intubation or tracheostomy. The typical pattern is one of fixed obstruction, although some lesions do vary with the phase of breathing. Granulomatous disease, such as sarcoidosis or tuberculosis, can occasionally cause upper airway obstruction. Extrinsic airway compression can also reduce airflow. Goiters or mediastinal masses are the most common culprits that compress the airways in this way.

Management of Upper or Large Airway Obstruction

Treatment of extrathoracic or intrathoracic large airway obstruction is aimed at reversing the process produced by the offending lesions. For VCD, stopping inappropriate therapy (e.g., steroids) is the first step. Speech therapy and breathing retraining have been demonstrated to reduce inspiratory obstruction. In severe cases, a mixture of helium and oxygen (80% He and 20% O_2) may be needed to alleviate dyspnea and interrupt the episode. Treatment of neuromuscular disease, such as myasthenia gravis, often reverses the associated airway obstruction. Tumors usually require resection. Some neoplasms can be managed by radiation or chemotherapy only. In either case, spirometry with flow-volume curves (see Chapter 2) is used to assess airway obstruction. Surgical repair of trauma to the upper or large airways directly relieves airway obstruction and reduces the work of breathing.

Restrictive Lung Disease

Restrictive lung disease is characterized by the reduction of lung volumes. The VC and TLC are both reduced below the LLN. Any process that interferes with the bellows action of the lungs or chest wall can cause restriction. Restriction is often associated with interstitial lung diseases, including idiopathic fibrosis, pneumoconiosis, and sarcoidosis, as well as the following:

- Disease of the chest wall and pleura
- Neuromuscular disorders
- Congestive heart failure (CHF)
- Obesity
- Lung resection

- Scarring (fibrosis) caused by radiation or chemotherapy
- Transient problems such as pleural effusions, abdominal ascites, or pregnancy

Pulmonary Fibrosis

Pulmonary fibrosis involves scarring of the lung with involvement at the alveolar level. Multiple causes have been identified, including environmental pollutants, smoking, radiation, and connective tissue diseases. Patients who have pulmonary fibrosis present with dyspnea that increases with exertion and a dry, nonproductive cough.

Pulmonary fibrosis can follow the use of medications such as bleomycin, cyclophosphamide, methotrexate, or amiodarone. It is also associated with several autoimmune diseases. Rheumatoid arthritis, systemic lupus erythematosus (SLE), and scleroderma all produce alveolar wall inflammation and fibrotic changes. As each disease progresses, lung volumes are reduced. These reductions in VC and TLC occur as fibrosis causes the lungs to become stiff. Measurement of pulmonary compliance (see Chapter 4) is sometimes helpful in quantifying the effects of the fibrosis. DLco (see Chapter 3) is often reduced because of loss of lung volume and ventilation-perfusion mismatching. The same processes also cause hypoxemia at rest that worsens with exertion.

When other causes of pulmonary fibrosis have been ruled out, this condition is called *idiopathic pulmonary fibrosis* (IPF). IPF is a chronic progressive interstitial lung disease of unknown etiology, characterized by alveolar wall inflammation, resulting in fibrosis. Vascular changes are usually associated with pulmonary hypertension. These patients also have increasing exertional dyspnea, usually with a nonproductive cough. Clubbing of the fingers and expiratory rales are common physical findings. On the chest x-ray film, infiltrates are visible, and advanced IPF shows a honeycombing pattern.

Management of pulmonary fibrosis relies primarily on corticosteroids (prednisone). Long-term therapy is usually indicated, with large initial doses followed by tapering and then maintenance. Immunosuppressive agents are sometimes used in conjunction with steroids in difficult cases. In the most severe presentations, lung transplantation may be required. Spirometry, lung volume measurements, and D_{LCO} are routinely used to monitor the patient's progress and response to therapeutic interventions. Blood gases and exercise tests may be needed to gauge the degree of oxygen desaturation that is known to occur.

Pneumoconiosis

Pneumoconiosis is lung impairment caused by inhalation of particulate material (e.g., dusts). Specific types of dust exposures have been shown to result in pneumoconiosis (Table 1.1). Dust particles in the size range between 0.5 and 5.0 microns are considered most dangerous because they are deposited throughout the lung. A carefully taken history of the patient's exposure, including work history, is essential. (See Pulmonary History in the Preliminaries to Patient Testing section.) Most cases of pneumoconiosis are characterized by pulmonary fibrosis and chest x-ray abnormalities. Pulmonary function studies typically reveal a restrictive pattern with a reduction in D_{LCO}.

Silicosis, caused by inhalation of silica dust, is common. Silica is found in sand, slate, granite, and other ores; sandblasters, miners, and ceramic workers are a few of the occupations commonly exposed to silica. Silica is deposited in the lung and ingested by macrophages. This results in the formation of nodules around bronchioles and blood vessels. As the silicosis advances, fibrosis occurs. The patient usually has cough and dyspnea, especially on exertion. In addition to restriction shown by pulmonary function studies, some airways may also be obstructed. As nodules increase in size to more than 1 cm, the condition is labeled *progressive massive fibrosis* (PMF). PMF is usually accompanied by hypoxemia and pulmonary hypertension. Treatment of silicosis is directed at relieving hypoxemia and managing right-sided heart failure.

Asbestosis results from inhalation of asbestos fibers. Asbestos has been commonly used in the manufacture of insulating materials, brake linings, roofing materials, and fire-resistant materials. As with most pneumoconiosis, the risk of developing asbestosis is related to the intensity and duration of exposure. The onset of symptoms is usually delayed for 20 years. Cigarette smoking has been shown to shorten the period between exposure and onset of symptoms. Inhaled asbestos fibers are engulfed by alveolar macrophages. Fibrosis in alveolar walls and around bronchioles develops. The visceral pleura may also show fibrous deposits. Plaques, made up of collagenous connective tissue, are often found on the parietal pleura. The patient experiences dyspnea on exertion. PFTs show restriction and impaired diffusion (D_{LCO}). The chest x-ray film may show irregular densities in the lower lung fields,

TABLE 1.1
Common Pneumoconiosis

Dust	Pneumoconiosis	Occupation
Iron	Siderosis	Welder, miner
Tin	Stannosis	Metal worker
Barium	Baritosis	Miner, metallurgist, ceramics worker
Silica	Silicosis (aka grinder disease or potter rot)	Sandblaster, granite worker, brick maker, coal miner
Asbestos	Asbestosis	Brake/clutch manufacturer, shipbuilder, steam fitter, insulator
Talc	Talcosis	Ceramics worker, cosmetics maker
Beryllium	Berylliosis	Alloy maker, electronic tube maker, metal worker
Coal	Coal worker pneumoconiosis	Coal miner

fibrotic changes (honeycombing), and diaphragmatic calcifications. COPD and lung cancer are also common in patients with asbestosis and are related to cigarette smoking. Treatment consists of assessment with PFTs (especially D$_{LCO}$) and relief of symptoms.

Coal worker's pneumoconiosis (CWP) is caused by an accumulation of coal dust (carbon particles) in the lungs. It should not be confused with *black lung*, which is a legal term used to describe any chronic respiratory disease in a coal miner. Some coal contains silica, but CWP begins with a reaction to an accumulation of dust called a *coal macule*. These macules are usually found in the upper lobes. The black coal pigment is deposited around the respiratory bronchioles. Diagnosis of CWP is made by history and chest x-ray film interpretation. Onset of symptoms caused by CWP usually occurs in advanced cases. Coal workers often have respiratory symptoms and physiologic findings consistent with COPD. These symptoms may be related more to cigarette smoking than to coal dust exposure. CWP causes fibrosis, restriction on PFTs, hypoxemia, and pulmonary hypertension. As in the case of other pneumoconiosis, treatment is aimed at relief of the symptoms.

Sarcoidosis

Sarcoidosis is a granulomatous disease that affects multiple organ systems. The lungs are often involved. The disease appears most often in the second through fourth decades of life. In the United States it occurs more commonly in African Americans, especially in women. The granulomas found in sarcoidosis are composed of macrophages, epithelioid cells, and other inflammatory cells. Sarcoidosis has an active phase and a nonactive phase. In the active phase, granulomas form and increase in size. These granulomatous lesions may resolve with little or no structural change, or they may cause fibrosis in the target organ. In the nonactive phase, inflammation subsides, but scar tissue usually remains.

Symptoms of sarcoidosis include fatigue, muscle weakness, fever, and weight loss. Other symptoms involve the specific organ system in which the granulomatous changes occur. The lungs and lymph nodes of the mediastinum are frequently involved in patients who have sarcoidosis. Dyspnea and a dry, nonproductive cough are the most common presenting symptoms. Chest x-ray films usually show enlargement of the hilar and mediastinal lymph nodes. Interstitial infiltrates may also be present. Other systems commonly involved in sarcoidosis include the skin, eyes, musculoskeletal system, heart, and central nervous system.

PFTs show a pattern of restriction with relatively normal flows. It is not unusual for sarcoidosis in the early stages to show completely normal lung function. D$_{LCO}$ may not be reduced except when there is advanced fibrosis of lung tissue. Arterial blood gas measurements may be normal, or there may be hypoxemia. Cardiopulmonary exercise testing may show worsened gas exchange. Diagnosis of sarcoidosis is sometimes made via clinical findings and chest x-ray examination, but biopsy of affected tissue is often necessary. This may involve mediastinoscopy or fiberoptic bronchoscopy.

Management of sarcoidosis includes medications to treat symptoms such as fever, skin lesions, or arthralgia. Serious complications involving worsening pulmonary function are usually treated with corticosteroids.

Diseases of the Chest Wall and Pleura

Several disorders involving the chest wall or pleura of the lungs result in restrictive patterns on pulmonary function studies. Conditions affecting the thorax include kyphoscoliosis and obesity. Pleural diseases include pleurisy, pleural effusions, and pneumothorax.

Kyphoscoliosis is a condition that involves abnormal curvature of the spine both anteriorly *(kyphosis)* and laterally *(scoliosis)*. The degree of curvature is usually determined by x-rays, with curvature greater than 40 degrees requiring surgery. Patients who have kyphoscoliosis show rib-cage distortion that can lead to recurrent infections, as well as blood gas abnormalities. Depending on the degree of spinal curvature, the patient may have normal lung function or restriction. Ventilation may be normal. Lung compression usually causes ventilation-perfusion mismatching and hypoxemia. In severe cases, there may be hypercapnia and respiratory acidosis. Treatment of the disorder involves prevention of infections and relief of hypoxemia if present. Surgical correction is necessary in many cases, and pulmonary function studies are used to evaluate patients both preoperatively and postoperatively.

Pectus excavatum (sunken chest) is a congenital abnormality affecting the development of the sternum and ribs of the anterior chest. It is found more frequently in boys than in girls (approximately 3:1) and occurs in about 1 in 300 to 400 births, making it the most common congenital abnormality of the chest. The caved-in chest is usually obvious in infants but often does not cause significant limitations until adolescence. Pectus excavatum varies in severity but typically results in a restrictive pattern on PFTs. Exercise testing or other tests of cardiac performance may be indicated to assess functional limitations in severe cases. Pulmonary function and exercise tests may also be used to assess improvements following corrective surgery.

Obesity restricts ventilation, especially when the obesity is severe. Obesity is usually categorized using body mass index (BMI). BMI equals body weight in kilograms divided by height in meters squared (BMI = kg/m^2). A BMI of 18.5 to 24.9 is normal, 25 to 29.9 is considered overweight, and 30 or greater is considered obese. A BMI of 40 or greater is sometimes referred to as *morbid obesity*. The increased mass of the thorax and abdomen interferes with the bellows action of the chest wall, as well as excursion of the diaphragm. TLC and VC are usually preserved in obese individuals, but FRC and expiratory reserve volume (ERV) are characteristically reduced. Obesity is also sometimes associated with asthma-like symptoms. It is not clear whether asthma is related to obesity or if the restriction caused by obesity contributes to airflow limitation that mimics asthma. The airflow limitation occurs secondary to the subject breathing at or near RV.

Obesity may also be associated with a more general syndrome that consists of hypercapnia and hypoxemia, sleep apnea, and decreased respiratory drive. The combination of these findings is sometimes called the *obesity-hypoventilation syndrome*. Chronic hypoxemia in this syndrome results in polycythemia, pulmonary hypertension, and cor pulmonale. Not all patients who are obese show the signs of obesity-hypoventilation syndrome. However, pulmonary function studies often show restriction in proportion to the excess weight. Weight reduction relieves many of the associated symptoms. Respiratory stimulants, tracheostomy, and continuous positive airway pressure (CPAP) are used to manage the obstructive sleep apnea component.

Pleurisy and pleural effusions can each result in restrictive ventilatory patterns. Pleurisy is characterized by the deposition of a fibrous exudate on the pleural surface. It is associated with other pulmonary diseases such as pneumonia or lung cancer. Pleurisy is often accompanied by chest discomfort or pain and may precede the development of pleural effusions. Pleural effusion is an abnormal accumulation of fluid in the pleural space. This fluid may be either a transudate or an exudate. Transudates occur when there is an imbalance in the hydrostatic or oncotic pressures, as occurs in CHF. Exudates are associated with infections or with inflammation, as in lung carcinoma. Patients with pleural effusions usually have symptoms that relate to the extent of the effusion. Small effusions often go unnoticed. If the effusion is large, there may be atelectasis from compression of lung tissue and associated blood gas changes. PFTs show restriction because of volume loss. In some cases, there is restriction caused by splinting because of pain. Treatment of pleurisy and pleural effusions is directed toward the underlying cause. Large or unresolved pleural effusions often require thoracentesis or chest tube drainage. Patients with painful pleural involvement may have difficulty performing spirometry or breath holding as required for D_{LCO}.

Pneumothorax is a condition in which air enters the pleural space. This air leak may be caused by a perforation of the lung itself or of the chest wall (e.g., chest trauma). A small pneumothorax may not cause any symptoms. A large pneumothorax can result in severe dyspnea and chest pain. Physical examination of the patient reveals decreased chest movement on the affected side. Breath sounds are usually absent. A chest x-ray study shows a shift of the mediastinum away from the pneumothorax. Small pneumothoraxes usually resolve without treatment as gas is reabsorbed from the pleural space. Large air leaks usually require a chest tube with appropriate drainage to allow lung reexpansion.

PFTs are usually contraindicated in the presence of pneumothorax. However, undiagnosed pneumothorax may present a risk if pulmonary function studies are performed. Maneuvers that generate high intrathoracic pressures (i.e., FVC, MVV, MIP/MEP) can aggravate an untreated pneumothorax. The potential for the development of a tension pneumothorax exists when these maneuvers are performed. In a tension pneumothorax, air enters the pleural space but cannot escape. Increasing pressure compresses the opposite lung as well as the heart and great vessels. Compression of the mediastinum interferes with venous return to the heart and can cause a rapid drop in blood pressure. A tension pneumothorax can be fatal if not treated immediately. ***Patients referred for pulmonary function studies who have a known or suspected pneumothorax should be tested very carefully or not at all.*** In many instances, the information obtained may not justify the risk to the patient.

Neuromuscular Disorders

Diseases that affect the spinal cord, peripheral nerves, neuromuscular junctions, and respiratory muscles can all cause a restrictive pattern of pulmonary function. Most of these disorders result in an inability to generate normal respiratory pressures. The VC and TLC are often reduced, whereas the RV may be preserved. Some chronic neuromuscular disorders are associated with decreased lung compliance. Blood gas abnormalities, particularly hypoxemia, may result if the degree of involvement is severe. Stiff lungs and rapid respiratory rates often result in respiratory alkalosis (**hyperventilation**). Progressive muscle weakness results in respiratory acidosis (**hypoventilation**) and respiratory failure.

Paralysis of the diaphragm may be bilateral or unilateral. Bilateral paralysis may be the end stage of various disorders. The most prominent finding is *orthopnea* or shortness of breath in the supine position. In the upright position, the patient has a marked increase in VC and improvement in gas exchange. Simple spirometry in the supine and sitting positions can demonstrate the functional impairment. Unilateral paralysis often results from damage to one of the phrenic nerves (e.g., trauma, surgery, or tumor). As with bilateral paralysis, there is a marked change in VC from supine to sitting position. Diagnosis of which side is involved may require a chest x-ray or examination under fluoroscopy. Reduced inspiratory pressures may suggest diaphragmatic involvement.

Amyotrophic lateral sclerosis (ALS), or Lou Gehrig disease, affects the anterior horn cells of the spinal cord (motor neurons). Progressive muscle weakness results in a gradual decrease in VC and TLC, which is invariably fatal. Pulmonary function studies may be done serially to assess the progression of the disease.

Duchenne muscular dystrophy is caused by a defective gene for dystrophin (a protein in the muscles). It occurs in about 1 out of every 3600 male infants and is an inherited disorder. Symptoms usually occur before age 6 and can appear in infancy. VC monitoring and respiratory muscle strength measurements (MIP, MEP) are commonly performed but may be challenging depending on the age of the patient.

Guillain–Barré syndrome is a progressive disease in which the body's immune system attacks the peripheral nerves. Lower extremity weakness ascends to the upper extremities and face. There may be marked respiratory muscle weakness, along with weakness of the pharyngeal and laryngeal muscles. Many patients eventually require mechanical support of ventilation. Serial measurements of the VC, MIP, and MEP, cough peak flow (CPF), or sniff nasal inspiratory pressures (SNIPs) are used to follow the disease progression (see Chapter 10).

Myasthenia gravis is a chronic autoimmune disease affecting neuromuscular transmission. In myasthenia gravis, antibodies produced by the body's immune system block or destroy the receptors for acetylcholine at the neuromuscular junction, which prevents the muscle contraction from occurring. It particularly affects muscles innervated by the bulbar nuclei (i.e., face, lips, throat, and neck). The patient with myasthenia gravis has pronounced fatigability of the muscles. Speech and swallowing difficulties can occur with prolonged exercise of the associated muscles. Administration of edrophonium chloride (Tensilon) is sometimes used to confirm the diagnosis of myasthenia gravis; the drug blocks acetylcholinesterase and temporarily increases muscle strength in patients who have myasthenia gravis. When the ventilatory muscles become involved, a myasthenic crisis occurs. Progression of a myasthenic crisis can be assessed using VC and respiratory pressures. Analysis of the flow-volume curve (see Chapter 2) may be helpful in detecting upper airway obstruction brought on by muscular weakness.

Congestive Heart Failure

CHF is often used synonymously with *left ventricular failure*. Failure of the left ventricle may be caused by systemic hypertension, coronary artery disease, or aortic insufficiency. CHF may also be associated with cardiomyopathy, congenital heart defects, and left-to-right shunts. In each case, fluid backs up in the lungs. The pulmonary venous system becomes engorged. Fluid may spill into the alveolar spaces (pulmonary edema) or the pleural space (effusion).

The patient who has CHF usually has shortness of breath on exertion, cough, and fatigue. If coronary artery disease is the cause of CHF, there may be chest pain *(angina)* as well. Exertional dyspnea is related to pulmonary venous congestion. The fluid overload in the lungs reduces lung volume and makes the lungs stiff (decreased compliance). Dyspnea is usually worse when the patient is supine (i.e., orthopnea). This orthopnea results from increased pulmonary vascular congestion, which happens when interstitial fluid becomes intravascular, causing an increase in volume, which in turn causes vascular engorgement, promoting capillary leak. Dyspnea brought on by CHF may be difficult to distinguish from other causes (e.g., chronic pulmonary disease); therefore patients are often referred for pulmonary function studies. The chest x-ray film usually shows increased pulmonary congestion. The heart (left ventricle) may appear enlarged, particularly if systemic hypertension is the cause.

Treatment of CHF is directed at the underlying cause. Relief of systemic hypertension can reduce the myocardial workload. This is usually accomplished by vasodilator therapy. Reducing fluid retention is also important in managing CHF. Diuretics such as furosemide (Lasix) are commonly used to reduce the afterload on the ventricle. Oxygen therapy may also help reduce myocardial workload, especially if there is hypoxemia. If the cause of CHF is an arrhythmia, *antiarrhythmic* agents are typically used. PFTs, particularly lung volumes and DLCO, may be used to monitor the effects of treatment.

Lung Transplantation

Lung transplantation has evolved as an effective treatment for end-stage lung disease. Lung transplantation has been used for patients with CF, primary pulmonary hypertension, and COPD (Table 1.2). Double-lung transplants are usually performed in patients who have CF, generalized bronchiectasis, or some types of COPD. Heart–lung transplants have been used for Eisenmenger syndrome, pulmonary hypertension with cor pulmonale, and end-stage lung disease coexisting with severe heart disease. Single-lung transplantation has been used effectively in patients with COPD who are younger than approximately 60 years old. Single-lung transplantation offers the benefit that two recipients can share a single donor's organs.

TABLE 1.2	
Indications for Lung Transplantation	
Transplant Type	**Disease State**
Heart–lung	Eisenmenger syndrome, severe cardiac defect Pulmonary hypertension, cor pulmonale End-stage lung disease, coexisting severe cardiac disease
Double lung	Cystic fibrosis Generalized bronchiectasis COPD with severe chronic bronchitis or extensive bullae
Single lung	Restrictive fibrotic lung disease Eisenmenger syndrome (less severe cardiac anomalies) COPD Primary pulmonary hypertension

COPD, Chronic obstructive pulmonary disease.
Modified from American Thoracic Society. (2014). International guidelines for the selection of lung transplant candidates. *American Journal of Respiratory and Critical Care Medicine, 158,* 335–339.

Survival rates for lung transplant recipients have steadily improved. Longer survival is mainly due to more potent antirejection drugs (e.g., *cyclosporine*) and better adjunctive therapy. PFTs are used to both assess potential transplant candidates and follow them postoperatively.

Preoperative evaluation consists of documentation of the severity of the specific disease process. Spirometry, lung volumes, D_{LCO}, and blood gas analysis are all used to rank the level of dysfunction. The same tests are also used to detect sudden worsening of lung function that might necessitate rapid intervention. Cardiopulmonary exercise testing may be indicated to determine the extent of the physiologic abnormality. For example, a patient with borderline pulmonary hypertension at rest may develop severe hypertension during even mild exertion.

Most transplantation programs list patients as prospective candidates when their pulmonary disease has advanced beyond predefined limits. An extended wait for lung transplantation is a direct result of the shortage of donor organs. Patients are often referred for transplant evaluation when a major decline in their condition is observed. The term *transplant window* has been used to describe the time during which the patient is sick enough to require transplantation but healthy enough to have a reasonable chance of survival.

Posttransplant follow-up relies heavily on PFTs. Spirometry has been used extensively to monitor improvements resulting from transplantation. Recipients of double-lung transplants often show lung function values approaching those of normal patients within a few months. Blood gas changes usually occur immediately after surgery. Single-lung transplant (SLT) recipients show similar gains. However, because SLT patients retain a native lung, improvement in pulmonary function is usually less than when both lungs are replaced. Interpretation of spirometry, lung volumes, and blood gases in SLT patients is often complicated by the presence of the native lung along with the transplanted lung.

Besides monitoring improved lung function, PFTs are used to detect rejection and the development of bronchiolitis obliterans (BO). Rejection may be difficult to distinguish from other pulmonary complications (e.g., pneumonia) in patients who are immunosuppressed. There is some evidence that changes in spirometry (FVC, FEV_1, $FEF_{25\%-75\%}$) or distribution of gas (as measured by the single-breath technique) may signal episodes of acute rejection. Chronic rejection is thought to be associated with the development of BO. This pattern is characterized by the development of severe airflow limitation in the transplanted lung. Spirometry, particularly indices of small airway function such as $FEF_{25\% \text{ to } 75\%}$, may provide the earliest signs of BO.

PRELIMINARIES TO PATIENT TESTING

Testing During a Pandemic

In 2020, the world was dealing with the global COVID-19 pandemic. This led to professional societies publishing recommendations on when to utilize pulmonary function testing because the virus may be spread during lung function procedures, which may induce cough. Even after the COVID-19 pandemic has subsided, future pandemics may be the new reality. The European Respiratory Society (ERS) published its recommendations based on three levels of a pandemic outbreak.*

Level I: High Community Prevalence
1. Establish a screening process and do not test patients with active disease.
2. Perform only essential testing, and limit testing to spirometry and D_{LCO}.
3. Reorganize waiting and testing rooms to reduce exposure.
4. Reorganize the testing schedule to allow for additional cleaning procedures.
5. Testing should be performed with high-efficiency bacterial/viral filters and utilize single-patient-use disposables (nose clips, mouthpieces).

*Adapted from the ERS Recommendation from ERS Group 9.1 (Respiratory Function Technologists/Scientists). (n.d.). *Lung function testing during COVID-19 pandemic and beyond.* https://ers.app.box.com/s/zs1uu88wy51monr0ewd990itoz4tsn2h.

6. **Personal protective equipment (PPE),** including facemasks, face shields and/or goggles, gowns, and gloves, is recommended for all the testing staff. Hand hygiene is critical and should be strictly followed by staff and the subject. The use of a hand sanitizer by the patient prior to entering and exiting the testing room should be required.

Level II: Low Community Prevalence

1. Essential infection control measures (e.g., cleaning, PPE) should be maintained even though the prevalence is reduced/
2. Exercise testing, nebulization, bronchial challenge testing, and other aerosol-generating procedures should be limited to specific equipment and testing rooms.
3. Use filters on the exhalation ports of nebulizers and exercise testing equipment.

Level III: Controlled

1. Return to prepandemic standards for the delivery of lung function tests.

Which tests the laboratory provides, when to expand diagnostic services beyond the basic tests, and the extra infection precaution steps put in place are the decision of the laboratory management team and the local infection control department. However, basic guidelines from the American Thoracic Society (ATS) and ERS can be used to assist in the decision-making process.

Before Patient Testing

To provide accurate patient data, the laboratory needs to have a defined quality assurance program in place. The Clinical and Laboratory Standards Institute (CLSI), an organization that provides guidance for medical laboratories, adapted the concepts found in the International Standards Organization (ISO) 9001 recommendations and applied them to the laboratory setting in a guideline titled "A Quality Management System; a Model for Laboratory Services (QMS01-A5)." Table 1.3 describes the various hierarchical stages of quality, where a quality management system is a systematic, "process-oriented" approach to quality. The quality system model describes, documents, implements, measures, and monitors the implementation and effectiveness of the work operations of the laboratory.

TABLE 1.3

Stages of Quality

The quality management system (QMS) is a major level in the health care quality hierarchy and forms the basis for this document. Also see Fig. 1.7.[a]

Stage	Activities Performed
Total quality management	Management approach centered on sustained high quality by focusing on long-term success through customer satisfaction
Quality cost management	Measurement system for the economic aspects of the "cost of quality"
Quality management system	Systematic, process-oriented approach to meeting quality objectives
Quality assurance	Planned and systematic activities to provide confidence that an organization fulfills requirements for quality
Quality control	Operational process-control techniques to fulfill quality requirements for regulatory compliance and accreditation[b]

[a]Cianfrani, C. A., Tsiakals, J. J., & West, J. E. (2002). *The ASQ ISO 9000:2000 handbook.* Milwaukee, WI: American Society for Quality.
[b]International Organization for Standardization. (2005). *Quality management systems: Fundamentals and vocabulary.* ISO 9000. Geneva, Switzerland: International Organization for Standardization.

The model is characterized by quality elements that are essential components of an organization or laboratory's quality system and are called the *quality system essentials,* or QSEs.

The 12 QSEs

1. Documents and records management
2. Organization and leadership
3. Personnel management
4. Equipment management
5. Supplier and inventory
6. Process management
7. Information management
8. Nonconforming event management
9. Assessments
10. Continual improvement
11. Customer focus
12. Facilities and safety management

In the CLSI's quality system model, these 12 QSEs are identified across the laboratory's "Path of Workflow." In the pulmonary function laboratory, the path of workflow (POW) would include pretest, test, and posttest activities. Chapter 12 will further detail the POW activities and how integrating these concepts into a laboratory's quality plan ensures quality testing results (Fig. 1.7).

Several preliminary steps precede any pulmonary function study. These include patient preparation, physical measurements and assessment, brief pulmonary history, and instructions to the patient in the performance of specific test maneuvers. In addition, PFTs are usually done in an ordered sequence. The testing sequence may be determined by laboratory policy, or it may be adapted for specific needs using a predefined protocol.

Patient Preparation (Pretest Instructions)

Patient preparation for pulmonary function studies consists mainly of instructions given to the patient in advance of the actual test session. These instructions focus on taking or withholding specific medications, refraining from smoking and eating, and other guidelines related to specific tests (e.g., exercise tests, blood gases).

Withholding Medications

Patients referred for evaluation of airflow limitation are often already taking bronchodilators or related drugs. If the response to bronchodilators is to be assessed, bronchodilators should be withheld before testing. The exact length of time to withhold a bronchodilator is dictated by the onset of action and how long it takes for the drug to be metabolized and/or excreted. Guidelines for withholding specific bronchodilators before simple spirometry are presented in detail in Chapter 2. Recommendations for withholding medications before a bronchial challenge test (methacholine, exercise, hyperventilation, etc.) are found in Chapter 9. Some patients may have difficulty withholding bronchodilators. In the case of simple spirometry, the test may be performed if necessary, with an operator comment describing the use of bronchodilators before testing. The patient should be instructed to take the bronchodilator when breathing problems require it. Patients scheduled for a bronchial challenge who inadvertently take their bronchodilators may need to be rescheduled because bronchodilators can significantly alter airway response and lead to false-negative results.

Care should be taken when instructing outpatients about withholding medications. Some patients may be unable to correctly identify all their medications. Therefore it may be difficult for them to correctly withhold bronchodilators only. Some patients incorrectly withhold all medications. This may cause serious problems for patients who rely on insulin (patients with diabetes), antiarrhythmics, or antihypertensives used for high blood pressure. If the patient is uncertain, it may be preferable not to withhold any medications.

Smoking Cessation

Patients referred for PFTs should be asked to refrain from smoking for 1 hour before the test. Smoking cessation is especially important if D_{LCO} tests or arterial blood gas tests are ordered. Smoking has been shown to directly reduce D_{LCO}. Smoking also raises the level of CO in the blood, which also interferes with the measurement of D_{LCO} (CO back pressure in blood). Increased CO in the blood (COHb) also makes it difficult to interpret O_2 saturation measured by pulse oximetry (see Chapter 6). Smoking has been shown to reduce the levels of eNO, which may artifactually reduce the level of NO in patients who have airway inflammation.

Other Patient Preparation Issues

Patients referred for PFTs should refrain from eating a large meal immediately before their appointment. Two hours is usually sufficient to avoid vomiting or gastric distress during routine testing. The same is true if the patient will be exercising as part of the evaluation. Patients scheduled for a bronchial challenge test (see Chapter 9) have further defined withholding schedules. Outpatients scheduled for metabolic studies may need to fast for 8 hours before testing to assure a stable baseline. Patients should refrain from alcohol consumption for at least 8 hours before testing (Box 1.8).

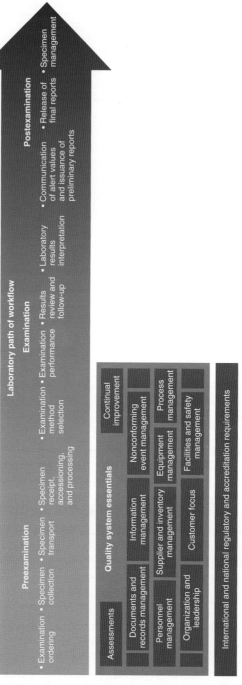

FIG. 1.7 The 12 quality system essentials (QSEs) function as building blocks that are necessary to support any laboratory's path of workflow and laboratory disciplines. This example represents how the 12 QSEs support a clinical laboratory's disciplines.(From Clinical and Laboratory Standards Institute. [2019]. CLSI document QMS01-A5. In *Quality management system: A model for laboratory services, approved guideline* [5th ed.]. Wayne, PA: Clinical and Laboratory Standards Institute.)

BOX 1.8   PRETEST INSTRUCTIONS FOR LUNG FUNCTION TESTING

- No smoking, vaping, or water pipe use 1 hour before the test.
- Do not consume intoxicants 8 hours prior to testing.
- Do not exercise (e.g., jogging, bicycling, fast walking, aerobics, etc.) for 1 hour before the test.
- Do not wear restrictive clothing that may interfere with taking a deep breath.

Patients should refrain from vigorous exercise immediately before testing and should be relaxed and comfortable during the test session. Exercise can result in circulating catecholamines, which affect airway tone. Depending on the time of exercise related to the testing time, exercise can also alter the subject's cardiac output, resulting in a change to carbon monoxide uptake. Tight-fitting clothing (e.g., neckties) may need to be loosened during testing. Dentures should be left in place; many patients find it easier to hold the mouthpiece using their dentures. However, if the dentures are loose, they may obstruct the mouthpiece, particularly during forced expiratory maneuvers.

Some patients may require special accommodations for PFTs to be performed safely and accurately. Patients, or those referring patients, should understand the requirements of the tests requested. Patients who are unable to sit or stand may require additional time or equipment for testing to be completed. Patients who have a permanent tracheostomy may also require special devices to allow connection to standard pulmonary function circuits. Patients who do not speak the primary language used in the laboratory may require an interpreter to be present during testing. Asking appropriate questions before the patient's appointment can identify each of these special needs.

Anthropometric Measurements

Various physical measurements are required for estimating each patient's expected level of pulmonary function. Age, height, and weight are usually recorded in addition to the patient's sex. Race or ethnic origin should also be recorded. Using the patient's declared ethnic origin is preferred. Basic physical assessment of the patient's respiratory status may be needed before and during testing.

The patient's age should be recorded as of the last birthday. Some computerized pulmonary function systems store the patient's birth date and calculate the age. This approach is helpful, especially when the patient returns periodically for serial testing. Care should be used when entering specially formatted data (e.g., dates) into a computerized system. Data-entry errors can result in gross overestimation or underestimation of the patient's expected values.

Standing height, in centimeters (within 1 decimal place), should be recorded with the patient barefoot or in stocking feet. A wall-mounted ruler (stadiometer) allows the patient to stand with the back against the wall and the head close to the ruler. If the patient is unable to stand upright, the arm span or other alternative methods (ulnar length) should be used. Patients who have a history of kyphosis, scoliosis, or related problems should also have the height estimated using their arm span. Arm span may be measured using a ruler placed on a wall or a tailor's tape measure (Fig. 1.8A–C). The patient should extend the arms horizontally on both sides, and the distance between the tips of the middle fingers is then measured. Alternately, the distance from the tip of the middle finger to the center of the vertebra at the level of the scapula is measured on each side and then summed. Height may then be estimated as arm span/1.06 or using regression equations that account for race, sex, and age in addition to arm span. Ulnar length is another method of estimating height in subjects. A measurement is made between the points of the elbow (olecranon process) and the midpoint of the prominent bone of the wrist (styloid process), on the left side if possible (Fig. 1.9).

A table is used to convert the ulnar length to an estimated height (Table 1.4). The patient's weight in pounds or kilograms (within 0.5 kg) should be measured with an accurate scale. Although body weight is typically not used in the calculation of predicted lung volumes, subjects who are morbidly obese may demonstrate a restrictive pattern. Measurement of weight and calculation of BMI

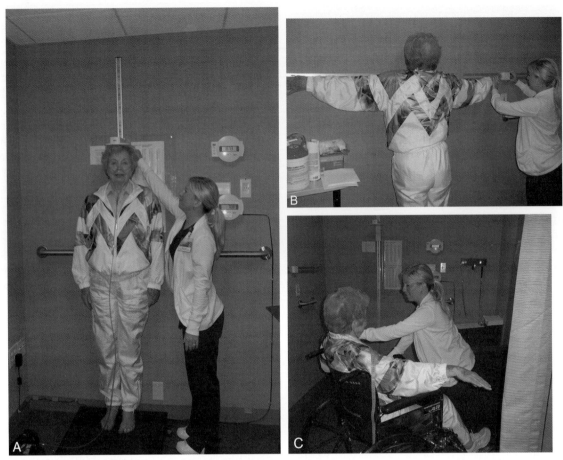

FIG. 1.8 (A) Measurement of height with stadiometer. (B) Measurement of arm span while standing. (C) Measurement of arm span with tailor's tape.

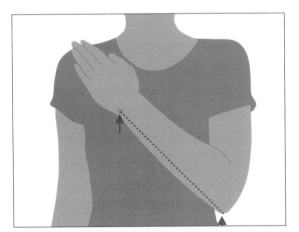

FIG. 1.9 The arm landmarks used to measure ulnar length to estimate standing height.

may be helpful for the interpretation of reduced lung volumes (e.g., FRC, ERV). Body weight is used to calculate other reference values (see Chapter 13). When weight is used to predict an expected value, the patient's ideal body weight should be used, unless noted otherwise. Using actual weight in patients who are obese may overestimate expected values if the reference set is based on subjects with normal weights. Weight is also used to express oxygen consumption (i.e., milliliter/kilogram) for exercise and metabolic measurements. The patient's weight may also be required when lung volumes are determined with the body plethysmograph. Weight is used to estimate body volume in the plethysmograph (see Chapter 4).

TABLE 1.4

Converting Ulnar Length to an Estimated Height

Height (m)														
Men (<65 years)	1.94	1.93	1.91	1.89	1.87	1.85	1.84	1.82	1.80	1.78	1.76	1.75	1.73	1.71
Men (>65 years)	1.87	1.86	1.84	1.82	1.81	1.79	1.78	1.76	1.75	1.73	1.71	1.70	1.68	1.67
Ulna length (cm)	32.0	31.5	31.0	30.5	30.0	29.5	29.0	28.5	28.0	27.5	27.0	26.5	26.0	25.5
Women (<65 years)	1.84	1.83	1.81	1.80	1.79	1.77	1.76	1.75	1.73	1.72	1.70	1.69	1.68	1.66
Women (>65 years)	1.84	1.83	1.81	1.79	1.78	1.76	1.75	1.73	1.71	1.70	1.68	1.66	1.65	1.63
Men (<65 years)	1.69	1.67	1.66	1.64	1.62	1.60	1.58	1.57	1.55	1.53	1.51	1.49	1.48	1.46
Men (>65 years)	1.65	1.63	1.62	1.60	1.59	1.57	1.56	1.54	1.52	1.51	1.49	1.48	1.46	1.45
Ulna length	25.0	24.5	24.0	23.5	23.0	22.5	22.0	21.5	21.0	20.5	20.0	19.5	19.0	18.5
Women (<65 years)	1.65	1.63	1.62	1.61	1.59	1.58	1.56	1.55	1.54	1.52	1.51	1.50	1.48	1.47
Women (>65 years)	1.61	1.60	1.58	1.56	1.55	1.53	1.52	1.50	1.48	1.47	1.45	1.44	1.42	1.40

PF TIP 1.2

Always measure the patient's height (without shoes) and weight. Height should be measured to the nearest centimeter and within 1 decimal place. Self-reported heights and weights are usually inaccurate. Arm span or other alternative measurements may be used to estimate standing height for patients who are unable to stand or who have significant spinal deformities.

Physical Assessment

Physical assessment of patients referred for pulmonary function studies may be needed to determine whether the individual can perform the test. Documentation concerning the physical assessment of the patient can also assist with the interpretation of test results. The physical assessment should focus on breathing pattern, breath sounds (if necessary), and respiratory symptoms (Box 1.9). These can be observed simply and noted as necessary. Assessment of the patient's oxygen status using pulse oximetry (see Chapter 6) may be required, especially if the subject presents to the laboratory using oxygen therapy. Some test modalities require the patient to be off oxygen, and if the patient is intolerant, that portion of the test will not be performed. Documenting operator comments regarding the patient's signs, symptoms, and oxygenation status at the time of the test is a useful adjunct, especially if test performance is less than optimal.

BOX 1.9 PHYSICAL ASSESSMENT DURING PULMONARY FUNCTION TESTING

- Breathing pattern
  - Is the respiratory rate excessive?
  - Are there any complaints of chest tightness or chest discomfort?
  - Are accessory muscles being used for breathing?
  - Is the patient using pursed lips?
- Breath sounds (with and without auscultation)
  - Are there audible breath sounds? Are breath sounds distant or absent?
  - Is there any wheezing? Over which lung fields?
  - Is there stridor, especially on inspiration?
  - Are there any other unusual breath sounds (e.g., crackles, rubs)?
- Respiratory symptoms
  - Is there obvious shortness of breath (mild, moderate, severe)?
  - Is the patient coughing? If so, is the cough productive?
  - Is there any cyanosis?
  - Is the patient receiving supplemental oxygen? If so, how much?
  - What is the patient's oxygen saturation (pulse oximetry reading)?

Pulmonary History

Accurate interpretation of pulmonary function studies—from simple screening spirometry to complete cardiopulmonary evaluation—requires clinical information related to possible pulmonary disease. An ordered array of questions that can be easily answered by the patient provides the most useful history. The interpreter of pulmonary function studies may have little clinical information other than that obtained at the time of testing. A pulmonary history should be taken routinely before pulmonary function testing (Box 1.10).

Most of these questions can be answered with *yes* or *no* or by circling an appropriate response. Space should be provided so that the patient or history taker can enter comments. Computerized pulmonary function systems often allow history data to be stored in a database along with the patient's test results. This is a useful feature but may limit the extent of the history that can be stored. In instances in which the physician performs the test, such history may be redundant if a medical history is available.

Interpretation of PFTs is best made if the clinical question asked of the test is considered. The clinician requesting the test should indicate the reason for the test. Examples of clinical questions asked of pulmonary function studies include, "Does the patient have airway obstruction?" or "Does the patient have hyperreactive airways?" The pulmonary history, including the reason for the test, should be used to decide what is normal or abnormal. Clinical information, as provided by the history, is especially

---

BOX 1.10   PULMONARY HISTORY

1. Age, sex, standing height, weight, race
2. Current diagnosis or reason for test
3. Family history: Did anyone in your immediate family (mother, father, brother, or sister) ever have the following?
   - Tuberculosis
   - Emphysema
   - Chronic bronchitis
   - Asthma
   - Hay fever or allergies
   - Lung cancer
   - Other lung disorders
4. Personal history: Have you ever had or been told that you had the following?
   - Tuberculosis
   - Emphysema
   - Chronic bronchitis
   - Asthma
   - Recurrent lung infections
   - Pneumonia or pleurisy
   - Allergies or hay fever
   - Chest injury (if so, what kind?) _____
   - Chest surgery (if so, what kind?) _____
5. Occupational/environmental exposure:
   - What is or was your occupation?
     _____
   - Have you ever been exposed to gases, dusts, or fumes that caused breathing problems? If so, what were they? _____
   - Do you have hobbies or other activities that cause breathing problems? If so, what are they?
     _____

6. Smoking habits: Have you ever smoked the following?
   - Cigarettes (how many packs per day?)
     _____
   - Cigars (how many per day?) _____
   - Pipe (how many bowls per day?) _____
   - How long? _____ years
   - Do you still smoke? Y/N If no, how long ago did you stop? _____ years
   - Do you live with a smoker? Y/N
7. Cough:
   - On most days, do you have a cough? Y/N
   - How long have you had this cough?
   - Is the cough productive or nonproductive?
8. Dyspnea: Do you get short of breath at the following times:
   - At rest? Y/N
   - On exertion? If so, what causes it? _____
   - At night? Y/N
9. Current medications (for heart, lung, blood pressure, other)

Medication	Last Taken

important when the patient's PFTs are near the lower or upper limits of normal. For example, an FEV_1 near the LLN would be interpreted differently in a healthy patient tested as part of a routine physical than it would be in a smoker who complained of increasing dyspnea.

PF TIP 1.3

A brief pulmonary history with the completion of a brief questionnaire can add significantly to the data provided by pulmonary function testing. Operators who are familiar with pulmonary pathophysiology can implement protocols that are appropriate for the purpose of the test.

TEST PERFORMANCE AND SEQUENCE

Pulmonary function laboratories should have written policies and procedures defining how each test is performed (see Chapter 12). An excellent resource is the ATS's *Pulmonary Function Laboratory Management and Procedure Manual,* 3rd edition (2016), which is available on the ATS website. Indications for performing a specific test should be related to the clinical question to be answered or to the patient's diagnosis. Testing protocols that can be modified for individual patients are usually the most cost-effective means of obtaining the required data. When the required tests have been determined, the exact sequence of tests can be selected. The sequence in which tests are performed may vary according to patient need and the test method used. For example, a patient with severe obstructive lung disease may not be able to perform an acceptable D_{LCO} maneuver until a bronchodilator has been administered.

Technologist-Driven Protocols (Operator-Driven Protocols)

As described previously, the basis for deciding which PFTs are needed is related to the clinical question being asked. The clinical question is often inappropriately stated as a diagnosis. In fact, many patients are referred for pulmonary function

studies to establish a diagnosis. For example, a patient may be referred with a diagnosis listed as "asthma." The clinical question is, "Does the patient have asthma?" Pulmonary function studies may be able to help answer this question, but the exact tests to be performed may not be defined. In this example, spirometry is indicated. Using an adaptive protocol, spirometry can be performed, and based on the results, appropriate additional tests can be selected (Fig. 1.10). Bronchial challenge tests may be performed if spirometry results are normal. Alternatively, additional tests such as lung volumes or D_{LCO} may be necessary.

The correct sequence (and timing) for performing tests is important. Many laboratories use a fixed order for component PFTs. This may include spirometry, followed by lung volumes and D_{LCO}. In some instances, the order of tests may need to be altered. The methodology used for some tests has definite effects on the results of subsequent procedures. For example, the multiple-breath N_2-washout test to determine FRC has the patient inhale 100% O_2 for several minutes. If this test is performed immediately before a D_{LCO} test, the elevated O_2 level in

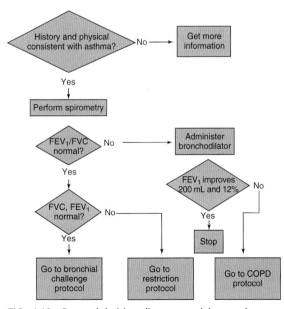

FIG. 1.10 Protocol-decision diagram used by a pulmonary function operator to select appropriate testing. The diagram shows routes to appropriate tests based on the results of simple spirometry.

the lungs (as well as in the blood and tissues) may reduce the measured D_{LCO}. Similarly, before repetition of the D_{LCO} maneuver or FRC determination by gas-dilution techniques, sufficient time must be allowed to wash out residual test gas.

Patient Instruction

Many PFTs depend on patient effort. To obtain valid data, patients must be instructed and coached for each maneuver. Instruction and coaching are particularly important for the FVC maneuver. Instruction should include a description of what the patient is expected to do, such as "You will take a deep breath in and then blow out as hard and as fast as possible." In addition to a description of the test, the maneuver should be demonstrated. During the actual test, vocal encouragement should be given so that the patient knows what is expected and continues for an appropriate interval. Any problems that occur with the first few efforts should be explained before the patient attempts the test again. For example, "That was a particularly good effort, but you stopped before blowing out for 6 seconds. Let us try that again, and keep blowing out until I signal you to relax." This type of feedback is important because patients may be uncertain of what is required. Patients should be instructed that some maneuvers will be repeated so that their best effort can be obtained. They should be assured that repeating some tests is required and does not necessarily reflect a problem on their part.

PF TIP 1.4

The most effective way to get good patient effort is to demonstrate each maneuver. For spirometry, this can be accomplished by using a mouthpiece and simulating the maneuver expected of the patient. Be sure to show what is meant by a maximal effort and how long the effort should last. Instructions such as "snap or blast" your air out after a maximal inspiration may help the patient understand the initial effort required during the maneuver.

Patients should also be carefully instructed for tests that require quiet breathing, such as lung volume determinations. Instructions about maintaining a good seal on the mouthpiece and continuing normal breathing can help reduce leaks or interrupted tests. Some maneuvers are complicated and may be difficult to describe to the patient. The D_{LCO} maneuver and panting in the body plethysmograph both consist of several steps. For these tests, a combination of demonstration and practice may be the most efficient means of instructing the patient.

Even after adequate instruction and demonstration, some patients may be unable to perform certain tests. This may be caused by a lack of coordination related to illness, pain because of their condition, or an inability to follow instructions. For example, a patient may experience uncontrollable coughing when asked to inspire deeply for an FVC maneuver. If the coughing prevents obtaining valid spirometry results, the fact should be noted in the operator's comments (see Chapter 2). Suboptimal effort by the patient can usually be detected as poorly repeatable results on effort-dependent tests (e.g., the FVC). Care should be taken that adequate instructions are given, and enough efforts recorded, before deciding that the patient did not give a maximal effort. If the patient cannot continue or refuses to continue a test, the exact reason should be documented in the operator's comments.

SUMMARY

- Tests are categorized as airway function tests (spirometry), lung volume tests, D_{LCO} tests, blood gases and gas exchange tests, cardiopulmonary exercise tests, and other specialized tests. Each of these groups contains a wide variety of tests and techniques.
- Indications are extremely important because they help the practitioner select appropriate tests. The clinical question asked of the test must be related to a valid indication for the test.
- The underlying pathology involved in common pulmonary diseases and the role of pulmonary function testing are discussed as they relate to the diagnosis and assessment of various diseases.

- Patient preparation for pulmonary function studies is covered in general terms. More detailed information for specific tests is presented in subsequent chapters. Many of the physical measurements and assessments, as well as the pulmonary history, are similar regardless of the tests being performed. Technologist-driven protocols are described. Algorithms for selecting only appropriate tests are becoming increasingly popular. Such tools improve the sensitivity of the tests to answer the clinical question, and they make tests more cost-effective.

CASE STUDY

CASE 1.1

Reason for test: Does the subject have asthma? (This case should be evaluated in conjunction with the protocol described in Fig. 1.10.)

HISTORY
The subject is a 22-year-old physical therapy student referred by the student health center at her college. She complains of cough and shortness of breath after vigorous exercise such as playing soccer. She describes a history of "sinus problems" and allergies. No one in her family has a history of pulmonary disease.

She has never smoked and has no history of unusual environmental exposure.

PULMONARY FUNCTION TESTING
Personal Data

Sex:	Female
Age:	22
Height:	175 cm
Weight:	55 kg
Ethnicity	Caucasian

Spirometry

	Before Drug					After Drug		
	Predicted	LLN	Actual	%	Z Score	Actual	%	% Change
FVC (L)	4.50	3.60	3.98	88.4	−0.94	4.21	95	6
FEV$_1$ (L)	3.88	3.12	2.71	69.8	−2.51	3.12	82	15
FEV$_1$/FVC	0.87	0.75	0.68	0.74	−2.43			

LLN, Lower limit of normal.

Technologist/Operator's Comments
All efforts met ATS/ERS criteria for acceptable spirometry. Subject had some coughing during prebronchodilator efforts.

QUESTIONS
1. What is the interpretation of the following?
   a. Prebronchodilator spirometry
   b. Response to a bronchodilator
2. What is the cause of the subject's symptoms?
3. What other tests might be indicated?

4. What treatment might be recommended based on these findings?

DISCUSSION
Interpretation
All spirometric efforts were performed acceptably. Prebronchodilator spirometry reveals mild obstruction. There is a significant improvement following an inhaled bronchodilator.

Impression: Reversible airway obstruction with significant response to a bronchodilator.

Cause of Symptoms

This subject's chief complaints of cough and shortness of breath following exertion are consistent with exercise-induced bronchospasm. The subject's FVC was above the LLN with a normal Z score, whereas her FEV_1 and FEV_1/FVC Z scores were both greater than –2. These findings are diagnostic of obstruction that is relatively mild. Posttesting following a β_2 agonist bronchodilator produced a 0.41-L (15%) increase in her FEV_1. This was a significant improvement in airflow. (The ATS/ERS recommends a 12% and 200-mL improvement as evidence of significant response to a bronchodilator.)

Other Tests

Using the sample protocol in Fig. 1.10, no additional tests are necessary to support the diagnosis of reversible airway obstruction. Bronchial challenge is not needed to document reversible obstruction.

Treatment

The subject was treated with a combination of ICS plus long-acting $\beta2$ agonist, which alleviated most of her symptoms. She was also given a short-acting bronchodilator for premedication before vigorous exercise.

SELF-ASSESSMENT QUESTIONS

Entry-Level

1. Measurement of airway resistance using the body plethysmograph was first described by
   a. Otis and McKerrow.
   b. Meneely and Kaltreider.
   c. DuBois and Comroe.
   d. August and Marie Krogh.
2. Indications for spirometry include which of the following?
   1. Preoperative evaluation for pneumonectomy
   2. Measurement of exercise capacity
   3. Determination of the beneficial effects of a bronchodilator
   4. Measurement of the effects of working in a dusty environment
   a. 1, 2, and 3
   b. 1, 3, and 4
   c. 2, 3, and 4
   d. 2 and 4 only
3. Measurement of lung volumes (TLC) is indicated
   a. to assess response to exercise training.
   b. whenever simple spirometry is performed.
   c. to diagnose restrictive lung disease.
   d. when hypoxemia is suspected.
4. Arterial blood gases would be indicated in which of the following patients?
   a. An adult with exercise-induced bronchospasm
   b. An adult with a suspected shunt
   c. An adolescent with myasthenia gravis
   d. An obese child

5. A 60-year-old male complains of dyspnea on exertion and when lying in bed; his FEV_1 and FVC are within normal limits. These symptoms are most consistent with which of the following?
   a. Emphysema
   b. CHF
   c. Sarcoidosis
   d. Interstitial pulmonary fibrosis
6. Which of the following diseases often results in an obstructive pattern when spirometry is performed?
   1. Asthma
   2. Emphysema
   3. Bronchiolitis obliterans
   4. Silicosis
   a. 1, 2, and 3
   b. 1, 3, and 4
   c. 2, 3, and 4
   d. 2 and 4 only
7. The most effective treatment for mild or moderate asthma is
   a. β_2-agonist bronchodilators.
   b. leukotriene receptor antagonists.
   c. ICSs.
   d. IgE blockers
8. Which of the following should a pulmonary function operator do before performing spirometry?
   a. Administer an anticholinergic bronchodilator.
   b. Ask the patient his or her current height and weight.

c. Demonstrate how to correctly perform the test maneuver.

d. Explain that the patient will be required to perform three maneuvers.

Advanced

9. Which of the following would be indicated for a patient who complains of dyspnea on exertion and chest tightness?
   a. D$_{LCO}$
   b. Cardiopulmonary exercise test
   c. Metabolic study
   d. eNO

10. Which of the following diseases is characterized by granulomatous changes and fibrosis in the lungs?
    a. Asthma
    b. CF
    c. Emphysema
    d. Sarcoidosis

11. Pulmonary function testing is usually contraindicated in which of the following conditions?
    a. ALS
    b. Eisenmenger syndrome
    c. Myasthenia gravis
    d. Untreated pneumothorax

12. Which of the following describes an appropriate physical measurement taken before pulmonary function testing?
    a. Actual body weight should be measured to calculate predicted values.

b. Standing height without shoes should be measured to the nearest decimal point in centimeters.

c. Arm span instead of height should be measured in children under age 12.

d. Sitting height × 1.32 may be used for patients who cannot stand.

13. A 25-year-old patient with suspected asthma performs spirometry. Her FVC is 3.2 L, and her FEV$_1$ is 2.2 L. Which of the following should the pulmonary function operator do next?
    a. Administer a bronchodilator.
    b. Evaluate for a possible restrictive disorder.
    c. Perform a bronchial challenge test.
    d. Check oxygen saturation by pulse oximetry.

14. A patient with COPD who is also a current smoker states that he has smoked within 1 hour before his scheduled PFT. Which of the following tests might produce inaccurate results because of this?
    1. FRC by He dilution
    2. D$_{LCO}$
    3. Pulse oximetry
    4. MIP and MEP
       a. 1, 2, and 3
       b. 2 and 3 only
       c. 2 and 4 only
       d. 3 and 4 only

SELECTED BIBLIOGRAPHY

General References

American Thoracic Society. (2016). *Pulmonary function laboratory management and procedure manual* (3rd ed.). New York: ATS. www.thoracic.org. Accessed 10.15.20.

Spriggs, E. A. (1978). The history of spirometry. *British Journal of Diseases of the Chest, 72,* 165–180.

Indications for Pulmonary Function Testing

Beydon, N., Davis, S., Lombardi, E., et al. (2007). An Official American Thoracic Society/European Respiratory Society Statement: Pulmonary function testing in preschool children. *American Journal of Respiratory and Critical Care Medicine, 175,* 1304–1345.

Graham, B., Brusasco, V., Burgos, F., Cooper, B., et al. (2017). 2017 ERS/ATS standards for single-breath carbon monoxide uptake in the lung. *Eur Respir J, 2017, 49.*

Graham, B., Steenbruggen, I., Miller, M., et al. (2019). Standardization of Spirometry 2019 Update. *Am J Respir Crit Care Med, Vol 200*(Iss 8), e70–e88. Oct 15, 2019.

Pauwels, R. A., Buist, S. A., Calverley, P. M. A., et al. (2001). GOLD Scientific Committee: Global strategy for the diagnosis, management, and prevention of chronic obstructive pulmonary disease. *American Journal of Respiratory and Critical Care Medicine, 163,* 1256–1276.

Raffin, T. A. (1986). Indications for arterial blood gas analysis. *Annals of Internal Medicine, 105,* 390–398.

Sietsema, K., Sue, D., Stringer, W., & Ward, S. (2020). *Wasserman and Whipp's Principles of exercise testing and interpretation* (6th ed.). Philadelphia, PA: Lippincott Williams & Wilkins.

Wanger, J., Clausen, J. L., Coates, A., et al. (2005). Standardisation of the measurement of lung volumes. *European Respiratory Journal, 26,* 511–522.

Patterns of Impaired Pulmonary Function

Aboussouan, L. S. (2005). Respiratory disorders in neurologic diseases. *Cleveland Clinic Journal of Medicine, 72*(6), 511–520.

Celli, B. R., MacNee, W., Agusti, A., et al. (2004). Standards for the diagnosis and treatment of patients with COPD: A summary of the ATS/ERS position paper. *European Respiratory Journal, 23,* 932–946.

Dundas, I., & Mckenzie, S. (2006). Spirometry in the diagnosis of asthma in children. *Current Opinion in Pulmonary Medicine, 12*(1), 28–33.

Enright, P. L. (2005). The diagnosis of asthma in older patients. *Experimental Lung Research, 31*(Suppl 1), 15–21.

Estenne, M., & Kotloff, R. M. (2006). Update in transplantation 2005. *American Journal of Respiratory and Critical Care Medicine, 173*(6), 593–598.

Flume, P., O'Sullivan, B., Robinson, K., et al. (2007). Cystic fibrosis pulmonary guidelines. *American Journal of Respiratory and Critical Care Medicine, 176,* 957–969.

Global Initiative for Asthma (GINA). www.ginaasthma. org. Accessed 10.01.2020.

Global Initiative for Chronic Obstructive Lung Disease (GOLD) 2020. www.goldcopd.org. Accessed 10.01.2020.

Lim, K., & Mottram, C. (2008). The use of fraction of exhaled nitric oxide in pulmonary practice. *Chest, 133,* 1232–1242.

National Asthma Education and Prevention Program. (2007). *Expert panel report 3: Guidelines for the diagnosis and management of asthma.* Bethesda, MD: Department of Health and Human Services. www.nhlbi.nih.gov/ guidelines/asthma/asthgdln.htm.

Putnam, M. T., & Wise, R. A. (1996). Myasthenia gravis and upper airway obstruction. *Chest, 109,* 400–404.

Raghu, G., Remy-Jardin, M., Myers, J., et al. (2018). An Official ATS/ERS/JRS/ALAT Statement: Diagnosis of Idiopathic pulmonary fibrosis: Evidence-based guidelines for diagnosis and management. *American Journal of Respiratory and Critical Care Medicine Volume 198 Number 5.*

Smith, A. D., Cowan, J. O., Filsell, S., et al. (2004). Diagnosing asthma: Comparisons between exhaled nitric oxide measurements and conventional tests. *American Journal of Respiratory and Critical Care Medicine, 169*(4), 473–478.

Spurzem, J. R., & Rennard, S. I. (2005). Pathogenesis of COPD. *Seminars in Respiratory and Critical Care Medicine, 26*(2), 142–153.

Weill, D., Benden, C., Corris, P., et al. (2015). A consensus document for the selection of lung transplant candidates: 2014—An update from the Pulmonary Transplantation Council of the International Society for Heart and Lung Transplantation. *Journal of Heart and Lung Transplantation, 34*(1), 1–15.

Preliminaries to Patient Testing

American Thoracic Society. (2016). Chapter 3: Quality system essentials for general operational issues. In *Pulmonary function laboratory management and procedure manual* (3rd ed.). New York: ATS.

Clinical and Laboratory Standards Institute (CLSI). (2019). *CLSI document QMS01-A5. Quality management system: A model for laboratory services, approved guideline* (5th ed.). Wayne PA: Clinical and Laboratory Standards Institute.

Disability Evaluation Under Social Security, 3.00 Respiratory Disorders – Adult. https://www.ssa.gov/ disability/professionals/bluebook/3.00-Respiratory-Adult.htm#3_00D4 (accessed 10.1.2020).

Recommendation from ERS Group 9.1 (Respiratory Function Technologists/Scientists). (n.d.). *Lung function testing during COVID-19 pandemic and beyond.* https://ers.app.box.com/s/ zs1uu88wy51monr0ewd990itoz4tsn2h. This statement is endorsed by ERS Assembly 4 and will be updated as evidence emerges.

Wilson, K. C., Kaminsky, D. A., Michaud, G., et al. (2020). Restoring Pulmonary and Sleep Services as the COVID-19 Pandemic Lessens: From an Association of Pulmonary, Critical Care, and Sleep Division Directors and American Thoracic Society-Coordinated Task Force. *Annals of the American Thoracic Society, 17*(11), 1343–1351.

Chapter 2

Spirometry

CHAPTER OUTLINE

LEARNING OBJECTIVES

After studying the chapter and reviewing the figures, tables, and case studies, you should be able to do the following:

Entry-level

1. Determine whether spirometry is acceptable, repeatable, and/or usable.
2. Identify airway obstruction using vital capacity (VC) and forced expiratory volume in 1 second (FEV_1).
3. Differentiate between obstruction and restriction as causes of reduced VC.
4. Determine whether there is a significant response to bronchodilators.

Advanced

1. Select the appropriate VC and FEV_1 for reporting from a series of spirometry maneuvers.
2. Quantify the degree of obstruction according to American Thoracic Society–European Respiratory Society (ATS-ERS) criteria.
3. Describe the characteristics of an intrathoracic or extrathoracic obstruction pattern.
4. Evaluate flow-volume curves.

KEY TERMS

body temperature, pressure, and saturation (BTPS)
expiratory reserve volume (ERV)

$FEF_{25\%-75\%}$
FEV_1/VC
forced expiratory volume (FEV_T)

forced vital capacity (FVC)
inspiratory capacity (IC)
isovolume correction

maximal expiratory flow volume
    (MEFV)
maximal inspiratory flow volume
    (MIFV)

maximal voluntary ventilation
    (MVV)
peak expiratory flow (PEF)
peak flow meter

start-of-test
transpulmonary pressure (Ptp)

The chapter begins with the measurement of the vital capacity (VC) using simple spirometry, followed by the most widely used pulmonary function test, the **forced vital capacity (FVC)** maneuver. Special emphasis is placed on the performance of each test. Criteria for judging the acceptability and repeatability of test data are provided based on the most recent guidelines published by the American Thoracic Society–European Respiratory Society (ATS-ERS) Task Force on Standardization of Lung Function Testing. Volume–time and flow–volume curves are described as the two most common presentations of spirometric data. Bronchodilator studies to determine the reversibility of airway obstruction are also presented. Other tests described include **peak expiratory flow (PEF)** and **maximal**

voluntary ventilation (MVV). Case studies and self-assessment questions are included at the end of the chapter.

VITAL CAPACITY

Description

The VC is the volume of gas measured from a slow complete expiration after a *maximal inspiration* without forced or rapid effort (Fig. 2.1). Alternately, VC may be recorded as a maximal inspiration after a complete expiration. VC is normally recorded in either liters (L) or milliliters (mL) and reported at **body temperature, pressure, and saturation (BTPS)**. VC is sometimes referred to as the *slow vital capacity*

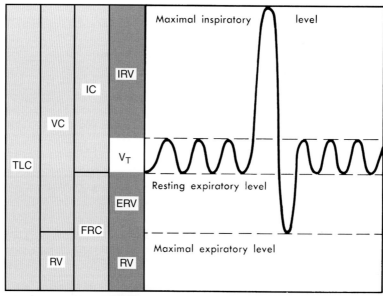

FIG. 2.1 Lung volumes and capacities. Diagrammatic representation of lung volumes and capacities based on a simple spirogram. Relationships between the subdivisions and relative sizes compared with TLC are shown *(shaded areas)*. Resting expiratory level is used as a starting point for FRC determinations because it remains more stable than other identifiable points during repeated measurements. *ERV,* Expiratory reserve volume; *FRC,* functional residual capacity; *IC,* inspiratory capacity; *IRV,* inspiratory reserve volume; *RV,* residual volume; *TLC,* total lung capacity; *VC,* vital capacity; *VT,* tidal volume. (Modified from Comroe, J. H. Jr., Forster, R. E., Dubois, A. B., et al. [1962]. *The lung: Clinical physiology and pulmonary function tests* [2nd ed.]. St. Louis, MO: Mosby.)

(SVC), distinguishing it from FVC. **Inspiratory capacity (IC)** and **expiratory reserve volume (ERV)** are subdivisions of the VC. IC is the largest volume of gas that can be inspired from the resting expiratory level (see Fig. 2.1). IC is sometimes further divided into the tidal volume (V_T) and inspiratory reserve volume (IRV). ERV is the largest volume of gas that can be expired from the resting end-expiratory level (see Fig. 2.1). Both the IC and ERV are recorded in liters or milliliters corrected to BTPS.

Technique

SVC is measured by having the patient inspire maximally and then exhale completely into a spirometer. (See Chapter 11 for a complete discussion of spirometers.) The patient is instructed to perform the maneuver slowly and completely. SVC can also be measured from maximal expiration to maximal inspiration. The spirometer does not need to produce a graphic display if only SVC is to be measured. However, if IC and ERV are to be determined (see Fig. 2.1), some means of recording volume change is required. The graphic display may be a computer screen or a recording device (see Chapter 11). A graphic display allows the technologist to determine that the test is performed correctly (Criteria for Acceptability 2.1). A graphic display is also usually required for reimbursement purposes.

CRITERIA FOR ACCEPTABILITY 2.1

Slow Vital Capacity

1. End-expiratory volume varies by less than 100 mL for three preceding breaths.
2. Volume plateau is observed at maximal inspiration and expiration.
3. Two acceptable VC maneuvers should be obtained—volumes agree within 150 mL.

Obtaining a valid SVC is important. The subdivisions of the SVC (IC and ERV) are used in the calculation of residual volume (RV) and total lung capacity (TLC). An excessively large V_T or an irregular breathing pattern during the SVC maneuver may alter ERV or IC. If either ERV or IC is erroneously recorded, other lung volumes may be incorrectly estimated (see Chapter 4).

IC is measured by having the patient breathe normally for three or four breaths and then inhale maximally. The volume inspired from the resting expiratory level is measured by the computer or from a spirogram. This is usually done as part of an SVC maneuver. IC may also be calculated by subtracting the ERV from the SVC. ERV is measured by having the patient breathe normally for three or four breaths and then exhale maximally. The change in volume from the end-expiratory level to the maximal expiratory level is the ERV. ERV may also be calculated by subtracting the IC from the SVC. IC and ERV are usually measured from the same VC maneuver. IC and ERV should be reported as the average of at least three acceptable maneuvers, whereas VC is reported as the largest of at least three acceptable maneuvers.

The accuracy of the IC and ERV measurements depends on the stability of the end-expiratory level, which should vary by less than 100 mL. Three or more tidal breaths should be recorded before the SVC maneuver is performed. If the end-expiratory volume is not consistent, IC and/or ERV may be measured incorrectly (i.e., too large or too small). Even if the end-expiratory level is constant, the V_T usually increases when the patient breathes through a mouthpiece with a nose clip in place. This increase in V_T may change the IC or ERV, depending on the patient's breathing pattern. Erroneous estimates of ERV may affect the calculation of RV, as described in Chapter 4.

Significance and Pathophysiology

Spirometry is indicated in a variety of situations (see Chapter 1). According to the 2019 ATS-ERS technical statement, there are no absolute contraindications to spirometry, but many relative contraindications should be considered (Box 2.1). Testing personnel should be aware of these conditions and have policies in place that guide decisions on whether or not to test the subject.

Normal SVC may vary as much as 20% above or below the predicted value in healthy individuals, but it must be above the bottom 5th percentile (lower limit of normal [LLN]; see Chapter 13) to be considered normal. The ATS-ERS guidelines recommend the use of the Global Lung Initiative (GLI) reference set. This predicted set has results from ages 3 to 95, with significantly stronger numbers than previously

---

BOX 2.1   RELATIVE CONTRAINDICATIONS TO SPIROMETRY

Attributable to increases in myocardial demand or changes in blood pressure
  Acute myocardial infarction within 1 wk
  Systemic hypotension or severe hypertension
  Significant atrial/ventricular arrhythmia
  Noncompensated heart failure
  Uncontrolled pulmonary hypertension
  Acute cor pulmonale
  Clinically unstable pulmonary embolism
  History of syncope related to forced expiration/cough
Attributable to increases in intracranial/intraocular pressure
  Cerebral aneurysm
  Brain surgery within 4 wk
  Recent concussion with continuing symptoms
  Eye surgery within 1 wk
Attributable to increases in sinus and middle ear pressures
  Sinus surgery or middle ear surgery or infection within 1 wk
Attributable to increases in intrathoracic and intraabdominal pressure
  Presence of pneumothorax
  Thoracic surgery within 4 wk
  Abdominal surgery within 4 wk
  Late-term pregnancy
Infection control issues
  Active or suspected transmissible respiratory or systemic infection, including tuberculosis
  Physical conditions predisposing to transmission of infections, such as hemoptysis, significant secretions, or oral lesions or oral bleeding

Adapted from 2019 ATS-ERS Spirometry Update.

---

in patients with diaphragmatic paralysis, neuromuscular disease, or symptoms that occur in the supine position that are not explained by other PF tests. Normal subjects typically have a decrease in VC of 3% to 8%, whereas subjects with diaphragm dysfunction would have a decrease of greater than 10%. Lechtzin and colleagues demonstrated that an FVC of less than 75% predicted was 100% sensitive and specific for predicting diaphragm weakness.

PF TIP 2.1

Normal values for lung function parameters are obtained by studying healthy subjects. The predicted or reference value for VC is computed using an equation, such as the following:

$$VC = x\,(Height) - y\,(Age) - z$$

where x, y, and z are constants
    Predicted values may be read from special diagrams called **nomograms** but are usually calculated by a computer. (See Chapter 13.) The LLN, representing the lower 5th percentile of the normal distribution curve, is recommended as the cutoff to judge normality.

---

published reference sets, which increased the statistical power of the reference (see Chapter 13).

In adults, VC varies directly with height and inversely with age; tall patients have larger VCs than short patients. VC increases up to approximately age 20 and then decreases each year thereafter, with an average decrease of about 25 to 30 mL/yr. It is usually smaller in women than in men because of differences in body size. Recent evidence indicates that lung volumes may differ significantly according to ethnic origin. VC also varies in individuals, depending on body position or time of day. Interpretation of lung function should consider the key factors of age, sex, height, and race (see Chapter 13).

VC can also be measured in the supine or prone position to characterize the effect the position has

As Dr. Hutchinson originally noted (see Chapter 1), a patient's VC is directly related to survival, and numerous studies have since supported his conclusion. In a study published in 2011 using data on spirometry and survival from the Atherosclerosis Risk in Communities (ARIC) data set, 7489 participants with usable spirometry data were compared against measures of ventilatory function after controlling for many other factors likely to be associated with survival. The study concluded that survival was strongly associated with the FVC over all other spirometry parameters.

There are numerous causes of a decreased VC (Box 2.2). In general, these fall into the categories of loss of distensible lung tissue (i.e., fibrosis), obstructive lung disease, and reduced chest wall expansion (i.e., neuromuscular, kyphosis).

When the VC is reduced, additional pulmonary function measurements may be indicated. Forced expiratory maneuvers (see the section Forced Vital

---

BOX 2.2   CAUSES OF REDUCED VITAL CAPACITY

Loss of Distensible Lung Tissue

Lung cancer
Pulmonary vascular congestion, pulmonary edema
Pneumonia
Atelectasis
Pulmonary fibrosis (e.g., from dust, drug toxicity, radiation, or idiopathic)
Pleural effusion or pleural scarring
Pneumothorax
Surgical removal (e.g., lobectomy)

Obstructive Lung Disease (caused by gas trapping, resulting in elevated residual volume [RV] but normal total lung capacity [TLC])

Reduced Chest Wall Excursion

Neuromuscular weakness (e.g., myasthenia gravis)
Chest wall deformity (e.g., kyphoscoliosis)
Obesity, pregnancy, ascites
Suboptimal patient effort (e.g., caused by pain, motivation)

Capacity in this chapter) can reveal whether the reduced VC is caused by obstruction. Reduced VC without slowing of expiratory flow is a nonspecific finding. Measurement of other lung volumes (see Chapter 4) may be indicated to determine whether a restrictive defect is present. Measurement of muscle pressures may help determine whether there is a problem with neuromuscular weakness (see Chapter 10).

In adults, VC less than the LLN (95% confidence limits; see Chapter 13) may be considered abnormal. Interpretation of the measured VC in relation to the reference value should consider the clinical question to be answered (Interpretive Strategies 2.1). The clinical question is often revealed in the history and physical findings of the patient (see Chapter 1). The terms *mild, moderate,* and *severe* may be used to qualify the extent of reduction of the VC in a manner similar to that described for FEV_1 (see the following section, Forced Expiratory Volume).

Artificially low estimates of the VC may result from poor patient effort. Similarly, inadequate patient instruction may affect the performance of the test maneuver. These errors may be eliminated by applying appropriate criteria (see Criteria for Acceptability 2.1). The values for at least two maneuvers should be reproducible within 150 mL.

IC and ERV are approximately 75% and 25% of the VC, respectively. Changes in IC or ERV usually parallel increases or decreases in the VC. Increased V_T caused by exertion or acid–base disorders (e.g., metabolic acidosis, respiratory alkalosis) may reduce IRV or ERV. This occurs because end-inspiratory and end-expiratory levels (see Fig. 2.1) are altered. A similar pattern is commonly seen when patients breathe into a spirometer through a mouthpiece with nose clips in place. Changes in IC or ERV are of minimal diagnostic significance when considered alone. Reduction of IC or ERV is consistent with restrictive defects. Obese patients typically show a decrease in ERV, usually resulting in a low VC. A reduced ERV is one of the earliest lung function changes in obese patients.

INTERPRETIVE STRATEGIES 2.1

Slow Vital Capacity

1. Was the test performed acceptably? Is it repeatable?
2. Are reference values correct? Age? Sex? Height? Ethnicity?
3. Is VC less than predicted? If so, to what extent? Is it less than the LLN?
4. How does SVC relate to the clinical question to be answered? Is SVC correlated to the history and physical findings?
5. Are additional tests indicated? Lung volumes? FVC?

FORCED VITAL CAPACITY, FORCED EXPIRATORY VOLUME, AND FORCED EXPIRATORY FLOW

Description

FVC is the maximum volume of gas that can be expired when the patient exhales as forcefully and rapidly as possible after a maximal inspiration. This procedure is often referred to as the *FVC maneuver.* A similar maneuver, beginning at maximal expiration and inspiring as forcefully as possible, is called *forced inspiratory vital capacity* (FIVC). The FVC and FIVC maneuvers are often performed in sequence to provide a continuous flow-volume loop (see the later section Flow-Volume Curve).

The **forced expiratory volume (FEV_T)** is the volume of gas expired over a given time interval (T) from the beginning of the FVC maneuver. The time interval is stated as a subscript of FEV. The FEV_1 measurement is the most widely used. Other intervals in common use are $FEV_{0.5}$, FEV_3, and FEV_6. The FVC and FEV_T are both reported in liters corrected to BTPS. $FEV_{T\%}$ is the ratio of FEV_T to FVC expressed as a percentage, where T is the interval from the start of the FVC. The $FEV_{1\%}$ (FEV_1/FVC × 100) is by far the most widely used of the various $FEV_{T\%}$ parameters. VC (slow vital capacity) may be used in place of FVC if the VC is significantly larger. Because a low value for the ratio of FEV_1 to FVC is used to detect obstruction, using the largest value obtained for vital capacity (either VC or FVC) for the denominator may be helpful and is currently recommended by the ATS-ERS guidelines.

Flows over specific intervals or at specific points in the FVC are expressed as FEF_X. The subscript X describes the point or interval in relation to the FVC maneuver. The **FEF25%–75%** is the average flow during the middle half (from the 25%–75% points) of an FVC maneuver. FEF_X values are usually recorded in liters per second, BTPS. $FEF_{25\%-75\%}$ was formerly designated the *maximum midexpiratory flow rate (MMFR)*. Other measures of average flow include the $FEF_{200-1200}$ (200- to 1200-mL portion of the FVC) and the $FEF_{75\%-85\%}$. FEF_X is also used to denote instantaneous flow at specific points in the FVC maneuver. Commonly reported flows are the $FEF_{25\%}$, $FEF_{50\%}$, and $FEF_{75\%}$. The subscript refers to the percentage of FVC that has been expired.

Technique

FVC is measured by having the patient, after inspiring maximally, expire as forcefully and rapidly as possible into a spirometer. The patient should inspire completely. The inhalation should be rapid but not forced. There should be little, if any, pause (<1 or 2 seconds) at maximal inspiration; a prolonged pause (4–6 seconds) may decrease flow during the subsequent expiration.

The volume expired may be displayed as volume–time tracing or (Fig. 2.2) flow-volume graph (Fig. 2.3). These tracings are typically shown on a computer monitor or small display screen. The computer analyzes the signal from the spirometer and then calculates and displays the FVC. A spirometer that produces a graphic tracing (either volume–time or flow volume) is essential for clinical laboratory purposes to allow a visual inspection of the maneuver (see Fig. 2.3). Devices providing only numeric data may be helpful for simple screening. Whether used for diagnosis or monitoring, all spirometers must meet the calibration and operational criteria proposed by the ATS-ERS (see Chapter 12). The FVC maneuver depends on patient effort. Not all patients may be able to perform it acceptably (Criteria for Acceptability 2.2).

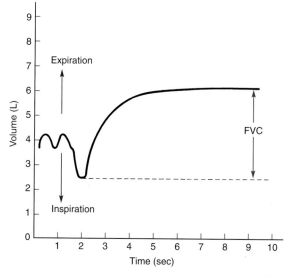

FIG. 2.2 Forced vital capacity (FVC). Typical spirogram plotting volume against time as patient exhales forcefully. In this tracing, expiration causes an upward deflection; in some systems, the tracing is inverted. The patient inspires to the maximal inspiratory level *(dashed line)*, at which point lung volume is close to total lung capacity (TLC). The patient then expires as forcefully and rapidly as possible to the maximal expiratory level, at which point the lungs contain the residual volume (RV) only (see text).

PF TIP 2.2

The FVC maneuver is extremely effort dependent and requires active coaching on the part of the operator. Some operators clap their hands, stomp their foot, or snap their fingers along with active vocalization ("blast," "snap," or "blow"), but whatever method is chosen should convey the urgency of blasting the air out fast and forcefully.

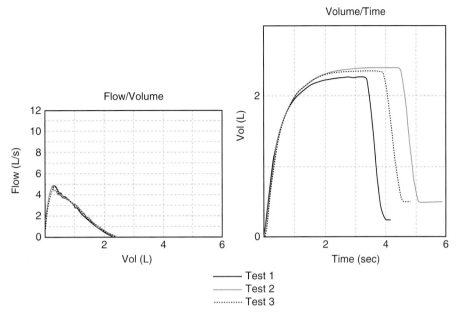

Flow/Volume

Volume/Time

FIG. 2.3   Three acceptable FVC maneuvers from a 10-year-old subject. Acceptability based on a fast start (no hesitation), a sharp peak flow, no cough or glottic closure in the first second, and meeting the end-of-test criteria.

2.1   How To ...

Perform an FVC Maneuver

1. Tasks common to all procedures:
   a. Calibrate and prepare equipment.
   b. Review order.
   c. Introduce yourself and identify patient according to institutional policies.
   d. Describe and demonstrate procedure.
2. Have the subject sit upright with feet flat on the floor.
3. Subject's chin should be upright, with the neck slightly extended.
4. The mouthpiece should rest on top of the tongue, with the patient gently biting down with the teeth and sealing the lips firmly around the mouthpiece. Nose clips are recommended, but the maneuver can often be performed without one.
5. With the spirometer hose or flow sensor in his or her hand, have the subject breathe quietly for several breaths on the mouthpiece (closed-circuit technique) and then take a maximal inspiration, or alternatively, have the subject take a maximal inspiration (open-circuit technique) and immediately place the mouthpiece in the mouth once TLC is reached. Some type of active encouragement (be a good coach/cheerleader) by the technologist may be helpful in conveying the necessity of the subject to take his or her deepest breath (e.g., "in, in, in"/"up, up, up"; raising the arms).
6. Instruct the subject to blast the air out forcefully. The technologist may wish to choose an action (e.g., clap the hands, snap the fingers, or stomp the foot) or a word (e.g., "blast," "snap") to convey the urgency of the maneuver.
7. Encourage the subject to continue to blow (verbal cues, "keep blowing"/"blow, blow, blow") until empty.
8. If performing a flow-volume loop, have the subject rapidly and forcefully inspire to TLC. The FIVC should match the FVC in volume as a quality indicator that the FVC maneuver began after a full inflation.
9. If the subject becomes lightheaded or complains of dizziness or shortness of breath, make sure to allow extra time between maneuvers.
10. Perform until acceptability and repeatability criteria are achieved (see Criteria for Acceptability 2.2).
11. Note comments related to test quality.

CRITERIA FOR ACCEPTABILITY AND REPEATABILITY 2.2

FVC Maneuver

1. Maximal effort; no cough in the first second; no leaks or obstruction of the mouthpiece
2. Good start-of-test; back-extrapolated volume less than 5% of FVC or 100 mL, whichever is greater, and a rise time from 10% to 90% of peak flow ≤ 150 ms
3. No glottic closure in the first second (FEV$_1$ useable criteria) or after the first second (acceptability criteria)
4. Must achieve one of these three indicators for the end of forced expiration (EOFE):
   1. Expiratory plateau (< 0.025 L in the last 1 s of expiration)
   2. Expiratory time > 15 seconds
   3. FVC is within the repeatability tolerance of or is greater than the largest prior observed FVC.
5. If the maximum inspiration after the EOFE is greater than the FVC, then the FIVC – FVC must be ≤ 100 mL or 5% of the FVC, whichever is greater.

Repeatability Criteria

1. In subjects > 6 years of age, the two largest acceptable FVC and FEV$_1$ values must be ≤ 150 mL.
2. In subjects ≤ 6, the two largest acceptable FVC and FEV$_1$ values must be ≤ 100 mL or 10%, whichever is greater.
3. Report the highest FVC and highest FEV$_1$, even if they come from separate maneuvers. The FEV$_1$/FVC ratio is derived from these values.

Adapted from ATS-ERS 2019 Spirometry Technical Statement.

FEV$_1$ (and other FEV$_T$ values) may be measured by timing the FVC maneuver over the described intervals. Historically, this was done by recording the FVC spirogram on graph paper moving at a fixed speed. The FEV for any interval could then be read from the graph, as shown in Fig. 2.4. Most modern spirometers time the FVC maneuver using a computer. The computer then calculates and displays the FEV$_1$ or other FEV$_T$ intervals. The spirometer should provide a volume–time display of each maneuver (Fig. 2.5). A graphic representation allows the monitoring of patient effort at the beginning of the test. Accurate measurement of FEV$_1$ (and other FEV$_T$ intervals) depends on the determination of the **start-of-test** (Fig. 2.6). Computerized spirometers detect the start-of-test as a change in flow or volume above a certain threshold. The computer then stores volume and flow data points in memory and calculates the FEV$_1$.

Open-circuit technique describes an FVC maneuver where the subject inhales maximally, places the mouthpiece or filter into the mouth, and then forcefully exhales until empty. Using this technique, the patient has to coordinate taking the deep breath, holding the breath at TLC, and placing the

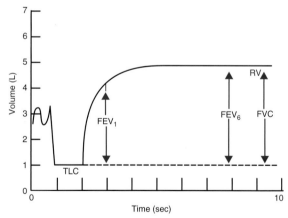

FIG. 2.4 Determination of forced expiratory volume (FEV$_T$) values from a forced vital capacity (FVC) maneuver. Various FEV$_T$ values can be measured from the volume–time display of an FVC effort. FEV at intervals of 1 and 6 seconds, along with the FVC, are shown *(arrows)*. FEV$_1$ is the most commonly used index of airflow. FEV$_6$ is sometimes used as a surrogate for FVC in patients with airway obstruction. Precise timing and acceptable start-of-test are required to determine FEV$_T$ values accurately (Criteria for Acceptability 2.2).

PF TIP 2.3

There are three key components to an FVC maneuver:
1. Deep breath
2. Blast
3. Meeting the EOFE test criteria ("keep blowing, keep blowing, keep blowing")
   All of these are important, but without the initial deep breath, the latter two are meaningless! This is why the 2019 ATS-ERS Spirometry Technical Statement added the FIVC as a quality check.

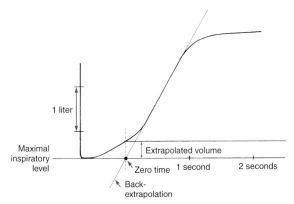

FIG. 2.5 Back-extrapolation of a volume–time spirogram. Back-extrapolation is a method for correcting measurements made from a spirogram that does not show a sharp deflection from the maximal inspiratory level. This occurs when a patient does not begin forced exhalation rapidly enough or hesitates at the start-of-test. A straight line drawn through the steepest part of a volume–time tracing is extended to cross the volume baseline (maximum inspiration). The point of intersection is the back-extrapolated *time zero*. To accurately determine the new time zero, the display should include at least 0.25 seconds and preferably at least 1 second before the start of the exhalation. Timed volumes, such as the forced expiratory volume in the first second (FEV_1), are measured from this point rather than from the initial deflection from the baseline or from the point of maximal flow. The perpendicular distance from maximal inspiration to the volume–time tracing at time zero defines the *back-extrapolated volume*. To accurately determine FEV_1, the back-extrapolated volume should be less than 5% of the forced vital capacity (FVC) or less than 150 mL, whichever is greater, and the rise time from 10% to 90% of peak flow should be ≤ 150 ms. FVC efforts with larger extrapolated volumes should be considered unacceptable.

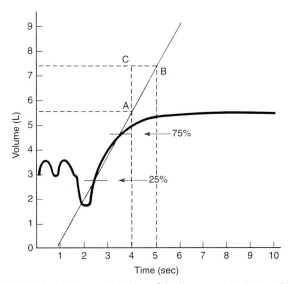

FIG. 2.6 $FEF_{25\%-75\%}$. The slope of the line connecting 25% and 75% points is the average flow over the middle half of the forced vital capacity (FVC) maneuver. Alternatively, a line connecting these points may be drawn to intersect two timelines 1 second apart (points *A* and *B*). The flow in liters per second can be read as the vertical distance between the points of intersection (*AC*)—in this case, approximately 2 L/sec.

$$FEV_{1\%} = \frac{FEV_1}{FVC} \times 100$$

$FEV_{1\%}$ is also commonly written as FEV_1/FVC. Both ratios are expressed as percentages, and this percentage is then related to normative values as a percentage of predicted. FEV_1 and FVC should be reported as the maximal values obtained from at least three acceptable FVC maneuvers. The FEV_1/FVC ratio based on these values may be different from the ratio obtained from any single maneuver. If both VC and FVC maneuvers have been performed, it is preferable to use the largest VC in the calculation. Some computerized spirometers calculate only the ratio obtained from FVC maneuvers.

The $FEF_{25\%-75\%}$ is measured from an FVC maneuver. The $FEF_{25\%-75\%}$ is the average flow during the middle half (from 25%–75%) of the VC. A computerized measurement of the $FEF_{25\%-75\%}$ requires storage of flow and volume data points for the entire maneuver. Calculation of the average flow over the middle portion of the exhalation is simply 50% of the volume expired divided by the time required to get

mouthpiece correctly, which can be a challenge for some subjects. *Closed-circuit technique* describes a maneuver where the subject breathes tidally on the spirometer, inhales maximally, forcefully exhales, and then may be instructed to inhale forcefully to measure the inspiratory flow and volume. Most computerized spirometers correct for a slow start-of-test by *back-extrapolation* (see Fig. 2.5). Visualization of the volume–time spirogram is the best means of identifying poor initial effort. Some portable spirometers report FEV_1 without a spirogram. Such measurements should be used with caution because it may be difficult to determine whether the maneuver was performed acceptably.

The ratio of the FEV_1 to FVC is expressed as follows:

from the 25% point to the 75% point. To manually calculate the $FEF_{25\%-75\%}$, a volume–time spirogram is used. The points at which 25% and 75% of the VC have been expired are marked on the curve (see Fig. 2.6). A straight line connecting these points can be extended to intersect two timelines 1 second apart. The flow (in liters per second) can then be read directly as the vertical distance between the points of intersection. Instantaneous flows, such as the $FEF_{50\%}$ or $FEF_{75\%}$, cannot be read directly from a volume–time display but can be measured using a flow–volume curve (see the later section Flow-Volume Curve).

The $FEF_{25\%-75\%}$ depends on the FVC. Large $FEF_{25\%-75\%}$ values may be derived from maneuvers that produce small FVC measurements because the "middle half" of the volume is actually gas expired at the beginning of expiration. This effect may be particularly evident if the patient terminates the FVC maneuver before exhaling completely. When the $FEF_{25\%-75\%}$ is used for assessing the response to bronchodilator or bronchial challenge, the effect of changes in the absolute lung volumes must be considered. Measuring the $FEF_{25\%-75\%}$ at the same lung volumes in the comparison tests is called the *isovolume technique*. **Isovolume corrections** are usually applied when the FVC changes by more than 10% (indicating a change in TLC or RV). This technique requires that lung volumes (see Chapter 4) be measured in conjunction with flows. The isovolume technique may also be used with other flow measurements that are dependent on FVC.

The largest $FEF_{25\%-75\%}$ is not necessarily the value reported. The $FEF_{25\%-75\%}$ is recorded from the maneuver with the largest sum of FVC and FEV_1. Flows must be corrected to BTPS.

Acceptability and Repeatability for Spirometry Results

1. Criteria used to judge the acceptability of test results from the FVC maneuver include the following: The tracing should show one of three indicators of EOFE: (1) There is less than 0.025 L volume over 1 second (a plateau). (2) The subject has achieved a forced expiratory time of 15 seconds. (3) The subject cannot blow out long enough to reach a plateau, but the FVC values are repeatable. This latter criterion is most commonly seen in children or smaller adults.

Patients with severe obstruction can often times exhale well past 15 seconds; however, multiple prolonged exhalations are rarely justified and may cause undue lightheadedness, and fatigue. Glottic closure will underestimate FVC; however, it may yield a "usable" FEV_1. In the event of glottis closure, reinforce the need to keep the chin elevated with the neck slightly extended. A simple trick might be to have the subject focus on an object located high on a wall, or instruct them to blow the air out as if he or she were "blowing at the stars." Another trick might be to have the subject focus on relaxing the throat or neck after the initial blast. If all these tricks fail to remedy the glottis closure, the FEV_1 can still be used if the closure happened after the first second.

2. The start-of-test should be abrupt and unhesitating. Each maneuver should have the back-extrapolated volume calculated. FEV_1 and all other flows must be measured after back-extrapolation (see Figs. 2.5 and Fig. 2.11C). The ATS-ERS guidelines recommend that the volume–time tracing must begin at least 0.25 seconds before the beginning of the exhalation to be able to measure the back-extrapolated volume. If the volume of back-extrapolation is greater than 5% of the FVC or 100 mL (whichever is greater) and the rise time from 10% to 90% of peak flow is > 150 ms, the maneuver is unacceptable and should be repeated. The patient should be shown the correct technique for performing the maneuver. Demonstration by the technologist is often helpful.

3. Performing a flow-volume loop (i.e., an FIVC) once the EOFE has been achieved is encouraged by the 2019 ATS-ERS Spirometry Technical Statement. A comparison of the FIVC to the FVC can then be used as a quality check on the completeness of the initial inspiration. If the FIVC – FVC is > 100 mL or 5% of the FVC, whichever is greater, the maneuver is unacceptable and should be repeated.

4. Other variables that make an effort unacceptable are leak, obstruction of the mouthpiece with the tongue, maneuvers conducted with zero-flow errors (see Figs. 2.11D and E), or maneuvers with an EOFE "sneak breath" (see Fig. 2.11F).

5. A minimum of three acceptable efforts should be obtained. The test may be repeated multiple times, and although eight maneuvers is generally

a reasonable upper limit in most adults, it may take more attempts. Children may require more than eight attempts because each maneuver may not be a complete maneuver. Regardless, the operator will need to be attentive to the child and his or her tolerance of the efforts being asked of him or her so as to not overwhelm the child. A grading system has been proposed for a spirometry testing session (Table 2.1). The medical director and laboratory manager should decide on a minimal grade achieved in order to post the results into the patient's medical record. A grade <D might result in reporting data that do not represent the subject's true lung function.

6. Ideally, the two largest values for both FVC and FEV_1 should be within 150 mL (for ages 2–6, within 100 mL or 10% of the largest). This is achieved by taking the largest FVC and FEV_1 and simply subtracting the second-largest values to determine repeatability. If the two largest FVC or FEV_1 values are not within 150 mL, the maneuver should be repeated up to a maximum of eight times or until the patient cannot or will not continue. The repeatability criteria should be applied only after the maneuver has been judged as acceptable. Individual spirometric maneuvers should not be rejected solely because they are not repeatable.

Bronchospasm or fatigue often affects repeatability. Interpretation of the test should include comments regarding repeatability or a lack of it. As a minimum, three acceptable satisfactory maneuvers should be saved for evaluation (see Fig. 2.3).

Data from all acceptable maneuvers should be examined. The largest FVC and the largest FEV_1 should be reported, even if the two values are from different test maneuvers. The reported FEV_1/FVC ratio is taken from these values. Flows that depend on the FVC (e.g., the $FEF_{25\%-75\%}$) should be taken from the single best test maneuver, which is the maneuver with the largest sum of FVC and FEV_1 (Table 2.2). The reported flow-volume curve is also taken from the single best test maneuver. One caveat to selecting the largest FEV_1 from *any* maneuver is when the peak flow is significantly less than that of another maneuver or maneuvers. A suboptimal blast may actually overestimate the FEV_1 in a subject with dynamic airway compression (see Fig. 2.11F).

A common problem may occur when using these criteria to produce a spirometry report. If a single volume–time or flow-volume tracing is included in the final report, it may not contain the FVC or FEV_1 that appears in the tabular data. It is advisable to maintain recordings or raw data for all acceptable maneuvers. Other methods of selecting the best test

TABLE 2.1

ATS-ERS Grading Scheme for Spirometry

Grade	Criteria for Adults and Older Children and for Children Aged 2–6 Years
A	>3 acceptable tests with repeatability within 0.150 L; ages 2–6, 0.100 L, or 10% of highest value, whichever is greater.
B	>2 acceptable tests with repeatability within 0.150 L; ages 2–6, 0.100 L, or 10% of highest value, whichever is greater
C	>2 acceptable tests with repeatability within 0.200 L; ages 2–6, 0.150 L, or 10% of highest value, whichever is greater
D	>2 acceptable tests with repeatability within 0.250 L; ages 2–6, 0.200 L, or 10% of highest value, whichever is greater
E	One acceptable test
F	No acceptable tests

ATS-ERS, American Thoracic Society–European Respiratory Society.

TABLE 2.2

Comparison of Spirometry Efforts

Test	Trial 1	Trial 2	Trial 3	Best Test Reported
FVC (L)	5.20	5.30	5.35[a]	5.35
FEV_1 (L)	4.41[a]	4.35	4.36[a]	4.41
FEV_1/FVC (%)	85	82	82	82
$FEF_{25\%-75\%}$ (L/sec)	3.87	3.92	3.94	3.94
$FEF_{50\%}$ (L/sec)	3.99	3.95	3.41	3.41
$FEF_{25\%}$ (L/sec)	1.97	1.95	1.89	1.89
PEF (L/sec)	8.39	9.44	9.89	9.89

FEF, Forced expiratory flow; *FEV,* forced expiratory volume; *FVC,* forced vital capacity; *PEF,* peak expiratory flow.

[a]These values are keys to selecting the best test results. The FEV_1 is taken from Trial 1 and the FVC from Trial 3, even though the largest sum of FVC and FEV_1 occurs in Trial 3. All FVC-dependent flows (average and instantaneous) come from Trial 3. The maximal expiratory flow-volume curve, if reported, would be the curve from Trial 3 as well. It should be noted that the $FEV_{1\%}$ (FEV_1/FVC) is calculated from the FEV_1 of Trial 1 and the FVC of Trial 3.

have been suggested and are sometimes used. PEF may be used to assess patient effort for an FVC maneuver. Selecting the effort with the largest PEF may cause errors if FVC and FEV_1 are not also evaluated.

Spirometry may be performed in either the sitting or standing position for adults and children, although the sitting position is recommended for safety, especially in adults. There is some evidence that FEV_1 may be larger in the standing position in adults and in children younger than 12 years of age. The position used for testing should be indicated in the final report. The patient should keep the head slightly elevated and keep false teeth in if they fit well. The use of nose clips is recommended for spirometric measurements that require rebreathing, even if just for a few breaths. Spirometers that record only expiratory flow may require the patient to place the mouthpiece into the mouth after maximal inspiration. If this is the case, nose clips are usually unnecessary. Care should be taken, however, that the patient places the mouthpiece into the mouth before beginning a forced expiration. Failure to do so may result in an undetectable loss of volume. It may be impossible to calculate the volume of back-extrapolation from a tracing that displays expiratory flow only.

PF TIP 2.4

The largest FVC and FEV_1 are reported, even if they come from different efforts, as long as the efforts are acceptable. Peak flow (PEF) is always the largest value from an acceptable effort. All of the other flows ($FEF_{25\%-75\%}$, etc.) are taken from the acceptable effort with the largest sum of FVC and FEV_1, as is the flow-volume loop.

Significance and Pathophysiology
Forced Vital Capacity

See Interpretive Strategies 2.2. FVC usually equals VC in healthy individuals. In patients without obstruction, FVC and SVC should be within 150 mL of each other. FVC and SVC may differ if the patient's effort is variable or if significant airway obstruction is present (i.e., $FEV_1/FVC < 0.70$). FVC is often lower than SVC in patients with obstructive diseases if forced expiration causes airway collapse. This pattern is often seen in emphysema because

of a loss of tethering support of the airways. Large pressure gradients across the walls of the airways during forced expiration collapse the terminal portions of the airways. Gas is trapped in the alveoli and cannot be expired. This causes the FVC to appear smaller than the SVC. The FVC can appear larger than the SVC if the patient exerts greater effort on the forced maneuver.

INTERPRETIVE STRATEGIES 2.2

FVC Maneuver

1. Were at least three acceptable spirograms obtained? Are FVC and FEV_1 repeatable (within 150 mL)?
2. Are reference values appropriate? Age? Sex? Height? Race?
3. Is $FEV_{1\%}$ (ratio) less than predicted? If so, obstruction is present.
   a. Is FVC also reduced? If so, is it caused by obstruction or restriction?
   b. If FVC is less than the LLN, lung volumes may be indicated.
   c. Is the obstruction reversible? Bronchodilators may be indicated.
4. Is $FEV_{1\%}$ equal to or greater than expected?
   a. Are FVC and FEV_1 both reduced proportionately? If so, restriction may be present; lung volumes and/or muscle pressures may be indicated.
   b. Are FVC and FEV_1 within normal limits? If so, spirometry is likely normal.
5. Are the spirometric findings consistent with the patient history and physical findings? Is bronchial challenge indicated to reveal obstruction?

FVC can be reduced by mucus plugging and bronchiolar narrowing, as is common in chronic bronchitis, chronic or acute asthma, bronchiectasis, and cystic fibrosis. Reduced FVC is also present in patients whose trachea or mainstem bronchi are obstructed. Tumors or diseases affecting the patency of the large airways can produce this result.

Some obstructed patients have a relatively normal FVC in relation to their predicted values. However, the time required to expire their FVC (forced expiratory time [FET]) is usually prolonged. Healthy adults can expire their FVC within 4 to 6 seconds. Normal children, adolescents, and many smaller adults may exhale their FVC in less than 4 seconds. Patients with severe obstruction (e.g., those with emphysema) may

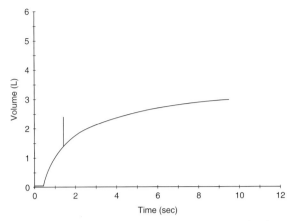

FIG. 2.7 Volume–time forced vital capacity (FVC) tracing from a patient with severe airway obstruction. A tick mark notes the point at which the patient exhaled his forced expiratory volume in the first second (FEV_1). A significant volume is exhaled after the first second, and the tracing does not show an obvious plateau.

require 15 seconds or more to exhale completely (Fig. 2.7). Accurate measurement of FVC in such individuals may be limited by how long the spirometer can collect exhaled volume. Some spirometers allow only 15 seconds of volume recording. This is usually long enough to diagnose airway obstruction. However, the FVC and $FEV_{1\%}$ may be inaccurate if the patient continues to exhale for a longer time. The ATS-ERS recommends that spirometers measure FVC for at least 15 seconds (see Chapter 11).

An alternative to measuring FVC in severely obstructed patients is to use FEV_6. Because normal patients can exhale their FVC in 6 seconds, substituting FEV_6 for FVC allows the FEV_1/FEV_6 to be used as an index of obstruction. Using FEV_6 in place of FVC eliminates the necessity of having the patient try to exhale for a long interval. Predicted values for FEV_6 and FEV_1/FEV_6 have been calculated. Because FEV_6 may underestimate FVC, the use of FEV_1/FEV_6 instead of FEV_1/FVC may reduce the sensitivity of spirometry to detect airway obstruction, especially in older patients and in those with mild obstruction.

Decreased FVC is seen in the same circumstances as described for reduced VC, discussed earlier. However, the reduction in FVC may be more evident than that of the slow VC in diseases that affect the bellows function of the chest, which is a key determinant of the force generation involved in the FVC compared with the VC maneuver. Such diseases include neuromuscular disorders and chest wall mechanical abnormalities, such as kyphoscoliosis and obesity. A reduction in FVC when going from sitting to supine has been shown to be a good indicator of diaphragmatic weakness.

Reduced FVC (or VC) is a nonspecific finding. Values below the 5th percentile are considered abnormal (see Chapter 13). A low FVC may be caused by either obstruction or restriction (see Box 2.2). Interpretation of the FVC in obstructive diseases requires correlation with flows. An FVC significantly lower than SVC suggests airway collapse and gas trapping. In restrictive patterns, low FVC may indicate the need to assess other lung volumes, particularly TLC (see Chapter 4). Interpretation of FVC values close to the LLN depends on the clinical question to be answered. An FVC at the 5th percentile would be interpreted differently in a healthy patient with no symptoms than in a patient with a history of cough or wheezing. An FVC much lower than expected is often accompanied by the complaint of exertional dyspnea.

A low value for FVC may also occur if the patient's effort is suboptimal. Patients who stop exhaling before achieving an obvious plateau (on a volume–time display) or who fail to take a maximal inhalation will typically have an underestimated FVC. These patients should be encouraged to inhale maximally at the start of the maneuver and then exhale completely for 6 seconds (3 seconds for children aged < 10) or until a plateau occurs. Premature termination of the FVC effort may cause the $FEV_{1\%}$ to be overestimated, masking the presence of obstruction.

An important quality issue to recognize is that a large FVC (and its derived parameters) derived from a flow sensor may result from improper zeroing or contamination of the sensor by condensation or mucus. This problem can usually be recognized by poor repeatability of measurements, characterized by progressively increasing test results within a single testing session.

Forced Expiratory Volume

FEV_1 measures the volume expired over the first second of an FVC maneuver. FEV_1 is reported as a volume, although it measures flow over a specific interval. FEV_1, like FVC, may be reduced in either

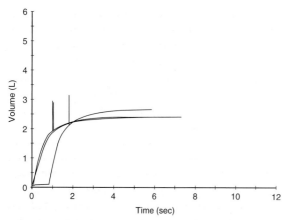

FIG. 2.8 All three maneuvers show relatively normal flows; most of the forced vital capacity (FVC) is expired in the first second. However, the FVC is much lower than the expected value of 3.5 L for the patient. Notice the delayed start to the effort with the highest FVC, for which determination of the back-extrapolated volume is necessary.

Mortality (likelihood of dying) caused by respiratory disease is similarly related to the degree of obstruction as measured by FEV_1. Patients with markedly reduced FEV_1 values are much more likely to die of chronic obstructive pulmonary disease (COPD), lung cancer, and even cardiovascular disease, including myocardial infarction and stroke. Although FEV_1 correlates with the prognosis and severity of symptoms in obstructive lung disease, outcomes for individual patients cannot be accurately predicted.

Whereas the ratio of FEV_1/VC defines obstruction, the severity of obstruction is defined by the degree to which the FEV_1 is reduced. The ATS-ERS Task Force suggests the following classifications of severity:

Severity	Z Score
Mild	$FEV_1 > -1.65 - < -2.5$
Moderate	$FEV_1 \geq -2.5$ and ≤ -4
Severe	$FEV_1 > 4$

The concept of grading severity based on FEV_1 applies best when the VC is in the normal range. Once the VC is below normal, a concomitant restrictive defect may also be present, and this can be determined only by further measurement of lung volumes, in particular TLC. Because the FEV_1 in restriction is reduced, in part, by the restrictive process itself, the decrement in FEV_1 resulting from the obstructive component of disease can no longer be assumed to reflect the severity of obstruction only. Thus the severity of obstruction in a combined restrictive and obstructive defect is typically overestimated when basing severity solely on the reduction in FEV_1.

Restrictive processes, such as fibrosis, edema, space-occupying lesions, neuromuscular disorders, obesity, and chest wall deformities, may all cause FEV_1 to be decreased. A reduction in FEV_1 occurs in much the same way as a reduction in VC. Unlike the pattern seen in obstructive disease, in which VC is preserved and FEV_1 is reduced, in restriction VC and FEV_1, values are proportionately decreased. Some patients with moderate or severe restriction have an FEV_1 nearly equal to the VC. The entire VC, because it is reduced, is exhaled almost completely in the first second. To distinguish between obstructive and restrictive causes of reduced FEV_1 values, the FEV_1/VC ratio ($FEV_{1\%}$) and other flow measurements are useful. Further definition of obstruction

obstructive or restrictive patterns (Fig. 2.8; see also Fig. 2.7). FEV_1 values may also be reduced because of poor effort or cooperation by the patient.

An obstructive ventilatory defect is characterized by the reduction of maximal airflow at all lung volumes (e.g., the classic concave shape to the flow-volume curve). Flow is limited by airway narrowing during forced expiration. Airway obstruction may be caused by mucus secretion, bronchospasm, and inflammation, such as in asthma or bronchitis. Airflow limitation may also result from a loss of elastic support for the airways themselves, as in emphysema. The earliest changes in obstructive patterns may occur in the small airways (i.e., those <2 mm), which may or may not be detected by changes in FEV_1.

FEV_1 may also be decreased in large airway obstruction (trachea and bronchi). Tumors or foreign bodies that limit airflow cause the FEV_1 to be reduced. These defects can be identified by flow reductions across the entire forced expiration (see the later section Flow-Volume Curve).

FEV_1 and **FEV_1/VC** are the most standardized indices of obstructive disease. An obstructive defect is defined best by a reduced FEV_1/VC ratio. The severity of obstructive disease may be gauged by the extent to which FEV_1 is reduced. The ability to work and function in daily life is related to FEV_1 and VC.

versus restriction may require the measurement of lung volumes (e.g., functional residual capacity [FRC] and TLC). However, studies have shown that when the FVC and FEV_1/VC ratio are both normal, restriction, as defined by a low TLC, is very unlikely.

FEV_1 is the most widely used spirometric parameter, particularly for the assessment of airway obstruction. FEV_1 is used in conjunction with VC for simple screening, assessment of response to bronchodilators, inhalation challenge studies, and the detection of exercise-induced bronchospasm (see Chapter 9). FEV_1 is the most robust pulmonary function test, making it the measurement of choice in evaluating lung function in general. In fact, the motto of the National Lung Health Education Program (NLHEP) is "Test your lungs. Know your numbers," and these numbers are the FEV_1 and FVC (or FEV_6). The NLHEP advocates for the widespread use of simple office spirometry to increase the awareness and detection of COPD, in addition to other respiratory disorders. In particular, the NLHEP recommends that all smokers age 45 years and older have spirometry done to detect airflow obstruction, even before the onset of clinical symptoms.

Forced Expiratory Volume Ratio

Normal $FEV_{T\%}$ ratios for healthy adults are as follows:

$FEV_{0.5\%}$ = 50% to 60%
$FEV_{1\%}$ = 75% to 85%
$FEV_{2\%}$ = 90% to 95%
$FEV_{3\%}$ = 95% to 98%
$FEV_{6\%}$ = 98% to 100%

These ratios may be derived by dividing predicted FEV_T by predicted VC. Some studies of normal patients derive equations for the ratio itself. The reported FEV_1/VC ratio is calculated from the highest FEV_1 and the highest FVC. The FEV_1/VC ratio decreases with increasing age, presumably because of a gradual loss of lung elasticity. For example, healthy older adults may have FEV_1/VC ratios in the 65% to 70% range. Thus the 5th percentile should be taken as the LLN when interpreting the FEV_1/VC, just as with the FEV_1 and VC separately.

Patients with unobstructed airflow can usually exhale their entire FVC within 4 seconds. Conversely, patients with obstructive disease have reduced $FEV_{T\%}$ for each interval (1 second, 2 seconds, etc.). The FEV_1/VC ratio is the most important measurement for distinguishing an obstructive impairment. A decreased FEV_1/VC ratio is the hallmark of an obstructive disease. As already mentioned, the ratio decreases with age, so care should be taken in interpreting the FEV_1/VC ratio in absolute terms. An absolute cutoff of 70% is considered to distinguish between normal and airflow obstruction in defining COPD by the Global Initiative for Chronic Obstructive Lung Disease (GOLD) and the ATS-ERS guidelines on COPD. However, this value may actually underestimate the presence of obstruction in younger adults (false negative) and overestimate it in older individuals (false positive) (see Chapter 13 for predicted values).

Diagnosis of an obstructive pattern based on spirometry should focus on three primary variables: VC, FEV_1, and FEV_1/VC. Measurements such as $FEF_{25\%-75\%}$ should be considered only after the presence and severity of obstruction have been determined using the primary variables. If the FEV_1/VC is borderline abnormal, additional flow measurements may suggest the presence of an obstructive pattern. Care should be taken when interpreting the FEV_1/VC ratio in patients who have VC and FEV_1 values greater than predicted. The FEV_1/VC ratio may appear to indicate an obstructive pattern because of the variability of the greater-than-normal VC and FEV_1 values.

Although a low FEV_1/VC ratio is the key to defining obstruction, the ATS-ERS guidelines also define obstruction in the subset of patients who have a normal FEV_1/VC ratio but a low VC and a normal TLC. This pattern has been hypothesized to be the result of small airway disease with resulting small airway closure and gas trapping. This is often termed a *parallel shift*.

PF TIP 2.5

Look at the FEV_1/FVC ratio first; if the FEV_1/FVC ratio is lower than expected (the LLN), obstruction is present. If the ratio is normal or elevated, check the percent predicted for FVC and FEV_1. If FVC and FEV_1 are both reduced compared with the expected values, restriction or muscle weakness may be present.

Patients who have a restrictive disease (e.g., pulmonary fibrosis) often have normal or increased $FEV_{T\%}$ values. Because airflow may be minimally affected in restrictive diseases, FEV_1 and VC are usually reduced in equal proportion. If the restriction is severe, FEV_1 may approach the VC value. In addition, the increased elastic recoil of fibrotic lungs may enhance expiratory airflow. As a result, $FEV_{1\%}$ appears to be higher than normal. The FEV_1/ VC ratio may be 100% if the VC is severely reduced. The presence of a restrictive disorder may be suggested by a reduced VC and a normal or increased FEV_1/VC ratio. Further studies (e.g., measurement of TLC) should be used to confirm the diagnosis of restriction.

Forced Expiratory Flow 25% to 75%

$FEF_{25\%-75\%}$ is measured from a segment of the FVC that includes flow from medium and small airways. Typical values for healthy young adults average 4 to 5 L/sec. These values decrease with age. $FEF_{25\%-75\%}$ is quite variable even in normal patients, with 1 standard deviation (SD) equal to approximately 1 L/sec. Values as low as 50% of predicted may be statistically within normal limits. This variability requires guarded interpretation of the $FEF_{25\%-75\%}$.

The $FEF_{25\%-75\%}$ may be indicative of the status of the medium to small airways. Decreased flows are common in the early stages of obstructive disease. Abnormalities in these measurements, however, are not specific for small airway disease. Although $FEF_{25\%-75\%}$ may suggest changes in the small airways, it should not be used to diagnose small airway disease in individual patients. In the presence of a borderline value for FEV_1/VC, a low $FEF_{25\%-75\%}$ may help confirm airway obstruction. Assessment of $FEF_{25\%-75\%}$ after bronchodilator use must consider changes in FVC as well. If FVC increases markedly, $FEF_{25\%-75\%}$ may actually decrease. Likewise, if the FVC decreases, the $FEF_{25\%-75\%}$ may increase. Isovolume correction can be used to compare $FEF_{25\%-75\%}$ before and after bronchodilator therapy. However, the inherent variability of $FEF_{25\%-75\%}$ and its dependence on FVC make it less useful than the FEV_1 for assessing bronchodilator response.

Reduced $FEF_{25\%-75\%}$ values are sometimes seen in cases of moderate or severe restrictive patterns. This is assumed to be caused by a decrease in the cross-sectional area of the small airways. $FEF_{25\%-75\%}$ depends somewhat on patient effort because it depends on the FVC exhaled. Patients who perform the FVC maneuver inadequately often show widely varying midexpiratory flow rates.

The $FEF_{25\%-75\%}$/FVC ratio is thought to reflect relative airway size to lung size, and as such, it has been found to be significantly associated with airway hyperresponsiveness. The clinical importance of this finding is unknown.

The validity of FVC maneuvers depends largely on patient effort and cooperation. Equally important are the instruction and coaching supplied by the technologist. Many patients need several attempts before performing the maneuver acceptably. Demonstration of the proper technique by the technologist helps the patient give maximal effort. Placement of the mouthpiece behind the teeth and lips, maximal inspiration, little if any pause, and maximal expiration should all be demonstrated. Emphasis should be placed on the initial burst of air and on continuing expiration for at least 6 seconds. The acceptability of each FVC maneuver should be evaluated according to specific criteria (see Criteria for Acceptability 2.2). The final report should include comments on the quality of the data obtained (see Chapter 12). These comments may be provided by the operator, physician, or both.

The validity of the FEV_1 also depends on cooperation and effort. Adequate instruction and demonstration of the maneuver by the technologist are essential. The target repeatability of FEV_1 should be within 150 mL for the two best of at least three acceptable maneuvers. Accurate measurement of FEV_1 requires an acceptable spirometer (see Chapter 11), preferably one that allows inspection of the volume–time curve and back-extrapolation.

The validity of the $FEV_{1\%}$ also depends on patient effort and cooperation. Because the values used to derive the ratio may be taken from separate maneuvers, both FEV_1 and FVC should be reproducible. Poor effort on an FVC test may result in an overestimate of $FEV_{T\%}$. If the patient stops prematurely, the FVC (i.e., denominator of the ratio) will appear smaller than it actually is. The $FEV_{1\%}$ will then appear larger than it actually is. Some clinicians prefer to use the VC to calculate the $FEV_{1\%}$. This may be useful if the VC is significantly larger than FVC because of airway compression.

Patients who have moderate or severe obstruction may require longer than 10 seconds to completely exhale. Although continuing to exhale increases measured FVC, the diagnosis of obstruction can be made with less-than-complete expiration. The FEV_6 may be a useful surrogate measurement in obstructed patients who have difficulty with prolonged exhalation. In some cases, prolonged effort may be difficult for the patient. The large transpulmonary pressure generated by a forced expiratory maneuver often reduces cardiac output. Patients may complain of dizziness, seeing "spots," ringing in the ears, or numbness of the extremities. A patient may occasionally faint as a result of decreased cerebral blood flow (termed *FVC-induced syncope*). This complication may be serious if it causes the patient to fall from a standing or sitting position.

FLOW-VOLUME CURVE

Description

The FVC graphs the flow generated during an FVC maneuver against volume change. The FVC may be followed by an FIVC maneuver, plotted similarly. Flow is usually recorded in liters per second, and the volume is recorded in liters, BTPS. The **maximal expiratory flow-volume (MEFV)** curve shows flow as the patient exhales from maximal inspiration (TLC) to maximal expiration (RV). The **maximal inspiratory flow volume (MIFV)** displays inspiratory flow plotted from RV to TLC. When MEFV and MIFV curves are plotted together, the resulting figure is called a *flow-volume (F-V) loop* (Fig. 2.9). The reported F-V loop is taken from the single best test maneuver (highest sum of FEV_1 and FVC).

Technique

The patient performs an FVC maneuver, inspiring fully and then exhaling as rapidly as possible. To complete the loop, the patient inspires as rapidly as possible from the maximal expiratory level

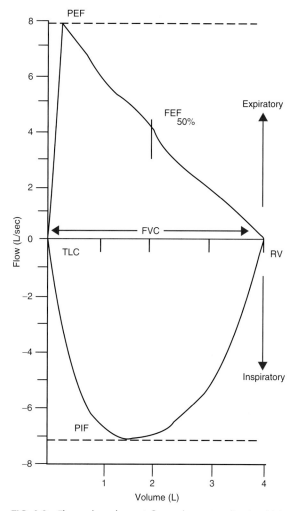

FIG. 2.9 Flow-volume loop. A flow-volume recording in which a forced vital capacity (FVC) and a forced inspiratory vital capacity (FIVC) maneuver are recorded in succession. Flow in liters per second is plotted on the *vertical axis*, and volume, in liters, is plotted on the *horizontal axis*. By convention, *expiratory* flow is plotted upward (positive), and *inspiratory* flow is plotted downward (negative). The maximal exhalation begins with the patient at total lung capacity (TLC) and continues until residual volume (RV) is reached; a maximal inspiration then returns to TLC. The FVC can be read from the tracing as the maximal horizontal deflection along the zero-flow line. Peak flows for expiration and inspiration (PEF and PIF) can be read directly from the tracing as the maximal deflections on the flow axis (positive and negative). The instantaneous flow (forced expiratory flow [FEF]) at any point in the FVC can also be measured directly. Abnormalities, such as small or large airway obstruction, may show up as characteristic changes in the maximal flow rates. The flow-volume loop is a graphic display of the maximal expiratory flow-volume (MEFV) and maximal inspiratory flow-volume (MIFV) curves combined.

back to maximal inspiration. Volume is plotted on the horizontal *x*-axis, and flow is plotted on the vertical *y*-axis. The F-V loop is usually displayed on a computer screen. Expired volume is usually plotted from left to right. Sometimes, when concomitant lung volumes have also been measured, an absolute lung volume scale is used, usually with TLC on the left and RV on the right. Airflow should be recorded at 2 L/sec/unit distance on the *y*-axis. Volume should be recorded at 1 L/unit distance on the volume axis. Scale factors should be at least 5 mm/L/sec for flow and 10 mm/L for volume. These factors are required so that manual measurements can be made from a printed copy of the maneuver. This one-to-two flow-volume relationship also ensures that the visual perspective of the graphic data is consistent regardless of the size of the display.

FVC, in addition to PEF and peak inspiratory flow (PIF), can be read directly from the F-V loop. Instantaneous flow at any lung volume can be measured directly from the F-V loop. Maximal flow at 75%, 50%, and 25% of the FVC is commonly reported as the $\dot{V}max_{75}$, $\dot{V}max_{50}$, and $\dot{V}max_{25}$. The subscript in these terms refers to the portion of the FVC remaining. The same flows are also reported as the $FEF_{25\%}$, $FEF_{50\%}$, and $FEF_{75\%}$, with the subscripts referring to the percentage of FVC exhaled. This latter terminology is now preferred by the ATS-ERS guidelines.

F-V loop data, stored in computer memory, can be easily manipulated. Multiple loops can be compared by superimposing them with contrasting colors. Bronchodilator or inhalation challenge F-V loops can be presented in a similar manner. A predicted MEFV curve can be plotted using points for PEF and maximal flows at 75%, 50%, and 25% of the FVC. A patient's flow-volume curve can then be superimposed directly over the expected values (Fig. 2.10). Superimpositions of multiple FVC maneuvers as F-V loops can be used to assess the reproducibility of the patient's effort. Positioning loops side by side or superimposing can also help detect decreasing flows with repeated efforts. This pattern may be seen because FVC maneuvers can induce bronchospasm (i.e., FVC-induced bronchospasm or FVC worsening). Storing tests in the order performed is

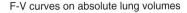

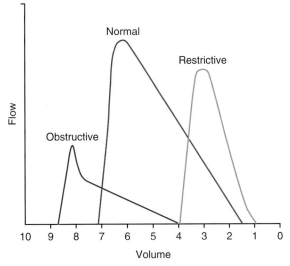

FIG. 2.10 Superimposed flow-volume loops on an absolute volume scale.

recommended. This allows a review of the test session and the detection of bronchospasm or fatigue.

Reproducible MEFV curves, particularly the PEF, are good indicators of adequate patient effort (Criteria for Acceptability 2.3). Assessing the start-of-test and determining whether exhalation lasted at least 6 seconds may be difficult if only the F-V loop is displayed. Simultaneous display of flow-volume and volume–time curves is useful (Fig. 2.11). Although computerized systems calculate the back-extrapolated volume, a volume–time tracing may be necessary to perform back-extrapolation manually (see Fig. 2.5). Common technical problems with volume–time tracings and F-V loops are shown in Fig. 2.11. These include cough in the first second (Fig. 2.11A); early termination or glottic closure (Fig. 2.11B); excessive back-extrapolated volume or "slow"/hesitative start (Fig. 2.11C); negative flow sensor drift, which would underestimate volumes (Fig. 2.11 D); positive flow sensor drift, which would overestimate volumes (Fig. 2.11E); a sneak breath at the end of exhalation (Fig. 2.11F); or a suboptimal blast, which might yield an overestimation of FEV_1 (Fig. 2.11G).

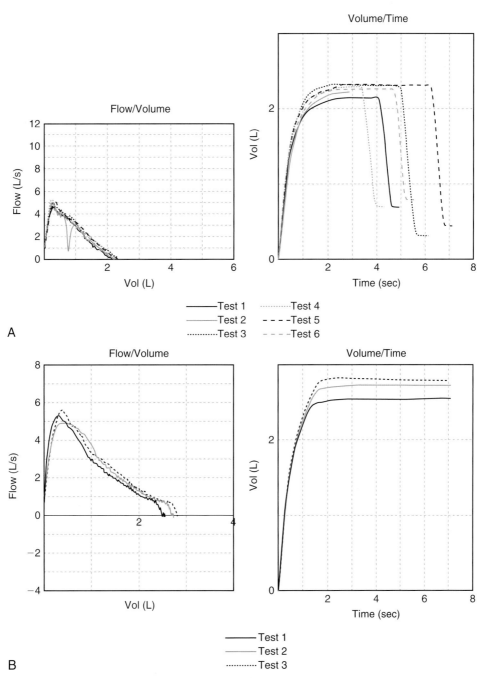

FIG. 2.11 Common technical problems identified with flow-volume loops. (A) Cough during the first second of exhalation will interfere with proper measurement of forced expiratory volume in the first second (FEV₁). (B) Glottic closure results in an abrupt termination of expiration and will affect accurate measurement of forced vital capacity (FVC).

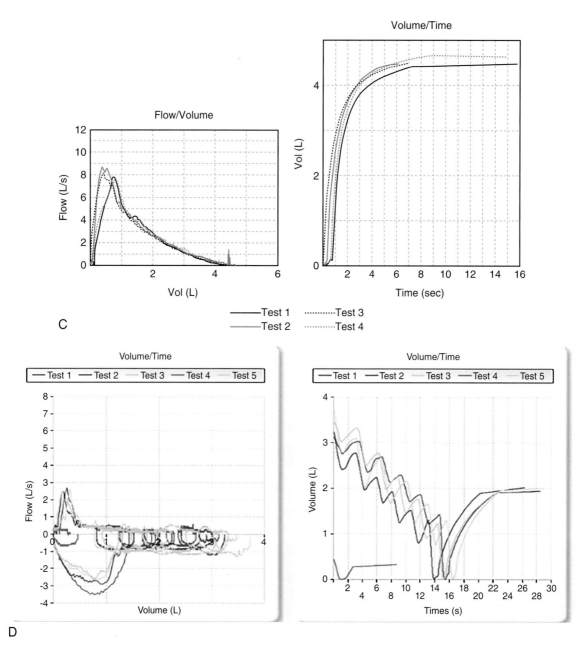

FIG. 2.11, CONT'D   (C) Test 1 demonstrates excessive back-extrapolation volume secondary to a slow start. This will cause an overestimation of the FEV$_1$. Look for the maneuver to "hug" the y-axis or not lean (Test 1 is a "leaning Tower of Pisa") (D) Negative flow sensor drift (all maneuvers slope downward).

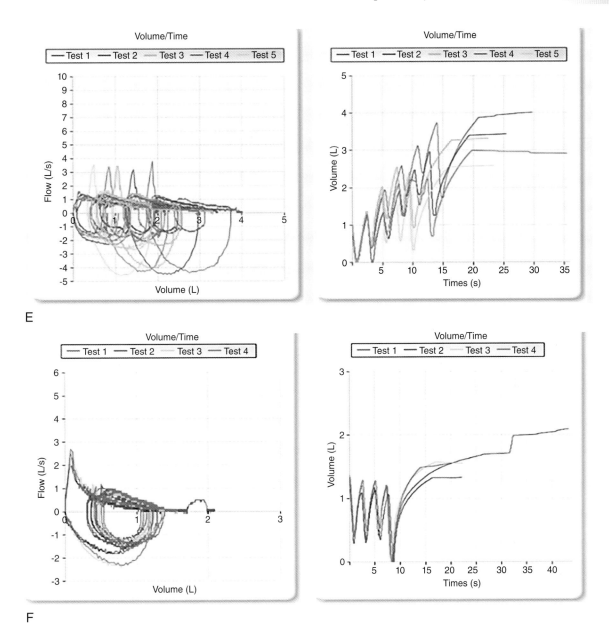

FIG. 2.11, CONT'D (E) Positive flow sensor drift (all maneuvers slope upward). (F) A sneak breath at the end of the exhalation.

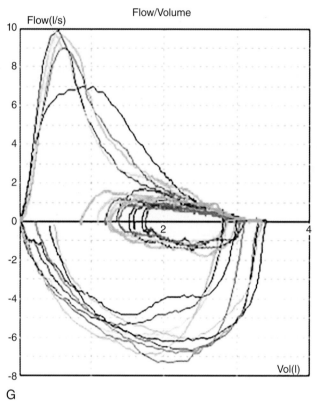

G

FIG. 2.11, CONT'D   (G) Maneuver with suboptimal blast (3L/sec less than the other maneuvers).

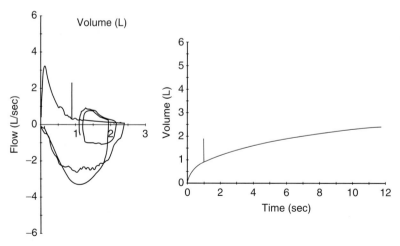

FIG. 2.12   Flow-volume loop and volume–time tracings from a patient with severe obstruction. The expiratory flow-volume curve shows severely reduced flows at all lung volumes; inspiratory flows are also markedly reduced. Note that the tidal breathing loop (recorded immediately before the forced effort) shows higher flows than the maximal expiratory flow-volume curve. This is consistent with *dynamic airway compression* during forced exhalation. The expiratory volume-time tracing reveals reduced flow with no obvious plateau even after 12 seconds of exhalation.

CRITERIA FOR ACCEPTABILITY 2.3

Flow-Volume Loop

1. Rapid rise from maximal inspiration to PEF (rise time of <150 ms)
2. Maximal effort until flow returns to zero baseline; no glottic closure or abrupt end of flow
3. No cough or artifact in the first second
4. Maximal inspiratory effort with return of volume to point of maximal inspiration. (Failure to close loop indicates that effort was not started from maximal inspiration, inspiratory effort was submaximal, or spirometer error.) Comparison of the FIVC – FVC is a recommended quality check. The values should be less than 100 mL.
5. At least three acceptable loops recorded; superimposed or side-by-side loops should be repeatable unless bronchospasm occurs.
6. Report the F-V loop from the single best test maneuver (highest sum of FEV_1 and FVC).

Significance and Pathophysiology

See Interpretive Strategies 2.3. Maximal flow at any lung volume during forced expiration or forced inspiration can be easily measured from the F-V loop (see Fig. 2.9). Significant decreases in flow or volume are easily detected from a single graphic display. Many clinicians prefer to include the F-V loop or MEFV curve as part of the patient's medical record.

The shape of an MEFV curve from approximately 75% of FVC to maximal expiration is largely independent of patient effort. Flow over this segment is determined by two properties of the lung: elastic recoil and flow resistance. The lung is stretched by maximal inspiration. Elastic recoil determines the pressure applied to gas in the lung during a forced expiration. This pressure is determined by the recoil of the lung and chest wall. Resistance to flow in the airways is the second factor affecting the shape of the flow-volume curve. Flow limitation occurs in the large and medium airways during the early part of a forced expiration. The site of flow limitation migrates "upstream" rapidly during forced expiration. Resistance to flow in small (<2 mm) airways is determined primarily by the cross-sectional area. This cross-sectional area can be affected by a number of factors. Destruction of alveolar walls, as in emphysema, reduces support of the small airways.

Bronchoconstriction and inflammation directly reduce the lumen of the small airways (Fig. 2.12).

INTERPRETIVE STRATEGIES 2.3

Flow-Volume Loop

1. Were at least three acceptable F-V loops obtained? Does the beginning of the expiratory curve show a sharp rise to PEF? If not, suspect patient effort or large airway obstruction.
2. Are the PEF and PIF values consistent? Do PEF or other expiratory flows fall with repeated efforts? If so, suspect hyperreactive airways.
3. Does the expiratory curve from PEF to maximal exhalation appear concave? If so, suspect airway obstruction.
4. Do either the expiratory or inspiratory portions of the curve show a "squared-off" pattern? If so, suspect large airway obstruction. If both, suspect a fixed obstruction.
5. Is the inspiratory curve repeatable? If not, suspect variable extrathoracic obstruction or suboptimal effort or fatigue.
6. Does the F-V loop show any other unusual patterns (sudden changes in flow that are reproducible or "sawtooth" pattern)?

In healthy patients, flow ($\dot{V}max$) over the effort-independent segment decreases linearly as lung volume decreases. Pressures around airways are balanced by gas pressures in the airways so that flow is limited at an "equal pressure point." As the lung empties, the equal pressure point moves upstream into increasingly smaller airways and continues until small airways begin to close, trapping some gas in the alveoli (the RV). This pattern of airflow limitation in healthy lungs causes the MEFV curve to have a linear or slightly concave appearance. This degree of concavity increases with age, presumably because of reduced flows secondary to loss of elastic recoil with aging.

Flow-Volume Loops in Small Airway Obstruction

Maximal flow is decreased in patients who have obstruction in small airways, particularly at low lung volumes. The effort-independent segment of the MEFV curve appears more concave or "scooped out." Values for $\dot{V}max_{50}$ and $\dot{V}max_{25}$ are characteristically decreased. Decreases in $\dot{V}max_{50}$ correlate well with the reduction in $FEF_{25\%-75\%}$ in patients with peripheral airway obstructive disease.

Because elastic recoil and resistance in small airways determine the shape of the MEFV tracing, different lung diseases can cause similar F-V patterns. Emphysema destroys alveoli, with a loss of elastic tissue and support for small airways. Flow through small airways decreases because of collapse of the unsupported walls. In contrast, bronchitis, asthma, and similar inflammatory processes increase resistance in the small airways. Increased resistance is caused by edema, mucus production, and smooth muscle constriction. Reduction in the cross-sectional area of the small airways reduces flow. Emphysema and chronic bronchitis are often found in the same individual because of their common cause—cigarette smoking. The MEFV curve thus presents a picture of the extent of obstruction without identifying its cause.

Flow-Volume Loops in Large Airway Obstruction

Obstruction of the upper airway, trachea, or mainstem bronchi also shows characteristic patterns. Both expiratory and inspiratory flow may be limited. The F-V loop is extremely useful in diagnosing these large airway abnormalities (Fig. 2.13). Comparison of expiratory and inspiratory flows at 50% of the FVC ($FEF_{50\%}$ and $FIF_{50\%}$, respectively) may help determine the site of obstruction. In healthy patients, the ratio of $FEF_{50\%}$ to $FIF_{50\%}$ is approximately 1.0 or slightly less. Fixed large airway obstruction causes equally reduced flows at 50% of the VC during inspiration and expiration (see Fig. 2.13). Obstructive lesions that vary with the phase of breathing also produce characteristic patterns. Variable extrathoracic obstruction usually shows normal expiratory flow but diminished inspiratory flow. The $FEF_{50\%}/FIF_{50\%}$ is often greater than 1.0 because the obstructive process

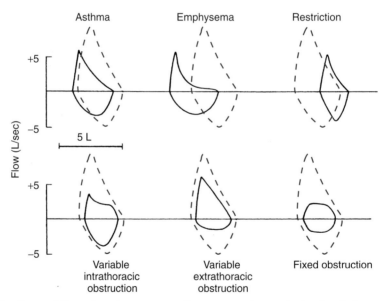

FIG. 2.13 Abnormal flow-volume loop patterns. Six curves are shown, plotting flow in liters per second against the forced vital capacity (FVC) on an absolute volume scale, with the expected curve shown as dashed lines. In patients who have asthma or emphysema, the expiratory curve is characteristically concave. The total lung capacity (TLC) and residual volume (RV) points are consistent with hyperinflation and/or air trapping. In patients with lung or chest wall restriction, the shape of the loop is preserved, but the FVC is decreased. The TLC and RV are displaced toward lower lung volume. The bottom three examples depict types of large airway obstructions. Variable intrathoracic obstruction shows reduced flows on expiration ("what's in is out") despite near-normal flows on inspiration. Variable extrathoracic obstruction shows an opposite pattern. Inspiratory flow is reduced, whereas expiratory flow is relatively normal ("what's out is in"). Fixed large airway obstruction is characterized by equally reduced inspiratory and expiratory flows.

is outside of the thorax; the MEFV portion of the curve appears as it would in a healthy individual, but the inspiratory portion of the loop is flattened. Inspiratory flow depends on how much obstruction is present. A common cause of variable extrathoracic obstruction, resulting in truncated inspiratory flow, is paradoxical vocal cord closure during inspiration, also known as *vocal cord dysfunction.* In variable intrathoracic obstruction, PEF is reduced.

Expiratory flow remains constant until the site of flow limitation reaches the smaller airways. This gives the expiratory limb a "squared-off" appearance (see Fig. 2.13). The inspiratory portion of the loop may be completely normal. The $FEF_{50\%}/FIF_{50\%}$ will typically be much less than 1.0, depending on the severity of obstruction. In patients with truncation of both the inspiratory and expiratory loops, a fixed obstruction may be present.

PF TIP 2.6

The classic analogy for an emphysematous lung is a balloon that has been blown up for several days and the air has escaped. The balloon (B), much like the emphysematous lung, is distended and floppy. It has lost its elastic recoil and is very compliant. The neck of the balloon is also affected and is collapsed. This gives the maximal expiratory flow-volume curve its characteristic obstructive concave or "scooped" appearance (A, C).

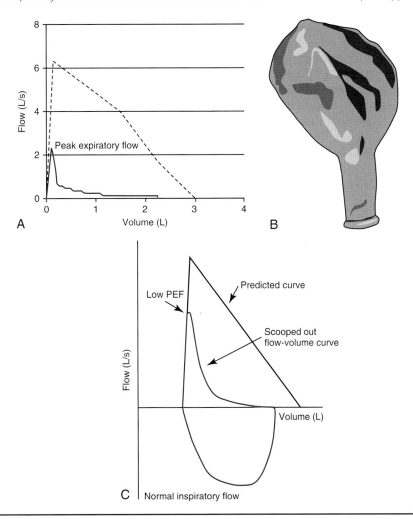

Airway obstruction associated with abnormality of the muscular control of the posterior pharynx and larynx sometimes produces a "sawtooth" pattern visible on the inspiratory and expiratory limbs of the MEFV curve (Fig. 2.14). This pattern is neither sensitive nor specific for patients with sleep apnea but is sometimes observed in this patient population. If this pattern is observed on the F-V curve and the subject complains of daytime hypersomnolence, a referral to a sleep center may be warranted. The interpretation of this noise is sometimes termed *redundant tissue of the upper airway*.

Peak inspiratory flow and the pattern of flow during inspiration are largely effort dependent. Poor patient effort may result in inspiratory flow patterns similar to variable extrathoracic obstruction. Instruction by the technologist should emphasize maximal effort during inspiration and expiration. If repeated efforts produce reduced inspiratory flows, an obstructive process should be suspected.

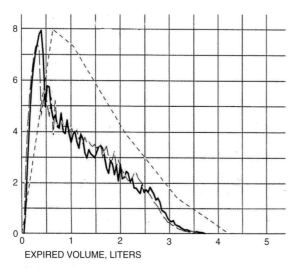

FIG. 2.14 The "sawtooth" pattern, sometimes termed *redundant tissue of the airway*, is sometimes seen in subjects with obstructive sleep apnea.

Flow-Volume Loops in Restrictive Disease

Restrictive disease processes may show normal or greater-than-normal peak flows with linear decreases in flow versus volume. The lung volume displayed on the *x*-axis is decreased. Moderate or severe

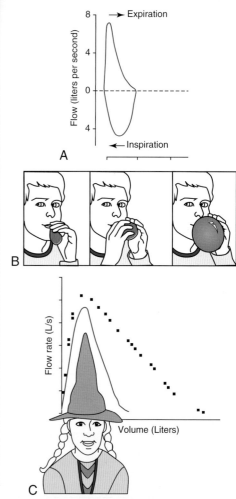

restriction demonstrates equally reduced flows at all lung volumes. Reduced flows are primarily caused by the decreased cross-sectional area of the small airways at low lung volumes. Simple restriction causes the F-V loop to appear as a miniature of the normal curve (see Fig. 2.10), often with supranormal flow, as evidenced by elevated FEV_1/VC.

In Bronchodilator Responsiveness Testing the F-V loops can be superimposed to measure changes in flow at specific lung volumes. The curves are usually positioned by superimposing at maximal inspiration. This method assumes that any increase in FVC occurs while TLC remains constant. If postbronchodilator lung volume tests are performed, the curves may be superimposed on an absolute volume scale (i.e., isovolume correction). This method shows bronchodilator-induced changes in lung volumes and flows. Sometimes, lung volumes will change after bronchodilator without any change in FEV_1. Inhalation challenge studies (see Chapter 9) can be displayed similarly to assess the reduction in flows at specific lung volumes.

Tidal breathing curves or MVV curves can also be superimposed on the F-V loop. The patient's ventilatory reserve can be assessed by comparing the areas enclosed under each of the curves. Patients who have obstructive lung disease may generate F-V loops only slightly larger than their tidal breathing curves. In severe obstruction, flow during tidal breathing may actually exceed flow during a forced expiration. Dynamic compression of small airways during forced expiration causes airway collapse, whereas tidal breathing may not. These patients have limited ventilatory reserve and shortness of breath with exertion.

F-V loops may also be measured during exercise (see Chapter 7). By superimposing a flow-volume curve during exercise over the maximal F-V loop, specific patterns of ventilatory response can be assessed. Patients who have airflow limitation are typically unable to increase ventilation during exercise when expiratory flow equals maximal flow. Exercise F-V curves can be used to demonstrate this phenomenon.

PEAK EXPIRATORY FLOW

Description

PEF is the maximum flow attained during an FVC maneuver. When reported in conjunction with other spirometric variables, PEF is expressed in liters per second, BTPS. When performed alone using a **peak flow meter**, PEF is usually reported in liters per minute, BTPS.

Technique

PEF can be easily measured from a flow-volume curve (MEFV). PEF may also be measured by using devices that sense flow directly (see Chapter 11) or by using volume-displacement spirometers and deriving the rate of volume change. Many portable devices (i.e., peak flow meters) are available to measure maximal flow during forced expiration. Most sense flow as movement of air against a turbine or through an orifice. PEF done in conjunction with spirometry is performed as described for F-V loops.

Measuring PEF with a peak flow meter may be done at the bedside, in the emergency department, in the clinic setting, or at home. In each setting, the individual performing the measurement must know how to operate the specific peak flow meter. The maneuver should be demonstrated to the patient. A return demonstration is essential when the patient is being trained to use the peak flow meter at home.

The peak flow meter should be set or zeroed, as required. When performed at home with a portable device as part of ambulatory monitoring, the standing position is usually recommended (if performed as part of a spirometry maneuver in the office or hospital setting, the patient should be sitting). The patient should inhale maximally; the inhalation should be rapid but not forced. The patient then exhales with maximal effort as soon as the teeth and lips are placed around the mouthpiece. The neck should be in a neutral position to avoid tracheal compression with neck flexion or extension because these will reduce PEF. As in the FVC maneuver, a long pause (4–6 seconds) at maximal inspiration may decrease the PEF; there should be no more than 1 second of hesitation. The expiratory effort needs to be only 1 to 2 seconds to record PEF.

At least three maneuvers should be performed and recorded, along with the order in which the values were obtained. All readings are recorded to detect effort-induced bronchospasm. The largest PEF obtained should be reported. The PEF is effort dependent and variable. It may be particularly variable in patients with hyperreactive airways (Criteria for Acceptability 2.4). Up to five attempts should be made to achieve adequate repeatability, defined as a difference of no more than 0.67 L/sec (40 L/min) between the largest of two out of three acceptable efforts.

When PEF is used to monitor patients with asthma, it is important to establish each person's best PEF (i.e., the largest PEF achieved). Best values can be obtained over 2 to 3 weeks. PEF should be measured twice daily (morning and evening). The personal best is usually observed in the evening after a period of maximum therapy. Daily measurements are then compared with the personal best. The personal best PEF should be reevaluated annually. This allows PEF to be adjusted for growth in children or for progression of disease. PEF should be periodically compared with regular spirometry results (FEV_1).

Portable peak flow meters need to be precise (low variability in the same instrument). Precision is more important than accuracy for detecting changes from serial measurements. Peak flow meters should have ranges of 60 to 400 L/min for children and 100 to 850 L/min for adults. Standards for peak flow monitoring devices have been published by the ATS-ERS (see Chapter 11).

may be limited. Peak flow is effort dependent. It primarily measures large airway function and muscular effort. Decreased PEF values should be evaluated for consistent patient effort. PEF values for patients without hyperreactive airways are usually similar with repeated efforts. Patients with asthma often have a pattern of decreasing PEF with repeated trials. Widely varying peak flows without a pattern of induced bronchospasm suggest poor effort or cooperation. However, PEF measurements alone are not sufficient to make a diagnosis of asthma. Spirometry, lung volumes, diffusing capacity, and airway resistance measurements may be required for a full evaluation of the associated physiologic impairment.

The effort dependence of PEF makes it a good indicator of patient effort during spirometry. Maximal **transpulmonary pressures (Ptp)** correlate well with maximal PEF. Patients who exert variable effort during FVC maneuvers are seldom able to reproduce their PEF. Some clinicians use PEF in addition to the FVC and FEV_1 to gauge maximal effort during spirometry. PEF measurements, when performed with a good effort, correlate well with the FEV_1 as measured by spirometry.

CRITERIA FOR ACCEPTABILITY 2.4

Peak Flow

1. Patient was standing or sitting up straight.
2. Patient inhaled maximally (rapid but not forced) and exhaled maximally without holding his or her breath.
3. At least three efforts were performed and recorded in order.
4. The largest two out of three efforts were repeatable within 0.67 L/s (40 L/min).
5. Largest PEF obtained is reported.

From ATS-ERS Task Force, 2005.

Significance and Pathophysiology

See Interpretive Strategies 2.4. The PEF attainable by healthy young adults may exceed 10 L/sec or 600 L/min, BTPS. Even when an accurate pneumotachometer is used, the value of PEF measurements

---

INTERPRETIVE STRATEGIES 2.4

Peak Flow

1. What is the patient's personal best PEF?
2. Is the current PEF the best of three trials? Was it obtained in the morning or evening? Was it obtained before or after inhaled bronchodilator therapy?
3. Zone system[a]:
   Green: 80% to 100% of personal best
   Signals good control. Take your medications as usual.
   Yellow: 50% to 79% of personal best
   Signals caution. Your asthma may not be under good control. Take your medicine as directed by your physician and follow your asthma plan, and/or ask your doctor whether you need to change or increase your daily medicines.
   Red: < 50% of personal best
   Signals a medical alert. You must take an inhaled short-acting β_2 agonist right away. Call your doctor or emergency room (ER) and ask what to do or go directly to the ER.

[a]From National Asthma Education and Prevention Program, EPR-3, 2007.

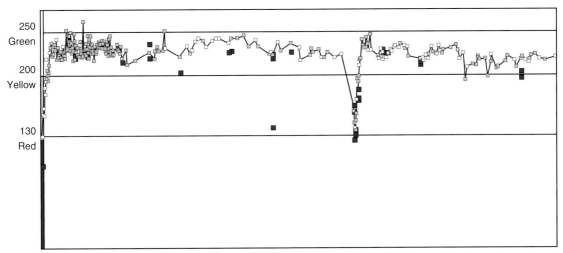

FIG. 2.15 Peak flow trend in a subject with asthma. The middle section of the trend data demonstrates an asthma exacerbation with a reduction in peak expiratory flow (PEF) that then responds to treatment.

Patients with early small airway obstruction may initially develop high flows during an FVC maneuver. Despite obstruction, these individuals show relatively normal PEF values. When small airway obstruction becomes severe, PEF also decreases. The reduction in PEF is often less than the decrease in $FEF_{50\%}$ or $FEF_{75\%}$ in patients with severe obstruction.

PEF measurements are particularly useful for monitoring patients with asthma at home. Daily monitoring of PEF can provide early detection of asthmatic episodes. It can be used to detect day-night patterns (circadian rhythms) related to airway reactivity. PEF monitoring provides objective criteria for treatment. It can help determine specific triggers (e.g., allergens) or workplace exposures that cause symptoms. Daily morning and evening readings are recommended. For patients taking inhaled bronchodilators, PEF may be measured before and after treatment. Significant variation from the personal best or from one reading to the next should be emphasized.

The NAEPP suggests a "zone" system based on the individual's personal best or predicted PEF (see Interpretive Strategy 2.4). The zone system uses green, yellow, and red as indicators for maintaining or altering therapy. Green (80%–100% of the personal best PEF) indicates a continuation of routine therapy. Yellow (50%–79% of the personal best PEF) indicates that an acute episode may be starting. Patients should be instructed to take their medi-

cation immediately according to their physicians' orders. Red (< 50% of the personal best PEF) indicates that an acute change has occurred. Immediate treatment is required, and the clinician should be notified, or after taking their medication, the patient should go to the ER. This approach dramatically improves the patient's ability to communicate symptomatic changes to the clinician (Fig. 2.15).

Uniformly decreased PEF is often associated with upper airway obstruction but is nonspecific. PEF assessed from F-V loops (along with PIF) helps define both the severity and site of large airway obstruction.

MAXIMUM VOLUNTARY VENTILATION

Description

MVV is the volume of air exhaled in a specific interval during rapid forced breathing. The maneuver should last at least 12 seconds. It is recorded in liters per minute, BTPS, by extrapolating the volume to 1 minute.

Technique

MVV is measured by having the patient breathe deeply and rapidly for a 12 to 15 seconds. Patients should set the rate but breathe rapidly and deeply.

The volume breathed should be greater than the V_T but less than the VC. Instruct the patient to move as much air as possible into and out of the spirometer. The technologist should encourage the patient throughout the maneuver. An ideal rate is 90 to 110 breaths per minute, and an ideal V_T is approximately 50% of the VC.

MVV is continued for at least 12 seconds but no more than 15 seconds. The patient is hyperventilating, so efforts longer than 15 seconds may exaggerate the sensation of lightheadedness. Even the 12-second interval may produce dizziness or syncope. The test may be performed with the patient in either a sitting or standing position. If done while standing, a chair should be available in case of dizziness. Some automated spirometers allow MVV to be terminated before 12 seconds. This accommodates patients who cannot continue because of coughing or lightheadedness. If MVV does not last 12 seconds, it should be noted in the technologist's comments (see Chapter 12). At least two MVV maneuvers should be performed. The two largest should be within 20% of each other. The largest value is reported (Criteria for Acceptability 2.5).

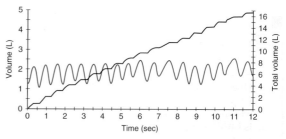

FIG. 2.16 Maximum voluntary ventilation (MVV). A composite MVV spirogram on which breath-by-breath volume change and accumulated volume are plotted against time. The undulating line shows the tidal volume (approximately 1 L in this test) moved during each breath over a 12-second interval. To calculate MVV, the volumes of individual breaths can be added and multiplied by a factor of 5 (i.e., 60 seconds/12 seconds = 5) because the MVV is reported in liters per minute.

The volume expired is measured by a spirometer. The spirometer must have an adequate frequency response over a wide range of flows (see Chapter 11). Historically, the volume of each breath was read from a volume–time spirogram or from a recording of accumulated volume (Fig. 2.16). Now volume data from each breath are summed by a computer for the interval measured. The MVV (for a 12-second test) is calculated as flow in liters per minute, as follows:

$$MVV = Vol_{12} \times \frac{60}{12}$$

where:

Vol_{12} = volume in liters expired in 12 seconds
60 = factor for extrapolation from seconds to minutes

For other intervals, the MVV is calculated similarly. The MVV must be corrected to BTPS.

PF TIP 2.9

You can quickly check the validity of the MVV by comparing it with the patient's FEV_1 multiplied by 40. If the MVV is significantly lower than $FEV_1 \times 40$, patient effort may be the cause. Neuromuscular disease may also cause a reduced MVV in relation to FEV_1.

CRITERIA FOR ACCEPTABILITY 2.5

MVV

1. Volume–time tracing shows continuous rhythmic effort for at least 12 seconds.
2. Volume is approximately 50% of VC, and the rate is 90 to 110 breaths per minute.
3. Two acceptable maneuvers are obtained; MVV values are within 20%.
4. Report the highest acceptable MVV and breathing rate.

From ATS-ERS Task Force, 2005.

Significance and Pathophysiology

See Interpretive Strategies 2.5. MVV tests the overall function of the respiratory system. It is influenced by airway resistance, respiratory muscles, compliance of the lung and/or chest wall, and ventilatory control mechanisms. Values in healthy young men average between 150 and 200 L/min. Values are slightly lower in healthy women. MVV decreases with age in both men and women and varies considerably in healthy patients. Only large reductions in MVV (25% or more) are considered significant.

MVV is decreased in patients with moderate or severe obstructive disease. This may be the result of the increased airway resistance caused by bronchospasm or mucus secretion. Reduction of MVV may also occur because of airway collapse and hyperinflation, as in emphysema. The MVV maneuver exaggerates air trapping and airflow limitation. Volume–time MVV tracings may show a shift if gas trapping occurs during the test. A slight shift is usually noted during the first few breaths, even in healthy patients. The patient adjusts to a lung volume that allows maximal airflow. These first few breaths are usually excluded from the MVV calculation.

The MVV maneuver also places a load on the respiratory muscles. Both inspiratory and expiratory muscles are used in the MVV maneuver. Weakness or decreased endurance of either system may result in low MVV values. Poor coordination of the respiratory muscles caused by a neurologic deficit may also cause a low MVV. Disorders such as paralysis or nerve damage reduce MVV as well.

A markedly reduced MVV correlates with postoperative risk for patients having abdominal or thoracic surgery. Patients who have low preoperative MVV values show an increased incidence of complications. Reduced strength or endurance of the respiratory muscles may be the factor that allows MVV to predict postoperative problems.

The MVV value may be helpful in estimating ventilation during exercise. Note, however, that the MVV maneuver does not mimic the true respiratory pattern during maximal exercise and thus is only an estimate of maximal breathing capacity during exercise (see Chapter 7). Airway-obstructed patients who have an MVV of less than 50 L/min often have a ventilatory limitation to exercise. Maximal exercise ventilation in healthy patients is usually less than 70% of their MVV. In airway-obstructed patients, maximal ventilation during exercise approaches or even exceeds their MVV. This pattern occurs partly because the MVV itself is reduced in obstruction. Highly conditioned healthy patients may also reach their MVV during maximal exercise (see Chapter 7).

MVV may be normal in patients who have restrictive pulmonary disease. Diseases that limit lung or chest wall expansion may not interfere significantly with airflow. Patients who have restrictive disease can compensate by performing the MVV maneuver with low V_T and high breathing rates.

The MVV maneuver depends on patient effort and cooperation. Low MVV values may indicate obstruction, muscular weakness, defective ventilatory control, or poor patient performance.

Patient effort during the MVV maneuver may be estimated by multiplying the FEV_1 by 40. For example, a patient with an FEV_1 of 2.0 L might be expected to ventilate approximately 80 L/min (40×2.0 L) during the MVV test. If the measured MVV is less than 80% of ($FEV_1 \times 40$), poor patient effort or neuromuscular weakness may be suspected. If the MVV exceeds ($FEV_1 \times 40$) by a large volume, the FEV_1 may be erroneous.

BRONCHODILATOR RESPONSIVENESS TESTING

Description

Spirometry can be performed before and after bronchodilator administration to determine the reversibility of airway obstruction. An $FEV_{1\%}$ of less than predicted is a good indication for bronchodilator studies. Patients whose FEV_1 and VC are within normal limits may have a low $FEV_{1\%}$. This happens when the VC is greater than 100% of predicted while the FEV_1 is slightly reduced. Even if the FEV_1 and $FEV_{1\%}$ are normal, one may still test for a bronchodilator response in patients for whom there is a high clinical suspicion of airflow obstruction because the normal range is defined for a population, not any one individual. In addition, airflow obstruction may not be reflected in the FEV_1 and $FEV_{1\%}$. Although any pulmonary function parameter may be measured before and after bronchodilator therapy, FEV_1 and specific airway resistance or conductance (sRaw, sGaw) are usually evaluated.

Technique

The patient may perform an array of tests, including spirometry, lung volumes, and diffusing capacity (D_{LCO}). Lung volumes should be recorded before bronchodilator administration. This provides a baseline for comparing lung volume changes after bronchodilator therapy. Even though indices of flow (FEV_1, $FEF_{25\%-75\%}$, and sGaw) usually show the greatest change, lung volumes and D_{LCO} may also respond to bronchodilator therapy.

Patients referred for spirometry testing should withhold routine bronchodilator therapy before the procedure (Table 2.3). Some patients may be unable to manage their symptoms if bronchodilators are withheld. These patients should be instructed to take their bronchodilator medication as needed. In these instances, the time when the medication was last taken should be noted. Some patients who use bronchodilators shortly before testing (within 4 hours) still show significant improvement after a repeated dose.

TABLE 2.3

Medication Withholding Schedule

Medication	Time to Withhold
Short-acting β_2 agonist (SABA; e.g., albuterol or salbutamol)	4–6 hours
Long-acting β_2 agonist (LABA; e.g., formoterol or salmeterol	24 hours
Ultra-LABA e.g., indacaterol, vilanterol, or olodaterol	36 hours
Short-acting muscarinic antagonist (SAMA; e.g., ipratropium bromide	12 hours
Long-acting muscarinic antagonist (LAMA; e.g., tiotropium, umeclidinium, aclidinium, or glycopyrronium)	36–48 hours

Adapted Table 8 from the American Thoracic Society/European Respiratory Society Standardization of Spirometry 2019 Update An Official American Thoracic Society and European Respiratory Society Technical Statement Graham BL, Steenbruggen I, Miller MR et al. Am J Respir Crit Care Med Vol 200, Iss 8, pp e70–e88, Oct 15, 2019.

Inhaled bronchodilators can be administered by a metered-dose inhaler (MDI) or a small-volume nebulizer. An MDI provides a reproducible means of administering the bronchodilator. Some patients are unable to coordinate activation of the MDI with slow, deep inspiration. For these patients, the use of an aerosol reservoir, or spacer, may provide a more consistent delivery of medication. If the patient is unfamiliar with the MDI, the technologist may need to activate the device (How To ... 2.2). Small-volume, jet-powered nebulizers may be used to administer more bronchodilator over a longer interval. Single-patient-use nebulizers (i.e., disposable nebulizers) are preferred and should never be reused.

β_2-agonist aerosols, such as albuterol, are most commonly used. Each of these drugs has a rapid onset of action, usually within 5 minutes. Maximum bronchodilatation usually takes longer. An interval of 10 to 15 minutes between administration and repeat testing is recommended for short-acting β_2 agonists and 30 minutes later for ipratropium bromide.

The ATS-ERS guidelines recommend a relatively high dose of bronchodilator be used to ensure that if a bronchodilator response exists, it will be seen. Thus the recommended dose of albuterol is 400 mcg delivered as four inhalations of 100 mcg each by MDI, separated by 30-second intervals. For ipratropium bromide, the recommended dose is 160 mcg delivered as four inhalations of 40 mcg each by MDI.

Bronchodilator administration often causes side effects. The most common side effect of β_2-agonist use is tachycardia. Increased blood pressure, flushing, dizziness, or lightheadedness is not unusual. Monitoring of pulse rate and possibly blood pressure may be recommended for susceptible patients. This includes patients with known cardiac arrhythmias or elevated blood pressure. Marked changes in heart rate, rhythm, or blood pressure or symptoms such as chest pain indicate a need to stabilize the patient. The test should be stopped and the referring physician or laboratory medical director should be notified immediately. Management of the patient's symptoms and continuation of testing are the decision of the physician.

2.2   **How To ...**

Use an MDI

1. Shake the MDI; activate once to prime and check contents. If empty, replace.
2. Hold the MDI mouthpiece slightly away from the patient's open mouth, or use a spacer or holding chamber (preferred method). The latter two should be attached when priming the MDI to eliminate the electrostatic properties of the device.
3. As the patient inspires slowly from the resting expiratory level, activate the MDI.
4. Have the patient continue slowly inhaling to maximal inspiration.
5. Have patient hold the breath for 5 to 10 seconds, followed by a slow exhalation.
6. Repeat inhalations as indicated (see text). Inhalations can be repeated at 30-second intervals.
7. Children may benefit from the use of a holding chamber and take up to 4 breaths after a single actuation of the MDI.

Measurements of FEV_1, FVC, $FEF_{25\%-75\%}$, PEF, and sGaw are commonly made before and after bronchodilator administration. In each case, the percentage of change is calculated as follows:

$$\%Change = \frac{Postdrug - Predrug}{Predicted\ value} \times 100,$$

where:

Postdrug = test parameter after administration
Predrug = test parameter before administration
Predicted Value = GLI predicted value

If the test value improves, the percentage of change will be positive. If the parameter worsens, a negative percentage results. Small prebronchodilator values (e.g., an FEV_1 of 0.5 L) may show large changes even though the improvement is minimal.

FEV_1 is the most commonly used test for quantifying bronchodilator response. If $FEF_{25\%-75\%}$ or flows such as $\dot{V}max_{50}$ are used, they should be isovolume-corrected for changes in the FVC. If FVC increases more than FEV_1 after bronchodilator therapy, $FEV_{1\%}$ may actually decrease. $FEV_{1\%}$ should not be used to judge bronchodilator response. sGaw may show a marked increase after bronchodilator therapy. Improved conductance may occur despite minimal change in FEV_1 or conventional measures of flow. Spirometry or plethysmography after bronchodilator therapy should meet the usual criteria for acceptability and repeatability (i.e., three acceptable and two repeatable maneuvers).

PF TIP 2.10

Patients who have a reduced FEV_1/FVC ratio may be candidates for a bronchodilator study, even if they have taken their own medication within 4 hours. Many patients with a history of asthma or COPD may show a significant improvement if they have been using their MDI incorrectly (see How To ... 2.2). Alternatively, some patients may have a bronchodilator response even with a normal baseline FEV_1 or FEV_1/FVC ratio.

Significance and Pathophysiology

See Interpretive Strategies 2.6. Reversibility of airway obstruction is considered significant for increases greater than 10% relative to the predicted value for FEV_1 or FVC (see Table 2.4). If the sGaw is assessed, an increase of 30% to 40% is usually considered significant. Some patients may show little or no improvement in FEV_1 but have a significant improvement in sGaw (see Chapter 4). Changes in $FEF_{25\%-75\%}$ of 20% to 30% are sometimes considered significant. However, flows that depend on the FVC should be volume-corrected (Case Study 2.2). If not corrected, $FEF_{25\%-75\%}$ may appear to decrease, although FEV_1 and FVC improve. Likewise, the $FEF_{25\%-75\%}$ may appear to increase even though there is no change in FEV_1. This tends to occur when the postbronchodilator FVC falls from the baseline value, often as a result of suboptimal technique or effort.

TABLE 2.4				
Illustration of Bronchodilator Responsiveness Test				
Test	Predicted	Prebronchodilator	Postbronchodilator	Absolute (%) Change
FVC (L)	3.30	2.80	3.25	+ 0.45 (14)
FEV_1 (L)	2.15	1.82	2.07	+ 0.25 (12)

FEV_1, Forced expiratory volume in the first second; *FVC,* forced vital capacity.

Diseases involving the bronchial smooth muscle usually improve most from "before" to "after." Increases greater than 50% in the FEV_1 may occur in patients with a clinical history of asthma. Patients with chronic obstructive diseases may show little improvement in flows. Poor bronchodilator response may be related to inadequate deposition of the inhaled drug because of poor inspiratory effort. Failure to show a significant improvement after inhaled bronchodilator therapy does not exclude a clinical trial. This is especially true if only the FEV_1 is being monitored. Changes in lung volumes, in particular, may occur without substantial change in FEV_1, but this may not be evident during spirometry. Such changes may still result in significant symptomatic improvement. Some patients have a significant response to one drug but little or no response to another. The efficacy of a specific drug may require repeat testing after a trial on the medication. Long-acting bronchodilators or inhaled corticosteroids may significantly improve a patient's lung function, even if there is no acute response to an inhaled β_2 agonist.

Some patients show a paradoxical response to bronchodilator therapy. In these individuals, flows may actually decrease after the bronchodilator therapy. Decreased flows after bronchodilator therapy may also be related to fatigue from multiple FVC efforts. Changes of less than 8% is within the variability of measurement of FEV_1. Such small changes may occur just with testing and are unlikely to be significant.

SUMMARY

- The chapter describes spirometry—the most commonly performed pulmonary function study.
- Various spirometry tests are identified. Techniques for performing the tests and criteria for acceptability are enumerated.
- Simple spirometry, F-V loops, and bronchodilator studies are discussed.
- Differentiation between obstructive and restrictive disorders is made by explaining the pathophysiologies involved.
- Other tests of respiratory mechanics related to airflow are discussed in related chapters (e.g., Chapters 4, 8, and 9).

INTERPRETIVE STRATEGIES 2.6

Bronchodilator Responsiveness Testing

1. Are the prebronchodilator and postbronchodilator measurements acceptable? Repeatable within 150 mL? If not, postbronchodilator changes may be erroneous.
2. Is there greater than 10% improvement in the percent predicted value for FEV_1 and FVC?
3. No significant improvement observed? Trial of bronchodilator therapy still may be recommended, if clinically indicated.

CASE STUDIES

CASE 2.1

HISTORY

The subject is a 21-year-old Caucasian male in good health who plays college football. His chief complaint is shortness of breath after wind sprints and similar vigorous exercises. He denies any other symptoms, including cough or sputum production. He has never smoked. His grandfather had lung problems, but there is no other history of pulmonary disease involving the family. He states that his brothers and sisters have hay fever.

There is no history of exposure to environmental pollutants.

PULMONARY FUNCTION TESTING
Personal Data

Sex:	Male
Age:	21 yr
Height:	73 in. (185 cm)
Weight:	180 lb (81.6 kg)

Spirometry

	Predrug	Pred	LLN	%Pred	Postdrug	%Pred	%Change
FVC (L)	6.85	6.08	4.93	113	6.73	111	− 2
FEV_1 (L)	4.65	5.10	4.14	0.91	5.45	107	16
FEV_1/FVC	0.70	0.85	0.74	—	0.81	—	

Pred, Predicted value.
Reference set = GLI 2012.

Technologist's Comments

All FVC efforts were performed acceptably. All tests met ATS-ERS criteria.

Interpretation

All spirometry efforts before and after bronchodilator therapy were performed acceptably. Spirometry results are within normal limits except for a decrease in the $FEV_{1\%}$. There is a significant increase in the FEV_1 after the administration of the bronchodilator.

Impression: Borderline obstruction with significant response to a bronchodilator. Evaluation for exercise-induced bronchospasm may be indicated.

Cause of Symptoms

This subject has normal or slightly above-average values for most of his lung function parameters. The exception is his FEV_1/FVC, which is below the expected value and consistent with borderline obstruction. Simply evaluating FVC and FEV_1 compared with predicted values might give the impression that he is normal. The FEV_1/FVC indicates that the subject, whose FVC is slightly larger than normal, expired a disproportionately small FEV_1. This pattern of supranormal volumes with lower-than-normal FEV_1/FVC is sometimes seen in healthy young adults. There is a 16% increase (0.8 L) in FEV_1 after the administration of a bronchodilator (see Spirometry results table % change column). This response is significant, in view of the subject's complaint of shortness of breath after exercise. He appears to have reversible airway obstruction triggered by exercise.

Other Tests

Further evaluation of the subject included an exercise test to demonstrate exercise-induced bronchospasm (EIB). He jogged for 6 minutes on a treadmill at 85% of his predicted maximal heart rate. Upon completing the exercise, the subject's FEV_1 began to decrease. Five minutes after stopping the test, his FEV_1 decreased to 3.81 L, a fall of 18% from the baseline value of 4.65 L. This extent of change (10% or greater fall in FEV_1) after exercise is diagnostic of exercise-induced bronchospasm. Scattered wheezes were heard on auscultation. The obstruction was readily reversed by an inhaled bronchodilator. Inhalation-challenge testing was deferred because the obstructive defect was obvious after the exercise test.

Treatment

The subject was given a regimen of inhaled short-acting β_2 agonist. He was given a portable peak flow meter to monitor his lung function. He reported a marked decrease in symptoms by pretreating himself with the inhaled medication 15 minutes before athletic activities.

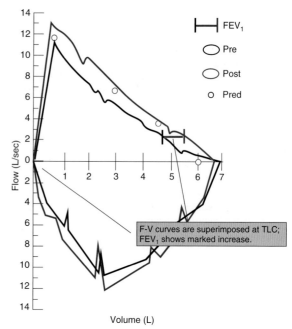

CASE STUDY 2.1   Flow-volume loops superimposed at total lung capacity (TLC).

CASE 2.2

HISTORY

The subject is a 47-year-old Caucasian carpenter whose chief complaint is shortness of breath on exertion. His dyspnea, although worse recently, has been present for several years. He smoked 1½ packs of cigarettes per day for 32 years (48 pack-years). He has a cough in the morning. He says that he produces a "small amount of grayish sputum." The subject's father had tuberculosis. A sister had asthma as a child and now as an adult. He denies any extraordinary exposure to environmental dusts or fumes.

PULMONARY FUNCTION TESTING
Personal Data

Sex:	Male
Age:	47 yr
Height:	70 in. (178 cm)
Weight:	190 lb (86.4 kg)

Spirometry

	Predrug	Pred	LLN	% Pred	Postdrug	% Pred	% Change
FVC (L)	4.01	5.09	4.00	79	4.49	90	9%
FEV_1 (L)	2.05	4.03	3.17	51	2.20	6	4%
FEV_1/FVC	0.51	0.74	0.69	—	0.49	—	—

Pred, predicted value.
Reference set = GLI 2012.

Technologist's Comments
All tests met ATS-ERS criteria.

QUESTIONS
1. What is the interpretation of the following?
   a. Prebronchodilator spirometry
   b. Response to bronchodilator
2. What is the cause of the subject's symptoms?
3. What other tests might be indicated?
4. What treatment might be recommended, based on these findings?

DISCUSSION
Interpretation
All spirometry efforts were acceptable. The subject has a reduced FEV_1, and his FVC was just above the LLN. There is only a slight increase in FEV_1 after inhaled bronchodilator therapy. FVC does not meet the 10% increase criteria.

Impression: Moderately severe airway obstruction without a significant improvement following inhaled bronchodilator.

Cause of Symptoms
The subject is a smoker who has developed moderately severe airway obstruction. His spirometry results reveal the extent of the obstruction with an FEV_1 that is 50% of predicted. The FVC is also just above the LLN and does increase with bronchodilator but does not meet the criteria for a positive response.

FEV_1 does not improve significantly after bronchodilator therapy. The $FEV_1/FVC_\%$ actually decreases as a result of the greater increase in FVC. This pattern is not unusual in subjects with obstructive airway disease. The improvement in FVC makes obstruction with air trapping the most likely cause of his improvement after a bronchodilator. The FV curves (Case Study 2.2 figure) plotted at absolute lung volumes (measured in the body box). Improvement in flow is evident by noting the curves at any particular lung volume.

Other Tests
The lung function of this subject is common in emphysema and chronic bronchitis. Air trapping is consistent with emphysematous changes but may also be present in bronchitis and asthma. Further evaluation of the subject included the measurement of lung volumes, D_{LCO}, and blood gas analysis. The findings from each of these additional tests were consistent with the results of his spirometry. He had some air trapping (elevated RV/TLC), which would explain the improved FVC after bronchodilator therapy. Blood gases and diffusing capacity were relatively normal, the latter finding making chronic bronchitis, not emphysema, the likely diagnosis.

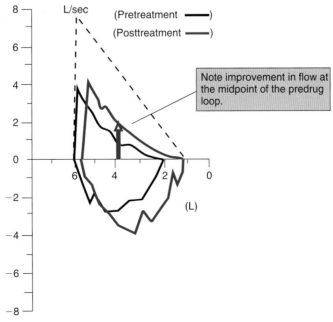

CASE STUDY 2.2   Flow-volume loops.

Each loop is plotted at the absolute lung volume at which it was measured. The increase in $FEF_{50\%}$ accurately describes the degree of bronchodilator response.

Treatment

A combination of bronchodilators and inhaled steroids was prescribed. The subject was also referred to a counselor for smoking cessation and successfully quit smoking. His cough gradually subsided during a 6-month period. He noted a marked improvement in his dyspnea.

CASE 2.3

HISTORY

The subject is a 27-year-old auto mechanic referred to the pulmonary function laboratory by his private physician. His chief complaint is "breathing problems." He describes breathlessness that occurs suddenly and then subsides. He has no other symptoms and no history of lung disease. None of his immediate family has any lung disease. He has smoked one pack of cigarettes per day for the past 10 years (10 pack-years). He has no unusual environmental exposure. He claims that gasoline fumes sometimes bring on the episodes of shortness of breath.

PULMONARY FUNCTION TESTS
Personal Data

Sex:	Male
Age:	27 yr
Height:	68 in. (173 cm)
Weight:	150 lb (68.2 kg)

Spirometry

	Before Drug	Predicted	LLN	% Predicted
FVC (L)	3.80	5.15	4.32	74
FEV_1 (L)	3.70	4.13	3.55	90
FEV_1/FVC	0.97	0.80	0.73	—
$FEF_{25\%-75\%}$ (L/sec)	4.62	4.49	2.94	103
$FEF_{50\%}$ (L/sec)	4.81	6.01	—	80
$FEF_{75\%}$ (L/sec)	3.12	3.33	—	94
MVV (L/min)	77	146	—	53

Reference set = National Health and Nutrition Examination Survey (NHANES) III.

Technologist's Comments

None of the FVC maneuvers was acceptable; they did meet the EOFE criteria. The best FVC value was also not repeatable (within 150 mL). In total, eight maneuvers were attempted. The subject had difficulty completing all maneuvers.

QUESTIONS

1. What is the interpretation of the following?
   a. Spirometry
   b. Variability of the subject's efforts
2. What is the cause of the subject's symptoms?
3. What other tests might be indicated?
4. What treatment might be recommended, based on these findings?

DISCUSSION
Interpretation

All spirometry maneuvers are unacceptable because of poor subject effort. The subject's best effort shows a reduced FVC. The FEV_1 was still usable and is within the normal limits. All other flows and the MVV are within normal limits.

Impression: Spirometry results are inconsistent. The FVC and FEV_1 are not repeatable. Overall, inadequate subject effort or technical errors are present. The FEV_1 was deemed "usable" and was within the normal limits.

Cause of Symptoms

This test shows poor repeatability, especially for effort-dependent measurements. The accompanying figure shows the variability for three FVC maneuvers. The tracings show incomplete exhalations and variability.

The low FVC is secondary to not meeting the EOFE criteria. However, the FEV_1, determined to be usable, is within the normal limits. If simple restriction were present, both FVC and FEV_1 should be reduced similarly. The subject's other flows are normal. Flows that depend on the FVC (e.g., the $FEF_{25\%-75\%}$) might also be in error if the FVC is incorrect. The FEV_1 and MVV do not depend on the FVC. The MVV is much less than 40 times the FEV_1, so the MVV is probably inaccurate secondary to subject effort.

Examination of the volume–time spirograms reveals that the subject terminated each FVC maneuver after approximately 2 seconds. The FVC values all varied by more than 150 mL, confirming poor subject cooperation. However, a lack of repeatability of the FVC maneuvers is not sufficient reason for discarding the test results. This subject's FVC maneuvers lasted only 2 seconds, despite repeated coaching by the operator. The efforts did not meet the EOFE criteria. Failure to exhale completely is one of the most common errors in spirometry. This error may be caused by a lack of cooperation on the part of the subject or the inability to continue exhalation because of cough. It may also occur if the technologist does not adequately explain or demonstrate the maneuver.

The operator performing this test repeated the FVC maneuver eight times. Only the three best efforts were recorded. Appropriate comments were added at the end of the test data. The poor quality of the data makes it impossible to determine whether his symptoms are real. He appears to be malingering— that is, not giving maximal effort on tests that are effort dependent. Poor repeatability in a subject who is free of symptoms at the time of the test suggests poor effort or lack of cooperation.

Other Tests

Alternative tests for this subject should be independent of the subject's effort. A simple blood gas analysis was performed. The results indicated normal oxygenation and acid–base status. Testing of lung volumes and diffusing capacity was postponed because both of these depend on subject effort and cooperation.

A bronchial challenge test (see Chapter 9) might have been indicated because he had asthma-like symptoms. However, bronchial challenge tests use spirometry, which this subject was unable or unwilling to perform acceptably.

Treatment

Before suggesting any treatment, the referring physician contacted the subject's employer to ask about possible environmental hazards that might cause the symptoms. He learned that the subject was facing possible termination for excessive absence from work. The subject's supervisor revealed that the subject claimed to have asthma, which caused his excessive absenteeism.

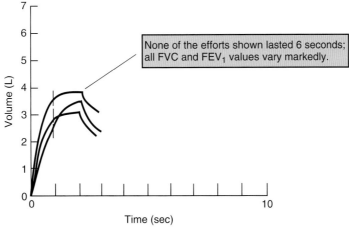

CASE STUDY 2.3   Volume–time graphs showing the lack of reaching a plateau, superimposed at total lung capacity (TLC).

SELF-ASSESSMENT QUESTIONS

Entry-Level

1. A patient performs three FVC maneuvers using a spirometer. The spirometer reports that all maneuvers had a back-extrapolated volume of less than 5% and 100 mL. The maneuvers met all other criteria for acceptability and repeatability. The technologist should do which of the following?
   a. Repeat all maneuvers.
   b. Correct the FEV_1 and all other flows by the amount of the back-extrapolated volume.
   c. Perform at least one more maneuver.
   d. Report the average of the three FVC values.

2. A 58-year-old man who complains of increased shortness of breath with exercise has the following spirometry results:

	Measured	Predicted	LLN	% Predicted
FVC (L)	5.11	4.93	4.19	104
FEV_1 (L)	2.57	3.95	3.38	65

These results are consistent with which of the following?
   a. Normal lung function
   b. Restrictive lung disease
   c. Obstructive lung disease
   d. Incorrect predicted values

3. An 81-year-old man performs three acceptable spirometry efforts and records these results:

	Measured	Predicted	LLN	% Predicted
FVC (L)	2.17	3.82	3.25	57
FEV_1 (L)	1.71	2.41	2.05	71

Which of the following is suggested by these values?
   a. Normal spirometry for an elderly man
   b. Obstructive lung disease
   c. Restrictive lung disease
   d. Erroneously measured FEV_1

4. Which of the following best describes the flow-volume curve shown?
   a. Normal forced expiratory flow pattern
   b. Variable intrathoracic obstruction
   c. Variable extrathoracic obstruction
   d. Fixed large airway obstruction

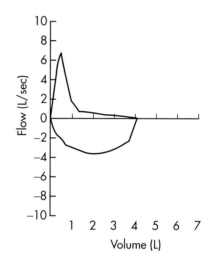

5. A 20-year-old man complains of shortness of breath with exercise. The following results of spirometry are obtained:

	Measured	Predicted	LLN	% Predicted	After Bronchodilator	% Change
FVC (L)	4.98	5.83	4.96	85	5.98	17
FEV_1 (L)	3.18	4.68	3.98	68	3.50	7

Which of the following statements best describes these findings?
   a. Results are of normal spirometry.
   b. There is moderate obstruction with significant response to bronchodilators.
   c. There is moderate obstruction without significant response to bronchodilators.
   d. Results are inconsistent and must be repeated.

6. A 33-year-old woman complains of increasing shortness of breath with exertion. Her spirometry results are as follows:

	Measured	Predicted	LLN	% Predicted
FVC (L)	2.25	3.09	2.62	73
FEV_1 (L)	1.84	2.62	2.23	70
PEF (L/s)	2.77	6.17	5.24	45
MVV (L/min)	45	104	—	43

Which of the following is most consistent with these results?
a. Moderate obstructive lung disease
b. Normal spirometry
c. Severe lung volume restriction
d. Muscle weakness or poor effort

7. How long should the pulmonary function operator wait after giving an inhaled β_2 agonist before conducting postbronchodilator testing?
a. 5 min
b. 15 min
c. 30 min
d. 45 min

8. A 60-year-old woman complains of increasing shortness of breath with exertion. Her spirometry results are as follows:

	Trial 1	Trial 2	Trial 3	Best	Predicted	LLN	% Predicted
FVC (L)	2.25	2.30	2.28	2.30	2.96	2.23	78
FEV_1 (L)	1.14	1.06	1.12	1.14	2.41	1.86	47
BE Vol (L)	0.230	0.145	0.09				

Which of the following is most consistent with these results?
a. Three acceptable and two repeatable maneuvers
b. The need to perform more maneuvers
c. Moderate obstructive disease
d. Severe obstructive lung disease

Advanced

	Trial 1	Trial 2	Trial 3
FVC (L)	3.01	2.99	3.12
FEV_1 (L)	1.99	2.01	1.95

9. A 14-year-old male with cystic fibrosis performs three spirometry trials:

The reported flow-volume loop should come from which data?
a. Trial 1
b. Trial 2
c. Trial 3
d. Average of all three trials

10. A healthy, physically fit patient performs spirometry, and the following values are recorded:

	Trial 1	Trial 2	Trial 3	Trial 4
FVC (L)	6.52	6.23	6.17	6.37
FEV_1 (L)	5.01	5.22	5.13	5.19

Which values of FVC, FEV_1, and $FEV_{1\%}$ should be reported for this patient?
a. FVC = 6.52 L, FEV_1 = 5.22 L, $FEV_{1\%}$ = 80%
b. FVC = 6.23 L, FEV_1 = 5.22 L, $FEV_{1\%}$ = 84%
c. FVC = 6.52 L, FEV_1 = 5.01 L, $FEV_{1\%}$ = 77%
d. FVC = 6.52 L, FEV_1 = 5.22 L, $FEV_{1\%}$ = 82%

11. A patient whose chief complaints are cough and hoarseness performs a series of FVC efforts, and flow-volume curves are recorded as shown. Which of the following diagnoses seems most likely?
a. Fixed airway obstruction
b. Variable intrathoracic obstruction
c. Variable extrathoracic obstruction
d. The patient was malingering

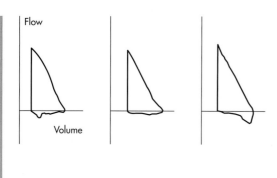

12. A patient performs the following test:

	Trial 1	Trial 2	Trial 3	Trial 4
FVC (L)	4.50	4.22	4.13	4.30
FEV_1 (L)	3.45	3.15	3.02	2.95

The data are consistent with which of the following?
a. Acceptable and repeatable spirometry
b. FVC-induced bronchospasm
c. Poor repeatability
d. Muscle weakness

SELECTED BIBLIOGRAPHY

General References

Ferguson, G. T., Enright, P. L., Buist, S. A., et al. (2000). Office spirometry for lung health assessment in adults: A consensus statement from the National Lung Health Education Program. *Chest, 117,* 1146–1161.

West, J. B. (2001). *Pulmonary physiology and pathophysiology: An integrated, case-based approach.* Baltimore, MD: Lippincott Williams & Wilkins.

Spirometry

Balfe, D. L., Lewis, M., & Mohsenifar, Z. (2002). Grading the severity of obstruction in the presence of a restrictive ventilatory defect. *Chest, 122,* 1365–1369.

Burney, P. G., & Hooper, R. (2011). Forced vital capacity, airway obstruction and survival in a general population sample from the USA. *Thorax, 66,* 49–54.

Eaton, T., Withy, S., Garrett, J. E., et al. (1999). Spirometry in primary care practice: The importance of quality assurance and the impact of spirometry workshops. *Chest, 116,* 416–423.

Enright, P. L., Linn, W. S., Avol, E. L., et al. (2000). Quality of spirometry test performance in children and adolescents: Experience in a large field study. *Chest, 118,* 665–671.

Hankinson, J. L., Odencrantz, J. R., & Fedan, K. B. (1999). Spirometric reference values from a sample of the general U.S. population. *American Journal of Respiratory and Critical Care Medicine, 159,* 179–187.

Hansen, J. E., Sun, X. G., & Wasserman, K. (2006). Should forced expiratory volume in six seconds replace forced vital capacity to detect airway obstruction? *European Respiratory Journal, 27,* 1244–1250.

Krowka, M. J., Enright, P. L., Rodarte, J. R., et al. (1987). Effect of effort on measurement of forced expiratory volume in one second. *American Review of Respiratory Disease, 136,* 829.

Leuallen, E. C., & Fowler, W. S. (1955). Maximal midexpiratory flow. *American Review of Tuberculosis, 72,* 783.

Milanzi1, E. B., Koppelman, G. H., Oldenwening, M., et al. (2019). Considerations in the use of different spirometers in epidemiological studies. *Environmental Health, 18,* 39.

Quanjer, P. H., Stanojevic, S., et al. (2012). Multi-ethnic Reference Values for Spirometry for the 3-95 Age Range: The Global Lung Function 2012 Equations. *European Respiratory Journal, 40,* 1324–1343.

Roberts, S. D., Farber, M. O., Knox, K. D., et al. (2006). FEV_1/FVC ratio of 70% misclassifies patients with obstruction at the extremes of age. *Chest, 130,* 200–206.

Stanojevic, S., Wade, A., Stocks, J., et al. (2008). Reference ranges for spirometry across all ages. *American Journal of Respiratory and Critical Care Medicine, 177,* 253–260.

Swanney, M. P., Beckert, L. E., Frampton, C. M., et al. (2004). Validity of the American Thoracic Society and other spirometric algorithms using FVC and forced expiratory volume at 6s for predicting a reduced total lung capacity. *Chest, 126,* 1861–1866.

Townsend, M. C., Hankinson, J. L., Lindesmith, L. A., et al. (2004). Is my lung function really that good? Flow-type spirometer problems that elevate test results. *Chest, 125,* 1902–1909.

Peak Expiratory Flow

Godfrey, S. (2001). Monitoring asthma severity and response to treatment. *Respiration, 68,* 637–648.

Hankinson, J. L. (2000). Beyond the peak flow meter: Newer technologies for determining and documenting changes in lung function in the workplace. *Occupational Medicine, 15,* 411–420.

Kennedy, D. T. (1998). Selection of peak flow meters in ambulatory asthma patients: A review of the literature. *Chest, 114,* 587–592.

Pesola, G. R., O'Donnell, P., Pesola, G. R., Jr., Chinchilli, V. M., & Saari, A. F. (2009). Peak expiratory flow in normals: Comparison of the mini Wright versus spirometric predicted peak flows. *Journal of Asthma, 46*(8), 845.

Wensley, D., & Silverman, M. (2004). Peak flow monitoring for guided self-management in childhood asthma: A randomized controlled trial. *American Journal of Respiratory and Critical Care Medicine, 170*(6), 606.

Before- and After-Bronchodilator Studies

Brocklebank, D., Ram, F., Wright, J., et al. (2001). Comparison of the effectiveness of inhaler devices in asthma and chronic obstructive airways disease: A systematic review of the literature. *Health Technology Assessment, 5,* 1–149.

Flow-Volume Curves

Hyatt, R. E., & Black, L. F. (1973). The flow volume curve. *American Review of Respiratory Disease, 107,* 191.

Lunn, W. W., & Sheller, J. R. (1995). Flow volume loops in the evaluation of upper airway obstruction. *Otolaryngologic Clinics of North America, 28,* 721–729.

Miller, R. D., & Hyatt, R. E. (1973). Evaluation of obstructing lesions of the trachea and larynx by flow volume loops. *American Review of Respiratory Disease, 108,* 475.

Standards and Guidelines

American Thoracic Society/European Respiratory Society Technical Standard on Interpretive Strategies for Routine Lung Function Tests (2021) Stanojevic S, Kaminsky DA, Miller M, *et al.* In press *Eur Respir.*

American Thoracic Society/European Respiratory Society Standardization of Spirometry 2019 Update An Official American Thoracic Society and European Respiratory Society Technical Statement Graham BL, Steenbruggen I, Miller MR et al. Am J Respir Crit Care Med Vol 200, Iss 8, pp e70–e88, Oct 15, 2019.

American Thoracic Society/European Respiratory Society Task Force. (2005). Standardization of Lung Function Testing. Number 2: Standardization of spirometry. *European Respiratory Journal, 26,* 319–338 (MVV resource).

American Thoracic Society/European Respiratory Society Task Force. (2005c). Standardization of Lung Function Testing. Number 5: Interpretative strategies for lung function tests. *European Respiratory Journal, 26,* 948–968.

Association of Respiratory Technology and Physiology (ARTP) statement on pulmonary function. testing 2020 Sylvester KP, Clayton N, Cliff N, et al. 2020. BMJ Open Resp Res 7:e000575.

National Asthma Education and Prevention Program. (2007). *Expert Panel Report III: Guidelines for the diagnosis and management of asthma.* Bethesda, MD: National Heart, Lung, and Blood Institute (NIH publication no. 08-4051).

Spirometry in Occupational Health–2020 = Townsend M. JOEM _ Volume 62, Number 5, May 2020.

Chapter 3

Diffusing Capacity Tests

CHAPTER OUTLINE

Carbon Monoxide Diffusing Capacity
  Description
  Techniques

Significance and Pathophysiology
Summary
Case Studies

LEARNING OBJECTIVES

After studying the chapter and reviewing the figures, tables, and case studies, you should be able to do the following:

Entry-level

1. Identify the steps for performing the single-breath D_{LCO}.
2. List at least two criteria for an acceptable single-breath D_{LCO} test.
3. Describe why D_{LCO} is often reduced in emphysema.

Advanced

1. Describe at least two nonpulmonary causes for reduced D_{LCO}.
2. Explain the significance of a reduced D_L/V_A.
3. Compare diffusion limitation caused by membranes and pulmonary capillary blood volume.
4. Explain the significance of the relationship between total lung capacity (TLC) and V_A.

KEY TERMS

alveolar sample
alveolar volume
alveolitis
breath hold
classic "discrete sample" systems
D_L/V_A
D_{LCO}
intrabreath method

Jones and Meade method
K_{CO}
membrane resistance
Müller maneuver
multigas analysis
O_2 desaturation
rapid gas analyzer (RGA) systems
rebreathing method

standard temperature, pressure, dry (STPD)
three-equation method
tracer gas
transfer factor (T_{LCO}; however, will be referred to as D_{LCO})
Valsalva maneuver
washout volume

The chapter describes measurement of diffusion in the lungs. Diffusing capacity (also referred to as **transfer factor**) is usually measured using small concentrations of carbon monoxide (CO) and is referred to as DLCO or DCO. DLCO is used to assess the gas-exchange ability of the lungs—specifically, oxygenation of mixed venous blood. Various methods, all of which use CO, have been described. The most-used method is the single-breath or breath-hold technique. The single-breath method is also the most widely standardized. The techniques section focuses on the single-breath method but also describes some of the other methods used for specific applications.

DLCO measurements are used in the diagnosis and management of most pulmonary disorders. The importance of standards and guidelines in the performance of DLCO tests and in the overall interpretation of results is highlighted. Interpretive strategies are presented in a format like those in previous chapters.

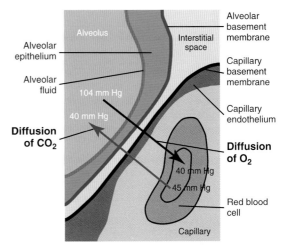

FIG. 3.1 Diffusing capacity is performed to evaluate the alveolar capillary interface where gas exchange occurs.

$$\frac{1}{D_{LCO}} = \frac{1}{Dm} + \frac{1}{\theta V_C}D$$

Diffusing capacity can be affected by factors that change the membrane component, as well as by alterations in Hb and the capillary blood volume.

A small amount of CO in inspired gas produces measurable changes in the concentration of inspired versus expired gas. Because little or no CO is normally present in pulmonary capillary blood, the pressure gradient causing diffusion is basically the alveolar pressure (P_ACO). If the partial pressure of CO in the alveoli and the rate of uptake of the gas can be measured, the DLCO of the lung can be determined. There are several methods for determining DLCO (Table 3.1). All methods are based on the following equation:

CARBON MONOXIDE DIFFUSING CAPACITY

Description

DLCO measures the transfer of a diffusion-limited gas (CO) across the alveolocapillary membranes. DLCO is reported in milliliters of CO/minute/millimeter of mercury at $0°C$, 760 mm Hg, dry (i.e., **standard temperature, pressure, dry [STPD]**).

Techniques

CO combines with hemoglobin (Hb) approximately 210 times more readily than oxygen (O_2). In the presence of normal amounts of Hb and normal ventilatory function, the primary limiting factor to diffusion of CO is the status of the alveolocapillary membranes. This process of conductance across the membranes can be divided into two components: membrane conductance (Dm) and the chemical reaction between CO and Hb (Fig. 3.1). Dm reflects the process of diffusion across the alveolocapillary membrane. Uptake of CO by Hb depends on the reaction rate (θ) and the pulmonary capillary blood volume (V_C). These two components occur in series, so the diffusion conductance can be expressed as follows:

$$D_{LCO} = \frac{\dot{V}_{CO}}{P_ACO - P_CCO}$$

where:

$\dot{V}_{CO}$ = milliliters of CO transferred/minute (STPD)
P_ACO = mean alveolar partial pressure of CO
P_CCO = mean capillary partial pressure of CO, assumed to be zero

DLCO is expressed in milliliters of gas/minute/unit of driving pressure at STPD conditions. It can also be expressed in SI units, mmol/min/kPal. The conversion from DLCO SI units to mm Hg is 2.986. Example DLCO 5.2 mmol/min/kPa = 15.5 mL/min/mm Hg.

TABLE 3.1

Advantages and Disadvantages of DLCO Testing Methods

Method	Technique	Advantages	Disadvantages	Applications
DLCOsb (breath hold)	CO and tracer gas analysis relatively simple; 10-sec breath hold	Easy calculations, simple, fast; highly standardized and automated; minimal COHb back-pressure effect; also utilized in DLNO technique	Sensitive to distribution of ventilation and matching; "nonphysiologic"; not practical for exercise testing	Screening and clinical applications
DLCOrb (rebreathing)	Rapid analysis of CO and tracer gas required; rebreathing must be controlled	Less sensitive to V_A than DLCOsb; less sensitive to $\dot{V}/\dot{Q}$ abnormalities; can be used to measure DLNO	Complex calculations (computerized); rapidly responding analyzers required; sensitive to COHb back-pressure	Clinical and research applications; provides most accurate DLCO
DLCOib (intrabreath)	Rapid analysis of CO and tracer gas during single controlled exhalation	Breath holding not required; can be used during exercise	Complex calculations (computerized); flow must be controlled; sensitive to uneven; not standardized	Screening and clinical applications; may be useful in patients who cannot hold the breath
$1/Dm + 1/\theta Vc$ (membrane diffusing capacity)	DLCOsb repeated at two different levels of alveolar P_{O_2}	Differentiates membrane transfer resistance from red cell uptake	Complex calculations; estimates of alveolar P_{O_2} are critical	Research with limited clinical applications

3.1   How To ...

Perform a DLCOsb Maneuver

1. Tasks common to all procedures:
   a. Calibrate and prepare equipment.
   b. Review order.
   c. Introduce yourself and identify patient according to institutional policies.
   d. Describe and demonstrate procedure.
2. Review spirometry data and adjust expired volume criteria if appropriate ($V_C < 2\,L$), if using a **classic "discrete sample" system.**
3. Enter recent Hgb and adjust for COHb if available.
4. Have the subject sit upright with feet flat on the floor and adjust the mouthpiece to the proper height.
5. The mouthpiece should rest on top of the tongue. Have the subject gently bite down with his or her teeth and seal lips firmly around the mouthpiece. Emphasize the need for tight lips without a leak. Place the nose clip securely.
6. Have the subject breathe quietly for several breaths and then empty completely to residual volume (RV; verbal cues such as "keep blowing until empty" are helpful; however, coaching subjects until "they are blue" is not necessary).
7. Once empty, have subject inhale rapidly as much as possible (verbal cues, "up, up, up") and hold the breath (verbal cues, "keep holding" or "hold it"). Counting down the last few seconds can be extremely helpful.
8. Have subject blow air out until empty or the system terminates the maneuver.
9. A wait period of 4 minutes is required between maneuvers.
10. Perform until acceptability and repeatability criteria are achieved or a maximum of five maneuvers. (See Criteria for Acceptability 3.1.)
11. Note comments related to test quality.

Single Breath-Hold Technique (Modified Krogh's Technique)

The patient exhales to RV and then inspires a vital capacity breath (referred to as the *IVC* or *VI*) from a system such as that in Fig. 3.2. A special diffusion gas mixture is delivered either from a spirometer, a reservoir bag, or by means of a demand valve. The diffusion mixture usually contains 0.3% CO, a "tracer" gas, 21% O_2, and the balance is N_2. The **tracer gas** is usually an insoluble inert gas such as helium (He), methane (CH_4), or neon (Ne). The tracer used depends on the type of analyzer implemented to analyze the exhaled gas. The traditional method uses He (usually about 10%) as the tracer gas. Rapidly responding infrared analyzers (see Chapter 11) have been used for continuous analysis of the small changes in CO. The same type of infrared analyzer can use CH_4 as the tracer, allowing a single analyzer can rapidly detect changes in both CO and the tracer.

After inspiring the vital capacity (VC) breath, the patient holds the breath at total lung capacity (TLC) for approximately 10 seconds. The patient then exhales. In a "classic system," a discrete sample of alveolar gas is collected after a suitable **washout volume** (750–1000 mL) has been discarded. The **alveolar sample** may be collected in a small bag (approximately 500 mL or less) or by continually aspirating a sample of the exhaled gas. In **rapid gas analyzer (RGA) systems,** which have a 0% to 90% response time of ≤ 150 ms, continuous gas analysis occurs, and a fixed washout or sample volume is not required.

Regardless of the specimen technology used, the sample is analyzed to obtain the fractional CO and tracer gas concentrations in alveolar gas, F_ACO_T (where T is the time of the breath hold), and $F_A$tracer, respectively. The concentration of CO in the alveoli at the beginning of the **breath hold** (F_ACO_0) must be determined as well. It is calculated as follows:

$$F_ACO_0 = F_ICO \times \frac{F_A\text{tracer}}{F_I\text{tracer}}$$

where:

F_ACO_0 = fraction of CO in alveolar gas at beginning of breath hold (time = 0)
F_ICO = fraction of CO in reservoir (usually 0.003)
$F_A$tracer = fraction of tracer in alveolar gas sample
$F_I$tracer = fraction of tracer in inspired gas (varies with tracer gas used)

The change in tracer gas concentration reflects the dilution of the inspired gas by the gas remaining in the lungs (i.e., RV). This change is used to determine the CO concentration at the beginning of the breath hold before diffusion from the alveoli into the pulmonary capillaries. The DLcosb (single breath) is then calculated as follows:

$$\text{DLCOsb} = \frac{V_A \times 60}{(P_B - 47) \times (T)} \times \text{Ln} \frac{F_ACO_0}{F_ACO_T}$$

where:

V_A = alveolar volume, mL (STPD)
60 = correction from seconds to minutes
P_B = barometric pressure, mm Hg
47 = water vapor pressure at 37°C, mm Hg
T = breath-hold interval, seconds
Ln = natural logarithm
F_ACO_0 = fraction of CO in alveolar gas at beginning of breath hold
F_ACO_T = fraction of CO in alveolar gas at end of breath hold

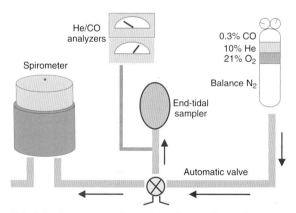

FIG. 3.2 DLco apparatus. Basic equipment for performing a DLco test (specifically the DLcosb). Gas is delivered to the automated valve from either a reservoir bag, spirometer, or a demand valve (not shown). The automated valve allows the patient to inhale the test gas rapidly. A computer usually displays a volume–time tracing, along with signals from the gas analyzer(s) (see Figs. 3.3, 3.4, and 3.5). Timing of the maneuver is usually performed by the computer.

V_A may be calculated from the single-breath dilution of the tracer gas:

$$V_A = (V_I - V_D) \times \frac{F_I tracer}{F_A tracer} \times STPD \text{ correction factor}$$

where:

V_I = volume of test gas inspired, mL (Fig. 3.3)
V_D = dead space volume (anatomic and instrumental), mL
$F_A tracer$ = fraction of tracer in alveolar gas sample
$F_I tracer$ = fraction of tracer in inspired gas (depends on tracer used)

Note that the V_A, usually expressed in body temperature, pressure, and saturation (BTPS) units, must be converted to STPD for the single-breath calculation. The dilution of tracer gas is used twice—to determine the CO concentration at the beginning of the breath hold and to determine the lung volume (i.e., V_A) at which the breath hold occurred.

Kco is the rate constant for carbon monoxide uptake from alveolar gas and the "measured" alveolar volume (V_A). Kco expressed per mm Hg multiplied by V_A equals DLco, thus DLco divided by V_A (DLco/V_A), is also termed Kco. It is the constant rate slope of the CO uptake during the breath-hold time (BHT; log $[F_A co_0/ F_A co_T]$/BHT; Fig. 3.4). The misinterpretation that DLco/V_A "corrects" DLco for reduced V_A is physiologically incorrect because DLco/V_A is not constant as V_A changes; thus the term Kco reflects the physiology more appropriately. The American Thoracic Society–European Respiratory Society (ATS-ERS) Standardized Pulmonary Function

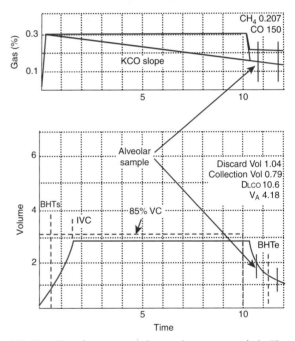

FIG. 3.4 DLcosb maneuver using continuous gas analysis. The top graph shows the slope of the constant uptake of CO (Kco) during the breath hold maneuver. Changes in gas concentrations are shown *(top)*. Test gases (CO and CH₄) rise rapidly to their initial values of 0.3% during the breath hold. During exhalation, both gas concentrations fall as dead space is washed out. The tracer gas, CH₄, shows a plateau as alveolar gas is exhaled. CO shows a similar pattern, but with a lower concentration because of uptake (diffusion). Gas concentration measurements are made from an alveolar window *(gray lines)* that can be adjusted. Simultaneous changes in lung volumes are shown on the bottom tracing. IVC indicates inspiratory volume (V_I). In this test, the patient failed to inspire at least 85% of the VC *(dashed gray line)*. Breath hold time start (BHTs) and breath hold time end (BHTe) indicate the breath-hold timing scheme. Calculated DLco and related measurements are displayed, allowing for inspection of changes as the alveolar sample "window" is adjusted.(Courtesy Vyaire, Mettawa IL.)

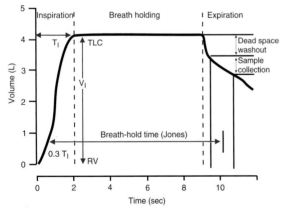

FIG. 3.3 DLcosb maneuver tracing. Tracing of a single-breath DLco maneuver proceeding from left to right *(heavy line)*. After exhaling to residual volume (RV; 0 L on the volume axis), the patient rapidly inspires a vital capacity breath (V_I) of the test gas and then holds the breath at total lung capacity (TLC) for approximately 10 seconds. At the end of the breath hold, the patient exhales rapidly. The dead-space washout volume is discarded, and an alveolar gas sample is analyzed. The breath-hold timing method used is Jones and Meade.

Reporting statement recommends reporting K_{CO} versus D_{LCO}/V_A to avoid any misinterpretation.

A simplification of the single-breath method described earlier is widely used. The tracer gas and CO analyzers may be calibrated to read full scale (100% or 1.000) when sampling the diffusion mixture and to read zero when sampling air (no tracer or CO). If the analyzers have a linear response to each other, the fractional concentration of the tracer gas in the alveolar sample is equal to the $F_A CO_0$. This technique assumes that both the tracer gas and CO are diluted equally during inspiration. Because no tracer gas leaves the lung during the breath hold, its concentration in the alveolar sample approximates that of the CO before any diffusion occurred. The exponential rate of CO diffusion from the alveoli can then be expressed as follows:

$$Ln\left(\frac{F_A tracer}{F_A CO_T}\right)$$

where:

$F_A tracer$ = fraction of tracer in alveolar gas, equal to $F_A CO_0$

$F_A CO_T$ = fraction of CO in alveolar gas at end of breath hold

Ln = natural logarithm of the ratio

This technique avoids the necessity of analyzing the absolute concentrations of the two gases. However, it requires that the analyzers be linear with respect to each other. Analysis of CO is often done using infrared analyzers (see Chapter 11), and their output is nonlinear. Care must be taken to ensure that corrected CO readings are used in the computation. These corrections are easily accomplished either electronically or via software in computerized systems. Systems that use the same detector for both CO and the tracer gas (e.g., infrared, gas chromatography) also need to provide linear output. The linearity of the system should be within 0.5% of full scale. This means that any drift or nonlinearity should cause no more than a 0.5% error when analyzing a known gas concentration (see Chapter 12).

D_{LCO} gas analysis is commonly performed with either a rapidly responding multigas analyzer or gas chromatography. **Multigas analysis** uses specialized infrared analyzers capable of detecting several gases simultaneously. These systems use methane (CH_4) as a tracer gas. One advantage of multigas analysis is that CO and CH_4 are measured rapidly and continuously (see Fig. 3.4) so that the calculated D_{LCO} is available as soon as the exhalation has been completed. Gas chromatography (see Chapter 11) can also be used for D_{LCO} gas analysis. Neon is used as the tracer gas (Fig. 3.5). Helium is used as a "carrier" gas for the chromatograph.

The resistance of the breathing circuit should be less than 1.5 cm H_2O/L/sec, at a flow of 6 L/sec. This is important in allowing the patient to inspire rapidly from RV to TLC. A demand valve may be used instead of a reservoir bag for the test gas. In a demand-flow system, the maximal inspiratory pressure to maintain a flow of 6 L/sec should be less than 10 cm H_2O. Increased resistance, in either a reservoir or a demand-valve system, may cause the patient to produce large subatmospheric pressures during inspiration. This has the effect of increasing pulmonary capillary blood volume and may falsely increase D_{LCO}.

The timing device for the maneuver should be accurate to within 100 msec over a 10-second interval (1%). Most computerized systems time the maneuver automatically. However, a means of verifying the accuracy of the BHT should be available. The **Jones and Meade method** of timing the breath hold should be used (see Fig. 3.5). The Jones and Meade method measures BHT from 0.3 of the inspiratory time (i.e., 0.7 of the inspiratory time) to the midpoint of the alveolar sample collection.

Corrections must be made for the patient's anatomic dead space (V_D) and for dead space in the valve (and sample bag, if used). Anatomic V_D should be calculated as 2.2 mL/kg (1 mL/lb) of ideal body weight. The equipment manufacturer should specify instrument V_D. Instrument V_D should not exceed 350 mL for adult subjects, including mouthpiece and any filters that might be used. Smaller-instrument V_D may be necessary for pediatric patients. Anatomic and instrument V_D are subtracted from inspired volume (V_I) before the **alveolar volume** (V_A) is calculated.

All gas volumes must be corrected from ambient temperature, ambient pressure, and saturated

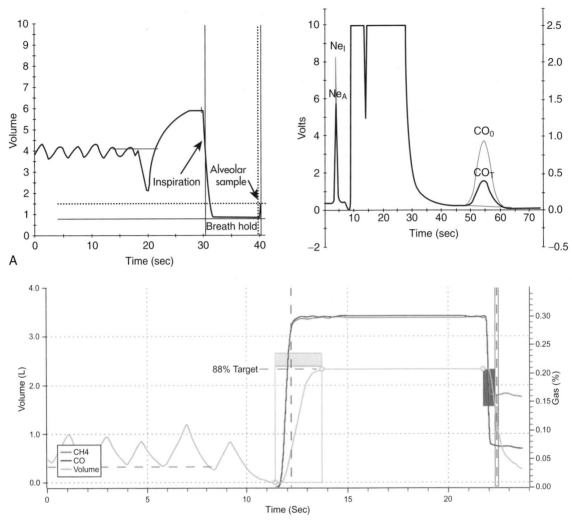

FIG. 3.5 (A) DLCOsb test using gas chromatography. (B) Rapid gas analyzer (RGA). (A) Volume–time tracing with inspiration, breath hold, and alveolar sampling is shown *(left graph)*. In this scheme, inspiration causes a downward deflection. The output of the gas chromatograph is shown *(right graph)*. Neon (the tracer gas, N_e) and CO show distinct peaks on the gas chromatograph tracing. The alveolar sample is superimposed over a preanalysis (calibration) curve of the test gas. NeI is the initial tracer concentration, and Ne_A is the concentration after the breath hold. CO concentrations of the undiluted test gas (CO_0) and end of the breath hold (CO_T) are superimposed. Calculated DLCO and related values for multiple efforts are shown at the top. (B) Volume–time tracing with inspiration, breath hold, and alveolar sampling using an RGA. Note that the inspiratory vital capacity (IVC) did not meet the 90% target. The maneuver would still be considered usable if the calculated V_A is within 200 mL or 5% of the largest V_A from acceptable maneuvers in the same test session. (Courtesy MGC Diagnostics, Inc., St. Paul, MN.)

with water vapor (ATPS) to STPD for the DLCO calculations. However, when the V_A is used to calculate the ratio of DLCO to lung volume (D_L/V_A), it is normally expressed in BTPS units. The new ATS-ERS specifically requires flow and volume

accuracy to be within 2% of expected. Using a 3-L calibration syringe (with ±0.5% tolerance), volume must be between 2.925 and 3.075 L. Volume-based spirometer systems must also be free from leaks.

Gas analyzers affected by carbon dioxide (CO_2) or water vapor require appropriate absorbers. Absorption of CO_2 is usually accomplished with a chemical absorber using $Ba(OH)_2$ (baralyme) or NaOH (sodium hydroxide, soda lye). Each of these reactions produces water vapor. Therefore CO_2 absorbers should be placed upstream of an H_2O absorber. Anhydrous $CaSO_4$ is commonly used to remove water vapor. Selectively permeable tubing (PERMA PURE) can also be used to establish a known water vapor content. Gas-conditioning devices must be routinely checked to ensure accurate gas analysis. Chemical absorbers typically add an indicator that changes color as the absorber becomes exhausted.

PF TIP 3.1

Watch the patient carefully during the $D_{LCO}sb$ effort to detect either a Valsalva or Müller maneuver. Widely varying results in two or more D_{LCO} measurements are often caused by the patient failing to relax during the breath hold. Some pulmonary function systems provide a pressure monitor to detect large positive or negative pressures during the breath hold.

$D_{LCO}sb$ maneuvers should be performed after the patient has been seated for at least 5 minutes. The patient should refrain from exertion immediately before the test; exercise increases cardiac output, which increases D_{LCO}. The patient should be instructed about the requirements of the maneuver and the technique demonstrated. Expiration to RV should be of a reasonable duration, usually 6 seconds or less. Patients who have airway obstruction may have difficulty exhaling completely in this interval. Inspiration to TLC should be rapid but not forced. Healthy subjects and patients with airway obstruction should be able to inspire 90% of their largest VC in the same test session or $\geq 85\%$ of the largest VC in the same test session *and* have a V_A within 200 mL or 5% (whichever is greater) of the largest V_A from other acceptable maneuvers (see Criteria for Acceptability 3.1). The single-breath calculation assumes instantaneous filling of the lung. Prolonged inspiratory times will decrease the actual time of breath holding at TLC, typically resulting

in a lower D_{LCO}. The breath hold should be relaxed, against either the closed glottis or a closed valve. The patient should avoid excessive positive intrathoracic pressure (**Valsalva maneuver**) or excessive negative intrathoracic pressure (**Müller maneuver**). A Valsalva maneuver reduces pulmonary capillary blood volume and may produce a falsely low D_{LCO}. A Müller maneuver increases pulmonary capillary blood volume and may falsely increase D_{LCO}. Expiration after the breath hold should be smooth and uninterrupted. Exhalation should take less than 4 seconds, and alveolar gas sampling should occur in less than 3 seconds (again because the calculations assume instantaneous emptying of the lung). Patients who have moderate or severe airway obstruction may have difficulty achieving these criteria. The BHT, measured using the Jones and Meade method (see Fig. 3.3), should be 10 seconds $\pm$ 2 seconds. Prolonged inspiratory or expiratory times may result in BHTs greater than 12 seconds. Adjustment of the shutter or valve closure time may be required to have the total BHT within the required time window.

CRITERIA FOR ACCEPTABILITY 3.1

$D_{LCO}sb$

1. System has passed calibration and quality control procedures.
2. Inspiration from RV to TLC should be rapid and should occur in less than 4 seconds.
3. $V_I \geq 90\%$ of largest VC in the same test session
   - OR $V_I \geq 85\%$ of largest VC in the same test session *and* V_A within 200 mL or 5% (whichever is greater) of largest VA from other acceptable maneuvers
4. BHT should be between 8 and 12 seconds, with no evidence of leaks or of Valsalva or Müller maneuver.
5. Exhalation should be rapid, with total exhalation lasting 4 seconds or less, with appropriate clearance of V_D and proper sampling/analysis of alveolar gas.
6. An interval of at least 4 minutes should elapse between repeated tests. No more than five single-breath maneuvers should be performed.
7. The V_A is consistent with the clinical presentation. In a normal subject, the TLC–V_A relationship should be remarkably close, if not the same, and TLC performed by any method in any disease state should be larger than V_A.
8. The average of two or more acceptable tests should be reported. Duplicate determinations should be within 2 mL/min/mm Hg (0.67 mmol/min/kPa).

To obtain an alveolar sample, dead space gas needs to be washed out (i.e., discarded). A washout of 0.75 to 1.0 L is usually sufficient to clear the patient and sampling device dead space. For patients with small vital capacities (> 2.0 L), the washout volume may be reduced to 0.5 L. A sample volume of 0.5 to 1.0 L should be collected, but a smaller sample may be necessary in patients whose VC is less than 1 L. In DLCOsb systems that use RGA technology to analyze expired gas continuously (see Fig. 3.4), inspection of the washout of the tracer gas may be used to select an appropriate alveolar sample. Rapidly RGAs that measure the CO and tracer gas simultaneously allow adjustment of washout volume (i.e., dead space) and sample volume after completion of the maneuver. These adjustments may be particularly useful in subjects who have small vital capacities (e.g., pediatric patients or adults with severe restrictive disease). Such adjustments assume that both the CO and tracer gas concentrations reflect changes occurring at the mouth. Alveolar sampling may be adjusted to begin at the point where the tracer gas and CO indicate an "alveolar plateau" (see Fig. 3.4). In patients who have uneven mixing or emptying of the lungs, there may not be a clear demarcation between dead space and alveolar gas. Adjustments to either washout (dead space) volume or sample volume should be noted on the report.

Two or more acceptable DLCOsb maneuvers (see Criteria for Acceptability 3.1) should be averaged. Duplicate determinations should be within 2 mL CO/min/mm Hg (0.67 mmol/min/kPa) of each other, obtained from acceptable efforts. No more than five repeated maneuvers should be performed

because of the effect of increasing carboxyhemoglobin (COHb) from inhalation of the test gas. There should be a 4-minute delay between repeated maneuvers to allow for washout of the tracer gas from the lungs.

The ATS-ERS DLCO technical statement describes a grading system (Table 3.2) that can be used in assessing the reliability of the results. This suggested grading system has not been validated, so its utility and impact have yet to be defined.

Hemoglobin Correction/Adjustment

Corrections for abnormal Hb concentrations should be applied with a current Hb value. The predicted DLCO should be corrected so that it reflects the DLCO at an Hb value of 14.6 g% for adult and adolescent males and to an Hb value of 13.4 g% for women and children of either sex younger than 15 years of age. The Hb-corrected predicted value for males may be calculated as follows:

$$DLCO(\text{predicted for Hb}) = DLCO(\text{predicted}) \times \frac{(1.7 \times Hb)}{10.22 + Hb}$$

Similarly, Hb correction of the predicted values for women and children younger than 15 years is calculated as follows:

$$DLCO(\text{predicted for Hb}) = DLCO(\text{predicted}) \times \frac{(1.7 \times Hb)}{(9.38 + Hb)}$$

Note that this scheme corrects the predicted value rather than the patient's measured value. For example, in an adult male patient with an Hb of 9.0 g/dL and a predicted DLCO of 25 mL/min/mm Hg, a measured

TABLE 3.2

DLCO Grading System

Grade	IVC/VC	BHT (seconds)	Sample Collection Time (seconds)
A	> 90%	8–12	< 4
B	> 85	8–12	< 4
C	> 80	8–12	< 5
D	< 80	< 8 or > 12	< 5
F	< 80	< 8 or > 12	> 5

BHT, Breath-hold time; *IVC,* inspiratory vital capacity; *VC,* vital capacity.

TABLE 3.3

Patient Results With and Without Hemoglobin Correction

	Actual	Predicted	%
DLCO mL/min/mm Hg	19.0	25.0	76
DLCO (Hb corrected) mL/min/mm Hg	19.0	19.9	95

DLCO of 19 mL/min/mm Hg would be reported as shown in Table 3.3.

Both uncorrected and corrected predicted DLCO values and the resulting percentages should be reported, along with the Hb value used for correction. Decreased Hb levels (anemia) will always reduce the predicted value, whereas elevated Hb (polycythemia) will increase the predicted value.

Carboxyhemoglobin Correction/Adjustment

Correction for the presence of COHb in the patient's blood is also recommended. The predicted DLCO may be adjusted as follows:

$$DLCO\,(predicted\,for\,COHb) = DLCO\,(predicted) \times (102\% - COHb\%)$$

PF TIP 3.3

DLCO is affected by both Hb and COHb levels in the patient's blood. A low Hb (anemia) or high COHb reduces the measured DLCO. A high Hb (polycythemia) causes the DLCO to appear elevated. As a "rule of thumb," a 10% COHb will reduce the measured DLCO by 10%.

The COHb% is the fraction of carboxyhemoglobin determined by hemoximetry expressed as a percentage. This method assumes that the predicted value already includes 2% COHb in healthy subjects. For subjects who have a COHb% greater than 2%, the predicted value will always be reduced using this method. Patients should be asked to refrain from smoking for 24 hours before the test to reduce the CO back-pressure in the blood. For patients who continue to smoke, the time of last exposure should be recorded.

Altitude Correction/Adjustment

DLCO varies inversely with changes in alveolar oxygen pressure (PAO$_2$). PAO$_2$ changes as a function of altitude, as well as with the partial pressure of oxygen in the test gas. DLCO increases approximately 0.35% for each mm Hg decrease in PAO$_2$, or about 0.31% for each mm Hg decrease in PIO$_2$. When test gas mixtures that produce an inspired O$_2$ pressure of 150 mm Hg (i.e., 21% at sea level) are used, DLCO values will be equivalent to those measured at sea level. Alternatively, standard test gas (FIO$_2$ = 0.21 is typical) can be used and the predicted DLCO corrected by adjusting PIO$_2$. For a gas with a PIO$_2$ of 150 mm Hg, the equation is as follows:

$$DLCO\text{ predicted for altitude} = DLCO\text{ predicted} / \left(1.0 + 0.0031\left[PIO_2 - 150\right]\right)$$

where:

$$PIO_2 = 0.21\left(P_B - 47\right)$$

and P_B is the local barometric pressure (at altitude). If the patient is breathing supplemental O$_2$ and the PAO$_2$ is measured, the predicted DLCO can be adjusted, assuming a PAO$_2$ of 100 mm Hg breathing air at sea level:

$$DLCO\text{ predicted for }PAO_2 = \frac{DLCO\text{ predicted}}{\left(1.0 + 0.0035\left[P_A - 100\right]\right)}$$

where:

$$PAO_2 = \text{measured or estimated alveolar oxygen partial pressure}$$

Note that corrections for altitude or elevated alveolar oxygen tensions are made to the predicted DLCO values.

Corrections for Hb, COHb, and altitude or elevated PAO$_2$ are recommended for all predicted DLCO values when the conditions for the corrections are known. Hb, COHb, and measured PAO$_2$ may not be available for all patients; correction for altitude (PIO$_2$) is easily performed for laboratories significantly above sea level. Previous guidelines recommended that corrections be applied to the patient's measured values rather than to the predicted values. Some laboratories may prefer to use the older method.

In some instances, it may be appropriate to correct the D_{LCO} for the lung volume at which it is measured. A common example would be when the subject inhales a volume substantially less than his or her known VC and breath holds at a V_A that is less than expected. The D_{LCO} may be corrected as follows:

$$D_{LCO}\left(at\ V_{Am}\right) = D_{LCO}\left(at\ V_{Ap}\right) \times \left(0.58 + 0.42\left(\frac{V_{Am}}{V_{Ap}}\right)\right)$$

where:

V_{Am} = measured alveolar volume
V_{Ap} = predicted alveolar volume (i.e., TLC – V_D)

A similar correction can be applied to the D_L/V_A:

$$\frac{D_L}{V_A}\left(at\ V_{Am}\right) = \frac{D_L}{V_A}\left(at\ V_{Ap}\right) \times \left(0.42 + 0.58\left(\frac{V_{Am}}{V_{Ap}}\right)\right)$$

These corrections are derived from healthy subjects whose D_{LCO} was measured at alveolar volumes less than the expected value. Such corrections may not be applicable in all disease states because D_L and V_A can be altered independently of one another (see the section on K_{CO}). In addition, some subjects may not exhale completely to RV, with the subsequent inspiration to TLC producing a V_I of less than 85% of their VC. In such an instance, the subject is actually breath holding at TLC, although the reduced V_I suggests otherwise.

Rebreathing Technique

The patient rebreathes from a reservoir containing a mixture of 0.3% CO, tracer gas, and air (or an O_2 mixture) for 30 to 60 seconds at a rate of approximately 30 breaths/min. The final CO, tracer, and O_2 concentrations in the reservoir are measured after this interval. An equation like that used for the single-breath technique is used (see Criteria for Acceptability 3.1):

$$D_{LCO}rb = \frac{V_s \times 60}{\left(P_B - 47\right)\left(T2 - T1\right)} \times Ln\left(\frac{F_{A}CO_{T1}}{F_{A}CO_{T2}}\right)$$

where:

V_S = volume of lung reservoir system (initial volume $\times\ F_I$tracer/$F_A$tracer)

60 = correction from seconds to minutes
P_B = barometric pressure, mm Hg
47 = water vapor pressure, mm Hg
T2 – T1 = rebreathing interval, seconds
Ln = natural logarithm
$F_{A}CO_{T1}$ = fraction of CO in alveolar gas at beginning of the rebreathing
$F_{A}CO_{T2}$ = fraction of CO in alveolar gas at the end of the rebreathing

The **rebreathing method** can also be implemented by using an RGA (for CO and tracer gas) and plotting the slope of the change in CO in relation to the slope of the tracer gas to estimate the rate of CO uptake. The rebreathing method can be used during exercise.

PF TIP 3.4

The V_A calculated from the single-breath D_{LCO} technique is essentially a "single-breath" helium-dilution measurement of lung volume and should never be larger than TLC calculated by any other method. If the V_A is larger, there is a technical issue with the measurement of either TLC or D_{LCO}, and the results should be questioned.

Slow Exhalation Single-Breath Intrabreath Method

The patient inspires a VC breath of test gas containing 0.3% CO, 0.3% CH_4 (methane), 21% O_2, and the balance N_2. Then the patient exhales slowly and evenly at approximately 0.5 L/sec from TLC to RV. A rapidly responding infrared analyzer monitors CO and CH_4 gas concentrations. The exponential rate of disappearance of CO can be calculated in a manner similar to the rebreathing method. The change in V_A is calculated from the change in the concentration of the CH_4 tracer gas. CH_4 is used as the tracer gas because it can be rapidly measured using an infrared analyzer. Multiple estimates of D_{LCO} can be made during a single exhalation, recording D_{LCO} as a function of lung volume. This is done using an equation like that used for the single-breath method. Instead of one estimate of V_A (equal to the lung volume at breath hold), multiple increments of V_A are made, and DLCO is plotted against lung volume. A single estimate of overall DLCO can also be obtained. The **intrabreath method** can also be used during exercise.

Membrane Diffusion Coefficient and Capillary Blood Volume

The patient performs two DLCOsb tests, each at a different level of alveolar P_{O_2}. The first DLCOsb test is performed as described previously. The patient then breathes an elevated concentration of O_2 (balance N_2) for approximately 5 minutes, exhales to RV, and performs the second DLCOsb maneuver. DLCO values are calculated for both the air- and oxygen-breathing maneuvers. The total resistance caused by the alveolocapillary membrane (Dm) and the resistance caused by the rate of chemical combination with Hb and transfer into the red blood cell (θV_C) are calculated as follows:

$$\frac{1}{D_{LCO}} = \frac{1}{Dm} + \frac{1}{\theta V_C}$$

where:

$1/D_{LCO}$ = reciprocal of diffusing capacity or resistance
$1/Dm$ = alveolocapillary membrane resistance
$1/\theta V_C$ = resistance of red blood cell membrane and rate of reaction with Hb
θ = transfer rate of CO/milliliter of capillary blood
V_C = capillary blood volume

Because CO and O_2 compete for binding sites on Hb, measurement of diffusion of CO at different levels of alveolar P_{O_2} can be used to distinguish resistance caused by the alveolocapillary membrane from resistance caused by the red blood cell membrane and Hb reaction rate. V_C is presumed to remain the same for both tests, but θ varies in response to changes in P_{O_2}. Resistance caused by the alveolocapillary membrane ($1/Dm$) can be calculated by plotting θ at two points against $1/D_{LCO}$ and extrapolating back to zero (as if no O_2 were present).

The membrane component of resistance to gas transfer can also be estimated by measuring the rate of uptake of nitric oxide (NO). DLNO has been suggested as a direct measure of the conductance of the alveolocapillary membrane. Because NO combines with Hb approximately 1500 times faster than CO, the rate of NO uptake by the blood (θ_{NO}) is large, although not infinite as previously understood. Therefore DLNO reflects the **membrane resistance** to gas diffusion in the lungs. DLNO can be measured with either a single-breath or rebreathing technique. A small amount of NO is added to the diffusion mixture, and the uptake is measured using a chemiluminescence analyzer (see Chapter 11). The ATS-ERS technical standard for the DLNO will not be review in this chapter.

Significance and Pathophysiology

See Interpretive Strategies 3.1. The average DLCO value for resting adult patients by the single-breath method is approximately 25 mL CO/min/mm Hg (STPD), with significant variability. Women have slightly lower normal values, presumably because of smaller normal lung volumes. The expected DLCO value in a healthy patient varies directly with the patient's lung volume. In some instances, it may be appropriate to adjust the predicted DLCO to account for decreased lung volume (see the section Techniques in this chapter). DLCO values can increase two to three times in healthy individuals during exercise in response to increased pulmonary capillary blood flow.

Most reference equations use age, height, sex, and race to predict DLCO. Some reference equations use body surface area (BSA) to calculate expected values. If the patient's weight is used (i.e., to calculate BSA), the ideal body weight is recommended. Using the actual body weight in obese patients can result in erroneously large predicted values unless similar subjects are included in the reference population. Significant differences exist among reference equations. These discrepancies result, in part, from different methods used to measure DLCO in various laboratories. Laboratories should check the appropriateness of their reference equations by comparing the results obtained from healthy subjects. They should measure DLCO in a sample of healthy patients of each sex and compare the results using several reference equations. If the reference equations used are appropriate, the differences between the measured and expected values (i.e., residuals) for the healthy patients should be minimal. Predicted values for DLCO and for DL/VA should be taken from the same reference set. Regression equations for the calculation of expected DLCO values are included in Chapter 13.

INTERPRETIVE STRATEGIES 3.1

DLCO

1. Were the test maneuvers performed acceptably? Were the tests repeatable within 2 mL/min/mm Hg of each?
2. Were all appropriate corrections made to the predicted values? Hb? COHb? Altitude? VA?
3. Are the reference values appropriate? Age? Height? Sex? (ATS-ERS guidelines recommend Global Lung Initiative [GLI] standards.)
4. Is DLCO less than the lower limit of normal (LLN) after appropriate corrections? If so, a gas exchange abnormality likely exists.
5. Is the KCO within normal limits? If so, the reduced diffusing capacity is likely related to parenchymal changes, pulmonary vascular disease, or pulmonary hypertension. Consider clinical correlation (e.g., patient's history, presentation, symptoms).
6. Is the KCO reduced? If so, reduced diffusing capacity is likely related to airway obstruction (uneven distribution of ventilation, V̇/Q̇ mismatch) or increased dead space. Compare VA and TLC; a large difference suggests an uneven distribution of ventilation. Look for a clinical correlation.
7. Is the DLCO increased after correction for Hb or altitude? If so, consider possible causes of increased pulmonary blood volume, hemorrhage, obesity, or left-to-right shunts. Also consider undiagnosed asthma. Look for clinical correlation.
8. Is DLCO less than 60% of predicted? If so, consider additional tests (blood gases, exercise desaturation study).

DLCO is often decreased in restrictive lung diseases, particularly those associated with pulmonary fibrosis. Fibrotic changes in the lung parenchyma are associated with asbestosis, berylliosis, and silicosis. Many other diseases caused by inhalation of dusts also result in fibrotic changes in lung tissue. Idiopathic pulmonary fibrosis, sarcoidosis, systemic lupus erythematosus, and scleroderma

are also commonly associated with a reduction in DLCO. Inhalation of toxic gases or organic agents may cause inflammation of the alveoli (**alveolitis**) and decrease DLCO. These disease states are sometimes categorized as diffusion defects. The decrease in DLCO is probably more closely related to the loss of lung volume, alveolar surface area, or capillary bed than to the thickening of the alveolocapillary membranes. DLCO also decreases when there is loss of lung tissue or replacement of normal parenchyma by space-occupying lesions such as tumors.

DLCO may also be reduced in the presence of pulmonary edema. Disruption of alveolar ventilation, reduction of lung volume, and congestion of the alveoli cause the reduction in DLCO in edema. In the early stages of congestive heart failure (CHF), DLCO may be normal or slightly increased. As the left ventricle decompensates, pulmonary vessels become engorged. The increased blood volume can cause DLCO to increase until the congestion becomes advanced. In most patients with heart failure, DLCO is decreased because of the restrictive ventilatory pattern. DLCO in patients who receive a heart transplant for CHF does not return to normal, as might be expected.

DLCO may also be decreased as a result of medical or surgical intervention for cardiopulmonary disease. Lung resection for cancer or other reasons typically results in decreased DLCO. The extent of reduction is usually directly proportional to the volume of lung removed. An exception to this pattern occurs in lung volume reduction surgery (LVRS) and in bullectomy. These surgical procedures typically resect areas of the lung that have little or no blood flow. Lack of perfusion is documented by a lung scan. Excision of tissue in such areas reduces lung volume without necessarily reducing the surface area available for diffusion. Improved ventilation-perfusion matching in the remaining lung often results in an improvement in DLCO.

Radiation therapy that involves the lungs usually causes a decrease in DLCO. Radiation causes pneumonitis that commonly results in fibrotic changes. Drugs used in chemotherapy (e.g., bleomycin) and those used to suppress rejection in organ transplantation may cause reductions in DLCO. These drugs appear to directly affect the alveolocapillary membranes. Some drugs used in the treatment of cardiac arrhythmias (e.g., amiodarone) have been shown to decrease DLCO. For this reason, DLCO is commonly used to monitor drug toxicity.

DLCO may also be helpful in evaluating disorders, such as hepatopulmonary syndrome, in which gas exchange and pulmonary vascular defects co-exist. Diseases that affect the pulmonary vascular bed also typically result in decreased DLCO. These include pulmonary vasculitis and pulmonary hypertension. Pulmonary vascular disease often manifests itself as a reduced diffusing capacity with otherwise-normal pulmonary function.

DLCO may be decreased in both acute and chronic obstructive lung disease. DLCO is decreased in emphysema for several reasons. Emphysematous lungs have a reduced surface area for gas exchange, with the loss of both alveolar walls and their associated capillary beds. As a result of the decreased surface area, less gas can be transferred per minute even if the remaining gas exchange units are structurally normal. In addition to a loss of surface area for gas exchange, the distance from the terminal bronchiole to the alveolocapillary membrane increases in emphysema. As alveoli break down, terminal lung units become larger. Gas must diffuse farther just to reach the alveolocapillary surface. There is also a mismatching of ventilation and pulmonary capillary blood flow in emphysema. Disruption of alveolar structures causes loss of support for terminal airways. Airway collapse and gas trapping result in ventilation-perfusion ($\dot{V}/\dot{Q}$) abnormalities (Fig. 3.6).

Other obstructive diseases (e.g., chronic bronchitis, asthma) may not reduce DLCO unless they result in markedly abnormal $\dot{V}/\dot{Q}$ patterns. DLCO is sometimes used to differentiate among these obstructive patterns. Low DLCO in the presence of

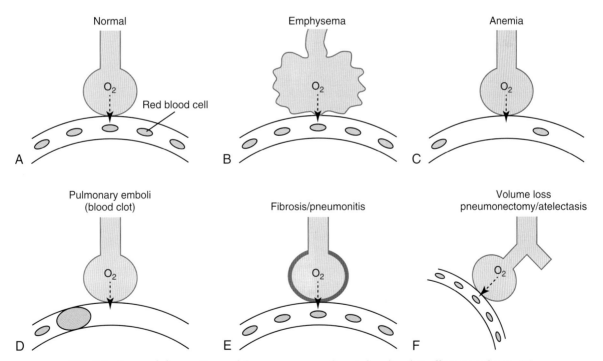

FIG. 3.6 DLCO and disease. Some of the more common disease disorders that affect gas exchange. (A) Depicts the normal alveolar capillary interface where gas exchange occurs. (B) Emphysema—destruction of the alveolar capillary interface and hyperinflation. (C) Anemia—reduction in oxygen-carrying capacity. (D) Pulmonary emboli and/or atrioventricular malformations affect oxygen transport. (E) Interstitial lung disease such as pulmonary fibrosis scars the alveolar membrane surface. (F) Alveolar volume loss from resection, alveolar collapse, or filling processes.

obstruction is sometimes assumed to be evidence of emphysema. However, $\dot{V}/\dot{Q}$ mismatching can cause D_{LCO} to appear to be decreased in asthma, chronic bronchitis, or emphysema. Some patients with asthma may have an increased D_{LCO}, but the cause is not completely understood.

D_{LCO} measurements at rest have been suggested to estimate the probability of **O2 desaturation** during exercise. A large retrospective study demonstrated that a D_{LCO} of less than 60% correlated with O_2 desaturation during exercise (75% sensitivity and specificity). Patients with restrictive lung disease and a low resting D_{LCO} are at risk of O_2 desaturation even with low levels of exercise. Low resting D_{LCO} may indicate the need for assessment of oxygenation during exercise.

D_{LCO} is directly related to lung volume (V_A) in healthy individuals. The D_L/V_A (also termed *KCO*) may be multiplied by the lung volume at which the measurement was obtained to express D_{LCO}. This calculation is simple because V_A must be measured to derive D_{LCO} (see Fig. 3.5). In healthy subjects, and even in those with mild to moderate restriction, V_A approximates the TLC minus the assumed dead space (V_D). Analysis of this relationship can be useful to differentiate whether decreased D_{LCO} is the result of loss of lung volume (as in restriction) or from some other cause. In healthy individuals, alveolar volume and D_{LCO} are proportional to body size (height). Two patients of different heights will have different D_{LCO} and V_A values, but their K_{CO} values will be similar. In healthy adults, K_{CO} is approximately 4 to 5 mL CO transferred/minute/liter of lung volume.

V_A is measured by the dilution of the tracer gas used (in the $D_{LCO}sb$) and reflects the same volume into which CO is distributed and diffuses across the pulmonary capillary membranes. Mismatching of ventilation and blood flow (as in obstructive disease) can cause a significant portion of the lung to not participate in gas exchange. This is usually characterized by a difference between the V_A measured during the D_{LCO} maneuver and the TLC measured by plethysmography or multiple-breath gas dilution. When the D_{LCO} is reduced but the K_{CO} is normal or near normal, the decrement in gas exchange can be assumed to be caused by an uneven distribution of ventilation rather than loss of lung volume.

In the presence of pulmonary disease, both D_{LCO} and V_A may be affected. D_{LCO} goes down as the lung empties but does so in a nonlinear fashion. In obstruction, low D_{LCO} without reduction in V_A results in a low ratio. In a purely restrictive process, a decrease in D_{LCO} reflects a loss of V_A, and the K_{CO} is preserved. For example, a patient who has a D_{LCO} of 12 mL CO/min/mm Hg (50% of predicted) and a V_A of 3.0 L would have a K_{CO} of 4. This reduction in D_{LCO} is roughly proportional to a loss of lung volume. Some pulmonary conditions (e.g., pneumonectomy) may result in an increased K_{CO}, where gas exchange is preserved and lung volume is decreased.

D_{LCO} and K_{CO} may also be affected if the patient performs the breath-hold maneuver at a lung volume of less than TLC. The predicted D_{LCO} may be corrected for the reduced V_A as described previously. There are important implications for the interpretation of diffusing capacity in the complex relationship between D_{LCO} and K_{CO}. Patients who fail to inspire fully during the maneuver will have a decreased D_{LCO}, but the K_{CO} may appear to increase. Correcting for V_A does not correct for poor inspiratory effort (< 85% of VC). In patients who have a low D_{LCO}, a "normal" K_{CO} should not be confused with normal gas exchange.

The $D_{LCO}sb$ is the most widely used method because it is relatively simple to perform, is noninvasive, and is more standardized than other methods. The rapidity with which repeated maneuvers can be performed also lends to its popularity. Most automated systems use the $D_{LCO}sb$, contributing a certain degree of standardization to the methodology. Large differences in reported D_{LCO} values exist among laboratories. This variability has been attributed to different testing techniques, problems in the gas analysis involved in the test, and differences in computations. Breath holding at TLC is not a physiologic maneuver. This and the fact that D_{LCO} varies with lung volume cause some concerns about $D_{LCO}sb$ as an accurate description of diffusing capacity. $D_{LCO}sb$ is not practical for use during exercise. Some patients have difficulty expiring fully, inspiring fully, or holding their breath. The

---

BOX 3.1   DLCOSB RECOMMENDATIONS

A. Equipment
   1. Volume accuracy same as for spirometry: $\pm 2.5\%$ over 8-L range, all gases and flow conditions (includes syringe accuracy of 0.5%); checked daily.
   2. Documented analyzer linearity from 0 to full span $\pm 0.5\%$ with minimal drift over test interval; checked quarterly.
   3. Circuit resistance less than $1.5\,cm\,H_2O$ at 6 L/sec.
   4. Demand valve sensitivity less than $10\,cm\,H_2O$ to generate 6-L/sec flow.
   5. Timing mechanism accurate to $\pm 1\%$ over 10 sec; checked quarterly.
   6. Instrument dead space (e.g., valves, filters) less than 0.200 L.
   7. Perform a 3-L syringe DLCO weekly in patient testing mode
   8. Perform a calibration syringe leak check monthly.
   9. Validate system weekly by testing healthy nonsmokers (biologic controls; see Chapter 12).
B. Patient preparation
   1. The patient should be instructed to refrain from smoking on the day of the test; time of last cigarette should be noted.
   2. Patient should be seated for DLCO maneuver.
   3. Patients on supplemental O_2 should be switched to breathing air for 10 minutes before testing, if clinically acceptable.
   4. The patient should be carefully instructed, and the procedure demonstrated.
C. Technique (see How To ... Box 3.1)
D. Calculations
   1. Average at least two acceptable tests; duplicate determinations should be within 2 mL/min/mm Hg.
   2. Use Jones and Meade method of timing the breath hold.
   3. Alveolar volume should be determined by single-breath dilution of tracer gas.
   4. Adjust for V_D volumes (instrument and patient).
   5. Determine inspired gas conditions (ATPS or ATPD).
   6. Correct for CO_2 and H_2O absorption.
   7. Report KCO in mLCO (STPD)/min/mm Hg per L (BTPS).
   8. Correct predicted value for Hb, COHb, and altitude (PIO_2).
   9. Consider adjusting predicted value for submaximal inspiration.
   10. Use reference equations appropriate to the laboratory method and patient population (ATS-ERS guidelines recommend GLI as the preferred reference set).

ATPD, ambient temperature, pressure, dry; *ATPS*, ambient temperature, pressure, and saturated with water vapor; *ATS-ERS*, American Thoracic Society–European Respiratory Society; *BTPS*, body temperature, pressure, and saturation; *GLI*, Global Lung Initiative; *STPD*, standard temperature, pressure, dry. Adapted from 2017 ATS-ERS standards for single-breath carbon monoxide uptake in the lung.

ATS-ERS guidelines aim to improve the standardization of the single-breath maneuver (Box 3.1).

The rebreathing method (DLCOrb) requires somewhat complicated calculations but offers the advantages of a normal breathing pattern without arterial puncture. DLCOrb is less sensitive to $\dot{V}/\dot{Q}$ abnormalities and uneven ventilation distribution than the DLCOsb. The rebreathing method is sensitive to the accumulation of COHb in the capillary blood and the resultant back-pressure. Capillary PCO is routinely assumed to be zero. The actual alveolocapillary CO gradient at the time of testing can be estimated, although with some difficulty. The rebreathing method can be used during exercise, provided the rebreathing interval is carefully controlled. An additional advantage is that acetylene can be added to the diffusion mixture to measure cardiac output simultaneously. Adding a small amount of nitric oxide (NO) to the diffusion mixture allows the DLNO to be measured during rebreathing as well.

Measurement of DLCO by the intrabreath method (DLCOib) offers the advantage of not requiring a breath hold at TLC. However, the patient must inspire a large enough volume of test gas so that the subsequent exhalation will clear the instrument and anatomic V_D. In addition, the single-breath exhalation must be slow and even. In some systems, a flow restrictor may be necessary to limit expiratory flow. The single-breath slow-exhalation method produces values similar to those obtained by the breath-hold method in healthy patients when flow is maintained at 0.5 L/sec. Uneven distribution of ventilation may produce intrabreath D_{LCO} values that are artificially elevated. Because the evenness of ventilation distribution can be assessed from the washout of CH_4, unacceptable D_{LCO} values can be detected. Table 3.1 compares some advantages and disadvantages of D_{LCO} testing methods.

Measurement of membrane (Dm) and red blood cell components (θV_c) of diffusion resistance in healthy patients reveals that each factor accounts for approximately half of the total resistance to gas exchange across the alveolocapillary membranes. Difficulty in quantifying the partial pressure of O_2 in the lungs (pulmonary capillaries) restricts the use of the membrane-diffusing capacity determination. Because the uptake of NO is limited almost entirely by the pulmonary capillary membranes, D_{LNO} can be measured to assess membrane resistance.

Numerous other physiologic factors can influence the observed D_{LCO}:

1. *Hemoglobin and hematocrit (Hct).* Decreased Hb or Hct reduces D_{LCO}, whereas increased Hb and Hct elevate D_{LCO}. D_{LCO} may be corrected if the patient's Hb is known. CO uptake varies approximately 7% for each gram of Hb. The predicted D_{LCO} may be corrected so that the value reported is compared with a standardized Hb level of 14.6 g% for men and 13.4 g% for women and children younger than 15 years. When this correction is applied, the predicted D_{LCO} will be reduced (and the percentage of predicted increased) if the patient's Hb is less than the standard value (14.6 g% or 13.4 g%, respectively). Conversely, the predicted D_{LCO} increases (and the percentage of predicted decreases) if the Hb is greater than the standard value. Both corrected and uncorrected D_{LCO} predicted values should be reported, along with the Hb value used for adjustment. Care should be taken to use Hb values representative of the patient's actual Hb level at the time of the D_{LCO} test.

2. *COHb.* Increased COHb levels, often found in smokers, reduce D_{LCO}. Smokers may have COHb levels of 10% or greater, causing significant CO back-pressure. The diffusion gradient for CO across alveolocapillary membranes is assumed to equal the alveolar pressure of CO. In healthy nonsmoking patients, little CO (usually <2% COHb) is present in pulmonary capillary blood. When there is carboxyhemoglobinemia, diffusion of CO is reduced because the gradient across the membrane is reduced. COHb also shifts the oxyhemoglobin dissociation curve, further altering gas transfer. Each 1% increase in COHb causes an approximate 1% decrease in the measured D_{LCO}. CO back-pressure corrections can also be made by estimating the partial pressure of CO in the pulmonary capillaries. This pressure can be used to correct the F_{ACO_0} and the F_{ACO_T}. More commonly, however, the predicted D_{LCO} is corrected for the presence of COHb in excess of 2% (see the section Techniques in this chapter).

3. *Alveolar P_{CO_2}.* Increased P_{CO_2} elevates D_{LCO} because the alveolar P_{O_2} is necessarily decreased. Significant increases in alveolar P_{CO_2} (i.e., moderate to severe hypoventilation) reduce the alveolar P_{O_2}.

4. *Pulmonary capillary blood volume.* Increased blood volume in the lungs (V_C) causes increased D_{LCO}. Increases in pulmonary capillary blood volume may result from increased cardiac output as occurs during exercise. Patients should be seated and resting for several minutes before D_{LCO} testing is performed. Pulmonary hemorrhage and left-to-right shunts may also cause an increase in blood volume in the lungs. In each of these cases, the increase in D_{LCO} is related to the increased volume of Hb available for gas transfer. Excessive negative intrathoracic pressure during breath holding can increase pulmonary capillary volume and elevate the D_{LCO}. Conversely, excessive positive intrathoracic pressure (Valsalva maneuver) can reduce pulmonary blood flow and decrease D_{LCO}.

5. *Body position.* The supine position increases D_{LCO}. Changes in body position affect the distribution of capillary blood flow.

6. *Altitude above sea level.* D_{LCO} varies inversely with changes in alveolar oxygen pressure (P_{AO_2}). At altitudes significantly greater than sea level, D_{LCO} increases unless corrections are made (see the section Techniques in this chapter).

7. *Asthma and obesity.* Asthma and obesity have been associated with an elevated D_{LCO} in some studies. Increased pulmonary capillary blood volume may explain these observations, but the exact physiology is unclear.

Several additional technical considerations may affect the measurement of D_{LCO} (particularly $D_{LCO}sb$). V_A is calculated from the dilution of a tracer gas during the single-breath maneuver. This technique typically underestimates lung volume in patients who have moderate or severe obstruction. A low estimated V_A results in low D_{LCO} values. Some clinicians prefer to use a separately determined lung volume to estimate V_A. RV, measured independently by plethysmography or one of the gas-dilution techniques, can be added to the inspired volume (V_I) to derive V_A. The V_A calculated by this method is usually larger in patients with airway obstruction than the V_A calculated from the single-breath dilution method. The resulting estimate of D_{LCO} is larger. The D_{LCO} calculation, however, is based on the volume of gas into which both the inspired CO and tracer gas are distributed but not the lung volume, in which gas mixing is minimal. Some laboratories report D_{LCO} values calculated by both methods. The ATS-ERS guidelines recommend the calculation of V_A using the single-breath tracer gas method. Comparison of the single-breath V_A measured during the D_{LCO} maneuver with lung volumes (i.e., TLC) measured by the standard methods is often helpful in elucidating the cause for a low D_{LCO}.

A simple method of evaluating the quality of the test is to compare the TLC–V_A relationship; the V_A should never be larger than the measured TLC, regardless of the TLC testing methodology.

RGAs allow for the calculation of anatomic dead space using the Fowler technique. This measured dead space (V_D) can then be used in the calculation of V_A versus using an estimated V_D.

The method of timing of breath hold also influences the calculation of D_{LCO} (see Fig. 3.3). Most systems measure BHT by one of three methods:

1. *Jones and Meade method:* Includes 0.7 of the inspiratory time to the midpoint of the alveolar sample.

2. *Epidemiology Standardization Project (ESP) method:* From the midpoint of inspiration (half of the V_I) to the beginning of alveolar sampling.

3. *Ogilvie method:* From the beginning of inspiration (V_I) to the beginning of alveolar sampling.

Theoretically, BHT is considered the time during which diffusion occurs. That is, the D_{LCO} equation assumes that the entire breath hold is at TLC. However, because some gas transfer takes place during inspiration and expiration, D_{LCO} will be influenced by the proportion of time spent in these two phases. A **three-equation method** has been proposed that uses separate equations for the three phases of the maneuver (i.e., inspiration, breath hold, expiration). This method has not been widely used, however. The timing method might become significant if the reference values used for comparison were generated by one of the other methods. The Jones and Meade method is the method recommended by the ATS-ERS guidelines (see Box 3.1). Rapid inspiration from RV to TLC and rapid expiration to the alveolar sampling phase reduce differences resulting from the timing methods (see Box 3.1). Conversely, patients who display prolonged inspiratory or expiratory times may have reduced D_{LCO} values.

The volume of gas discarded before collecting the alveolar sample may affect the measured D_{LCO}. Most classic discrete sampling systems allow the washout volume to be adjusted, with 0.75 to 1.0 L most used. Washout volume may need to be reduced to 0.5 L if the patient's VC is less than 2.0 L. In patients who have obstructive disease, reducing the washout volume may result in increased dead-space gas being added to the alveolar sample. Because dead-space gas resembles the diffusion mixture, D_{LCO} may be underestimated.

The alveolar sampling technique also affects D_{LCO} measurement. Alveolar samples should be collected within 4 seconds, including washout and alveolar sampling. A sample volume of 0.5 to 1.0 L is recommended. Patients with a small VC (i.e., <2.0 L) may require a smaller volume, just as with the washout. When only a small sample is obtained, the gas may not accurately reflect alveolar concentrations of CO and tracer gas, particularly in the presence of $\dot{V}/\dot{Q}$ abnormalities. Continuous analysis of the expired air using RGA technology allows identification of alveolar gas. Infrared analyzers that can simultaneously analyze the tracer gas and CO will allow the entire breath to be analyzed. These instruments permit adjustment of the alveolar sampling window so that a representative gas sample can be obtained (see Fig. 3.4).

SUMMARY

· The chapter addresses the measurement of diffusing capacity (D_{LCO}), also referred to as *transfer factor* (T_{LCO}). D_{LCO} can be measured by various techniques, including the single-breath, rebreathing, and intrabreath methods.
· The single-breath method, or D_{LCO}sb, is most used. D_{LCO}sb is noninvasive and can be repeated easily to obtain multiple measurements. Many automated D_{LCO}sb systems are common.

· The ATS-ERS and others have published standardization guidelines for D_{LCO}sb. Careful attention to these standards can reduce the variability in D_{LCO}sb measurements in different laboratories.
· D_{LCO} measurements are used diagnostically for a variety of diseases. Because D_{LCO} assesses gas exchange, it is useful in both obstructive and restrictive disease patterns.
· D_{LCO} measurements may be affected by a variety of factors, such as Hb level, COHb, or altitude. Techniques for correcting D_{LCO} for these factors include adjusting the predicted values used for interpretation.

CASE STUDIES

CASE 3.1

HISTORY

A 55-year-old woman is referred to the pulmonary function laboratory because of shortness of breath on exertion. She has a 38-pack-year smoking history but stopped smoking 6 months ago. She still coughs each morning, but her sputum volume has decreased since she stopped smoking. She has no significant environmental or family history of pulmonary disease. She had been using an inhaled β_2 agonist but withheld it for 12 hours before the test.

PULMONARY FUNCTION TESTING
Personal Data

Age:	55
Height:	65 in. (165 cm)
Weight:	137 lb (62.3 kg)
Race:	African American

Spirometry							
			Prebronchodilator			Postbronchodilator	
	Predicted	LLN	Actual	% Predicted	Actual	% Predicted	% Change
FVC (L)	2.89	2.16	2.77	96	2.82	98	2
FEV$_1$ (L)	2.30	1.67	1.91	83	2.01	87	5
FEV$_{1\%}$ (%)	80	70	69		71		
FEF$_{25\%-75\%}$ (L/sec)	2.33	0.92	1.44	62	1.51	65	5
PEF (L/min)	6.08	4.01	4.01	66	5.13	84	28

FEF, Forced expiratory volume; *FEV$_1$,* forced expiratory volume in the first second; *PEF,* peak expiratory flow.

Lung Volumes

	Predicted	LLN	Actual	% Predicted
TLC (L)	4.39	3.42	4.97	113
FRC (L)	2.45		3.10	127
RV (L)	1.58		2.20	139
VC (L)	2.89	2.16	2.77	96
IC (L)	1.94		1.87	96
ERV (L)	0.87		0.90	103
RV/TLC (%)	36		44	

ERV, Expiratory reserve volume; *FRC,* fractional reserve capacity.

Diffusing Capacity

	Predicted	Actual	% Predicted
DLcosb (mL CO/ min/mm Hg)	19.7	10.0	51
DLcosb corr (mL CO/min/ mm Hg)	18.1	10.0	55
V_A (L)	4.39	3.99	91
Kco	4.49	2.51	46
Hb (g/dL)		11.0	

Technologist's Comments

Spirometry maneuvers met ATS-ERS criteria. Lung volumes by body plethysmography were performed acceptably and met ATS-ERS criteria. All DLco maneuvers met ATS-ERS criteria (two tests were averaged). DLco was corrected for an Hb of 11 g/dL.

QUESTIONS

1. What is the interpretation of the following?
   a. Prebronchodilator and postbronchodilator spirometry
   b. Lung volumes
   c. DLco
2. How are the pulmonary function test results related to the subject's symptoms?
3. What other tests might be indicated?
4. What treatment might be recommended based on these findings?

DISCUSSION

Interpretation

All maneuvers were performed acceptably. FVC and FEV_1 are within normal limits, but the $FEV_{1\%}$ is below the LLN, consistent with airway obstruction. After inhaled bronchodilator, there is only a minimal change in FEV_1 and FVC. Lung volumes reveal a slightly increased functional residual capacity and moderately increased RV. The RV/TLC ratio is increased, consistent with air trapping. DLco is markedly decreased even after correction for Hb. Kco is decreased, consistent with an obstructive process.

Impression: Mild obstruction with minimal response to bronchodilator; this should not preclude a therapeutic trial if clinically indicated. Lung volumes suggest air trapping. DLco is severely decreased, even when corrected for Hb.

Cause of Symptoms

This subject has symptoms characteristic of airway obstruction that has progressed to the point where dyspnea on exertion prompted a visit to the physician. Her obstruction appears mild. Her FEV_1 is still above the LLN for her age and height. Her response to bronchodilator therapy seems to indicate obstruction caused by inflammation rather than reversible bronchospasm. Lung volume testing confirms that the obstruction appears to have caused some air trapping. This pattern is not unusual for subjects with chronic bronchitis and emphysema.

Her gas exchange, as measured by DLco, is markedly impaired. Emphysema reduces DLco by reducing the alveolocapillary surface area available for diffusion. Chronic bronchitis can reduce DLco by causing a ventilation-perfusion mismatch. The subject may have both disease processes disrupting gas transfer. Her V_A measured by the single-breath inhalation of tracer gas during the DLco maneuver is about a liter less than her TLC measured in the body plethysmograph. This discrepancy suggests poor distribution of inspired gas and is typical in subjects with some degree of airway obstruction.

Subjects who have reduced DLco values seldom have normal blood gases. Exertion or exercise often aggravates the gas exchange impairment. Many subjects with markedly reduced DLco (<50%–60% of predicted) display exercise desaturation. That is, their Pao_2 falls to levels of 55 mm Hg or less with exercise. The decrease in DLco does not, however, accurately predict the degree of desaturation that will occur.

Other Tests

An obvious additional test for this subject would be measuring resting arterial blood gases while she breathes room air. Resting hypoxemia would explain dyspnea on exertion. The subject returned to have a blood gas sample drawn. Her Pa_{O_2} while breathing air was 63 mm Hg, with a saturation of 91%. Because this value did not qualify her for supplemental O_2, an exercise test was performed with an arterial catheter in place (see Chapter 7). At a low workload on the treadmill, her Pa_{O_2} decreased to 51 mm Hg. She was then retested while breathing O_2 via nasal cannula at 1 L/min. She then tolerated more exercise, and her Pa_{O_2} never decreased below 68 mm Hg.

Treatment
Based on the results of the exercise evaluation, supplemental O_2 was prescribed for the subject to use during exertion. Because she showed little response to bronchodilators, her inhaled β_2 agonist was discontinued. However, a trial of inhaled steroids (beclomethasone) resulted in a noticeable improvement of symptoms.

CASE 3.2

HISTORY
The subject is a 63-year-old woman with a history of cardiomyopathy, hypertension, and pernicious anemia. She has had episodes of ventricular tachycardia that have been managed by means of an implantable cardiac defibrillator (ICD). She has never smoked and denies cough or sputum production. She experiences shortness of breath with exertion. Her family history includes a sister who had asthma and chronic bronchitis. She has no history of environmental toxin exposure. To manage her arrhythmias, her physician

prescribed amiodarone. To monitor the effects of this medication, she was referred for tests before starting the drug and again after 3 months of therapy.

PULMONARY FUNCTION TESTING
Personal Data

Sex:	Female
Age:	63
Height:	62 in. (157 cm)
Weight:	131 lb (59.5 kg)
Race:	Caucasian

Spirometry

		Pretreatment			3 Months	
	Predicted	LLN	Actual	% Predicted	Actual	% Predicted
FVC (L)	2.96	2.31	2.50	84	1.97	67
FEV$_1$ (L)	2.27	1.72	2.09	92	1.81	80
FEV$_{1\%}$ (%)	77	68	84		92	
FEF$_{25\%-75\%}$ (L/sec)	2.09	0.94	2.82	135	2.77	133

FEF, forced expiratory flow.

Lung Volumes (He Dilution)

		Pretreatment			3 Months	
	Predicted	LLN	Actual	% Predicted	Actual	% Predicted
TLC (L)	4.88	3.66	3.92	87	3.50	78
FRC (L)	2.54		2.26	89	2.23	88
RV (L)	1.71		1.50	87	1.52	89
VC (L)	2.96	2.31	2.42	82	1.97	67
IC (L)	1.94		1.66	85	1.26	65
ERV (L)	0.83		0.76	91	0.71	85
RV/TLC (%)	38		38		44	

Diffusing Capacity (D$_{LCO}$sb)

	Pretreatment			3 Months	
	Predicted	Actual	% Predicted	Actual	% Predicted
D$_{LCO}$ (mL/min/mm Hg)	18.0	12.6	69	9.7	54
D$_{LCO}$sb corr (mL/min/mm Hg)	16.7	12.6	75	9.7	58
V$_A$ (L)	4.48	3.26	72	3.31	95
K$_{CO}$	4.0	3.9		2.9	
Hb (g/dL)	13.4	11.3		11.4	

Technologist's Comments

Pretreatment: Spirometry and lung volumes by He dilution met ATS-ERS criteria. The inspiratory volume during the D$_{LCO}$ maneuver was less than 85% of the VC.

3 Months: Spirometry, lung volumes, and D$_{LCO}$ all met ATS-ERS criteria.

QUESTIONS

1. What is the interpretation of the following?
   a. Pretreatment spirometry, lung volumes
   b. D$_{LCO}$ before treatment
   c. D$_{LCO}$ after 3 months of treatment
2. What is the cause of change in the subject's D$_{LCO}$?
3. What technical problems might have affected the interpretation of the D$_{LCO}$ before treatment?

DISCUSSION

Interpretation

Pretreatment, FVC is normal, as are FEV$_1$ and FEV$_{1\%}$. Lung volumes by He dilution are normal. The diffusing capacity was substandard in performance because the subject could not inspire fully. The best efforts show mildly reduced D$_{LCO}$ at the LLN after correction for the subject's Hb of 11.3.

After 3 months, FVC is decreased, but FEV$_1$ is normal. This makes the FEV$_{1\%}$ appear greater than expected. Lung volumes by He dilution show a TLC that is mildly decreased but with a normal FRC and RV. D$_{LCO}$ is moderately decreased even when corrected for an Hb of 11.4 g%. Since the previous test, the subject's VC has decreased slightly, and the D$_{LCO}$ has decreased significantly.

Cause of Changes in Diffusing Capacity

This case presents a good example of one application of D$_{LCO}$: monitoring drug therapy. The subject had essentially normal lung function. Initially, her D$_{LCO}$ was slightly reduced. However, because she had a history of anemia, her Hb level was checked. The Hb-adjusted D$_{LCO}$ was at the LLN (approximately 75% for the reference equation used). Because amiodarone has been shown to cause changes to the lung parenchyma, her cardiologist requested pulmonary function studies, including D$_{LCO}$.

On her return visit after 3 months of antiarrhythmic therapy, some significant changes had occurred. As described in the interpretation of the 3-month follow-up, her FVC had decreased slightly. TLC also decreased by a similar volume (400–500 mL). Her other lung volumes (FRC, RV) remained largely unchanged. These changes suggest that something happened that primarily affected her VC.

The subject's D$_{LCO}$ showed the greatest decrease during the 3-month period. Her D$_{LCO}$ decreased by approximately 30%. The Hb-corrected percentage of predicted fell from 75% to 58%. The K$_{CO}$ also decreased slightly. The K$_{CO}$ is often preserved when D$_{LCO}$ decreases simply because of loss of lung volume. When the K$_{CO}$ decreases in conjunction with a low D$_{LCO}$, factors other than loss of lung volume are assumed to be responsible for the change. In this subject, it appears that drug therapy did affect D$_{LCO}$. However, a pattern of pneumonitis and fibrosis causing reduced lung volumes is not clear. Because of the changes in D$_{LCO}$, amiodarone therapy was discontinued.

Technical Factors Influencing D$_{LCO}$

A second factor is that the subject's pretreatment D$_{LCO}$ tests did not meet established criteria for acceptability. She was unable to inspire at least 85% of her VC in any of the maneuvers. This information is documented in the technologist's comments for the test. When the subject fails to inspire maximally, the breath hold may not occur at TLC. Therefore D$_{LCO}$ may appear low compared with predicted values. This technical difficulty may have influenced the pretreatment test results. The subject's measured V_A (3.26 L) was significantly less than the TLC assessed by He dilution (3.92 L). In this instance, it may be appropriate to correct the predicted DLCO for the effect of the reduced lung volume using the equation described previously:

$$DLCO\left(at\ V_{Am}\right)=DLCO\left(at\ V_{Ap}\right)\times\left(0.58+0.42\left(\frac{V_{Am}}{V_{Ap}}\right)\right)$$

Substituting the subject's measured alveolar volume (V_{Am}) and the predicted alveolar volume (V_{Ap}) along with the Hb-corrected predicted DLCO (16.7 mL/min/mm Hg, in this case) for the right-hand terms in the equation gives the following:

$$DLCO\left(at\ V_{Am}\right)=14.8\,mL\,/\,min\,/\,mm\,Hg$$
$$\left(predicted\,at\,the\,measured\,V_A\right)$$

$$DLCO\left(at\ V_{Am}\right)=16.7\times\left(0.58+0.42\left(\frac{3.26}{4.48}\right)\right)$$

When the subject's measured DLCO of 12.6 mL/min/mm Hg is compared with 14.8 mL/min/mm Hg as the expected value, the percent predicted becomes 85%. Correcting for Hb and the effect of a substandard inspired volume suggests that the subject's diffusing capacity was well within normal limits before beginning the antiarrhythmic therapy.

SELF-ASSESSMENT QUESTIONS

Entry-Level

1. Correct performance of the DLCOsb requires that the subject inspire at least
   a. 90% of the VC.
   b. 85% of the TLC.
   c. 80% of the IC.
   d. 2 to 3 times the V_T.

2. In which DLCO method does the patient perform slow exhalation of the VC after inspiring?
   a. DLCOrb (rebreathing)
   b. DLNO (nitric oxide)
   c. DLCOsb (single breath)
   d. DLCOib (intrabreath)

3. A patient with a VC of 2.0 L performs several DLCOsb maneuvers, with the following results:

Trial	DLCO	KCO	V_I
1	8.0	4.0	1.8
2	7.4	3.8	1.4
3	7.3	3.6	1.4
4	6.9	4.0	1.0

The pulmonary function technologist should
   a. average the first two trials and report the result.
   b. report the DLCO as 8.0.
   c. average all trials and report the result.
   d. perform one more trial.

4. In which of the following conditions would an increased DLCO be expected?
   1. Pulmonary hemorrhage
   2. Sarcoidosis
   3. Pneumonectomy
   4. Polycythemia
   a. 1 and 3
   b. 1 and 4
   c. 2 and 3
   d. 2 and 4

5. DLCO is often reduced in emphysema because of which of the following?
   1. Fibrotic granulomas
   2. Destruction of alveolar walls
   3. Anemia
   4. Increased distance from the terminal bronchiole to alveolocapillary membrane
   a. 1 and 2
   b. 1 and 3
   c. 2 and 4
   d. 3 and 4

Advanced

6. A 52-year-old female patient has a DLCO of 15.0 mL/min/mm Hg with a predicted value of 20.0. If her Hb is 9.5 g/dL, what is her corrected percentage of predicted diffusing capacity?
   a. 64%
   b. 75%
   c. 88%
   d. 91%

7. A 25-year-old male has an uncorrected D_{LCO} of 24.9 mL/min/mm Hg (69% of predicted) but no history of pulmonary disease. Which of the following might explain these findings?
   1. Left-to-right shunt
   2. Carboxyhemoglobin
   3. Congestive heart failure
   4. Anemia
      a. 1 and 2 only
      b. 3 and 4 only
      c. 1, 2, and 3
      d. 2, 3, and 4

8. An adult patient whose TLC is 6.5 L (by plethysmography) performs two acceptable $D_{LCO}sb$ maneuvers and records the following results:
   $D_{LCO}sb$ 9.1 mL/min/mm Hg
   V_A 4.5 L
   Which of the following interpretive statements is most consistent with these values?
   a. Normal diffusing capacity corrected for lung volume
   b. Reduced D_{LCO} consistent with airway obstruction
   c. Reduced D_{LCO} consistent with a restrictive defect
   d. Reduced D_{LCO} consistent with obesity

9. A healthy adult male has his D_{LCO} measured at two different levels of inspired oxygen to estimate his membrane-diffusing capacity. Which of the following results would be expected in this subject?
   a. $1/Dm$ and $1/\theta V_c$ approximately equal
   b. $1/Dm$ approximately 2 times larger than $1/\theta V_c$
   c. $1/\theta V_c$ approximately 2 times larger than $1/Dm$
   d. $1/Dm$ 5 to 10 times larger than $1/\theta V_c$

10. A patient has a $D_{LCO}sb$ of 10.6 mL/min/mm Hg (STPD), which is 50% of his predicted value. His K_{CO} is 1.6. Which of the following is most consistent with these values?
    a. Pulmonary hemorrhage
    b. Pneumonectomy
    c. Pulmonary emphysema
    d. Obesity

SELECTED BIBLIOGRAPHY

General References

Crapo, R. O., Jensen, R. L., & Wanger, J. S. (2001). Single-breath carbon monoxide diffusing capacity. *Clinics in Chest Medicine, 22,* 637–649.

Hadeli, K. O., Siegel, E. M., Sherrill, D. L., et al. (2001). Predictors of oxygen desaturation during submaximal exercise in 8,000 patients. *Chest, 120,* 88–92.

Hsia, C. W. (2006). Recruitment of lung diffusing capacity. *Chest, 1222,* 1774–1783.

Jensen, R. L., & Crapo, R. O. (2003). Diffusing capacity: How to get it right. *Respiratory Care, 48,* 777–782.

Johnson, D. C. (2000). Importance of adjusting carbon monoxide diffusing capacity (D_{LCO}) and carbon monoxide transfer coefficient (KCO) for alveolar lung volume. *Respiratory Medicine, 94,* 28–37.

Plummer, A. L. (2008). The carbon monoxide diffusing capacity clinical implications, coding, and documentation. *Chest, 134,* 663–667.

Saydain, G., Beck, K. C., Decker, P. A., et al. (2004). Clinical significance of elevated diffusing capacity. *Chest, 125,* 446–452.

Stam, H., Splinter, T. A. W., & Versprille, A. (2000). Evaluation of diffusing capacity in patients with a restrictive lung disease. *Chest, 117,* 752–757.

$D_{LCO}sb$

Drummond, M. B., Schwartz, P. F., Duggan, W. T., et al. (2008). Intersession variability in single-breath diffusing capacity in diabetics without overt lung disease. *American Journal of Respiratory and Critical Care Medicine, 178,* 225–232.

Hughes, J. M. B., & Pride, N. B. (2012). Examination of the Carbon Monoxide Diffusing Capacity (DLCO) in Relation to Its KCO and VA Components. *American Journal of Respiratory and Critical Care Medicine Vol, 186,* 132–139.

Jones, R. S., & Meade, F. (1961). A theoretical and experimental analysis of anomalies in the estimation of pulmonary diffusing capacity by the single breath method. *Quarterly Journal of Experimental Physiology and Cognate Medical Sciences, 46,* 131–143.

Mohsenifar, Z., & Tashkin, D. P. (1979). Effect of carboxyhemoglobin on the single breath diffusing capacity: Derivation of an empirical correction factor. *Respiration, 37*, 185–188.

Punjabi, N. M., Shade, D., Patel, A. M., et al. (2003). Measurement variability in single breath diffusing capacity of the lung. *Chest, 123*, 1082–1089.

Wise, R. A., Teeter, J. G., Jensen, R. L., et al. (2007). Standardization of the single-breath diffusing capacity in a multicenter clinical trial. *Chest, 132*, 1191–1197.

DLcorb

Barazanji, K. W., Ramanathan, M., Johnson, R. L., Jr., et al. (1996). A modified rebreathing technique using an infrared gas analyzer. *Journal of Applied Physiology, 80*, 1258–1262.

Hsia, C. C. W., McBrayer, D. G., & Ramanathan, M. (1995). Reference values of pulmonary diffusing capacity during exercise by a rebreathing technique. *American Journal of Respiratory and Critical Care Medicine, 152*, 658–665.

DLcoib

Huang, Y. C., & MacIntyre, N. R. (1992). Real-time gas analysis improves the measurement of single-breath diffusing capacity. *American Review of Respiratory Disease, 146*, 946–950.

Huang, Y. C., O'Brien, S. R., & MacIntyre, N. R. (2002). Intrabreath diffusing capacity of the lung in healthy individuals at rest and during exercise. *Chest, 122*, 177–185.

Wilson, A. F., Hearne, J., Brennan, M., et al. (1994). Measurement of transfer factor during constant exhalation. *Thorax, 49*, 1121–1126.

Standards and Guidelines

Graham, B. L., Brusasco, V., Burgos, F., Cooper, B. G., Jensen, R., Kendrick, A., et al. (2017). ERS/ATS standardisation of the single-breath carbon monoxide uptake in the lung. *European Respiratory Journal, Eur Respir J, 49*.

Zavorsky, G. L., Hsia, C. W., Hughes, M. B., Borland, C. D., & Guénard, H., et al. (2017). Standardisation and application of the single-breath determination of nitric oxide uptake in the lung. *Eur Respir J, 49*.

Chapter 4

Lung Volumes, Airway Resistance, and Gas Distribution Tests

JEFFREY M. HAYNES, RRT, RPFT, FAARC

CHAPTER OUTLINE

Lung volumes: functional residual capacity, residual volume, total lung capacity, and residual volume/total lung capacity Ratio
Description
Technique
Significance and Pathophysiology
Airway Resistance and Conductance
Description
Technique
Significance and Pathophysiology

Gas Distribution Tests: Single-Breath Nitrogen Washout, Closing Volume, and Closing Capacity
Description
Technique
Significance and Pathophysiology
Multiple-Breath Nitrogen Washout, Lung Clearance Index, And Phase III Slope Analysis
Description
Technique
Significance and Pathophysiology
Summary
Case Studies

LEARNING OBJECTIVES

After studying the chapter and reviewing the figures, tables, and case studies, you should be able to do the following:

Entry-level

1. Describe the measurement of lung volumes using gas-dilution/washout methods.
2. Explain two advantages of measuring lung volumes using the body plethysmograph.
3. Calculate residual volume and total lung capacity from functional residual capacity (FRC) and the subdivisions of vital capacity (VC).
4. Identify a restricted disease process from measured lung volumes.
5. Describe the measurement of airway resistance using the body plethysmograph.

Advanced

1. Calculate FRC using helium-dilution and nitrogen-washout methods.
2. Describe the correct technique for measuring thoracic gas volume using body plethysmography.
3. Identify air trapping and hyperinflation using measured lung volumes.
4. Describe the differences between Raw, sGaw, and sRaw.
5. Identify uneven distribution of gas in the lungs by either single- or multiple-breath techniques.

KEY TERMS

airway resistance (Raw)
Boyle's law

closed-circuit, multiple-breath
helium dilution (FRC$_{He}$)

closing capacity (CC)
dilutional lung volumes

distribution of ventilation	open-circuit, multiple-breath nitrogen-	specific airway conductance
end-expiratory level	washout technique (FRCN$_2$)	(sGaw)
FRC$_{pleth}$ (FRC measured with the	residual volume (RV)	specific airway resistance
body plethysmograph)	RV/TLC ratio	(sRaw)
functional residual capacity (FRC)	single-breath nitrogen-washout	"switch-in" error
hyperinflation	test (SBN$_2$)	thoracic gas volume (V$_{TG}$)
lung volume reduction surgery (LVRS)	slope of phase III	total lung capacity (TLC)

The chapter introduces the measurement of absolute lung volumes beyond the inspired and expired lung volumes measured by spirometry. The gas volume remaining in the lungs after the vital capacity (VC) has been exhaled must be measured indirectly. Several methods can accomplish this. Each method has its own advantages and disadvantages. Two methods—helium (He) dilution and nitrogen (N$_2$) washout—involve having the patient breathe gases or gas concentrations not normally present in the lungs: He or 100% oxygen (O$_2$). These techniques are sometimes referred to as **dilutional lung volumes**. The gas-dilution techniques can also provide information about the distribution of gas in the lungs.

A third method uses the body plethysmograph to measure the **thoracic gas volume (VTG)**. The use of the body plethysmograph also allows the measurement of **airway resistance (Raw)** and the volume-associated parameters of **specific airway conductance (sGaw)** and **specific airway resistance (sRaw)**. Conventional radiographs, nuclear medicine imaging of the lungs, computerized tomography (CT), and magnetic resonance imaging (MRI) may also provide an estimate of lung volumes, especially in patients with a limited ability to cooperate. However, these methods are more complex, may involve radiation, can be quite costly, and at present are not used routinely in clinical care.

LUNG VOLUMES: FUNCTIONAL RESIDUAL CAPACITY, RESIDUAL VOLUME, TOTAL LUNG CAPACITY, AND RESIDUAL VOLUME/TOTAL LUNG CAPACITY RATIO

Description

Functional residual capacity (FRC) is the volume of gas remaining in the lungs at the end of a quiet breath. On a simple spirogram, this point is termed the **end-expiratory level** (see Fig. 2.1). **Residual volume (RV)** is the volume of gas remaining in the lungs at the end of a maximal expiration, regardless of the lung volume at which exhalation was started (see Fig. 2.1). **Total lung capacity (TLC)** is the volume of gas contained in the lungs after maximal inspiration. FRC, TLC, and RV are reported in liters (L) or milliliters (mL) corrected to body temperature, pressure, and saturation (BTPS). The **RV/TLC ratio** defines the fraction of TLC that cannot be exhaled (RV), expressed as a percentage.

Thoracic gas volume (V$_{TG}$) is the absolute volume of gas in the thorax at any point in time and any level of alveolar pressure. V$_{TG}$ is only measured when using a body plethysmograph to measure lung volumes. V$_{TG}$ is usually measured at the end-expiratory level and is therefore usually close to the FRC. V$_{TG}$ is not a physiologic measure like FRC; it is simply the lung volume where closed-shutter breathing is performed to calculate FRC. The V$_{TG}$ is reported in liters or milliliters, BTPS.

Technique

There are a variety of methods for measuring absolute lung volumes (Table 4.1). FRC is measured directly with the open-circuit multiple-breath N$_2$-washout, closed-circuit multiple-breath He-dilution, and body plethysmographic techniques. Once FRC and VC have been measured, RV and TLC can be calculated. TLC can be estimated directly with the single-breath N$_2$ washout and single-breath He dilution as part of the diffusing capacity (DLCO) test and by chest imaging techniques. RV can only be measured indirectly once FRC or TLC has been determined.

Open-Circuit, Multiple-Breath Nitrogen Washout

Determination of FRC with the **open-circuit multiple-breath nitrogen-washout technique (FRCN$_2$)** is based on washing out the N$_2$ from the lungs while the patient breathes 100% O$_2$ for several

TABLE 4.1		
Methods for Measurement of Lung Volumes		
Method	**Lung Volume**	**Advantages/Disadvantages**
Multiple-breath He dilution	FRC	Simple, relatively inexpensive; affected by distribution of ventilation in moderate or severe obstruction; multiple-breath; requires IC and ERV to calculate other lung volumes. Requires more time to repeat measurements.
Multiple-breath N_2 washout	FRC	Simple, relatively inexpensive; affected by distribution of ventilation in moderate or severe obstruction; multiple-breath; requires IC and ERV to calculate other lung volumes. Requires more time to repeat measurements.
Single-breath N_2 washout	TLC	Calculated from single-breath N_2 distribution test; may underestimate lung volume in the presence of obstruction.
Single-breath He (or other inert gas; e.g., neon) dilution	TLC	Calculated as part of D_{LCO} (V_A); may underestimate lung volume in the presence of obstruction.
Plethysmography	V_{TG} (FRC_{pleth})	Plethysmographic method more complex but very fast; tends to be more accurate in the presence of airway obstruction than gas dilution techniques.
Chest radiograph	TLC	Requires posterior-anterior and lateral chest x-ray films; must breath hold at TLC; not accurate in the presence of diffuse, space-occupying diseases.
Chest computerized tomography (CT)	TLC	Involves radiation exposure and increased cost; must breath hold at TLC. Must be performed in the supine position which may affect lung volumes. Underestimates lung volumes in the presence of airway obstruction.
Magnetic resonance imaging (MRI)	TLC	No radiation exposure; very costly; research tool only. Must be performed in the supine position which may affect lung volumes.

D_{LCO}, Diffusing capacity; *ERV*, expiratory reserve volume; *FRC*, functional reserve capacity; *IC*, inspiratory capacity; N_2, nitrogen; *TLC*, total lung capacity; V_A, alveolar volume; *VTG*, thoracic gas volume.

minutes. At the start of the test, the N_2 concentration in the lungs is approximately 75% to 80%. As the patient breathes 100% O_2, the N_2 in the lungs is gradually washed out, and the total expired volume is measured. At the end of the test, the N_2 concentration in the lungs is approximately 1.5%. The initial N_2 concentration, amount of N_2 washed out, and final N_2 concentration are measured and can then be used to calculate the volume of air in the lungs at the start of the test (FRC) using the following formula:

$$FRC = \frac{F_E N_{2final} \times Expired\ volume - N_{2tissue}}{F_A N_{2alveolar1} - F_A N_{2alveolar2}}$$

where:

$F_E N_{2final}$ = fraction of N_2 in volume expired
$F_A N_{2alveolar1}$ = fraction of N_2 in alveolar gas initially
$F_A N_{2alveolar2}$ = fraction of N_2 in alveolar gas at end (from an alveolar sample)
$N_{2tissue}$ = volume of N_2 washed out of blood/tissues

A correction must be made for N_2 washed out of the blood and tissue. For each minute of O_2 breathing, approximately 30 to 40 mL of N_2 is removed from blood and tissue. $N_{2tissue}$ = 0.04 times T (where T is the time of the test). This value is subtracted from the total volume of N_2 washed out.

The original N_2-washout technique lasted 7 minutes. However, not all the N_2 in the lungs may be washed out even after 7 minutes of 100% O_2 breathing. The $F_A N_{2alveolar2}$ is measured at the end of the test and subtracted from the initial N_2 concentration. Correction for the "switch-in" error should also be made (see Correcting for the Switch-in Error section later in this chapter). The final FRC is then corrected to BTPS, and the volume of the equipment dead space (including filters) must be subtracted (see the Sample Calculations on the Evolve website, http://evolve.elsevier.com/Mottram/Ruppel/).

To obtain RV, the expiratory reserve volume (ERV) measured immediately after the acquisition of FRC as a "linked" maneuver (i.e., without the patient coming off the mouthpiece) is subtracted from the FRC:

$$RV = FRC - ERV\ (expiratory\ reserve\ volume)$$

To obtain TLC, the calculated value for RV is added to the "linked" inspiratory vital capacity (IVC):

$$TLC = RV + IVC$$

Some available commercial systems use a rapid N_2 analyzer in combination with a spirometer to provide a "breath-by-breath" analysis of expired N_2 (Fig. 4.1A). An alternative approach is to use fast-response O_2 and carbon dioxide (CO_2) analyzers

to calculate the concentration of N_2 in expired gas during the washout:

$$N_2 = 1 - F_E O_2 - F_E CO_2$$

where:

F_{EO_2} = fraction of O_2 in expired gas (dry)
F_{ECO_2} = fraction of CO_2 in expired gas (dry)

In these fast methods, the patient, wearing a nose clip, breathes through a mouthpiece-valve

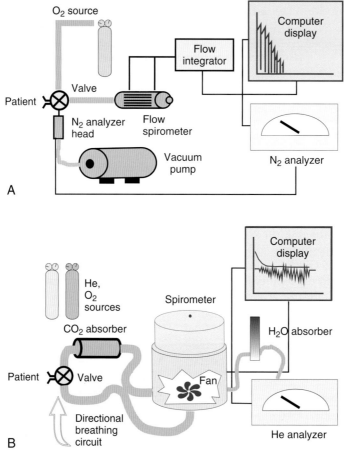

FIG. 4.1 Open-circuit and closed-circuit functional residual capacity (FRC) systems. (A) Open-circuit equipment used for N_2-washout determination of FRC. The patient inspires O_2 from a regulated source and exhales past a rapidly responding N_2 analyzer into a pneumotachometer. FRC is calculated from the total volume of N_2 exhaled and the change in alveolar N_2 from the beginning to the end of the test (Fig. 4.2 and open-circuit method). (B) Closed-circuit equipment used for He-dilution FRC determination includes a directional breathing circuit with a volume-based spirometer, He analyzer, CO_2 absorber, O_2 source, and water absorber. A breathing valve near the mouth allows the patient to be "switched in" to the system after He has been added and the system volume determined. Tidal breathing and the He-dilution curve are displayed on the computer.

system. Precisely at end expiration, a valve is opened to allow 100% O_2 breathing to begin. Each breath of 100% O_2 washes out some of the residual N_2 in the lungs. Analog signals proportional to N_2 concentration and volume (or flow) are integrated to derive the volume of N_2 exhaled for each breath. Values for each breath are summed to provide a total volume of N_2 washed out (Fig. 4.2). The test is continued until the N_2 in alveolar gas has been reduced to approximately 1.5% (Criteria for Acceptability 4.1). Some older systems terminate the test at 7 minutes. However, the O_2 breathing should be continued until alveolar N_2 falls to less than 1.5% for at least three consecutive breaths. A change in inspired N_2 concentration of greater than 1% or sudden large increases in expiratory N_2 concentrations indicate a leak, in which case the test should be stopped and repeated.

At least one technically satisfactory FRC_{N_2} determination should be made. If additional washouts are performed, a waiting period of at least 15 minutes is recommended to allow normal concentrations of N_2 to be reestablished in the lungs, blood, and tissues. If more than one FRC measurement is obtained, the mean of the technically acceptable results that agree within 10% should be reported.

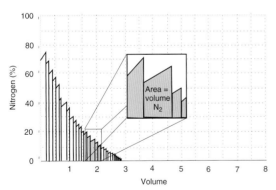

FIG. 4.2 Open-circuit (N_2 washout) determination of functional residual capacity (FRC). The concentration (or log concentration) of N_2 is plotted against time or against the volume expired as the patient breathes through a circuit (Fig. 4.1A). The volume of N_2 expired with each breath is measured by integrating flow and N_2 concentration to determine the area under each curve (see inset). FRC is determined by dividing the volume of N_2 expired by the change in alveolar N_2 from the beginning to the end of the test, with corrections, as described in the text.

CRITERIA FOR ACCEPTABILITY 4.1

N_2-Washout FRC

1. The washout tracing or display should indicate a continually falling concentration of alveolar N_2.
2. The test should be continued until the N_2 concentration falls to 1.5% for three consecutive breaths.
3. Washout times should be appropriate for the type of subject tested. Healthy subjects should wash out N_2 completely within 3 to 4 minutes.
4. The washout time should be reported. Failure to wash out N_2 within 7 minutes should be noted.
5. Multiple measurements should agree within 10%; the average FRC from acceptable trials should be used to calculate lung volumes. At least 15 minutes of room-air breathing should elapse between repeated trials.

4.1   How To …

Perform Nitrogen-Washout Maneuver

1. Tasks common to all procedures:
   a. Calibrate and prepare equipment.
   b. Review order.
   c. Introduce yourself and identify patient according to institutional policies.
   d. Describe and demonstrate procedure.
2. Arrange the chair so that the patient is at a comfortable height relative to the mouthpiece, sitting up straight.
3. Nose clips on, mouthpiece in mouth, tight seal with lips.
4. At the end of a normal exhalation, after about four steady breaths, open the valve to begin breathing 100% oxygen.
5. Continue *relaxed breathing* until end-tidal N_2 concentration is less than 1.5%.
6. Perform SVC maneuver from FRC; either ERV to RV followed by inhaled VC to TLC or IC to TLC followed by exhaled VC to RV, or both.
7. At least one technically acceptable trial is required; if needed, you may repeat after a resting period on room air of at least 15 minutes; FRC should agree within 10%.
8. Review data and note comments about test quality.

Some pulmonary function systems use pneumotachometers that may be sensitive to the composition of expired gas. These devices correct for changes in the viscosity of the gas as O_2 replaces N_2

in the expirate. Such corrections are easily accomplished by software or electronic correction of the analyzer output.

Closed-Circuit, Multiple-Breath Helium Dilution

FRC can also be determined by equilibrating the gas in the lungs with a known volume of gas containing He (**closed-circuit, multiple-breath helium dilution [FRC$_{He}$]**). A spirometer is filled with a known volume of air, and then a volume of He is added so that a concentration of approximately 10% is achieved (see Fig. 4.1B). The exact concentration

of He and spirometer volume are measured and recorded before the test is begun. The patient breathes through a valve that allows a connection to a rebreathing system. The valve is opened at the end of a quiet breath (i.e., the end-expiratory level). Then the patient rebreathes the gas in the spirometer with a CO$_2$ absorber and desiccant (absorbs H$_2$O produced from CO$_2$ absorption) in place until the concentration of He falls to a stable level (Fig. 4.3). A fan or blower mixes the gas within the spirometer system. O$_2$ is added to the spirometer system to maintain the F$_{IO_2}$ near or above 0.21 and to keep the system volume relatively constant.

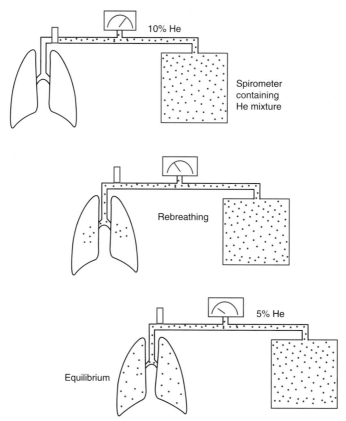

FIG. 4.3 Closed-circuit (He dilution) determination of functional residual capacity (FRC). At the beginning of the test, the patient's lungs contain no He. The spirometer contains a known concentration of He in a known volume (see text). The patient then rebreathes the He mixture from this system (Fig. 4.1B). He is diluted until equilibrium is reached. At the end of the test, the known volume of He has been diluted in the rebreathing system and the lungs. FRC is calculated from the change in He concentration and the known system volume. The patient must be switched from breathing air to the He mixture at the end-expiratory level for accurate measurement of FRC. RV is derived by subtracting the ERV. (Modified from Comroe, J. H. Jr., Forster, R. E., Dubois, A. B., et al. [1962]. *The lung: Clinical physiology and pulmonary function tests* [2nd ed.]. St. Louis, MO: Mosby.)

An older method (i.e., the bolus method) added a large volume of O_2 to the spirometer at the beginning of the test. The patient then rebreathed and gradually consumed the O_2. Because of the possibility of equilibrium not being attained before the added O_2 was depleted, this method is no longer used.

Equilibration between normal lungs and the rebreathing system takes place in approximately 3 minutes when a 10% He mixture in a system volume of 6 to 8 L is used (Fig. 4.4). The final concentration of He is then recorded. The system volume is computed first. System volume is the volume of the spirometer, breathing circuitry, and valves before the patient is connected. It can be calculated as follows:

$$\text{System volume (L)} = \frac{\text{He}_{added}(L)}{F_{\text{He initial}}}$$

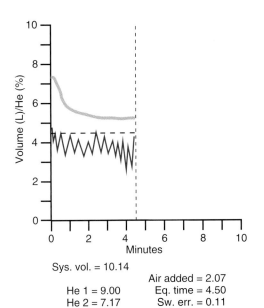

where:

He_{added} = volume of He placed in the spirometer in liters (L)

$F_{\text{He initial}}$ = % He converted to a fraction (%He/100)

When the system volume is known, FRC can be computed as follows:

$$\text{FRC} = \frac{\%\text{He}_{initial} - \%\text{He}_{final}}{\%\text{He}_{final}} \times \text{System volume}$$

Either percent or fractional concentration of He may be used because the FRC calculation is based on a ratio.

Some automated systems use a similar method to calculate the system volume; a small amount of He is added to the closed system, followed by a known volume of air. The change in He concentration after the addition of the air is used to determine the system volume. Rebreathing is continued until the He concentration changes by no more than 0.02% in 30 seconds (Criteria for Acceptability 4.2).

Sys. vol. = 10.14

	Air added = 2.07
He 1 = 9.00	Eq. time = 4.50
He 2 = 7.17	Sw. err. = 0.11
He 3 = 5.71	FRC = 3.81

FIG. 4.4 Computer-generated recording of closed-circuit, multiple-breath functional residual capacity (FRC) determination in a healthy patient. Graph shows He concentration from the beginning of rebreathing until equilibrium is achieved *(upper line)*. The system volume of the spirometer and the patient's tidal breathing is also shown *(lower line)*. A CO_2 absorber removes carbon dioxide produced by the patient. A computerized valve system replaces O_2 to keep the system volume constant. Measurements of He concentrations and system variables are also displayed.

CRITERIA FOR ACCEPTABILITY 4.2

He Dilution FRC

1. A tracing or display of spirometer volume should indicate that no leaks are present (system baseline flat). He concentration should be stable before testing.
2. The rebreathing pattern should be regular. If recorded, successive tidal breaths should show a gradually falling end-tidal level as O_2 is consumed. The addition of O_2 should return breathing to close to the system baseline.
3. The test should be continued until the He readings change by less than 0.02% in 30 seconds.
4. The addition of O_2 should be appropriate for quiet tidal breathing (i.e., 200–400 mL/min).
5. The He equilibration curve, if plotted or displayed, should show a smooth and regular fall of He concentration until equilibrium is achieved.
6. Multiple measurements of FRC (only practical for children) should agree within 10%; the average of acceptable multiple measurements should be reported.

4.2   How To ...

Perform Helium Dilution Maneuver

1. Tasks common to all procedures:
   a. Calibrate and prepare equipment.
   b. Review order.
   c. Introduce yourself and identify patient according to institutional policies.
   d. Describe and demonstrate procedure.
2. Arrange the chair so that the patient is at a comfortable height relative to the mouthpiece, sitting up straight.
3. Nose clips on, mouthpiece in mouth, tight seal with lips.
4. At the end of a normal exhalation, after approximately four steady breaths, open the valve to begin closed-circuit rebreathing.
5. Continue *relaxed breathing* until helium concentration stabilizes at a minimum level, no more than 0.02% in 30 seconds or a maximum of 10 minutes.
6. Perform SVC maneuver from FRC—either ERV to RV followed by inhaled VC to TLC or IC to TLC followed by exhaled VC to RV, or both.
7. At least one technically acceptable trial is required; if needed, you may repeat after a resting period on room air of at least 5 minutes; FRC should agree within 10%. (See Criteria for Acceptability Box 4.2.)
8. Review data and note comments about test quality.

At least one technically satisfactory measurement should be obtained. If additional dilutions are performed, a waiting period of at least 5 minutes is recommended between repeated tests. If more than one measurement of FRC_{He} is obtained, it is recommended that the mean of the technically acceptable results that agree within 10% be reported.

Although a small volume of He dissolves in the blood during the test, it results in a negligible increase in FRC, and it is recommended that no correction be made. The volume of the equipment dead space (including filters) must also be subtracted from the measured FRC.

Correcting for the "Switch-In" Error

Most manufacturers provide **"switch-in" error** correction when the patient begins the test at a point either above or below the actual end-expiratory level (FRC). Depending on the patient's breathing pattern, a volume difference of several hundred milliliters may result. The effect of the switch-in error may be insignificant, especially with the closed-circuit method. Equilibrium does not occur instantaneously at switch-in. The total volume of the spirometer and lungs is constantly changing with tidal breathing, the removal of CO_2, and the addition of O_2. If the switch-in error is large or the end-expiratory level appears to change during the maneuver, the test may need to be repeated.

Additional Comments on FRC by Gas-Dilution Techniques

In the gas-dilution techniques, RV is measured indirectly as a subdivision of the FRC. This method is preferred because the resting end-expiratory level depends less on patient effort than on maximal inspiration or expiration. The end-expiratory level (and the ERV) must be accurately measured. If tidal breathing is irregular, ERV may be overestimated or underestimated. Subtraction of an ERV value that is too large from the FRC will cause the RV to appear smaller than it actually is. Similarly, a small ERV will produce a larger-than-actual RV. For this reason, the patient's tidal breathing pattern must be carefully monitored during the VC measurement.

The accuracy of the gas-dilution techniques depends on all parts of the lung being well ventilated. In patients who have an obstructive disease, some lung units are poorly ventilated. In these patients, it is often difficult to wash N_2 out or mix He to a stable level in poorly ventilated parts of the lungs. Thus FRC, RV, and TLC may all be underestimated, usually in proportion to the degree of obstruction. Extending the time of these tests improves their accuracy. However, prolonging the test may not measure completely trapped gas, such as is found in bullous emphysema.

The graphic method of displaying breath-by-breath N_2 washout provides a means of quantifying the evenness of ventilation. Some systems plot the logarithm of the N_2 concentration against time or volume exhaled. The slope of the washout curve is determined by the FRC, tidal volume, dead-space volume, and frequency of breathing. If N_2 is washed out of the lungs evenly, the log N_2 plot appears as a straight line. Because the lung is not perfectly symmetric, the washout curve is slightly concave. The deviation from the expected curve indicates the extent to which ventilation is uneven. Washout should be complete within 3 to 4 minutes in healthy patients. The time to reach He equilibrium during the closed-circuit FRC determination can also be used as an index of **distribution of ventilation**. By simply recording the time to reach equilibrium and plotting the dilution curve, an estimate of the evenness of ventilation is obtained. The use of gas-dilution techniques to assess the distribution of ventilation is more commonly performed using radioisotope imaging and CT scanning.

PF TIP 4.1

The gas-dilution techniques of measuring lung volumes sometimes underestimate lung volumes in the presence of moderate or severe obstruction. Both methods (N_2 washout and He dilution) are also subject to leaks in their respective breathing circuits. Leaks usually cause the measured lung volume to be overestimated.

In either of the gas-dilution techniques, a leak will cause erroneous estimates of FRC. Leaks may occur in breathing valves or circuitry or at the patient connection. Some patients have difficulty maintaining an adequate seal at the mouthpiece throughout the test. Failure to properly apply nose clips can also result in a leak. Leaks usually result in an overestimate of lung volume. A leak in the open-circuit N_2-washout system allows room air to enter, increasing the volume of N_2 washed out. A leak in the closed-circuit He dilution system allows air to dilute the He concentration or He to escape. Each situation causes the test gas concentration to change more than it should. Leaks during the N_2 washout can usually be identified by an inspection of the graphic display or recording (Fig. 4.5). Inaccuracy or malfunction of the gas analyzers in either method often causes errors. Leaks or analyzer problems should be considered whenever lung volume values are inconsistent with spirometry

results, for example, an extremely high TLC and RV/TLC ratio with normal spirometry (Interpretive Strategies 4.1).

INTERPRETIVE STRATEGIES 4.1

Dilutional Lung Volumes

1. Was the FRC determination performed acceptably? Were multiple trials performed? If so, were they within 10%?
2. Was the VC maneuver acceptable? Were the ERV and IC measurements within 5% or 60 mL?
3. Were other lung volumes calculated appropriately (TLC, RV)?
4. Are the reference values appropriate? Age, height, sex, race?
5. Is the TLC less than the lower limit of normal (LLN)? If so, restriction is present. Are other lung volumes (FRC, RV) reduced in similar proportion?
6. Is the TLC greater than the upper limit of normal (ULN)? If so, suspect hyperinflation.
7. If the RV/TLC ratio is greater that the ULN, suspect air trapping
8. Are lung volumes consistent with spirometric findings in regard to obstruction or restriction? Are they consistent with the history and physical findings?
9. Are additional tests indicated (plethysmographic lung volumes)?

Body Plethysmography

FRC measured with the body plethysmograph (**FRC$_{pleth}$**) (Fig. 4.6) refers to the volume of intrathoracic gas measured when airflow occlusion occurs at end expiration (FRC) during shutter closure. The technique is based on **Boyle's law** relating pressure to volume. A volume of gas varies in inverse proportion to the pressure to which it is subjected if the temperature remains constant (isothermal). The patient has an unknown volume of gas in the lungs at the end of a normal expiration (i.e., at FRC). The airway is occluded momentarily at or near FRC; the patient is asked to gently breathe at a frequency between 0.5 and 1.0 Hz (0.5–1.0 cycles per second), allowing the air in the chest to be gently compressed and decompressed. The breaths are shallow and should not create pressure changes > 10 cm H_2O. The closed-shutter breathing causes a change in

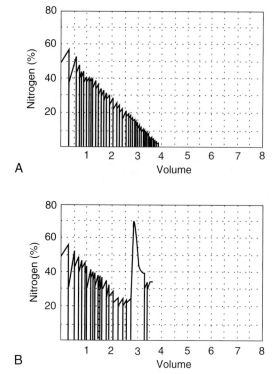

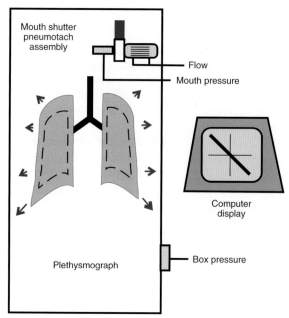

FIG. 4.5 Open-circuit, multiple-breath N_2-washout tracings. (A) A computer-generated recording of an N_2-washout test in a healthy patient. The tracings show a continuous decrease in end-tidal N_2 concentration with successive breaths. The test is continued until the N_2 concentration falls to less than 1.5% for three consecutive breaths or for 7 minutes total. (B) A similar plot of N_2 washout from a healthy patient, but in this instance, a leak occurs during the test. Leaks may occur if the patient does not maintain a tight seal at the mouthpiece. Leaks are usually easy to detect because room air enters the system and causes an abrupt increase in N_2 concentration.

FIG. 4.6 Components of the body plethysmograph used to measure thoracic gas volume (V_{TG}). Boyle's law states that volume varies inversely with pressure if temperature is held constant. A pressure-type (constant volume) plethysmograph, with pressure transducers for measurements of box pressure and mouth (alveolar) pressure, is shown. A pneumotachometer measures flow to track lung volumes. The mouth shutter occludes the airway momentarily so that alveolar pressure can be estimated. The patient breathes shallowly against the closed shutter. Gas in the lungs is alternately compressed and decompressed. Changes in lung volume are reflected by changes in box pressure. These changes are displayed as a sloping line on a computer display. When the original pressure (P), the new pressure (P + ΔP), and the new volume (V + ΔV) are known, the original volume (V or V_{TG}) can be computed from Boyle's law (see the section on the technique of thoracic gas volume, and see the Evolve website, http://evolve.elsevier.com/Mottram/Ruppel/).

volume and pressure. The changes in pressure are easily measured at the mouth (PMOUTH) with a pressure transducer. Mouth pressure theoretically equals alveolar pressure when there is no airflow. Changes in pulmonary gas volume are estimated by measuring pressure changes in the plethysmograph. The pressure in the plethysmograph is measured by a sensitive transducer. This transducer is calibrated by a small piston that moves a small volume of gas into and out of the sealed box and relates the pressure change to the known volume (PBOX). The calibration factor is then applied to measurements made on human patients. The term

panting is used to describe the gentle, shallow breathing pattern just discussed; however, in some patients, the use of the term *panting* may elicit fast breathing (e.g., >1 breath per second). Breathing too quickly may result in an overestimation of lung volume.

The display of the shallow breathing maneuver is a graph with PMOUTH and PBOX. PMOUTH is plotted on the vertical axis, and PBOX is plotted on the horizontal axis (Fig. 4.7). The resulting figure appears as a sloping line equal to ΔP/ΔV, where ΔP equals the change in alveolar pressure, and ΔV equals the

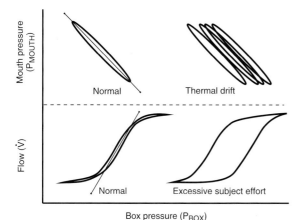

FIG. 4.7 Normal and abnormal plethysmograph recordings. *Top left,* Normal closed-shutter maneuver in which mouth pressure is plotted against box pressure. The loop should be closed, or nearly so. If thermal equilibrium has not been achieved, the loop (shown on the *top right*) tends to be open and to drift across the screen. *Bottom left,* Normal open-shutter measurement in which flow is plotted against box pressure. If the patient breathes near functional residual capacity (FRC), the loop takes on a nearly closed S-shaped appearance. If the patient breathes too rapidly or too deeply, the tracing becomes open and flattened (shown on the *bottom right*). Thermal drift can also cause the open-shutter tracing to resemble excessive patient effort.

change in alveolar volume (V_A). The change in V_A is measured indirectly by noting the reciprocal change in plethysmograph volume.

The V_{TG} can then be obtained from the slope of the tracing by applying a derivation of Boyle's law:

$$V_{TG} = \frac{P_B}{\lambda V_{TG}} \times \frac{P_{BOX}cal}{P_{MOUTH}cal} \times K$$

where:

V_{TG} = thoracic gas volume

P_B = barometric pressure minus water vapor pressure

λV_{TG} = slope of the displayed line equal to DP/DV

$P_{BOX}cal$ = box pressure transducer calibration factor

$P_{MOUTH}cal$ = mouth pressure transducer calibration factor

K = correction factor for volume displaced by the patient

For the complete derivation of the equation and sample calculations, see the Evolve website at http://evolve.elsevier.com/Mottram/Ruppel/.

Computerized plethysmograph systems permit the monitoring of tidal breathing in conjunction with the V_{TG} maneuver. Instantaneous changes in lung volume can be monitored by continuously integrating the flow through the plethysmograph's pneumotachometer. The end-expiratory level can be determined from tidal breathing. The patient then breathes shallow with the mouth shutter open. The computer records the change in lung volume above or below the resting level (FRC). When asked to breathe shallowly, most patients do so slightly above FRC. The shutter then closes automatically, the patient continues to breathe shallowly, and V_{TG} is measured as described. The computer then adds or subtracts the change in volume from the end-expiratory level (before shallow breathing began) to calculate the true FRC. This computerized technique allows the patient to breathe at the correct frequency and depth before the shutter is closed. It also eliminates the necessity of closing the shutter precisely at end expiration. Raw and sGaw can also be measured simultaneously during the open-shutter breathing (see following text). It should be noted that the correct breathing frequencies for measuring Raw and V_{TG} are slightly different. Raw measurements should be made with the patient breathing shallow at about 1.5 to 2.5 Hz (1.5–2.5 cycles per second, or 90–150 breaths/min), whereas V_{TG} should be measured with the patient breathing at a slower rate of 0.5 to 1 Hz. Many computerized systems display the breathing frequency so that the technologist can coach the patient to achieve the correct rate.

A VC maneuver, along with its subdivisions (ERV and IC), should be performed immediately after the acquisition of FRC$_{pleth}$. The American Thoracic Society-European Respiratory Society (ATS-ERS) Task Force recommends that a linked ERV maneuver to RV followed by an IC maneuver to TLC be performed. An alternative method is to perform linked maneuvers with an IC first to TLC followed by a VC breath to RV. Most plethysmograph systems allow these measurements using the built-in pneumotachometer. The same standards for accuracy should be applied to a slow VC measured in the plethysmograph as for any other spirometer. When FRC$_{pleth}$ has been determined, the remaining lung volumes can be calculated as described for the gas-dilution techniques.

Measurement of FRC_{pleth} is a complex procedure. Each patient must be carefully instructed in the required maneuvers. Allowing the patient to sit in the box with the door open is helpful. A few patients may experience claustrophobia in the plethysmograph. The shallow-breathing maneuver should be demonstrated by the technologist and then practiced by the patient. The patient should be instructed to place both hands against the cheeks. This prevents unwanted pressure changes in the mouth when the patient pants against the closed shutter. If practical, the shutter may be closed so the patient knows what to expect during the test. The door of the plethysmograph can then be closed. The patient should understand that the plethysmograph can be opened if he or she becomes uncomfortable. The patient should be instructed on how to open the door from within the box. If the plethysmograph is equipped with a communication device, it should be adjusted so that the patient can hear instructions.

Depending on the construction of the plethysmograph, venting to the atmosphere is usually required to establish thermal equilibrium. Equilibrium takes about 30 to 60 seconds and can be presumed when the flow-volume recording stabilizes (i.e., does not drift). Some systems compensate for thermal drift, so waiting for equilibrium is not necessary. The patient is then instructed to breathe shallowly. When the correct breathing frequency and depth have been established, the shutter may be closed. Some plethysmograph systems require tidal breathing before shutter closure to establish the patient's end-expiratory level. In either type of system, the patient should breathe shallowly against the closed shutter until a stable tracing is produced. Two to four breaths are usually sufficient. If the patient breathes too hard, the tracing may drift or appear as an "open" loop (see Fig. 4.7). The recorded pressure changes should be within the range over which the transducers were calibrated. The entire tracing should be visible on the display. If the tracing goes off-screen, the pressure changes probably exceed the calibration ranges.

4.3   **How To**

Perform Body Plethysmography ("Body Box") Maneuvers

1. Task common to all procedures:
   a. Calibrate and prepare equipment.
   b. Review order.
   c. Introduce yourself and identify patient according to institutional policies.
   d. Describe and demonstrate procedure.
2. Place the patient in a body box; adjust height of mouthpiece so the patient is sitting up straight; nose clips on; mouthpiece in mouth, tight seal with lips.
3. Patient can practice breathing and shallow-breathing maneuvers.
4. Close door; allow temperature stabilization.
5. Have the patient place hands on cheeks and breathe normally.
6. At end of a normal exhalation, after approximately four steady breaths, begin open shutter breathing; frequency = 1.5 to 2.5 breaths per second. Demonstrate and say "in-out-in-out" or "1-2-1-2-1-2." This will allow the determination of Raw. Allow time for the subject to reestablish a stable FRC baseline.
7. Warn the patient that the shutter is about to close. Then close the shutter and continue to coach shallow breathing at a slightly slower rate (0.5–1 breath per second). This will allow the determination of V_{TG} and sGaw.
8. Alternatively, after recording open- then closed-shutter breathing, repeat closed-shutter breathing alone to obtain V_{TG}.
9. Open shutter, perform SVC maneuver from end exhalation—either ERV to RV followed by inhaled VC to TLC (ATS-ERS preferred method) or IC to TLC followed by exhaled VC to RV (ATS-ERS alternative method).
10. Repeat maneuver until you obtain at least three technically acceptable trials; FRC (V_{TG}) should agree within 5% (Criteria for Acceptability 4.3).
11. Open door; test ends.
12. Review data and make adjustments in slopes if needed.
13. Note comments about test quality.

A minimum of three technically satisfactory maneuvers should be recorded, each followed by ERV and IVC maneuvers (see Criteria for Acceptability 4.3). At least three FRC_{pleth} values that agree within 5% should be obtained and the mean value reported. The technologist's comments should note the acceptability of the maneuvers. Most computerized plethysmographs automatically measure the slope of the $\Delta P/\Delta V$ tracings. This is done by using the least-squares method to calculate a "best-fit" line through the recorded data points. The technologist may need to correct computer-generated tangents depending on data quality from the breathing maneuvers.

PF TIP 4.2

Plethysmography offers several advantages over other methods of measuring lung volumes. FRC_{pleth} is less affected by the distribution of ventilation. Multiple measurements can be made quickly and averaged. It may provide a more accurate estimate of lung volumes in patients who have airway obstruction. In addition, Raw, sGaw, and sRaw can be measured in the same testing session.

CRITERIA FOR ACCEPTABILITY 4.3

FRC_{pleth}

1. The shallow-breathing maneuver shows a closed loop without drift or another artifact.
2. Pressure changes are within calibration ranges; the tracing does not go off-screen.
3. Breathing frequency should be between 0.5 and 1.0 Hz.
4. A minimum of three technically satisfactory shallow-breathing maneuvers should be recorded.
5. At least three FRC_{pleth} values that agree within 5% should be obtained.
6. Reported FRC_{pleth} is averaged from the three acceptable and repeatable panting maneuvers.

Additional Comments on FRC by Plethysmography

The plethysmographic method is a quick and accurate means of measuring lung volumes. It can be used in combination with simple spirometry to derive all lung volume compartments. The plethysmograph's primary advantage is that it measures all gas in the thorax, whether in ventilatory communication with the atmosphere or not. The plethysmographic measurement of FRC is often larger than that measured by He dilution or N_2 washout. This is the case in emphysema and other diseases characterized by air trapping, as well as in the presence of an uneven distribution of ventilation. When gas-dilution tests are continued for more than 7 minutes, the results for FRC determinations approach the V_{TG} value. See Interpretive Strategies 4.2.

It may be useful, albeit impractical for a busy laboratory, to compare FRC values obtained by plethysmography with values obtained by gas-dilution methods, particularly in patients with obstructive disease. The ratio of $FRC_{pleth}/FRCN_2$ or FRC_{pleth}/FRC_{He} can be used as an index of gas trapping. This ratio is usually near 1.0 in patients with normal lungs or even those with a restrictive lung disorder. Values greater than 1.0 indicate gas volumes detectable by the plethysmograph but hidden to the gas-dilution techniques. Care must be taken that lung volumes determined by the two separate methods are reliable before the values can be expressed as a ratio. Patients with severe bullous emphysema may have a difference in TLC of more than 1 L between FRC_{pleth} and the gas-dilutional methods of measuring FRC.

Although it is conventional wisdom that dilution techniques may underestimate lung volumes in patients with airflow obstruction, there is evidence suggesting that in severe airway obstruction, FRC may be overestimated when the plethysmographic technique is used. This occurs primarily because P_{MOUTH} (measured when the shutter is closed) may not equal alveolar pressure if the airways are severely obstructed. Rapid breathing rates aggravate this inaccuracy. Care should be taken that patients with spirometric evidence of obstruction breathe at a rate of 0.5 to 1 Hz (30–60 breaths per minute).

Spirometry (e.g., forced vital capacity [FVC], forced expiratory volume in the first second [FEV_1], and VC) may be performed with the patient in the plethysmograph. The pneumotachometer must be capable of accurately measuring the entire range of gas flows required (i.e., up to 12 L/sec).

Two varieties of body boxes are commonly used: pressure-based and flow-based boxes (see Chapter 11). Flow boxes allow a slightly different type of flow-volume curve to be recorded. Normal spirometry plots airflow at the mouth against volume at the mouth (as detected by the spirometer). With the patient in a flow box, flow at the mouth can be plotted against actual lung volume changes as detected by the box. This may be particularly useful in patients with severe airway obstruction. It is possible to detect a significant compression volume during forced expiration and plot it against the flow generated. Spirometry, lung volumes, and airway resistance can all be obtained in a single sitting with either type of plethysmograph.

INTERPRETIVE STRATEGIES 4.2

FRC$_{pleth}$

1. Was the closed-shutter breathing maneuver performed acceptably? Was the breathing frequency appropriate (0.5–1.0 Hz)? If not, interpret results cautiously.
2. Were at least three maneuvers averaged to obtain FRC? Were individual values repeatable (within 5%)? If not, interpret cautiously.
3. Are reference values appropriate? Age, height, weight, race? Were they obtained plethysmographically?
4. Were other lung volumes (TLC) calculated appropriately? Were VC, ERV, and IC acceptable? If not, evaluate FRC only.
5. If the TLC is less than the LLN, suspect restriction.
6. If the TLC is greater than the ULN, suspect hyperinflation.
7. If the RV/TLC ratio is greater than the ULN, suspect air trapping
8. Are lung volumes consistent with spirometric findings? If not, evaluate carefully for combined obstruction and restriction.

Total Lung Capacity and Residual Volume/Total Lung Capacity Ratio

TLC is calculated by combining other lung volume measurements once FRC is measured by either a gas-dilution method or body plethysmography. The two most common methods to calculate TLC are as follows:

$$TLC = RV + VC$$

or

$$TLC = FRC + IC$$

Each method requires accurate measurement of the subdivisions of the VC. TLC can also be calculated with single-breath techniques (i.e., single-breath He dilution or single-breath N_2 washout). Single-breath measurements of lung volumes are usually done as part of other tests, such as the diffusing capacity (DLCO) test (see Chapter 3). Single-breath lung volumes correlate well with multiple-breath techniques in healthy patients. However, single-breath lung volumes tend to underestimate true values in moderate to severe obstruction. TLC can also be measured from standard chest x-ray films, as well as from CT scans of the thorax.

The RV/TLC ratio is calculated by dividing the RV by the TLC. This ratio is expressed as a percentage. Either ambient temperature, pressure, saturation (ATPS) or BTPS values may be used in the ratio, but both RV and TLC must be expressed in the same units.

The FRC, RV, and TLC should be reported in liters or milliliters, BTPS. Barrier filters must be used during lung volume determinations. The filter volume is subtracted from the lung volumes measured via dilution methods by the software.

Significance and Pathophysiology

FRC varies with body size, change in body position, and time of day (i.e., diurnal variation). However, unlike TLC and RV, FRC is an effort-independent maneuver determined by the balance of lung and chest wall recoil at relaxed end expiration. As with other lung volumes, normal FRC may be affected by racial or ethnic background (see Interpretive Strategies 4.1 and 4.2). Equations for calculating predicted FRC can be found on the Evolve website, http://evolve.elsevier.com/Mottram/Ruppel/.

Increased FRC is considered pathologic. FRC values greater than the ULN represent **hyperinflation**. Hyperinflation may result from emphysematous changes or from obstruction caused by asthma or bronchitis. Compensation for surgical removal of lung tissue or thoracic deformity can also cause increased FRC. Elevated FRC usually results in muscular and mechanical inefficiency of the respiratory apparatus. As lung volume increases, the chest wall and lungs themselves become "stiffer." This causes an increase in the work of breathing. FRC can increase dynamically; patients with airway obstruction may increase their end-expiratory lung volume (EELV) during exercise. This change in lung volume with increased ventilatory demand often results in a sensation of breathlessness and reduces exercise time. Reduction in the rate of air trapping is one of the primary benefits of bronchodilator therapy in chronic obstructive pulmonary disease (COPD).

The TLC is the maximal volume of inspired air. TLC is determined by the balance of lung recoil plus chest wall recoil, on the one hand, and muscle strength and effort, on the other hand. Thus diseases that reduce lung recoil will result in increased TLC; those that increase lung recoil may reduce TLC. Likewise, muscle weakness or suboptimal effort may reduce TLC.

The RV is the volume left in the lungs after the VC is exhaled. An increased RV indicates that despite maximal expiratory effort, the lungs contain a larger volume of gas than normal. Increased RV often results in an equivalent decrease in VC (Fig. 4.8). Elevated RV may occur during an acute asthmatic episode but is usually reversible. Increased RV is characteristic of emphysema and bronchial obstruction; both may cause chronic air trapping. RV and FRC usually increase together. As RV becomes larger, increased ventilation is needed to adequately exchange O_2 and CO_2 in the lung. This requires an increase in the tidal volume, respiratory rate, or both. Because of altered pressure–volume characteristics of the lung, the work of breathing is also increased. Patients with increased RV often display gas exchange abnormalities such as hypoxemia or CO_2 retention. Because RV is effort dependent, elevated RV may also be caused by muscle weakness or suboptimal effort.

Measuring lung volumes is critical to understanding changes in FVC. A normal FVC almost always excludes significant restriction. But because decrements in FVC can be from restriction, neuromuscular weakness, suboptimal effort, or severe

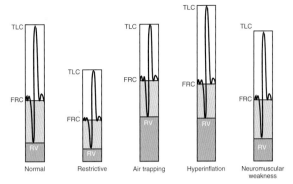

FIG. 4.8 Lung volumes in normal, restrictive, obstructive, and neuromuscular weakness patterns. A comparison of changes in lung volume compartments and vital capacity (VC) *(superimposed)* shows the following: In restrictive patterns, functional residual capacity (FRC), residual volume (RV), and VC are all decreased proportionately, resulting in a decrease in the total lung capacity (TLC), which defines restriction (see text). In obstruction (with air trapping), FRC and RV are both increased at the expense of the VC, and therefore TLC remains relatively unchanged. Similar increases in RV and FRC may occur without reduction of VC, in which case the TLC increases (hyperinflation). In neuromuscular weakness, the FRC is normal, but the TLC is reduced, and the RV/TLC is too high.

obstruction, knowledge of TLC, FRC, and RV is invaluable in sorting out these possibilities.

FRC, RV, and TLC are typically decreased in restrictive diseases. Decreased lung volumes are seen in interstitial diseases associated with extensive fibrosis (e.g., sarcoidosis, asbestosis, and idiopathic pulmonary fibrosis). Restrictive disorders affecting the chest wall include kyphoscoliosis, neuromuscular disorders, and obesity. Diseases that impair the diaphragm often result in reduced lung volumes, particularly TLC. Lung volumes may also be decreased in diseases that occlude many alveoli, such as pneumonia. Congestive heart failure causes pulmonary congestion and pleural effusions, which can also reduce lung volume. Any disease process that occupies volume in the thorax (e.g., tumors) can reduce lung volume.

Table 4.2 lists comparative lung volumes for a healthy adult male and for patients with air trapping (as in emphysema), hyperinflation, restriction (as in sarcoidosis), and neuromuscular weakness (as in amyotrophic lateral sclerosis [ALS]).

Restrictive processes usually cause lung volumes to be reduced equally. Proportional relationships

TABLE 4.2

Comparative Lung Volumes for a Healthy Adult Male and Patients With Air Trapping, Hyperinflation, Restriction, and Neuromuscular Weakness

Value	Normal	Air Trapping	Hyperinflation	Restriction	Neuromuscular Weakness
VC (L)	4.80	3.00	4.80	3.00	3.50
FRC (L)	2.40	3.60	3.60	1.50	2.40
RV (L)	1.20	3.00	3.00	0.75	1.50
TLC (L)	6.00	6.00	7.80	3.75	5.00
RV/TLC (%)	20	50	38	20	30

between lung volume compartments, such as the RV/TLC ratio, may be relatively normal in restrictive diseases. In various forms of extrapulmonary restriction, such as kyphoscoliosis, or pleural effusion, RV is often less reduced than TLC, resulting in a relatively elevated RV/TLC ratio despite a low TLC. Obesity usually affects ERV and FRC earlier more significantly than TLC.

In obstruction, two different patterns may be observed. RV is usually increased. This increase may be at the expense of a reduction in VC (see Fig. 4.6) with TLC remaining close to normal, in which case the elevated RV/TLC ratio reflects *air trapping.* Elevated TLC is referred to as *hyperinflation,* which is usually accompanied by air trapping. TLC may be either normal or increased in obstructive processes such as asthma, chronic bronchitis, bronchiectasis, cystic fibrosis, and emphysema. TLC does not appear to change dynamically, even though FRC may increase acutely during exercise (dynamic hyperinflation).

The RV/TLC ratio describes the percentage of total lung volume that cannot be emptied during expiration. In healthy adults, the RV/TLC ratio may vary from 20% in young adults to 35% in older patients. Values greater than 35% may result from absolute increases of RV (as in emphysema) or from a decrease in TLC because of a loss of VC. As mentioned previously, an elevated RV/TLC in the presence of increased TLC is often indicative of both hyperinflation and air trapping. An increased RV/TLC with a normal TLC indicates that air trapping is present. As an indicator of air trapping, the RV/TLC ratio is a weak but statistically significant in-

dicator of outcome after **lung volume reduction surgery (LVRS)**.

In neuromuscular weakness, FRC is typically normal because lung and chest wall recoil are not specifically affected. However, TLC is low, and RV is high, relative to FRC, because of the reduced muscle strength required to reach these upper and lower limits of lung volume, respectively.

Processes that occupy space in the lungs, such as edema, atelectasis, neoplasms, or fibrotic lesions, may decrease TLC. Other diseases that commonly result in decreased TLC include pulmonary congestion, pleural effusions, pneumothorax, and thoracic deformities. Pure restrictive defects show proportional decreases in most lung compartments, as described for FRC and RV. When the TLC value is less than the LLN, a restrictive process is present. Reduced VC, along with a normal or increased FEV_1/FVC ratio, is suggestive of restriction, but a measurement of TLC is needed to confirm the diagnosis of a restrictive defect.

PF TIP 4.3

TLC is an important diagnostic tool in both obstructive and restrictive lung diseases. In restriction, the TLC is usually less than the LLN. In obstruction, the TLC is either normal or increased (hyperinflation).

A less common pattern is mixed obstructive-restrictive lung disease, characterized by a low FEV_1/FVC ratio and a low TLC. This is suggested by simple spirometry when both FEV_1/FVC and

FVC are reduced but can only be confirmed by measuring TLC. Measuring the reduction in TLC may allow for more accurate characterization of the concomitant degree of airway obstruction. Another interesting pulmonary function test (PFT) pattern is the so-called "nonspecific" pattern characterized by a reduced FEV_1 and FVC, normal FEV_1/FVC ratio, and normal TLC. This pattern may represent lung volume decruitment occurring in the presence of airway disease or thoracic restriction such as obesity. Obesity is typically characterized by larger decrements in FRC and ERV than in TLC.

AIRWAY RESISTANCE AND CONDUCTANCE

Description

The forces governing maximal airflow are the elastic recoil pressure of the lung and airway resistance upstream from the equal pressure point. This section addresses the measurement of airway resistance, which is accomplished by examining the relationship between alveolar pressure and flow during open-loop shallow breathing in the body plethysmograph.

Airway resistance (Raw) is the pressure difference per unit flow as gas flows into or out of the lungs. Raw is the difference between mouth pressure and alveolar pressure, divided by flow at the mouth. This pressure difference is caused primarily by the friction of gas molecules in contact with the airways. Raw is recorded in centimeters of water per liter per second (cm H_2O/L/sec).

Gaw is the flow generated per unit of pressure drop across the airways. It is the reciprocal of Raw (1/Raw) and is recorded in liters per second per centimeter of water (L/sec/cm H_2O). Gaw is not commonly reported because it changes with lung volume. Instead, specific airway conductance (sGaw), which is Gaw divided by the lung volume (in liters) at which the measurement was made, is usually calculated. It is reported in liters per second per centimeter of water per liter of lung volume (L/sec/cm H_2O/L). The lung volume at which Raw is measured is determined during the closed-shutter maneuver to calculate V_{TG}. However,

the closed-shutter maneuver may be difficult to perform in some individuals, especially children, so V_{TG} cannot be measured. It is possible to derive sRaw by comparing flow to the small shifts in lung volume that occur during tidal breathing without closed-shutter breathing, but this is rarely done, and few manufacturers offer this option. Mathematically, sRaw = Raw × V_{TG}. Because sRaw encompasses lung volume, and Raw and lung volume vary inversely, sRaw is relatively stable with respect to changes in lung volume (i.e., as lung volume decreases, Raw increases, so the product sRaw remains the same, and vice versa). In this way, sRaw is similar to sGaw because it takes lung volume into account. However, whereas sGaw reflects Raw only, sRaw reflects both Raw and lung volume.

Technique

Raw can be measured as the ratio of alveolar pressure (P_A) to airflow ($\dot{V}$). Gas flow at the mouth is measured with a pneumotachometer (see Chapter 11). P_A is measured in the body plethysmograph (Fig. 4.9A). For gas to flow into the lungs during inspiration, P_A must fall below atmospheric pressure (mouth pressure). During expiration, P_A rises above atmospheric pressure. Changes in V are plotted against plethysmograph pressure changes. Changes in plethysmograph pressure are proportional to V_A changes. The patient breathes with a small V_T at a rate of about 1.5 to 2.5 breaths/sec (1.5–2.5 Hz). Shallow rapid breathing may produce an S-shaped pressure–flow curve (see Fig. 4.9B). A tangent (the slope) is measured from this curve. Traditionally, the tangent is drawn to pass through zero flow and connects the +0.5 L/sec and −0.5 L/sec flow points. The slope of this line is the ratio of $\dot{V} / P_{BOX}$. $\dot{V}$ is flow at the mouth, and P_{BOX} is plethysmograph pressure.

Problems with the open-shutter breathing technique are illustrated by the loops seen in Fig. 4.10. The most common problems are thermal drift and breathing at too high or low of a frequency or volume.

To measure V_{TG} in association with Raw, the shutter at the mouthpiece is closed immediately after the open-shutter breathing, and the patient continues to breathe shallowly. The optimal rate for closed-shutter breathing is about 0.5 to 1.0 Hz,

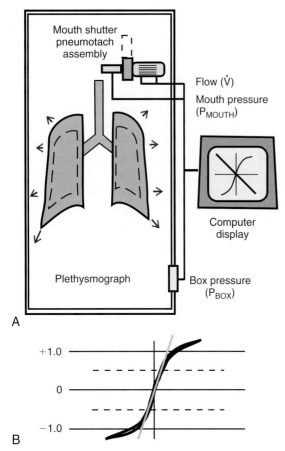

FIG. 4.9 Measurement of airway resistance (Raw) using the body plethysmograph. (A) Diagrammatic representation of airway resistance measurement: Raw = Atmospheric pressure-alveolar pressure/Flow. Flow ($\dot{V}$) is measured directly by means of the pneumotachometer. As the patient breathes with the shutter open, flow is plotted against box pressure (PBOX) as it occludes the airway momentarily, usually at end expiration, and a sloping line representing the ratio of mouth pressure to box pressure (PMOUTH/PBOX) is recorded in a manner similar to that used for measurement of thoracic gas volume (V_{TG}). In this example, the flow tracing (shutter open) and volume tracing (shutter closed) are superimposed on the computer display. The PMOUTH/PBOX tangent is measured as for the V_{TG}. (B) The flow tangent is measured from the steep portion of the flow tracing, from −0.5 to +0.5 L/sec. Airway resistance is then calculated as the ratio of these two tangents, using appropriate calibration factors (see text and Evolve website, http://evolve.elsevier.com/Mottram/Ruppel/).

slightly slower than open-shutter panting. Changes in PBOX are then plotted against PMOUTH. Because there is no flow into or out of the lungs, PMOUTH equals P_A. A second tangent is measured from this curve. The slope of this line is P_A/PBOX, where P_A

equals alveolar pressure. Computerized plethysmographs usually calculate a "best-fit" line to measure the open-shutter and closed-shutter tangents. The technologist should visually inspect all computer-fitted lines. PFT systems allow the technologist to adjust computer-generated tangents manually. Problems with the closed-shutter breathing technique are similar to those that plague the open-shutter breathing measurement and also include leak around the mouth or nose.

Raw is then calculated by taking the ratio of these two slopes, as follows:

$$Raw = \frac{P_A / P_{BOX}}{\dot{V} / P_{BOX}} \times \frac{Mouth\ cal}{Flow\ cal}$$

where:

$\dot{V}$ = airflow
P_A = alveolar pressure
PBOX = plethysmographic pressure, measured with the shutter open and closed
Mouth cal = calibration factor for the mouth pressure transducer
Flow cal = calibration factor for the pneumotachometer

This formula shows how Raw is calculated from the ratio of P_A and $\dot{V}$, as PBOX cancels out. Calibration factors for the flow and mouth pressure transducers are included in the previous equation (see the Sample Calculations on the Evolve website, http://evolve.elsevier.com/Mottram/Ruppel/).

Shallow breathing eliminates several artifacts from the tracing. Small rapid breaths (1.5–2.5 per

---

CRITERIA FOR ACCEPTABILITY 4.4

Raw and sGaw

1. Pressure-flow loops should be closed; pressure and flow should be within the calibrated range of the respective transducers.
2. Thermal equilibrium should be established; no drift during recording.
3. Shallow breathing frequency should be 1.5 to 2.5 Hz for each maneuver.
4. Raw and sGaw should be calculated for each maneuver; do not average tangents.
5. Mean of three or more acceptable efforts should be reported; individual values should be within 10% of mean.

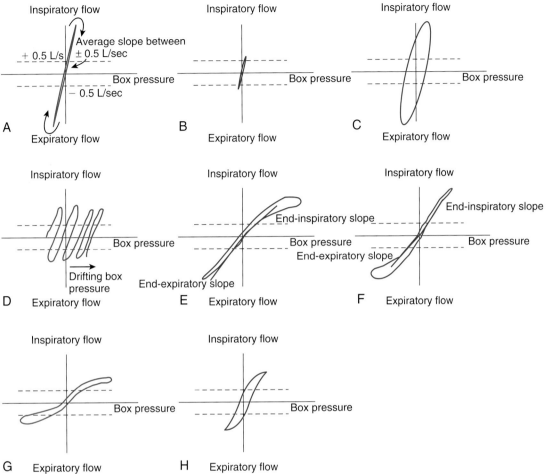

FIG. 4.10 Normal and abnormal open shutter tracings. (A) Normal tracing showing narrow loop and consistent slope on both inspiration and expiration. (B) Small narrow loop caused by a breathing frequency that is too high or volume that is too small. (C) Wide large loop (hysteresis) caused by a breathing frequency that is too low or volume that is too large. (D) Thermal drift caused by the failure of body plethysmograph to come to a steady temperature before obtaining shallow breathing loops. (E) High inspiratory resistance causing hysteresis and flattening of inspiratory portion of the shallow breathing loop. Notice that separate inspiratory and expiratory tangents (slopes) can be obtained. (F) High expiratory resistance causing hysteresis and flattening of expiratory portion of the shallow-breathing loop. (G) High inspiratory and expiratory resistance caused by fixed airway obstruction causing flattening of both inspiratory and expiratory portions of the shallow loops. (H) Typical loop seen in asthma with slight widening and flattening of the loop indicative of overall increased resistance.

second) reduce thermal drift, both in the box and in the pneumotachometer. Shallow breathing helps keep the glottis open, allowing measurement of alveolar pressure. Shallow breathing also allows measurements to be made near FRC. The resistances of the mouthpiece and pneumotachometer are subtracted from the patient's Raw.

Gaw can be calculated as the reciprocal of Raw. Specific conductance is calculated by dividing Gaw by the lung volume at which it was measured, which is V_{TG} calculated from the closed-shutter maneuver. sGaw should be calculated separately for each Raw maneuver because the lung volume at which measurements are made influences Raw and Gaw. After three to five acceptable trials are obtained, calculated Raw and sGaw are averaged. Individual values should be within approximately 10% of the mean (Criteria for Acceptability 4.4).

sRaw is calculated from the ratio of change in box volume (measured through changes in box pressure) to flow during tidal breathing, which is done in practice by taking the slope of the flow-pressure (or specific resistance) loop. The slope may be drawn through the $+0.5\,L/s$ and $-0.5\,L/s$ fixed flow rates or may be drawn between the points of maximal change in box pressure. Measurements should be made at breathing frequencies of 30 to 45 breaths per minute, which is usually near spontaneous breathing frequency for very young children. The final value is taken as the median of five technically valid specific resistance loops.

Computerized plethysmographs permit thoracic gas volume (V_{TG}), Raw, and sGaw to be measured from a combined maneuver. The patient breathes through the pneumotachometer with the plethysmograph sealed. Tidal breathing is recorded with the patient breathing near FRC. The computer stores this end-expiratory volume as a reference point. Then the patient pants, and the open-shutter slope of $\dot{V}/P_{BOX}$ is recorded. The mouth shutter is then closed, and P_{MOUTH}/P_{BOX} is recorded as described previously. The V_{TG} in this maneuver does not equal the FRC because the shutter is closed at a volume different from the FRC. However, the change in volume from the tidal breathing level was stored at the beginning of the maneuver. This volume is the "switch-in" volume described earlier and can be added to or subtracted from the V_{TG} to determine FRC. Most patients pant above their FRC, so the V_{TG} in this combined method is usually slightly greater (Fig. 4.11). Because of this issue, a separate test to measure FRC for use in calculating absolute lung volumes may need to be done and is often recommended.

Significance and Pathophysiology

Reference equations for indices of airway resistance are very limited. Normal values of Raw in adults may range from 0.6 to 2.4 cm $H_2O/L/sec$. Gaw in healthy adults may range between 0.42 and 1.67 L/sec/cm H_2O. sGaw varies in a manner similar to Gaw. sGaw values of less than 0.11 L/sec/cm H_2O/L are consistent with airway obstruction. Measurements are standardized at flow rates of ± 0.5 L/sec, as described previously. Normal values for sRaw in children may range between 9.2 to 17.3 cm H_2O/sec.

Raw in healthy adults is divided across the airway as follows: Nose, mouth, upper airway = 50%
Trachea and bronchi = 30%
Small airways = 20%

Small airways (less than 2 mm in diameter) contribute only approximately one-fifth of the total resistance to flow. Significant obstruction can develop in the small airways with little increase in Raw or decrease in sGaw. Early or mild obstructive processes are not usually identified by abnormal Raw or sGaw. Raw may be increased in an acute asthmatic episode by as much as 3 times the normal values. Inflammation, mucus secretion, and

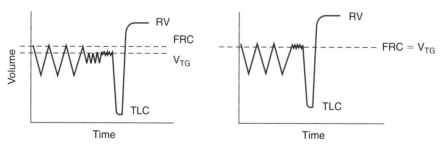

FIG. 4.11 Difference in thoracic gas volume (V_{TG}) and functional residual capacity (FRC) measured in a combined maneuver. On the *left,* a combined open-shutter followed by closed-shutter maneuver was performed to obtain both Raw and V_{TG}. Inhalation is down and exhalation is up. Because V_{TG} drifted above FRC (downward in the tracing) during the open-shutter breathing maneuver, V_{TG} is higher than FRC. V_{TG}, in this case, is still necessary to calculate sGaw, but it is a poor approximation of FRC. On the *right,* only a closed-shutter maneuver was performed to measure V_{TG}, which closely approximates FRC. In this case, a separate open-shutter maneuver is needed to measure Raw followed by a closed-shutter maneuver to calculate sGaw. *RV,* residual volume; *TLC,* total lung capacity.

bronchospasm all increase Raw in the small and medium airways. Raw is increased in advanced emphysema because of airway narrowing and collapse, especially in the bronchioles. Other obstructive diseases (e.g., bronchitis) may cause increases in Raw proportionate to the degree of obstruction in medium and small airways.

Lesions obstructing the larger airways (e.g., tumors, traumatic injuries, or foreign bodies) may also cause a significant increase in Raw. Large airway obstruction is often accompanied by increased work of breathing and dyspnea on exertion. Airflow in the trachea and mainstem bronchi is predominantly turbulent. Any large airway obstruction can exaggerate this turbulent flow. For this reason, Raw and sGaw may be more sensitive to elevations in central airway resistance than FEV_1. Breathing low-density gas mixtures (e.g., helium + oxygen) reduces Raw and therefore the work of breathing. The shapes of the open-shutter breathing loops may give clues as to the underlying pathophysiology, as seen in Fig. 4.10.

Because some patients have changes in sGaw without changes in FEV_1 or FVC after a bronchodilator, and such changes are thought to be clinically significant, measuring bronchodilator response by sGaw may be more sensitive than relying on spirometric indices only. Part of the reason for this may be caused by the anatomic location of airway obstruction, and part may relate to the bronchodilating ability of the deep breath necessarily associated with measuring spirometry, which occurs in healthy subjects and those with mild airway obstruction. Because of this increased sensitivity, sGaw may be less specific for patients with asthma compared with healthy subjects.

Raw is decreased at increased lung volume. The airways (particularly large and medium airways) are distended slightly, and their cross-sectional area increases. For this reason, the V_{TG} is obtained with Raw to derive sGaw. This allows a comparison of values in different patients or in the same patient after treatment. sGaw is particularly useful for assessing changes in airway caliber after bronchodilator therapy or inhalation challenge. sGaw may change significantly after a bronchodilator or inhalation challenge even though other measures of flow (i.e., FEV_1) vary only slightly. The primary site of airway obstruction (i.e., large versus small airways) may determine which parameters reflect changes in airway caliber.

sRaw is similar to sGaw because it considers lung volume. However, sGaw reflects only Raw, whereas sRaw reflects both Raw and lung volume. This may be illustrated by considering an obstructed patient with hyperinflation versus an obstructed patient without hyperinflation. In the former, Raw is elevated and sRaw is increased (increased work to move air through a higher lung volume), but the increased V_{TG} associated with hyperinflation corrects conductance back to normal (normal sGaw). In the latter, Raw is increased and sRaw is increased (increased work to move air through an increased resistance), but sGaw is reduced (elevated Raw is not reduced by altered lung volume).

Raw and sGaw measurements are not influenced by the degree of patient effort, so Raw and sGaw measurements may be useful for determining airway status in patients who are unable or unwilling to exert maximum effort. However, acceptable shallow-breathing maneuvers in the plethysmograph require a certain degree of patient coordination. Not all patients may be able to perform these maneuvers. Patients with severe obstruction may produce pressure–flow curves during shallow breathing that are difficult to measure. Such curves may be flat (see Fig. 4.10) or show widening (hysteresis). Inspiratory and expiratory flows may produce different resistances, causing the curve to appear as a loop (see Fig. 4.10). In these cases, inspiratory flow resistance is usually reported.

In addition to resistance caused by flow through conducting airways, some frictional resistance is caused by the displacement of the lungs, rib cage, and diaphragm. In healthy patients, this tissue resistance is only approximately one-fifth of the total resistance, and therefore total pulmonary resistance is approximately 20% greater than the measured Raw.

In addition to measuring Raw by use of the body plethysmograph, measurement of Raw by means of the forced oscillation technique is becoming increasingly common. For further discussion, see Chapter 10. Another method, more popular outside the United States, especially in children, is the use of the interrupter technique to measure Raw. Both methods do not require special breathing maneuvers and are conducted during quiet tidal breathing, thus making them appealing from the standpoint of ease of performance on the part of the patient.

GAS DISTRIBUTION TESTS: SINGLE-BREATH NITROGEN WASHOUT, CLOSING VOLUME, AND CLOSING CAPACITY

Description

The **single-breath nitrogen-washout test (SBN₂)** measures the distribution of ventilation. Distribution is analyzed by measuring the change in N_2 concentration during expiration of the VC after a single breath of 100% O_2. The evenness of distribution is assessed by two parameters: the change in percentage of N_2 between the 750- and 1250-mL portion of the SBN_2 test ($\Delta\%N_{2\,750-1250}$) and the **slope of phase III** of the expiratory tracing. Each of these indices is recorded as a percentage. Closing volume (CV) is the portion of the VC that can be exhaled from the lungs after the onset of airway closure. CV is also measured from the SBN_2 maneuver and is usually expressed as a percentage of the VC. A related measurement, **closing capacity (CC),** is the sum of the CV and RV. CC is expressed as a percentage of the TLC.

Technique

The test is performed with equipment like that used for the open-circuit $FRCN_2$ determination (see Fig. 4.1A). The patient exhales to RV and then inspires a VC breath of 100% O_2 from a reservoir or demand valve. The 100% O_2 dilutes the N_2 present in the lungs. Without holding the breath, the patient exhales slowly and evenly at a flow of 0.3 to 0.5 L/sec. The N_2 concentration is measured by an N_2 analyzer, and the exhaled volume is measured by the spirometer. The volume expired is plotted against the N_2 concentration on a graph (Fig. 4.12). This washout curve can be divided into four phases:

Phase I: Upper airway gas from the anatomic dead space (V_{Danat}), consisting of 100% O_2.

Phase II: Mixed dead space gas in which the relative concentrations of O_2 and N_2 change abruptly as the V_{Danat} volume is expired.

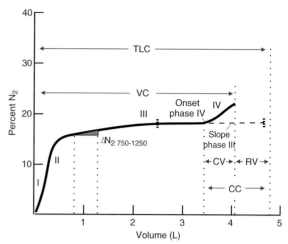

FIG. 4.12 Single-breath nitrogen elimination (SBN_2). A plot of increasing N_2 concentration on expiration after a single VC breath of 100% O_2. The curve is divided into four phases. Phase I is the extreme beginning of the expiration when only O_2 is being exhaled. Phase II shows an abrupt rise in N_2 concentration as mixed bronchial and alveolar air is expired. Phase III is the alveolar gas plateau. N_2 concentration changes slowly as long as ventilation is uniformly distributed. Phase IV is an abrupt increase in N_2 concentration as basal airways close and a larger proportion of gas comes from the N_2-rich lung apices. Several useful parameters are derived from the SBN_2 tracing. The $\Delta N_{2\,750-1250}$ and slope of phase III are indices of the evenness of ventilation distribution. CV can be read directly from the onset of phase IV until RV is reached; VC can also be read directly. RV, TLC, and CC can be calculated if the area under the curve is determined either by planimetry or electronic integration (see text).

Phase III: A plateau caused by the exhalation of alveolar gas in which relative O_2 and N_2 concentrations change slowly and evenly.

Phase IV: An abrupt increase in the concentration of N_2 that continues until RV is reached.

The initial 750 mL of expired gas contains deadspace gas from phases I and II and is not used to assess the distribution of ventilation. The difference in the N_2 concentration between the 750-mL and 1250-mL points is called the $\Delta N2$ ($\%N_{2\,750-1250}$).

The slope of phase III is the change in N_2 concentration from the point at which 30% of the VC remains up to the onset of phase IV. It is recorded as $\Delta\%N_2$ per liter of lung volume.

The volume expired after the onset of phase IV is the CV. CV may be added to the RV, if the RV has been determined, and expressed as the CC. CV is reported as a percentage of VC:

$$\frac{CV}{VC} \times 100$$

CC is recorded as a percentage of TLC:

$$\frac{CC}{TLC} \times 100$$

TLC can be determined from the SBN_2 test by integrating the area of the washout curve. When the volume of N_2 is known, a dilution equation can be used to calculate RV. RV is then added to the measured VC to derive TLC. RV is calculated as follows:

$$RV = VC \times \frac{F_{E\text{-}}N_2}{F_A N_2 - F_{E\text{-}}N_2}$$

where:

$F_E\text{-}N_2$ = mean expired N_2 concentration determined by integration of the area under the curve

$F_A N_2$ = N_2 concentration in the lungs at the beginning of inspiration, approximately 0.75 to 0.79

This method is accurate only in patients who do not have significant obstruction or dead-space–producing disease. CV and CC measurements may be in error if the patient does not perform an acceptable VC maneuver (Criteria for Acceptability 4.5). The inspired and expired VC should be within 5%. The VC during the SBN_2 should match the FVC or VC within 5% or 200 mL. Expiratory flow should be maintained between 0.3 and 0.5 L/sec.

CRITERIA FOR ACCEPTABILITY 4.5

SBN_2

1. Inspired and expired VC should be within 5% or 200 mL.
2. The VC during SBN_2 should be within 200 mL of a previously determined VC.
3. Expiratory flow should be maintained between 0.3 and 0.5 L/sec.
4. The N_2 tracing should show minimal cardiac oscillations.

Significance and Pathophysiology

See Interpretive Strategies 4.3.

INTERPRETIVE STRATEGIES 4.3

SBN_2

1. Was the test performed acceptably? Was the VC reproducible within 5% or 200 mL? Is expiratory flow appropriate?
2. Are reference values appropriate? Age, height, sex, race?
3. Is $\Delta\%N_2$ 750–1250 greater than 1.5%? If so, suspect uneven distribution of ventilation.
4. Is the slope of phase III greater than 1.0% to 1.5%? If so, there is an uneven distribution of ventilation.
5. Is CV/VC% greater than 20% (or age-related expected value)? If so, suspect small airway abnormalities. Correlate with clinical findings.

$\Delta\%N_2$ 750–1250

The normal $\Delta\%N_2$ 750–1250 is 1.5% or less for healthy young adults and slightly higher for healthy older adults (up to approximately 3%). Increased $\Delta\%N_2$ 750–1250 is found in diseases characterized by uneven distribution of gas during inspiration or unequal emptying rates during expiration, such as asthma, COPD, or cystic fibrosis. In patients with severe emphysema, $\Delta\%N_2$ 750–1250 may exceed 10%.

Slope of Phase III

A best-fit line is drawn through the phase III segment of the tracing from the point where 30% of the VC remains above RV to the onset of phase IV. The slope of this line is an index of gas distribution, similar to the $\Delta\%N_2$ 750–1250. Values in healthy young adults range from 0.5% to 1.0% N_2/L of lung volume, with wide variability. Very slow expiratory flow rates may cause oscillations in the tracing of phase III, making the accurate measurement of $\Delta\%N_2$ difficult. These oscillations are attributed to changes in alveolar N_2 concentrations as blood pulses through the pulmonary capillaries during cardiac systole. Increasing the expiratory flow rate slightly eliminates this artifact. Patients who have small VC values may have difficulty exhaling enough gas to make the $\Delta\%N_2$ or slope of phase III meaningful.

Other gases, such as He or sulfur hexafluoride (SF_6), may also be used to assess the distribution of ventilation. The slope of the alveolar phase using these gases may be useful in detecting early changes in the small airways. Detecting these changes may identify bronchiolitis obliterans in recipients of double-lung transplants.

Closing Volume and Closing Capacity

After maximal expiration by an upright patient, more RV remains at the apices of the lungs than at the bases. Gravity causes this difference. When the test gas (O_2) is inspired, the apices receive the gas occupying the patient's dead space, which consists mostly of N_2. O_2 then goes preferentially to the bases of the lungs. Gas concentrations in the lungs become widely different. The apices contain RV gas plus dead-space gas rich in N_2. The bases of the lungs contain a higher concentration of the test gas O_2. Compression of the airways during the subsequent expiration causes the airways to narrow and then close as lung volume approaches RV. The airways at the bases close first because of gravity and the weight of the lung in patients sitting upright. As the airways at the bases close, proportionately more gas comes from the apices (known as the "first in, last out" phenomenon). This appears as an abrupt rise in the concentration of N_2—the onset of phase IV.

The onset of phase IV marks the lung volume at which airway closure begins. The point at which this occurs in the VC depends on the caliber of the small airways. In healthy young adults, airways begin closing after 80% to 90% of the VC has been expired. This equates to a CC in healthy young adults of approximately 30% of the TLC with wide variations. CV and CC may be increased, indicating an earlier onset of airway closure, in the following:

· Elderly patients
· Restrictive disease patterns in which the FRC becomes less than the CV
· Smokers and other patients with early obstructive disease of small airways
· Congestive heart failure when the caliber of the small airways is compromised by edema

Patients with moderate or severe obstructive disease may have no sharp inflection separating phases III and IV of the SBN$_2$. This lack of a clear point of airway closure is the result of the grossly uneven distribution of gas in the lungs. Patients who have airway obstruction typically show greater-than-normal values for the $\Delta\%N_{2\ 750-1250}$ and slope of phase III.

In some patients with no pulmonary disease, the onset of phase IV cannot be accurately determined. Because of the variability in both the CV and CC, the mean of three tests is usually reported. Because of its poor reproducibility, the CV test is not widely used. Although it appears to be a sensitive indicator of abnormalities in the small airways, particularly in smokers, an increased CV/VC ratio is not highly predictive of which individuals will have chronic airway obstruction. To calculate normal values for CV/VC and CC/TLC according to age and sex, see the Evolve website at http://evolve.elsevier.com/Mottram/Ruppel/.

Of note, another commonly available global assessment of the distribution of ventilation is the comparison of the single-breath V_A to the TLC as measured by multiple-breath inert gas washout or by body plethysmography. The V_A is obtained as part of the single-breath diffusing capacity (discussed in Chapter 3) and is the volume of gas at TLC minus the estimated anatomic dead space. As such, the VA is very close to the TLC, with the normal V_A/TLC ratio being greater than or equal to 85%. If the V_A/TLC is less than 85%, this implies there is too much gas maldistribution such that the 10-second breath hold made during the measurement of V_A is not adequate to allow full distribution of the inert gas throughout the lung.

MULTIPLE-BREATH NITROGEN WASHOUT, LUNG CLEARANCE INDEX, AND PHASE III SLOPE ANALYSIS

Description

Another gas distribution test that can be used to assess the distribution of ventilation is the multiple-breath nitrogen washout (MBNW). This test measures inert gas clearance over multiple tidal breaths as the patient breathes pure oxygen and washes out the ambient nitrogen in the lung. The patient essentially performs the same nitrogen-washout test for measuring FRC, except the data are analyzed to also allow a global indication of gas distribution, termed the *lung clearance index* (LCI), and a more specific analysis of the convection- and diffusion-dependent components of the phase III slope. Outside the United States, the multiple-breath washout test can also be performed with inhalation (wash-in phase) and subsequent exhalation (wash-out phase) of inert gases such as helium or sulfur hexafluoride (SF_6).

Technique

The MBNW test is performed in the same manner as described for the open-circuit multiple-breath nitrogen-washout described previously. However, to accurately measure the LCI and components of the phase III slope, the ATS-ERS has recommended specific criteria of acceptability. In particular, these specify a regular breathing pattern with tidal volumes of 1.0 to 1.3 L, if feasible, with test termination indicated by at least three consecutive breaths with the end-tidal nitrogen concentration below one-fortieth of the starting concentration.

Significance and Pathophysiology

The LCI is defined as the number of FRC lung volume turnovers (cumulative expired volume/FRC) required to drive the nitrogen concentration down to one-fortieth of the starting nitrogen concentration. The normal LCI is in the range of 6 to 9, depending on patient age and equipment used. Clinical studies have suggested that LCI may be a more sensitive indicator of airway disease than FEV_1, and some clinical trials are now using LCI as a primary outcome measure in response to intervention. For the phase III slope analysis, several steps are performed to determine the convection and diffusion-convection interaction-dependent components of ventilation inhomogeneity, termed the *conductive slope* (S_{cond}) and the *acinar slope* (S_{acin}), respectively. S_{cond} and S_{acin} are thought to roughly correspond to the terminal conducting airways and acinar airways, respectively. These slopes are currently used as research tools; for example, in asthma, both slopes are abnormal, implicating peripheral lung dysfunction.

SUMMARY

- To measure TLC, the FRC is measured first. FRC can be measured with N_2-washout ($FRCN_2$), He-dilution (FRC_{He}), or body plethysmograph (FRC_{pleth}) techniques.
- TLC is calculated by adding the inspiratory capacity (measured from simple spirometry) to the FRC.
- The ERV (measured by simple spirometry) may be subtracted from FRC to derive RV.
- The addition of RV and VC (from spirometry) also provides an estimate of TLC.
- The plethysmographic technique is the preferred method because it is largely independent of gas distribution in the lungs.
- The plethysmographic technique also allows the measurement of airway resistance (Raw) and its volume-associated parameters, sGaw and sRaw.
- Gas-dilution techniques may underestimate lung volumes in the presence of significant airway obstruction.
- Analysis of expired N_2 after a single breath of oxygen (SBN_2) provides a means of assessing gas distribution in the lungs. A more sophisticated analysis is possible by analyzing the breath-by-breath nitrogen washout that occurs during the MBNW test.

CASE STUDIES

CASE 4.1

HISTORY

The subject is a 27-year-old male high school teacher whose chief complaint is dyspnea on exertion. He states that his breathlessness has worsened over the past several months. He has smoked one pack of cigarettes per day for 10 years (10 pack-years). He denies a cough or sputum production. No one in his family ever had emphysema, asthma, chronic bronchitis, carcinoma, or tuberculosis. There is no history of exposure to extraordinary environmental pollutants.

PULMONARY FUNCTION TESTING
Personal Data

Sex:	Male
Age:	27 yr
Height:	65 in.
Weight:	297 lb
Body surface area (BSA):	2.28 m^2

Spirometry and Airway Resistance

	Measured	Predicted	% Predicted
FVC (L)	2.9	4.7	62
FEV$_1$ (L)	2.47	3.86	64
FEV$_1$/FVC (%)	85	82	–
FEF$_{25\%-75\%}$ (L/sec)	4.62	4.35	106
FEF$_{50\%}$ (L/sec)	4.94	5.82	85
MVV (L/min)	178	130	137
Raw (cm H$_2$O/ L/sec)	2.33	0.6–2.4	–
sGaw (L/sec/cm H$_2$O/L)	0.23	0.12–0.50	–

MVV, Maximal voluntary ventilation.

Lung Volumes (by Plethysmograph)

	Measured	Predicted	% Predicted
VC (L)	2.9	4.7	62
IC (L)	1.96	2.91	67
ERV (L)	0.94	1.8	59
FRC (L)	1.87	3.29	57
RV (L)	0.93	1.49	57
TLC (L)	3.83	6.2	62
RV/TLC (%)	24	24	–

Technologist's Comments

Spirometry results met all ATS-ERS acceptability and repeatability recommendations. Good subject cooperation and effort.

QUESTIONS

1. What is the interpretation of the following?
   a. Spirometry
   b. Lung volumes
   c. Airway resistance
2. What is the cause of the subject's symptoms?
3. What other tests might be indicated?
4. What treatment might be recommended based on these findings?

DISCUSSION
Interpretation

All data from spirometry and lung volumes are acceptable. Spirometry shows a decreased FVC and FEV$_1$. The FEV$_{1\%}$ is normal. Flows are within normal limits, as is the MVV. Raw is near the ULN, but sGaw is normal. Lung volumes are decreased, with the RV/TLC ratio preserved.

Impression: Moderate restrictive lung disease without evidence of obstruction. The restrictive pattern may be related to the subject's weight. Recommend arterial blood gas testing to evaluate gas exchange abnormalities.

Cause of Symptoms

This case is a good example of what might be considered a pure restrictive defect. A proportional decrease in all lung volumes, including FVC and FEV$_1$, is characteristic of a restrictive process. Flows such as FEF$_{25\%-75\%}$ or FEF$_{50\%}$ show little or no decrease (see subject's flow-volume curve). In addition, characteristic of simple restriction is the well-preserved ratio of FEV$_1$ to FVC. The volume expired in the first second was in correct proportion to the VC despite decreases in their absolute volumes. The MVV demonstrates the subject's ability to move a normal maximal volume. This may be accomplished, despite moderately severe restriction, by an increase in the rate rather than the tidal volume.

The explanation for the restrictive pattern lies in the subject's weight of 297 pounds. His actual weight

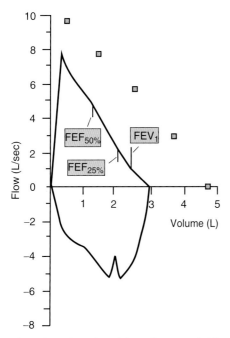

Flow-volume loop from the subject. The upward tick mark superimposed on the loop denotes the FEV_1, whereas downward tick marks show $FEF_{50\%}$ and $FEF_{25\%}$, respectively. The small shaded boxes represent the subject's reference values.

is approximately 200% of his ideal weight. Obesity commonly causes restrictive patterns.

Other Tests

The subject returned for analysis of arterial blood gases, which revealed resting hypoxemia and slightly elevated Pa_{CO_2}. Blood gas measurements confirmed the degree of impairment caused by the moderately severe restrictive pattern. Other tests that might be considered include ventilatory response tests for hypoxemia or hypercapnia (Chapter 5). Studies to diagnose sleep apnea might be indicated if the subject had symptoms of disordered breathing during sleep or excessive daytime sleepiness. This subject's borderline Raw suggests upper airway involvement, which might predispose him to obstructive sleep apnea. Obesity is also associated with an increased risk of asthma, which may indicate the need for challenge testing (e.g., methacholine) if the patient reports suggestive symptoms.

Treatment

The subject was referred to a dietician for counseling in weight management.

CASE 4.2

HISTORY

The subject is a 37-year-old pipefitter whose chief complaint is shortness of breath at rest and with exertion. His dyspnea has worsened in the past 6 months, so much so that he is no longer able to work. Additional symptoms include a dry cough. He admits some sputum production when he has a chest cold. He has smoked one pack of cigarettes per day for 19 years (19 pack-years). He quit smoking approximately 3 weeks before the tests. His father died of emphysema and his mother of lung cancer. His brother is in good health. His occupational exposure includes working for the past 13 years in the assembly room of a boiler plant. He admits to seldom using the respirators provided at work despite a dusty environment.

PULMONARY FUNCTION TESTS
Personal Data

Sex:	Male
Age:	37 yr
Height:	69 in.
Weight:	143 lb

Spirometry

	Pre BD	Predicted	% Predicted	Post BD	% Predicted	% Change
FVC (L)	3.04	5.05	60	3.1	61	+2%
FEV_1 (L)	2.03	3.90	52	2.26	58	+11%
FEV_1/FVC (%)	67	77	–	73	–	+9%
$FEF_{25\%-75\%}$ (L/sec)	1.3	4.09	32	1.60	39	+23%
$FEF_{50\%}$ (L/sec)	2.12	5.78	37	2.42	42	+14%
$FEF_{25\%}$ (L/sec)	0.78	2.95	26	1.2	41	+54%
MVV (L/min)	83	141	59	91	65	+10%
Raw (cm H_2O)/L/sec)	2.51	0.6–2.4	–	2.47	–	-2%
sGaw (L/sec/cm H_2O/L)	0.14	0.11–0.44	–	0.15	–	+7%

Lung Volumes (by N_2 Washout)

	Measured	Predicted	% Predicted
VC (L)	3.04	5.05	60
IC (L)	1.62	3.18	51
ERV (L)	1.42	1.87	76
FRC (L)	2.75	3.81	72
RV (L)	1.33	1.94	69
TLC (L)	4.37	6.99	63
RV/TLC (%)	30	28	–

Technologist's Comments

Spirometry results met all ATS-ERS recommendations, prebronchodilator and postbronchodilator. Lung volumes by N_2 washout: All maneuvers were performed acceptably. Duplicate measurements were averaged. Raw and sGaw efforts were performed appropriately.

QUESTIONS

1. What is the interpretation of the following?
   a. Prebronchodilator spirometry
   b. Response to bronchodilator
   c. Airway resistance and conductance
   d. Lung volumes
2. What is the cause of the subject's symptoms?
3. What other tests might be indicated?
4. What treatment might be recommended based on these findings?

DISCUSSION

Interpretation

All data from spirometry and lung volumes are acceptable. Spirometry shows a reduced FVC and FEV_1. The $FEF_{25\%-75\%}$, $FEF_{50\%}$, and $FEF_{25\%}$ are all reduced. The MVV is low. Raw and sGaw are close to their respective limits of normal. Response to bronchodilators is borderline, with an increase in the FEV_1 of 230 mL (11%). The $FEF_{25\%}$ improved somewhat more than the other flows. The subject's lung volumes are all decreased. His RV/TLC ratio is normal.

Impression: There is mild airway obstruction combined with a restrictive pattern. The response to inhaled bronchodilator medication is borderline. A trial of bronchodilators should be considered. Arterial blood gas testing to evaluate possible hypoxemia is recommended.

Cause of Symptoms

He typifies a patient who has combined obstructive and restrictive disease. His spirometry results indicate that a mild obstructive component is present, as revealed by his FEV_1 (52% of predicted) and the other flows. His FEV_1/FVC, however, is close to normal because his FVC is also reduced. His symptoms of cough and sputum suggest an obstructive process. His smoking and family history place him at risk. Because FVC can be reduced in either obstructive or restrictive processes, spirometry alone would not have adequately defined the subject's disease.

Lung volume measurements (see subject's N_2-washout curve) confirm the presence of a restrictive component (see Fig. 4.8). All lung volumes are reduced in similar proportions. The reduction in VC matches decreases in FRC, RV, and TLC. The patient's history and symptoms suggest the possibility of restrictive or obstructive disease or both. The obstructive component may be related to the subject's smoking history, but the etiology of the restrictive component is less clear. On further inquiry, it was learned that the patient's occupation involved exposure to asbestos,

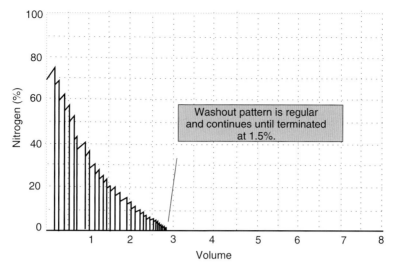

Open-circuit multiple-breath N$_2$-washout graph. Tracing shows a normal pattern of washout with N$_2$ concentration plotted against lung volume (functional reserve capacity [FRC]). The test was terminated when N$_2$ concentration fell to less than 1.5%.

which can cause fibrosis and/or carcinoma. Chest radiographs revealed linear calcifications of the diaphragmatic pleura and pleural thickening, as well as fibrotic changes. These findings are all consistent with asbestos exposure.

Other Tests

A sputum examination was performed, and asbestos bodies were identified from the subject's sputum. Open-lung biopsy was deferred because both the obstructive and restrictive components seemed to be appropriately identified. Analysis of resting arterial blood gases is probably indicated because the subject has a significant degree of restriction. Diffusing capacity (D$_{LCO}$) could also be used to identify possible gas exchange abnormalities.

Because of his dyspnea on exertion, the patient returned for an exercise evaluation. He walked on a treadmill with an arterial catheter in place. His Pa$_{O_2}$ fell from 65 mm Hg (rest) to 55 mm Hg after only 2 minutes of walking at 2 miles per hour. The desaturation was corrected when the subject breathed O$_2$ by nasal cannula at 1 L/min. A baseline 6-Minute Walk Test would allow future assessments of the patient's functional capacity and prognosis.

Treatment

The patient was given a trial of bronchodilators and reported significant symptomatic improvement. He began using supplemental O$_2$ via a portable system and was able to return to work in a position modified to accommodate his abilities.

CASE 4.3

HISTORY

A 68-year-old white woman, whose chief complaint is worsening dyspnea, was seen by a pulmonologist in the office. She admitted to having been a heavy smoker (90 pack-years) but recently quit. She has a productive cough and trouble sleeping at night. She had worked in the meat department of a grocery store for many years, and there was no history of exposure to extraordinary environmental pollutants. She is 62 inches tall and weighs 110 pounds. Her chest radiograph had an emphysematous appearance with increased diameters.

DOCTOR'S OFFICE PULMONARY FUNCTION TEST

Spirometry

	Pre-BD	Predicted	% Predicted	Post-BD	% Predicted	% Change
FVC (L)	2.18	3.63	60	2.38	66	+9%
FEV_1 (L)	1.09	2.57	42	1.19	46	+9%
FEV_1/FVC (%)	50	71	—	50	—	0%
$FEF_{25\%-75\%}$ (L/sec)	0.65	2.38	26	0.71	30	+9%

BD, Bronchodilator.

Lung Volumes (by N_2 Washout)

	Measured	Predicted	% Predicted
VC (L)	2.55	3.63	70
IC (L)	2.05	2.02	101
ERV (L)	0.50	0.89	56
$FRCN_2$ (L)	2.58	2.80	92
RV (L)	2.08	1.91	109
TLC (L)	4.63	4.82	96
RV/TLC (%)	45	40	—

After seeing the results of the office pulmonary function test, the doctor ordered another pulmonary function test at the area hospital.

HOSPITAL PULMONARY FUNCTION TEST

Spirometry and D_{LCO}

	Pre-BD	Predicted	% Predicted	Post-BD	% Predicted	% Change
FVC (L)	2.30	3.63	63	2.45	67	+6%
FEV_1 (L)	1.12	2.57	44	1.30	51	+16%
FEV_1/FVC (%)	49	71	—	53	—	+8%
$FEF_{25\%-75\%}$ (L/sec)	0.59	2.38	25	0.83	35	+41%
Raw (cm H_2O/L/sec)	2.89	0.6–2.4	—	—	—	—
sGaw (L/sec/cm H_2O/L)	0.06	0.12–0.50		—	—	—
D_{LCO} (mL/min/mm Hg)	17.4	23.5	74	—	—	—
K_{CO} (mL/min/mm Hg/L)	3.66	4.88	75	—	—	—

Lung Volumes (by Plethysmography)

	Measured	Predicted	% Predicted
VC (L)	2.66	3.63	73
IC (L)	1.80	2.02	89
ERV (L)	0.86	0.89	97
FRC_{pleth} (L)	3.99	2.80	142
RV (L)	3.13	1.91	164
TLC (L)	5.79	4.82	120
RV/TLC (%)	54	40	—

QUESTIONS

1. What is the interpretation of the pulmonary function tests done in the doctor's office?
2. What is the interpretation of the pulmonary function tests done in the hospital laboratory?
3. Why is there such a difference?

DISCUSSION

Interpretation of Tests from Doctor's Office

Pulmonary function test data from the doctor's office reveal normal lung volumes (TLC, FRC, and RV) and a reduced VC. The results also reveal severe airflow limitation with a small but clinically insignificant response to the bronchodilator (9%, 100-mL improvement in FEV_1). The interpretation of these data would be a severe obstructive disorder.

Interpretation of Tests from Hospital Laboratory

Pulmonary function data from the hospital pulmonary function laboratory, which used a body plethysmograph, reveal severe airflow limitation, decreased diffusing capacity, but markedly increased lung volumes. There is a larger bronchodilator response (16%, 180-mL improvement in FEV_1). The interpretation of these data is that of severe airflow limitation.

Why the Difference?

The major difference between the two pulmonary function tests is the measurement of FRC. In the doctor's office, the $FRCN_2$ value was 2.58 L. In the hospital laboratory, the body plethysmography was used in determining an FRC_{pleth} of 3.99 L. The difference between these values can be explained by the presence of trapped gas or poorly communicating airways. In subjects with significant airway obstruction, the gas-dilutional methods (i.e., N_2 washout and He dilution) will likely underestimate true lung volume, and the body plethysmograph is a better instrument to use.

CASE 4.4

HISTORY

A 38-year-old man is referred to the pulmonary function testing lab for testing for asthma. The subject has classic symptoms of intermittent shortness of breath, especially after exercise, and a bronchodilator relieves the symptoms, but spirometry in the primary care office reveals normal FEV_1, FVC, and FEV_1/FVC, with no bronchodilator response.

	Pre-BD			Post-BD		
	Measured	Predicted	% Predicted	Measured	% Predicted	% Change
FVC (L)	4.17	4.89	85	4.23	86	+1%
FEV_1 (L)	3.46	3.79	91	3.49	92	+1%
FEV_1/FVC (%)	83	77	—	83	—	0%

The pulmonologist reviews these data and orders lung volumes and airway resistance to be measured pre- and postbronchodilator. The results are as follows:

	Measured	Predicted	% Predicted	Measured	% Predicted	% Change
TLC (L)	6.13	6.76	91	5.55	82	−9%
FRC (box) (L)	2.97	3.70	80	2.28	62	−23%
RV (L)	2.09	1.87	112	1.44	77	−31%
Raw (cm H_2O/L/sec)	2.30	0.2–2.5		1.18		−49%
sGaw (L/sec/cm H_2O)	0.14	0.11–0.40		0.32		+128%

Technologist's Comments

Lung volumes and airway resistance and conductance measurements met all ATS-ERS criteria for repeatability and acceptability. The subject gave good effort and cooperation.

QUESTIONS

1. How do you interpret the spirometry, lung volume, and airway resistance measurements?
2. Do you think this information is sufficient to explain the subject's symptoms?
3. How would you treat this subject?

DISCUSSION

Interpretation

1. The lung function tests show normal spirometry with no bronchodilator response based on the change in FEV_1 or FVC. Baseline lung volumes are normal, with a slightly elevated RV/TLC, suggesting the possibility of air trapping. Following the bronchodilator, the FRC and RV significantly decrease, suggesting less air trapping after the bronchodilator. Baseline airway resistance and conductance are normal, but after the bronchodilator, resistance falls substantially, and conductance increases. Because resistance measurements are volume dependent and lung volumes changed here, one must use the sGaw to assess any bronchodilator response, which, in this case, increased by more than 100%.

2. The subject's symptoms can definitely be explained by these findings because dyspnea is strongly associated with air trapping, which the subject has at baseline and is markedly reduced after the bronchodilator.

3. Although there was no bronchodilator response on spirometry, the subject had clinical improvement with bronchodilator therapy and clearly has a bronchodilator response in lung volumes and airway resistance. A reasonable significant response in lung volumes is a decrease of approximately 20% or more, and in sGaw, it is an increase of approximately 25% or more. The reason spirometry did not change is that an "isovolume shift" in airflow caused by the bronchodilator, such that under conditions of less hyperinflation, flows are greater at any given absolute lung volume. In fact, approximately 15% of subjects with suspected obstructive airway disease may be missed by spirometry testing alone, but most will be identified by performing additional measurements of volumes or airway resistance. This subject should continue to be treated with the bronchodilator.

SELF-ASSESSMENT QUESTIONS

Entry-Level

1. Which of the following *cannot* be used to measure FRC?
   a. Single-breath nitrogen washout
   b. Open-circuit multiple-breath nitrogen washout
   c. Closed-circuit multiple-breath helium dilution
   d. Body plethysmography
2. In patients with obstructive lung disease, the gas-dilution methods for FRC determination
   a. overestimate FRC.
   b. equal body plethysmography FRC.
   c. underestimate FRC.
   d. equal radiographic FRC.
3. Standardizing the measurement of lung volumes, the N_2-washout test is considered complete when the
   a. N_2 concentration has decreased to less than 2.5% after 7 minutes.
   b. N_2 concentration has decreased to less than 1.5% for at least three consecutive breaths.
   c. N_2 concentration changes by less than 0.02% in 30 seconds.
   d. N_2 concentration has reached equilibrium.
4. A patient has the following results from a pulmonary function test:

VC	4.35 L
IC	3.15 L
ERV	1.20 L
FRC_{He}	3.40 L

What is the patient's RV, and what is the RV/TLC ratio?
   a. 4.60 L and 70%
   b. 1.80 L and 27%

c. 2.20 L and 34%
d. 1.95 L and 26%

5. A patient has the following lung volumes measured using a body plethysmograph:

	Measured	Predicted	% Predicted
VC (L)	3.50	4.30	81
FRC_{pleth} (L)	3.80	3.00	127
RV (L)	3.00	2.00	150
TLC (L)	7.20	6.30	114

These values are most consistent with
a. normal lung volumes.
b. a restrictive pattern as in pulmonary fibrosis.
c. an obstructive pattern such as emphysema.
d. a mixed obstructive and restrictive pattern.

6. The calculation of FRC with the body plethysmograph is based on
a. Charles' law.
b. Poiseuille's law.
c. Boyle's law.
d. Dalton's law.

7. Which is the correct formula for sGaw?
a. sGaw = Raw × TLC
b. sGaw = Raw × V_{TG}
c. sGaw = (1/Raw)/V_{TG}
d. sGaw = (1/Raw)/TLC

8. Which of the following are true about the measurement of lung volumes using the body plethysmograph?
1. The plethysmograph measures all gas in the thorax.
2. Gas in the thorax that does not communicate with the mouth is not measured by the plethysmograph.
3. FRC_{pleth} is often larger than gas-dilutional FRC determinations.
4. FRC_{pleth} can overestimate true FRC in severe airway obstruction.
   a. 1, 2, 3, and 4
   b. 1 and 2
   c. 1, 3, and 4
   d. 2 and 3

9. A 53-year-old woman has the following measurements obtained during pulmonary function testing:

FVC	2.55 L
FEV_1	1.20 L
FEV_1/FVC	47%
FRC_{He}	2.32 L
FRC_{pleth}	3.59 L

Which of the following best explains these findings?
a. A leak during the FRC_{He} determination
b. Normal pulmonary function
c. Airflow obstruction with air trapping
d. Poor patient effort

10. In measuring FRC by body plethysmography, which of the following is most correct?
1. The patient should pant at a rate between 0.5 and 1 Hz.
2. The patient should pant at about 90 breaths/min.
3. The largest of three acceptable tests is reported.
4. The average of three acceptable tests that agree within 5% is reported.
   a. 1 and 3 only
   b. 2 and 4 only
   c. 1 and 4 only
   d. 1, 2, and 3

11. A 25-year-old patient performs an SBN_2 test and records a slope of phase III of 2.9%. This value is
a. consistent with increased physiologic dead space.
b. indicative of uneven distribution of gas within the lungs.
c. within normal limits.
d. consistent with a gas analyzer malfunction.

12. A patient with alpha-1 antitrypsin deficiency and severe airway obstruction has lung volumes measured with the open-circuit N_2-washout method and by plethysmography, with the following results:

FRCN$_2$	2.99 L
FRC$_{pleth}$	4.58 L
VC	2.77 L
IC	1.54 L
FRC predicted	3.67 L

The volume of trapped gas is
a. 0.91 L.
b. 3.04 L.
c. 1.81 L.
d. 1.59 L.

13. A patient with an FEV$_1$ of 1.24 L and an FVC of 3.10 L performs the FRC$_{He}$ test. The He concentration between 6 and 6.5 minutes changed by 0.1%, and between 7 and 7.5 minutes, it changed by 0.08%. The technician correctly concludes that equilibration has not been reached. Which is the most likely explanation?
a. The patient is malingering.
b. The N$_2$ analyzer has malfunctioned.
c. The CO$_2$ absorber is contaminated.
d. This is consistent with severe airway obstruction.

14. A 30-year-old man is being tested for asthma but has normal spirometry at baseline and no change after a bronchodilator. Which of the following parameters could be used to assess whether the patient has a bronchodilator response?
a. sGaw
b. TLC
c. Raw
d. FEV$_1$/FVC

SELECTED BIBLIOGRAPHY

General References

Crapo, R. O., Morris, A. H., Clayton, P. D., et al. (1982). Lung volumes in healthy nonsmoking adults. *Bulletin European de Physiopathologie Respiratoire, 18*, 419.

Forster, R. E. (1988). *The lung: Clinical physiology and pulmonary function tests* (3rd ed.). St. Louis, MO: Mosby.

Goldman, H. I., & Becklake, M. R. (1959). Respiratory function tests: Normal values at median altitudes and the prediction of normal results. *American Review of Tuberculosis Pulmonary Disease, 79*, 457.

Hibbert, M. E., Lanigan, A., Raven, J., et al. (1988). Relation of arm span to height and the prediction of lung function. *Thorax, 43*, 657.

Jones, R. L., & Nzekwu, M. M. (2006). The effects of body mass index on lung volumes. *Chest, 130*, 827–833.

Ries, A. (1989). Measurement of lung volumes. *Clinics in Chest Medicine, 10*, 177–186.

Ruppel, G. L. (2012). What is the clinical value of lung volumes? *Respiratory Care, 57*, 26–38.

Spirometry and Lung Volumes

Dykstra, B. J., Scanlon, P. D., Kester, M. M., Beck, K. C., & Enright, P. L. (1999). Lung volumes in 4,774 patients with obstructive lung disease. *Chest, 115*(1), 68–74.

Gardner, Z., Ruppel, G., & Kaminsky, D. A. (2011). Grading the severity of obstruction in mixed obstructive-restrictive lung disease. *Chest, 140*, 598–603.

Hyatt, R. E., Cowl, C. T., Bjoraker, J. A., & Scanlon, P. D. (2009). Conditions associated with an abnormal nonspecific pattern of pulmonary function tests. *Chest, 135*(2), 419–424.

Smith, H. R., Irvin, C. G., & Cherniack, R. M. (1992). The utility of spirometry in the diagnosis of reversible airways obstruction. *Chest, 101*, 1577–1581.

Plethysmographic Lung Volumes

Begin, P., & Peslin, R. (1984). Influence of panting frequency on thoracic gas volume measurements in chronic obstructive pulmonary disease. *American Review of Respiratory Diseases, 130*, 121.

Borg, B. M., & Thompson, B. R. (2012). The measurement of lung volumes using body plethysmography: a comparison of methodologies. *Respiratory Care, 57*, 1076–1083.

Criee, C. P., Sorichter, S., Smith, H. J., et al. (2011). Body plethysmography—Its principles and clinical use. *Respiratory Medicine, 105*, 959–971.

Dubois, A. B., Bothelo, S. Y., Bedell, G. H., et al. (1956). A rapid plethysmographic method for measuring thoracic gas volume: A comparison with a nitrogen washout method for measuring functional residual capacity. *Journal of Clinical Investigation, 35*, 322.

Habib, M. P., & Engel, L. A. (1978). Influence of the panting technique on the plethysmographic measurement of thoracic gas volume. *American Review of Respiratory Diseases, 117*, 265.

Jones, R. L., & Nzekwu, M. M. (2006). The effects of body mass index on lung volumes. *Chest, 130*(3), 827–833.

Lourenco, R. V., & Chung, S. Y. K. (1967). Calibration of a body plethysmograph for measurement of lung volume. *American Review of Respiratory Diseases, 95*, 687.

O'Donnell, C. R., Bankier, A. A., Stielbellehner, L., et al. (2010). Comparison of plethysmographic and helium dilution lung volumes: Which is best in COPD? *Chest, 137*(5), 1108–1115.

Rodenstein, D. O., Stanescu, D. C., & Francis, C. (1982). Demonstration of failure of body plethysmography in airway obstruction. *Journal of Applied Physiology, 52*, 949.

Airway Resistance

Bisgaard, H., & Nielsen, K. G. (2005). Plethysmographic measurements of specific airway resistance in young children. *Chest, 128*, 355–362.

Blonshine, S., & Goldman, M. D. (2008). Optimizing performance of respiratory airflow resistance measurements. *Chest, 134*, 1304–1309.

Kaminsky, D. A. (2012). What does airway resistance tell us about lung function? *Respiratory Care, 57*, 85–99.

Khalid, I, Morris, Z. Q., & DiGiovine, B. (2009). Specific conductance criteria for a positive methacholine challenge test: are the American Thoracic Society guidelines rather generous? *Respiratory Care, 54*, 1168–1174.

Gas Dilution Lung Volumes

Hathirat, S., Renzetti, A. D., & Mitchell, M. (1970). Measurement of the total lung capacity by helium dilution in a constant volume system. *American Review of Respiratory Diseases, 102*, 760.

Kaminsky, D. A. (2013). Multiple breath nitrogen washout profiles in asthmatic patients: What do they mean clinically? *Journal of Allergy and Clinical Immunology, 131*, 1329–1330.

McMichael, J. (1939). A rapid method of determining lung capacity. *Clinical Science, 4*, 16.

Meneely, G. R., Ball, C. O., Kory, R. C., et al. (1960). A simplified closed-circuit helium dilution method for the determination of the residual volume of the lungs. *American Journal of Medicine, 28*, 824.

Robinson, P. D., Goldman, M. D., & Gustafsson, P. M. (2009). Inert gas washout: Theoretical background and clinical utility in respiratory disease. *Respiration, 78*, 339–355.

Robinson, P. D., Latzin, P., Verbanck, S., et al. (2013). Consensus statement for inert gas washout measurement using multiple- and single-breath tests. *European Respiratory Journal, 41*, 507–522.

Rodenstein, D. O., & Stanescu, D. C. (1982). Reassessment of lung volume measurements by helium dilution and by body plethysmography in chronic airflow obstruction. *American Review of Respiratory Diseases, 126*, 1040.

Schaaning, C. G., & Gulsvik, A. (1973). Accuracy and precision of helium dilution technique and body plethysmography in measuring lung volume. *Scandinavian Journal of Clinical and Laboratory Investigation, 32*, 271.

Gas Distribution

Berend, N., Glanville, A. R., & Grunstein, M. M. (1984). Determinants of the slope of phase III of the single-breath nitrogen test. *Bulletin Européen de Physiopathologie Respiratoire, 20*, 521.

Buist, A. S., & Ross, B. B. (1973). Quantitative analysis of the alveolar plateau in the diagnosis of early airway obstruction. *American Review of Respiratory Diseases, 108*, 1078–1087.

Estenne, M., Van Muylem, A., Knoop, C., et al. (2000). Detection of obliterative bronchiolitis after lung transplantation by indexes of ventilation distribution. *American Journal of Respiratory and Critical Care Medicine, 162*, 1047–1051.

Fowler, W. S. (1949). Lung function studies. III. Uneven pulmonary ventilation in normal subjects and in patients with pulmonary disease. *Journal of Applied Physiology, 2*, 283.

Hathirat, S., Renzetti, A. D., & Mitchell, M. (1970). Intrapulmonary gas distribution: A comparison of the helium mixing time and nitrogen single-breath test in normal and diseased subjects. *American Review of Respiratory Diseases, 102*, 750.

Standards and Guidelines

American Association for Respiratory Care. (2001). Clinical practice guidelines: Body plethysmography: 2001 revision and update. *Respiratory Care, 46*, 506–513.

American Association for Respiratory Care. (2001). Clinical practice guidelines: Static lung volumes: 2001 revision and update. *Respiratory Care, 46,* 531–539.

American Thoracic Society. (1991). Lung function testing: Selection of reference values and interpretive strategies. *American Review of Respiratory Diseases, 144,* 1202.

American Thoracic Society. (2016). *Pulmonary Function Laboratory Management and Procedure Manual,* Third Edition: American Thoracic Society.

British Thoracic Society and Association of Respiratory Technicians and Physiologists. (1994). Guidelines for the measurement of respiratory function. *Respiratory Medicine, 88,* 165–194.

Martin, R., & Macklem, P. T. (1973). Suggested standardization procedures for closing volume determinations (nitrogen method). *DHD-NHLBI.*

Quanjer, P. H., Tammeling, G. J., Cotes, J. E., et al. (1993). Lung volumes and forced ventilatory flows. Report Working Party Standardization of Lung Function Tests, European Community for Steel and Coal. Official Statement of the European Respiratory Society. *European Respiratory Journal Supplement, 16,* 5–40.

Wanger, J., Clausen, J. L., Coates, A., et al. (2005). Standardisation of the measurement of lung volumes. *European Respiratory Journal, 26,* 511–522.

Chapter 5

Ventilation and Ventilatory Control Tests

CHAPTER OUTLINE

LEARNING OBJECTIVES

After studying the chapter and reviewing the figures, tables, and case studies, you should be able to do the following:

Entry-level

1. Describe the measurement of tidal volume and minute ventilation.
2. Identify at least two causes of decreased minute ventilation.
3. Calculate the V_D/V_T ratio using the modified Bohr equation.

Advanced

1. Compare the calculation of V_D/V_T using Pa_{CO_2} and $P_{ET_{CO_2}}$.
2. List at least two causes for an increased V_D/V_T ratio.
3. Explain the function of a variable CO_2 scrubber in a circuit for measuring ventilatory response to hypoxia.
4. Describe the high-altitude simulation test (HAST).

KEY TERMS

alveolar dead space
alveolar ventilation ($\dot{V}_A$)
anatomic dead space
Bohr equation
end-tidal P_{CO_2}
high-altitude simulation test (HAST)

hypercapnia
hypoxemia
occlusion pressure (P_{100} or $P_{0.1}$)
recruitment
respiratory dead space (V_D)
respiratory exchange ratio (RER)

respiratory frequency (f_b)
tidal volume (V_T)
V_D/V_T ratio
ventilatory response

The chapter discusses the measurement of ventilation and its components: tidal volume (V_T), respiratory frequency (f_b), and minute ventilation ($\dot{V}_E$). Wasted or dead-space ventilation is defined, and techniques for estimating dead space (V_D) and alveolar ventilation ($\dot{V}_A$) are described. Because a variety of diseases can increase dead space, measurements of V_D and the V_D/V_T **ratio** are used to evaluate many disorders. Ventilation and V_D measurements are used in several different clinical situations. These parameters may be measured in the critical care unit and in the pulmonary function or exercise laboratory.

Assessment of ventilatory responses is closely related to the measurement of resting ventilation. The responses to two stimuli, carbon dioxide (CO_2) and oxygen (O_2), are commonly evaluated. **Ventilatory response** is usually assessed by measuring the change in ventilation that occurs with elevated CO_2 (**hypercapnia**) or decreased O_2 (**hypoxemia**). The output of the central respiratory centers is also sometimes measured as the pressure developed during the first tenth of a second when the airway is blocked (P_{100} or $P_{0.1}$). Another related test that has recently become clinically significant is the **high-altitude simulation test (HAST).** This test uses a reduced inspiratory oxygen concentration to mimic elevation, but instead of measuring the ventilatory response, the patient's oxygen status is evaluated.

TIDAL VOLUME, RATE, AND MINUTE VENTILATION

Description

Tidal volume (V_T) is the volume of gas inspired or expired during each respiratory cycle (see Fig. 2.1). It is usually measured in liters or milliliters and corrected to body temperature, pressure, and saturation (BTPS). Conventionally, the volume expired is expressed as V_T. The respiratory rate is the number of breaths per minute (sometimes called *breathing frequency* or *respiratory frequency* or f_b). The total volume of gas expired per minute is $\dot{V}_E$, or minute ventilation. $\dot{V}_E$ includes alveolar and dead-space ventilation and is recorded in liters per minute, BTPS.

Technique

V_T can be measured directly by simple spirometry (see Fig. 2.1). The patient breathes into a volume-displacement or flow-sensing spirometer (see Chapter 11). Volume change may be measured directly from the excursions of a volume spirometer. V_T may also be measured from an integrated flow signal (see Chapter 11). A graphic representation of tidal breathing can be displayed on a computer screen. Because no two breaths are the same, inhaled or exhaled tidal breaths should be measured for at least 1 minute and then divided by the rate to determine an average volume:

$$V_T = \frac{\dot{V}}{f_b}$$

where:

$\dot{V}$ = volume expired or inspired per minute (usually the $\dot{V}_E$)

f_b = number of breaths for the same interval (i.e., the respiratory rate)

The inspired minute volume ($\dot{V}_I$) and V_T are normally slightly greater than the $\dot{V}_E$ because at rest, the body produces a slightly lower volume of CO_2 than the volume of O_2 consumed. This exchange difference is termed the **respiratory exchange ratio (RER).** It is calculated as $\dot{V}CO_2 / \dot{V}O_2$, where $\dot{V}co_2$ is the volume of CO_2 produced, and $\dot{V}O_2$ is the volume of O_2 consumed per minute. It is assumed that RER is approximately 0.8 in resting patients. For most clinical purposes, expired volume is measured to calculate V_T.

V_T may also be estimated by means of respiratory inductive plethysmography (RIP). RIP uses coils of wire as transducers that respond to changes in the cross-sectional area of the rib cage and abdominal compartments. With appropriate calibration, inductive plethysmography can be used to measure V_T. This method allows the measurement of V_T and minute ventilation without a direct connection to the patient's airway.

PF TIP 5.1

Not all spirometers allow bidirectional breathing (i.e., breathing in and out of the spirometer). For flow-based spirometers that do not measure flow in both directions, a one-way breathing circuit may be used. To measure ventilation with a volume-based spirometer, the subject rebreathes; CO_2 must be removed and O_2 added for prolonged measurements.

Respiratory frequency (f_b) may be determined by counting chest movements, noting the excursions of a volume displacement spirometer (Criteria for Acceptability 5.1), or most commonly by measuring flow changes while the subject breathes through a flow-sensing spirometer. Counting the rate for several minutes and taking an average produces a more accurate value than shorter measurements. Prolonged measurement of V_T and rate with a volume-displacement spirometer requires a means of removing CO_2. This is called a *rebreathing system* and uses a chemical CO_2 absorber (see Fig. 4.1B). Sodium hydroxide crystals (Sodasorb) or barium hydroxide crystals (Baralyme) are commonly used to scrub CO_2 from rebreathing systems. Flow-sensing spirometers usually do not require a chemical absorber.

The $\dot{V}_E$ may be measured by allowing the patient to breathe into or out of a volume-displacement or flow-sensing spirometer for at least 1 minute. A shorter breathing interval can be used with minute volume extrapolated but may give a misleading estimate of ventilation if the patient's breathing rate is irregular. If a rebreathing system is used, a CO_2 absorber must be included, as well as a means of replenishing O_2. Measuring expired gas volume for several minutes and dividing by the time gives an average $\dot{V}_E$. $\dot{V}_E$, measured from expired gas, is usually slightly smaller than $\dot{V}_I$ because of the RER, as described previously. For most clinical purposes, this difference is negligible. BTPS corrections should be made.

Significance and Pathophysiology

See Interpretive Strategies 5.1. Average V_T for healthy adults at rest ranges between 400 and 700 mL, but there is considerable variation. Decreased V_T occurs in many types of pulmonary disorders, particularly those that cause severe restrictive patterns. Pulmonary fibrosis and neuromuscular diseases (e.g., myasthenia gravis) often cause a reduced V_T. Decreased tidal breathing usually accompanies changes in the mechanical properties of the lungs or chest wall (i.e., compliance and resistance). These changes usually produce an increased respiratory rate (f_b) required to maintain an adequate $\dot{V}_A$. Decreases in both V_T and respiratory rate are often associated with respiratory center depression because of drugs or pathologic conditions affecting the brainstem. Low V_T and rate usually result in alveolar hypoventilation.

Some patients who have pulmonary disease may exhibit increased V_T, particularly at rest. The V_T alone is not a good indicator of the adequacy of **alveolar ventilation** ($\dot{V}_A$). Tidal volume should always be considered in conjunction with respiratory rate and $\dot{V}_E$. Many healthy patients display increased V_T simply because of breathing into the pulmonary function apparatus with the nose occluded. Estimates of resting ventilation may be artifactually increased when measured during pulmonary function testing. Some subjects adopt unusual breathing strategies (e.g., large tidal volumes

---

CRITERIA FOR ACCEPTABILITY 5.1

Tidal Volume, Rate, Minute Ventilation

1. V_T averaged from at least 60 seconds of ventilatory data; either accumulated volume divided by respiratory rate or multiple breaths summed and averaged.
2. $\dot{V}_E$ measured for at least 60 seconds; one-way breathing circuit or appropriate rebreathing system used. Repeated measurements should be within 10%.
3. Respiratory rate measured for at least 15 seconds; longer intervals may be necessary for patients with disordered breathing patterns.

INTERPRETIVE STRATEGIES 5.1

Tidal Volume, Rate, Minute Ventilation

1. Were V_T, respiratory rate, and $\dot{V}_E$ measured appropriately? Was the data collection adequate? Did the ventilatory pattern (i.e., rate or tidal volume) change during the measurements? If so, suspect breathing circuit problems.
2. Is the pattern of ventilation consistent with the patient's clinical status?
3. Is V_T, respiratory rate, and/or $\dot{V}_E$ excessive? If so, suspect hyperventilation. Arterial blood gases (pH and $Paco_2$) may be necessary to document respiratory alkalosis.
4. Is V_T, respiratory rate, and/or $\dot{V}_E$ decreased? If so, suspect hypoventilation. Arterial blood gases (pH and $Paco_2$) may be necessary to document respiratory acidosis.

with slow respiratory rate or small tidal volumes with rapid breathing rates) during exercise or stress for nonphysiologic reasons.

The normal respiratory rate (f_b) ranges from 10 to 20 breaths/min in adults. Increased demand for ventilation, such as during exercise, usually results in increases in both the rate and depth of breathing (i.e., the tidal volume). Increases or decreases in the respiratory rate are indications of a change in the ventilatory status. Breathing frequency, when evaluated with the V_T, may be used as an index of ventilation. Hypoxia, hypercapnia, metabolic acidosis, decreased lung compliance, and exercise can all result in increased respiratory rate. Rapid breathing rates and small tidal volumes may suggest increased V_D or hypoventilation but must be correlated with arterial pH and P_{CO_2} values to confirm those conditions. Decreased breathing frequency is common in central nervous system depression and in CO_2 narcosis. Respiratory rate may be falsely elevated in patients connected to unfamiliar breathing circuits, with or without a nose clip.

Normal $\dot{V}_E$ ranges from 5 to 10 L/min in healthy adults, with wide variations in normal patients. The $\dot{V}_E$, when used in conjunction with blood gas values, indicates the adequacy of ventilation. $\dot{V}_E$ is the sum of the $\dot{V}_D$ (dead-space ventilation per minute) and $\dot{V}_A$. Because the relative proportions of these components can change, absolute values for $\dot{V}_E$ do not necessarily indicate either hypoventilation or hyperventilation. In other words, low minute ventilation does not necessarily indicate hypoventilation. Similarly, elevated $\dot{V}_E$ does not indicate hyperventilation. To make these diagnoses, arterial pH and P_{CO_2} must be measured.

A large $\dot{V}_E$ at rest (> 20 L/min) may result from an enlarged V_D because an increase in total ventilation is required to maintain adequate $\dot{V}_A$. $\dot{V}_E$ increases in response to hypoxia, hypercapnia, metabolic acidosis, anxiety, and exercise. Hyperventilation is ventilation at a rate that is higher than what is needed to adequately remove CO_2, resulting in respiratory alkalosis.

Decreased ventilation may result from hypocapnia, metabolic alkalosis, respiratory center depression, or neuromuscular disorders that involve the ventilatory muscles. Hypoventilation is

defined as inadequate ventilation to maintain a normal arterial P_{CO_2}, with respiratory acidosis as the result. The diagnosis of either hyperventilation or hypoventilation requires blood gas analysis (see Chapter 6).

RESPIRATORY DEAD SPACE AND ALVEOLAR VENTILATION

Description

Respiratory dead space (VD) is the lung volume that is ventilated but not perfused by pulmonary capillary blood flow. V_D can be divided into the conducting airways or **anatomic dead space** and the nonperfused alveoli or **alveolar dead space.** The combination of alveolar and anatomic dead space is respiratory (or physiologic) dead space. V_D is recorded in milliliters or liters, BTPS.

$\dot{V}_A$ is the volume of gas that participates in gas exchange in the lungs. It can be expressed as follows:

$$\dot{V}_A = \dot{V}_E - \dot{V}_D$$

where:

$\dot{V}_A$ = alveolar ventilation
$\dot{V}_E$ = minute ventilation
$\dot{V}_D$ = dead-space ventilation per minute

For a single breath, the $\dot{V}_A$ equals the $\dot{V}_T$ minus the $\dot{V}_D$. $\dot{V}_A$ is usually expressed in liters per minute, BTPS.

Technique
Dead Space

Anatomic dead space is sometimes estimated from an individual's body size as 1 mL/lb of ideal body weight. The actual respiratory dead space, however, is of greater clinical importance. V_D can be calculated in two ways. The first uses the Enghoff modification of the Bohr equation defining V_D:

$$V_D = \frac{F_A CO_2 - F_{\bar{E}} CO_2}{F_A CO_2} \times V_T$$

where:

V_T = tidal volume

$F_{A}CO_2$ = fraction of CO_2 in alveolar gas
$F_{\bar{E}}CO_2$ = fraction of CO_2 in mixed expired gas

Because the fractional concentration of alveolar CO_2 is difficult to measure, the partial pressure of CO_2 may be substituted, and the equation is written as follows:

$$V_D = \frac{\left(Paco_2 - P_{\bar{E}}co_2\right)}{Paco_2} \times V_T$$

where:

$Paco_2$ = arterial Pco_2
$P_{\bar{E}}co_2$ = Pco_2 of mixed expired gas sample

Note that the $Paco_2$ is substituted for the alveolar Pco_2. This substitution presumes perfect equilibration between alveoli and pulmonary capillaries. This may not be true in certain diseases. The test also assumes that little CO_2 is in the atmosphere. Therefore the Pco_2 in expired gas is inversely proportional to the V_D. Exhaled gas is collected over a short interval, and arterial blood is obtained simultaneously to measure $Paco_2$. V_D is calculated by applying the previous equation. The estimate usually becomes more representative as more expired gas is collected. Accuracy depends on measurement of V_T (usually derived from $\dot{V}_E$ and f_b) and on the precision of the partial pressures of CO_2 measured in expired gas and arterial blood. The mixed expired gas sample is usually collected in a bag or balloon after filling and emptying it several times with expired gas to wash out room air from the valves, tubing, and bag itself. The volume of gas in the bag can be measured during collection by including a flow-sensing spirometer in the circuit. If $\dot{V}_E$ and the respiratory rate are recorded, the volumes of V_D and V_T can be determined. If expired volume is not measured, only a dilution ratio can be determined; this is called the V_D/V_T *ratio*.

The V_D/V_T ratio can be calculated if arterial and mixed-expired Pco_2 values are known. It can also be estimated noninvasively. **End-tidal Pco_2** (see the section on capnography in Chapter 6) can be used to estimate $Paco_2$. The main advantage of this method is that it is not necessary to obtain an arterial blood sample. This technique is often used in systems that monitor expired CO_2 continuously and in breath-by-breath metabolic measurement devices. V_D/V_T may be estimated as follows:

$$\frac{V_D}{V_T} = \frac{PETCO_2 - P_{\bar{E}}CO_2}{PETCO_2}$$

where:

$PETCO_2$ = end-tidal Pco_2
$P_{\bar{E}}CO_2$ = Pco_2 of mixed-expired gas sample

PF TIP 5.2

Dead space consists of anatomic and alveolar components. Anatomic dead space is usually estimated from body weight (2 mL/kg ideal body weight). Respiratory dead space measured using mixed-expired and arterial CO_2 measures both components.

In some patients, particularly those with severe obstruction, $PETCO_2$ may not accurately reflect $Paco_2$. Consequently, the V_D/V_T ratio may be estimated incorrectly. $Paco_2$ should be used in the V_D calculation whenever possible.

Alveolar Ventilation

$\dot{V}_A$ can be calculated in two ways:

$$\dot{V}_A = f_b \left(V_T - V_D\right)$$

where:

V_T = tidal volume
V_D = respiratory dead space
f_b = respiratory rate

For convenience, V_D is often estimated as equal to anatomic dead space. This method is valid only when there is little or no alveolar dead space, as in individuals who do not have pulmonary disease.

Because atmospheric gas contains almost no CO_2, $\dot{V}_A$ can be calculated based on CO_2 elimination from the lungs. A volume of expired gas may be collected in a bag, balloon, or spirometer and analyzed to determine the volume of CO_2. The following equation can then be used:

$$\dot{V}_A = \frac{\dot{V}CO_2}{F_A CO_2}$$

where:

$\dot{V}CO_2$ = volume of CO_2 produced in liters per minute (standard temperature, pressure, dry [STPD])
$F_A CO_2$ = fractional concentration of CO_2 in alveoli

If an end-tidal CO_2 monitor (i.e., a capnograph) is used, a close approximation of the concentration of alveolar CO_2 is easily obtained, and the equation is simplified as follows:

$$\dot{V}_A = \frac{\dot{V}CO_2}{\%alveolar CO_2} \times 100$$

End-tidal CO_2 may not equal alveolar CO_2 in patients with grossly abnormal patterns of ventilation-perfusion (see Chapter 6).

The same equation can be used substituting $Paco_2$ for the alveolar Pco_2 (i.e., $P_A CO_2$), again presuming that arterial blood and alveolar gas are in equilibrium. The equation is then as follows:

$$\dot{V}_A = \frac{\dot{V}CO_2}{PaCO_2} \times 0.863$$

where:

$\dot{V}CO_2$ = CO_2 production in mL/min (STPD)
$Paco_2$ = partial pressure of arterial CO_2
0.863 = conversion factor (concentration to partial pressure, correcting $\dot{V}co_2$ to BTPS)

Significance and Pathophysiology

See Interpretive Strategies 5.2. Measurement of V_D yields important information regarding the ventilation-perfusion characteristics of the lungs. Anatomic dead space is larger in men than in women because of differences in body size. It increases along with the V_T during exercise, as well as in certain forms of pulmonary disease (e.g., bronchiectasis). It may be decreased in asthma or in diseases characterized by bronchial obstruction or mucus plugging. Because of the difficulty in measuring the anatomic dead space, estimates based on age, sex, functional residual capacity, or body size may be used. For clinical purposes, anatomic dead space in milliliters is sometimes considered equal to the patient's ideal body weight in pounds or twice their weight in kilograms.

INTERPRETIVE STRATEGIES 5.2

V_D and $\dot{V}_A$

1. Was dead space determination based on $Paco_2$? If not, interpret cautiously.
2. Was $\dot{V}_E$ or V_T measured? If not, then interpret V_D/V_T only.
3. Is the V_D/V_T ratio greater than 0.40? If so, elevated dead space is likely. Consider clinical correlation, especially pulmonary embolism or pulmonary hypertension.
4. Is the V_D/V_T ratio less than 0.20 with the patient at rest? Is there an elevated level of ventilation? Consider technical problems.
5. Is $\dot{V}_A$ (if measured) consistent with the patient's clinical signs and symptoms?

Of greater clinical significance is the measurement of respiratory dead space, which is accomplished reasonably well by applying the **Bohr equation.** The portion of ventilation wasted on the conducting airways and poorly perfused alveoli is usually expressed as the V_D/V_T ratio. The normal value for V_D/V_T in spontaneously breathing adults is about 0.3 (with a range of 0.2–0.4). V_D/V_T is also commonly expressed as a percentage (e.g., 30%). Expressing dead space in this way eliminates the need to measure the volume of expired gas in the Bohr equation. However, if V_T or $\dot{V}_E$ is known, the dead-space volume can be easily calculated. Physiologic dead-space measurements are a good index of ventilation–blood flow ratios because all CO_2 in expired gas comes from perfused alveoli (see Chapter 6). If there were no dead space in the lung, arterial and mixed-expired CO_2 would be equal. As the difference between arterial and mixed-expired CO_2 increases, the volume of "wasted" ventilation rises.

The V_D/V_T ratio decreases in healthy subjects during exercise. As cardiac output increases, perfusion of alveoli at the lung apices also increases. This increased perfusion is referred to as **recruitment.** Alveoli at the apices are poorly perfused at rest, accounting for some of the normal resting dead space. Both V_D and V_T increase with exercise. In healthy individuals, the V_T increases more than V_D; thus the ratio decreases.

Increased dead space and V_D/V_T ratio may be observed in pulmonary embolism and in pulmonary hypertension. In pulmonary embolism, large numbers of arterioles may be blocked, resulting in little or no CO_2 removal in the associated alveoli. In pulmonary hypertension, increased pulmonary arterial pressure causes most alveoli to be perfused, so there is little or no recruitment of underperfused gas exchange units. This is most notable during exercise, when the V_D/V_T ratio normally decreases. In both pulmonary embolism and hypertension, the patient may be noticeably short of breath (i.e., dyspneic) because of the increased dead space.

The $\dot{V}_A$ at rest is approximately 4 to 5 L/min, with wide variations in healthy adults. The adequacy of $\dot{V}_A$ can be determined by arterial blood gas studies only. Low $\dot{V}_A$ associated with acute respiratory acidosis ($Pa_{CO_2} > 45$ and pH < 7.35 in healthy patients) defines hypoventilation. Excessive $\dot{V}_A$ ($Pa_{CO_2} < 35$ and pH > 7.45 in healthy patients) defines hyperventilation. Chronic hypoventilation and hyperventilation are associated with abnormal Pa_{CO_2} values but near-normal pH values (see Chapter 6). Decreased $\dot{V}_A$ can result from absolute increases in dead space and decreases in $\dot{V}_E$.

VENTILATORY RESPONSE TESTS FOR CARBON DIOXIDE AND OXYGEN

Description

The ventilatory response to CO_2 is a measurement of the increase or decrease in $\dot{V}_E$ caused by breathing various concentrations of CO_2 under normoxic conditions ($Pa_{O_2} \approx 100$ mm Hg). It is recorded as L/min/mm Hg P_{CO_2}.

The ventilatory response to O_2 is a measurement of the increase or decrease in $\dot{V}_E$ caused by breathing various concentrations of O_2 under isocapnic conditions ($Pa_{CO_2} \approx 40$ mm Hg). The change in ventilation (in liters per minute) may be recorded in relation to changes in Pa_{O_2} or saturation as monitored by oximetry.

Occlusion pressure (P_{100} or $P_{0.1}$) is the pressure generated at the mouth during the first 100 msec of an inspiratory effort against an occluded airway. Changes in P_{100} are related to changes in the ventilatory stimulant (hypercapnia or hypoxemia). P_{100} is usually measured in centimeters of water (cm H_2O).

Technique

Ventilatory Response to CO_2

The response to increasing levels of CO_2 (hypercapnia) can be measured in two ways:

1. *Open-circuit technique.* The patient breathes increasing concentrations of CO_2 (1%–7%) in air or O_2 from a demand valve or reservoir until a steady state is reached. Measurements of Pet_{CO_2}, Pa_{CO_2}, P_{100}, and $\dot{V}_E$ may be made at each concentration.
2. *Closed-circuit or rebreathing technique.* The patient rebreathes from a reservoir (usually an anesthesia bag) filled with a gas mixture of 5% to 7% CO_2 and the balance oxygen (Figs. 5.1 and 5.2). The breathing circuit usually includes ports for pressure monitoring (P_{100}) and for extracting gas samples (Pet_{CO_2}). A pneumotachometer is placed in the rebreathing circuit to record $\dot{V}_E$. Alternatively, the gas reservoir bag may be placed in a rigid container or box and volume change measured by connecting a spirometer to the container (i.e., "bag-in-box" setup). The patient rebreathes until the concentration of Fet_{CO_2} (x100) exceeds 9% or until 4 minutes have elapsed (Fig. 5.3). The rebreathed gas may be analyzed to ensure that the Fi_{O_2} remains above 0.21.

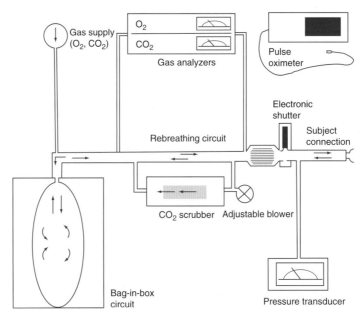

FIG. 5.1 Closed-circuit system for the rebreathing O_2 response test. The circuit allows the patient to rebreathe from a bag to which CO_2 or O_2 can be added. Gas analyzers allow continuous monitoring of gas concentrations in the circuit during testing. Ventilation is measured by integrating flow from the pneumotachometer or by attaching a spirometer to the bag-in-box setup. A pressure transducer and mouth shutter allow the measurement of P_{100}, and a pulse oximeter provides data on the patient's saturation. A CO_2 scrubber with an adjustable blower allows the level of CO_2 in the system to be maintained at baseline levels (isocapnia). Increases in ventilation caused by the gradual consumption of O_2 in the circuit can be measured by scrubbing just enough of the exhaled CO_2 to maintain a near-normal alveolar P_{CO_2}. A similar circuit can be used to measure response to CO_2 by rebreathing. The bag is filled with 5% to 7% CO_2 in O_2, and the scrubber is removed from the circuit.

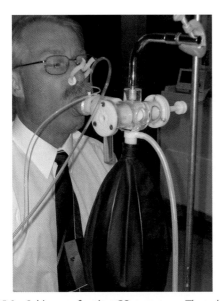

FIG. 5.2 Subject performing CO_2 response. The subject is placed on the breathing valve with 10-L rebreathing bag partially filled with a 5–7% CO_2, balance O_2 gas mixture. After 3 to 5 minutes of monitoring quiet breathing, the subject is switched into the rebreathing system. The test is terminated when the concentration of F_{ETO_2} (x100) exceeds 9% or until 4 minutes have elapsed and/or subject intolerance.

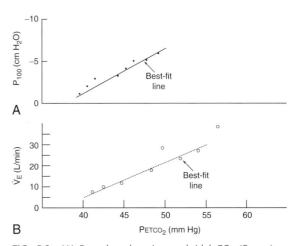

FIG. 5.3 (A) P_{100} plotted against end-tidal CO_2 (P_{ETCO_2}) as might be obtained during a CO_2 rebreathing study. (B) Minute ventilation plotted against P_{ETCO_2} during the same study. Individual points may be plotted, and a "best-fit" line constructed by statistical methods. The slope of the best-fit line is the rate at which ventilation or occlusion pressure increases with increasing stimulation from the rebreathed CO_2.

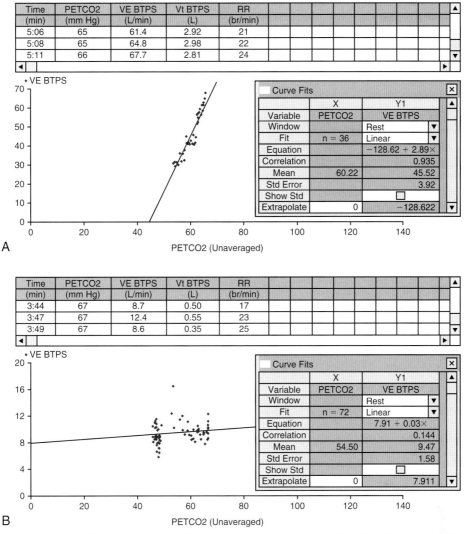

Time	PETCO2	VE BTPS	Vt BTPS	RR								▲
(min)	(mm Hg)	(L/min)	(L)	(br/min)								
5:06	65	61.4	2.92	21								
5:08	65	64.8	2.98	22								
5:11	66	67.7	2.81	24								▼

Curve Fits

	X	Y1
Variable	PETCO2	VE BTPS
Window		Rest
Fit	n = 36	Linear
Equation		−128.62 + 2.89×
Correlation		0.935
Mean	60.22	45.52
Std Error		3.92
Show Std		☐
Extrapolate	0	−128.622

A

PETCO2 (Unaveraged)

Time	PETCO2	VE BTPS	Vt BTPS	RR								▲
(min)	(mm Hg)	(L/min)	(L)	(br/min)								
3:44	67	8.7	0.50	17								
3:47	67	12.4	0.55	23								
3:49	67	8.6	0.35	25								▼

Curve Fits

	X	Y1
Variable	PETCO2	VE BTPS
Window		Rest
Fit	n = 72	Linear
Equation		7.91 + 0.03×
Correlation		0.144
Mean	54.50	9.47
Std Error		1.58
Show Std		☐
Extrapolate	0	7.911

B

PETCO2 (Unaveraged)

FIG. 5.4 (A) Normal CO_2 response test with minute ventilation increasing 2.89 L/min/unit increase in CO_2. (B) A patient diagnosed with central apnea with a flat response curve.

The patient's Sp_{O_2} may also be monitored by means of a pulse oximeter. Changes in $\dot{V}_E$ are monitored and plotted against P_{ETCO_2} to obtain a response curve (Fig. 5.4). A plot of $\dot{V}_E$ versus P_{ETCO_2} may be used to determine a slope or response curve. The CO_2 response curve may be extrapolated backward to determine the P_{CO_2} at which ventilation would be zero. This P_{CO_2} is termed the *threshold* and is sometimes used as a measure of sensitivity to the ventilatory stimulant.

5.1	How to

Perform a CO_2 Response Test

1. Tasks common to all procedures:
   a. Calibrate and prepare equipment.
   b. Review order.
   c. Introduce yourself and identify patient according to institutional policies.
   d. Describe and demonstrate procedure.
2. Inform the subject that he or she may or may not experience shortness of breath, dizziness, or headache during or following the test.
3. Place pulse oximeter and ensure a quality signal; optionally monitor the subject's electrocardiogram (ECG).
4. Some laboratories play music or dim the lights to facilitate quiet breathing.
5. Collect 3 to 5 minutes of resting ventilation. Assess breathlessness using the rating of perceived exertion (RPE) scale (also known as the *Borg scale*).
6. Switch the subject into the system (open or closed technique).
7. The patient rebreathes until the concentration of $FETCO_2$ (x100) exceeds 9% or until 4 minutes has elapsed and/or subject intolerance. Activate shutter if measuring P_{100}.
8. Once the end of test criteria is achieved, have the subject come off the system. Assess end-test RPE, heart rate, and SpO_2.
9. Calculate the slope of the $\dot{V}_E$ versus $PETCO_2$ response.
10. Report results and note comments related to test quality.

CRITERIA FOR ACCEPTABILITY 5.2

Ventilatory Response Tests

1. CO_2 response—Appropriate concentrations of CO_2 (i.e., 5–7% CO_2 in O_2 for rebreathing studies) must be used.
2. CO_2 response—Normoxia maintained; subject's SpO_2 should remain greater than 95% during testing.
3. O_2 response—FIO_2 appropriate to induce hypoxic response; isocapnia demonstrated by monitoring $PETCO_2$.
4. P_{100}—Pressure transducer and monitor capable of recording up to 50 cm H_2O with a recorder speed of 50 to 100 mm/sec. Occlusion device should be hidden from the patient.
5. Ventilatory responses (O_2, CO_2) should be reproducible within 10%; average of two trials should be reported if clinically practical.
6. Reported P_{100} should be the average of three or more occlusions at each level of challenge.

Ventilatory Response to O_2

Response to decreasing levels of O_2 (hypoxemia) can also be measured by either open-circuit or closed-circuit techniques:

1. *Open-circuit technique.* The patient breathes gas mixtures containing O_2 concentrations from 12% to 20%, to which CO_2 is added to maintain alveolar PCO_2 ($PaCO_2$) at a constant level. When a steady state is reached, PaO_2, $\dot{V}_E$, and P_{100} can be measured. This procedure, often called a *step test,* is repeated with decreasing O_2 concentrations to produce the response curve. Continuous monitoring of $PETCO_2$ is necessary to titrate the addition of CO_2 to the system to maintain isocapnia. Pulse oximetry may be used to monitor changes in saturation. CO_2 response curves are sometimes measured at widely varying PaO_2 levels, and the subsequent difference in ventilation or P_{100} at any particular PCO_2 is attributed to the response to hypoxemia.

2. *Closed-circuit technique (progressive hypoxemia).* The patient rebreathes from a system similar to that used for the closed-circuit CO_2 response, but the system contains a CO_2 scrubber. CO_2 can be added to the inspired gas to maintain isocapnia, or an adjustable blower may be used to direct a portion of the rebreathed gas through the scrubber to maintain isocapnia (see Fig. 5.1). The response to decreasing inspired PO_2 is monitored by recording $\dot{V}_E$ or P_{100}, and the PaO_2 or saturation is measured either directly by indwelling catheter or by pulse oximetry.

> **PF TIP 5.3**
>
> To measure the response to hypoxemia, it is necessary to maintain a constant level of CO_2 (isocapnia). To measure the response to hypercapnia, it is necessary to maintain normoxia (Pa_{O_2} of 80–100 mm Hg).

P_{100} is measured with a system similar to that in Fig. 5.1. A port at the mouth records pressure changes versus time by means of a computer or high-speed recorder. A large-bore stopcock or electronic shutter mechanism is included in the inspiratory line so that inspiratory flow can be randomly occluded. The stopcock or shutter can be closed so that inspiration occurs against a complete occlusion near functional residual capacity. The entire apparatus is usually hidden so that the patient is unaware of the impending airway occlusion. A pressure–time curve is recorded. P_{100} is usually measured at varying P_{ETCO_2} values or levels of desaturation to assess the effect of changing stimuli to ventilation. P_{100} and $\dot{V}_E$ are usually graphed against P_{ETCO_2} (see Fig. 5.3) or versus O_2 saturation (for O_2 response tests). See Criteria for Acceptability 5.2 for ventilatory response measurements.

The normal response to a decrease in Pa_{O_2} varies depending on the level of P_{CO_2} at which the measurement is made. There is little change in ventilation until the Pa_{O_2} falls to less than 60 mm Hg. The response appears to be exponential once the Pa_{O_2} has fallen to the range of 40 to 60 mm Hg, and it varies widely among individuals on a genetically determined basis. The hypoxic response is increased in the presence of hypercapnia and decreased in hypocapnia. Patients who have severe chronic obstructive pulmonary disease (COPD) with CO_2 retention receive their primary respiratory stimulus from the hypoxemic response. This group of patients may experience severe or even fatal respiratory depression if that response is obliterated by uncontrolled O_2 therapy.

Some patients with minimal intrinsic lung disease show a markedly decreased response to hypoxemia or hypercapnia. These include patients with myxedema, obesity-hypoventilation syndrome, obstructive sleep apnea, central apnea, and idiopathic hypoventilation. CO_2 and O_2 response measurements, along with tests of pulmonary mechanics, may be particularly valuable in the evaluation and treatment of these types of patients.

The P_{100} ($P_{0.1}$) has been suggested as a measurement of ventilatory drive independent of the mechanical properties of the lungs. Because no airflow occurs during occlusion of the airway, significant interference from mechanical abnormalities (e.g., increased resistance or decreased compliance) is omitted. Reflexes from the airways and chest wall are also of little influence during the first 100 msec of the occluded breath. Therefore the pressure generated can be viewed as proportional to the neural output of the medullary centers that drive the rate and depth of breathing. This proportionality may be influenced by other factors, however, such as body position and the contractile properties of the respiratory muscles.

Individuals with normal Pa_{CO_2} values have P_{100} values in the range of 1.5 to 5 cm H_2O. P_{100} has been shown to increase in hypercapnia and hypoxia and appears to correlate well with the observed ventilatory responses. Increasing P_{CO_2}, and thereby inducing hypercapnia, in healthy patients typically results in an increase in the occlusion pressure of 0.5 to 0.6 cm H_2O/mm Hg P_{CO_2}, with as much as 20% variability. Healthy subjects increase their P_{100} when breathing through artificial resistance on challenge with high P_{CO_2} or low P_{O_2}. Some patients who have chronic airway obstruction demonstrate no increase in P_{100} in response to increasing P_{CO_2} even with increased airway resistance. This failure to respond to increased resistance in the airways may predispose individuals with COPD to respiratory failure when lung infections occur. Similarly, patients supported by mechanical ventilation may be difficult to wean if their ventilatory drive is compromised, as demonstrated by the failure to increase P_{100} when challenged with increased P_{CO_2}. Determination of P_{100} may prove helpful in determining the effects of treatment in patients who have abnormal ventilatory responses.

Significance and Pathophysiology

See Interpretive Strategies 5.3. The response to an increase in Pa_{CO_2} in a normal individual is a linear increase in $\dot{V}_E$ of approximately 3 L/min/mm Hg (P_{CO_2}). The normal range of response varies from 1 to 6 L/min/mm Hg P_{CO_2}. Some variation is present in repeated testing of the same individual. The response to CO_2 in patients who have obstructive disease may be reduced. This is partially attributable to increased airway resistance, which has been shown to reduce ventilatory drive in healthy individuals. It is unclear why some patients who have obstructive disease increase ventilation to maintain a normal $Paco_2$, whereas others tolerate an increased $Paco_2$. Genetic variation in drive may explain some of the differences in blood gas tensions in patients with COPD. Lesions in the central nervous system may also cause a decreased sensitivity to CO_2 (see Fig. 5.4A and B). Some individuals who have no respiratory muscle weakness, mechanical ventilatory problems, or neurologic disease have a decreased sensitivity to CO_2. This condition is described as primary alveolar hypoventilation. These patients can lower their Pco_2 by voluntary hyperventilation.

INTERPRETIVE STRATEGIES 5.3

Ventilatory Response Tests

1. CO_2 response—Were appropriate levels of elevated CO_2 attained? If rebreathing was used, was test terminated at 4 minutes or a $Fetco_2$ of 0.09 (9%)?
2. CO_2 response—Was normoxia maintained? Did Spo_2 demonstrate adequate saturation? If not, interpretation may be compromised.
3. CO_2 response—Did ventilation increase by at least 1 L/mm Hg change in $Petco_2$? If not, decreased ventilatory response to CO_2 is likely.
4. O_2 response—Were appropriate low levels of Fio_2 attained? Was isocapnia maintained as demonstrated by $Petco_2$? If not, interpretation may be compromised.
5. O_2 response—Did ventilation increase exponentially at Spo_2 levels less than 90%? If not, suspect decreased ventilatory response to hypoxia.
6. P_{100}—Was the occlusion pressure appropriate for the baseline $Paco_2$ (1.5–5.0 cm H_2O at a $Paco_2$ of 40 mm Hg)? Did P_{100} increase by at least 0.5 cm H_2O/mm Hg change in $Petco_2$? If not, a decreased central ventilatory drive is likely.

HIGH-ALTITUDE SIMULATION TEST

Description

The HAST, also known as the *hypoxia inhalation test (HIT)* or *hypoxic challenge test (HCT),* is used to emulate high altitude in subjects susceptible to hypoxia during air travel or travel to high elevation

(i.e., those with COPD, pulmonary fibrosis). The standard for aircraft cabin pressurization is administered by the Federal Aviation Administration (FAA). The FAA standard ARP1270B notes that cabin altitude pressure should not exceed more than 8000-ft altitude in normal conditions. The HAST involves breathing a hypoxic gas mixture for 20 minutes, with the aim of predicting hypoxemia at the target altitude of 8000 ft with a reduced Fio_2 versus the change in altitude.

Technique

To replicate the in-flight Pio_2 at sea-level pressure (760 mm Hg), the Fio_2 would need to be 0.15 in a nitrogen balance. To estimate the target Fio_2 at an altitude other than sea level, a factor is calculated to use in the alveolar air equation (Fig. 5.5):

$$Factor = \left(1 - 6.873E^{-6} \times Alt[Feet]\right)^{5.256}$$

$$Bag\,FIO_2 = \left([760 \times factor]/local\,PBaro\right) \times 0.21$$

The desired Fio_2 can be delivered via a specialized tank mixture administered with a demand valve, a mixed gas (100% nitrogen and room air added to a Douglas bag, analyzed to desired Fio_2 and delivered via directional valve), a blender attached to 100% nitrogen supply and compressed air tanks, or a Ventimask driven by a 100%

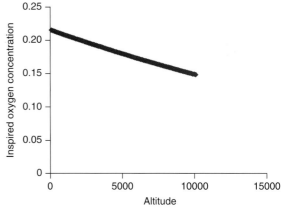

High-altitude simulation

FIG. 5.5 Graph calculating the reduction in Fio_2 to emulate an increasing altitude.

nitrogen source (40% setting = 14%–15% F_{IO_2}; 35% setting = 15%–16% F_{IO_2}) (Fig. 5.6). The various interfaces were evaluated via patient feedback, with the mask and canopy being the preferred methods. Once the desired F_{IO_2} is established and the mode of delivery determined, the subject can be tested. It is typical to monitor the patient's electrocardiogram (five leads at a minimum) during the procedure.

The Borg or RPE scale may also be used to assess dyspnea or breathlessness during the study. The patient oxygen level is monitored with pulse oximetry. Some laboratories assess end-of-test oxygen status using arterial blood gas, whereas others rely on the oximetry readings if the signal quality is acceptable. The subject breathes the hypoxic gas mixture for 20 minutes. The test is terminated early if the patient's

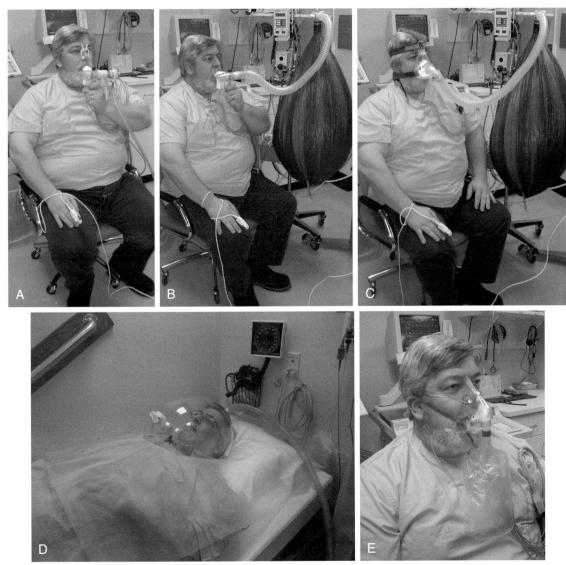

FIG. 5.6 High-altitude simulation test methods. Desired F_{IO_2} delivered via different methods: (A) directional valve with demand valve; (B) directional valve with reservoir bag; (C) continuous positive airway pressure (CPAP) mask with reservoir bag; (D) canopy with gas source; (E) Ventimask driven with 100% nitrogen source.

SpO_2 is less than 80%, there is a change in the ECG rhythm, ST-T wave depression/elevation is greater than 1.0 mm, or the patient develops symptoms suggesting intolerance.

Using a nasal cannula to supplement or titrate oxygen under a facemask application has been shown to underestimate the desired liter flow resulting from mixing of the gases in the nasal-oral pharyngeal and device space. Supplemental oxygen is recommended if the test results yield an SaO_2 or SpO_2 of less than 84%. In most cases, an oxygen flow of 2 L/min via nasal cannula is adequate to correct for the altitude effect. Incrementing the current oxygen flow rate by 2 L/min in a subject already receiving therapy might also be warranted during flight.

Significance and Pathophysiology

Air travel causes significant hypobaric hypoxemia in patients at risk. The British Thoracic Society recommends an evaluation before airline travel in subjects with severe COPD or asthma (forced expiratory volume in the first second [FEV_1] < 30%), severe restrictive disease (vital capacity [VC] < 1.00 L), cystic fibrosis, and comorbidity conditions worsened by hypoxemia (coronary artery disease, congestive heart failure, etc.). A HAST should be performed if the screening process yields a resting SpO_2 between 92% and 95% with additional risk factors (Table 5.1).

Equations are available to predict in-flight hypoxemia; however, several authors have concluded that equations do not accurately predict altitude PaO_2 and favor a hypoxia altitude test (see Criteria for Acceptability 5.2 and Interpretive Strategies 5.3).

TABLE 5.1

HAST Initial Assessment

Screening Result	Recommendation
Sea-level SpO_2 > 95%	Oxygen not required [B]
Sea-level SpO_2 92%–95% and no risk factor[a]	Oxygen not required [C]
Sea-level SpO_2 92%–95% and additional risk factor[a]	Perform hypoxic challenge test with arterial or capillary measurements [B]
Sea-level SpO_2 < 92%	In-flight oxygen [B]
Receiving supplemental oxygen at sea level	Increase the flow while at cruising altitude [B]

Grade types of recommendations:

A. Requires at least one randomized controlled trial as part of the body of literature of overall good quality and consistency addressing the specific recommendation

B. Requires availability of well-conducted clinical studies but no randomized clinical trials on the topic of recommendation

C. Requires evidence from expert committee reports or opinions and/or clinical experience of respected authorities; indicates absence of directly applicable studies of good quality

[a]Additional risk factors: hypercapnia; forced expiratory volume in the first second (FEV_1) < 30% predicted; lung cancer; restrictive lung disease (vital capacity [VC] < 1 L) involving the parenchyma (fibrosis), chest wall (kyphoscoliosis) or respiratory muscles; ventilator support; cerebrovascular or cardiac disease; within 6 weeks of discharge for an exacerbation of chronic lung or cardiac disease. From British Thoracic Society Standards of Care Committee. (2002). Managing passengers with respiratory disease planning air travel: British Thoracic Society recommendations. *Thorax, 57,* 289–304.

5.2	How To ...

Perform a High-Altitude Simulation Test

1. Tasks common to all procedures:
   a. Calibrate and prepare equipment.
   b. Review order.
   c. Introduce yourself and identify patient according to institutional policies.
   d. Describe and demonstrate procedure.
2. Calculate the desired FIO_2 and select the delivery system.
3. Place pulse oximeter and ensure a quality signal (optional: monitor the subject's ECG).
4. Have the subject breathe the hypoxic gas mixture for 20 minutes. In the last minute, record ECG, RPE, and SpO_2 (optional end-test arterial blood gases may be obtained).
5. Early termination criteria include SpO_2 less than or equal to 80%, a change in ECG rhythm, or ST-T wave depression/elevation greater than 1.0 mm or patient develops symptoms suggesting intolerance.
6. Report results and note comments about test quality.

SUMMARY

· The chapter discusses measurement of $\dot{V}_E$, V_T, respiratory rate, alveolar ventilation, dead space, and the ventilatory responses to hypercapnia and hypoxemia.

· Resting ventilatory measurements can be used in conjunction with blood gases to evaluate respiratory status.

· One of the most important parameters is the respiratory or physiologic dead space. An estimate of wasted ventilation can be made by comparing expired CO_2 with arterial PCO_2. Dead space and reduced $\dot{V}_A$ are common in many pulmonary disorders. When dead space increases, ventilation must increase to maintain a normal acid–base status.

· Disorders of ventilatory control are also common to many diseases. Evaluation of responses to hypoxemia and hypercapnia are often useful in characterizing types of ventilatory response disorders. Different techniques of assessing responses have been described.

· The rebreathing techniques for O_2 and CO_2 are used most often. P_{100} can discriminate central ventilatory drive problems from other causes of abnormal responses.

· HAST, also known *HIT*, is used to emulate high altitude in subjects susceptible to hypoxia during air travel (i.e., those with COPD, pulmonary fibrosis). If the subject desaturates significantly (SpO_2 or SaO_2 < 84%), the clinician can order supplemental oxygen during the flight.

CASE STUDIES

CASE 5.1

HISTORY

A 45-year-old man is admitted to the hospital for acute shortness of breath. He has never smoked but has a family history of heart disease. His lungs are clear during auscultation. He becomes breathless just moving around his hospital room. He denies any recent respiratory infections. Because of his rapid respiratory rate, his attending physician requested an arterial blood gas test using room air and a V_D/V_T ratio determination.

PULMONARY FUNCTION STUDIES
Personal Data

Age:	45
Height:	67 in. (170 cm)
Weight:	175 lb. (80 kg)
Race:	Caucasian

Blood Gas Analysis

pH	7.49
PCO_2 (mm Hg)	29
PO_2 (mm Hg)	102
HCO_3^- (mEq/L)	21
Hb (g/dL)	14.2
SaO_2 (%)	98

Exhaled Gas Analysis

$\dot{V}_A$ (L / min)	24.20
f_b (breaths/min)	20
$P_{P\bar{E}CO_2} - CO_2$ (mm Hg)	14

QUESTIONS

1. Determine the following for this subject:
   a. V_T
   b. VD/VT
2. $\dot{V}_A$ What is the interpretation of the subject's ventilation?
3. What other tests might be indicated?
4. What treatment might be indicated based on these findings?

DISCUSSION

Calculations

$$V_T = \frac{\dot{V}_E}{f_b}$$

$$= \frac{24.2}{20}$$

$$V_T = 1.21 L$$

$$= \frac{PaCO_2 - P_{\bar{E}}CO_2}{PaCO_2}$$

$$= \frac{(29-14)}{29}$$

$$\frac{V_D}{V_T} = 0.517$$

$$\dot{V} = f_b(V_T - V_D)$$

where:

$$V_D = \frac{V_D}{V_T}(V_T) = 0.517(1.21)V_D = 0.626$$

Substituting this value in the alveolar ventilation equation gives the following:

$$V_A = 20(1.21 - 0.626) = 20(0.584)\dot{V} = 11.68.$$

Ventilation

This subject has a rapid respiratory rate and a large V_T. The result of this is a large $\dot{V}_E$ (i.e., 24.2 L/min). The blood gas analysis shows hyperventilation (respiratory alkalosis) consistent with excessive ventilation. The V_D/V_T ratio is increased at 52% (0.517 as a fraction). Healthy subjects have V_D/V_T ratios of 30% to 40% at rest. In effect, this subject is wasting more than half of each breath. Calculation of the $\dot{V}_A$ similarly reveals that less than half of his $\dot{V}_E$ is actually available for gas exchange. To maintain a normal $PaCO_2$ (or in this case, to hyperventilate), subjects who have increased dead space must increase their total ventilation. Large increases in dead space can occur as a result of obstruction of pulmonary arterial vessels by blood clots or similar lesions. Congestion of pulmonary vessels (resulting from pulmonary hypertension) can also cause imbalances in ventilation-perfusion ratios, especially during exercise.

Other Tests

Other diagnostic procedures that might be indicated include perfusion or ventilation-perfusion scanning of the lungs. Perfusion scans can identify areas of the lung in which there is little or no blood flow. $\dot{V}/\dot{Q}$ scans can detect which areas of the lungs have decreased blood flow in relation to their ventilation. These imaging tests are often used when pulmonary emboli are suspected. Ventilation-perfusion scans of subject indicated multiple areas of decreased perfusion in both lower lobes, consistent with multiple pulmonary emboli.

Treatment

The subject had been given O_2 therapy after the blood gas test results were obtained. Because there was adequate oxygenation on room air, the O_2 therapy was inappropriate and was discontinued. After the lung scans, the subject was started on anticoagulant therapy (heparin). During the next week, the pattern of pulmonary embolization gradually resolved. His ventilation and V_D/V_T ratio returned to normal.

CASE 5.2

HISTORY

The subject is a 37-year-old Caucasian male. He is 69 inches tall and weighs 275 pounds (body mass index [BMI] = 40.6 kg/m^2). He was referred to the pulmonary function laboratory after an evaluation in the sleep laboratory revealed obstructive sleep apnea (OSA). He admits to daytime somnolence. Baseline pulmonary function studies revealed the following:

	Actual	% Predicted
FVC (L)	3.2	72
FEV$_1$ (L)	2.7	81
TLC (L)	4.1	71
RV/TLC	22%	

FVC, Forced vital capacity; RV, residual volume; TLC, total lung capacity.

Baseline blood gas results were as follows:

pH	7.36
PCO_2 (mm Hg)	47
PO_2 (mm Hg)	77
HCO$_3^-$ (mEq/L)	28
SaO_2 (%)	93

A CO_2 response test (rebreathing method) was performed to assess the subject's respiratory drive. The subject rebreathed a mixture of 7% CO_2 in O_2 for 4 minutes. Triplicate measurements of P$_{100}$ were made at intervals throughout the test with a pneumatically operated occlusion valve. The following data were obtained:

P$ETCO_2$ (mm Hg)	$\dot{V}_E$ (L/min)	P$_{100}$ (cm H$_2$O)
43	4.5	2.2
46	4.4	—
50	5.9	—
54	7.9	7.8
57	15.1	—
59	17.1	12.0

QUESTIONS

1. What is the interpretation of the following?
   a. Ventilatory response to CO_2 stimulation
   b. Respiratory drive response to CO_2 stimulation
2. What is the cause of the subject's daytime somnolence?
3. What treatment(s) might be indicated, based on these findings?

DISCUSSION

Interpretation

All data obtained during the CO_2 rebreathing test were acceptable. The P$ETCO_2$ increased appropriately, and the test was terminated after 4 minutes of rebreathing. P$_{100}$ was obtained at baseline, after 2 minutes, and near the end of the test. All pressures were repeatable, and the average values were reported. Ventilatory response was diminished at 0.8 L/mm Hg PCO_2. P$_{100}$ appeared to increase appropriately.

Impression: Markedly reduced ventilatory response to CO_2 with a normal occlusion pressure.

Cause of Symptoms

This subject, who has documented sleep apnea, also displays a reduced sensitivity to increasing levels of CO_2. His spirometry and total lung capacity show a restrictive pattern. His baseline blood gases indicate mild CO_2 retention. His slightly elevated HCO$_3^-$ suggests that this is a chronic condition. The PO_2 is mildly reduced as a result of hypoventilation.

The CO_2 rebreathing test documents that the subject does not increase his ventilation appropriately in response to an increasing load of CO_2 (see accompanying patient graphs). At the same time, the subject's P$_{100}$ shows a relatively normal response to hypercapnia. This pattern suggests that the subject does not increase ventilation, although his respiratory center is signaling otherwise. These findings are consistent with his obstructive sleep apnea. Subjects who retain CO_2 because of large airway or small airway obstruction often have reduced sensitivity to elevated CO_2. This subject might be suspected of having obesity-hypoventilation syndrome. However, subjects with obesity-hypoventilation typically have a decreased central drive to ventilation along with their daytime hypercapnia. Obesity-hypoventilation is often associated with obstructive sleep apnea or central apnea and usually involves severe hypoxemia and hypercapnia. This subject has less severe blood gas abnormalities and a normal respiratory drive (P$_{100}$), suggesting a different cause for the reduced ventilatory response to CO_2.

Treatment

This subject treatment was nasal continuous positive airway pressure (CPAP) at night. Nasal CPAP alleviates much of the obstruction occurring in the upper airway. The subject reported a marked decrease in daytime hypersomnolence. He was also referred for weight-loss counseling because his increased weight and reduced ventilatory response placed him at increased risk for pulmonary and cardiac complications.

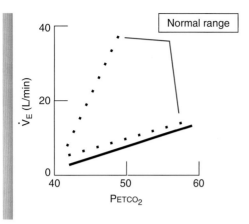

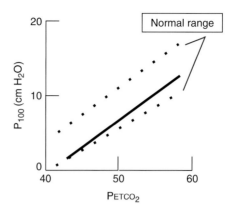

SELF-ASSESSMENT QUESTIONS

Entry-Level

1. During a rebreathing test, a patient with COPD has his ventilation measured for 3 minutes, with the following results:
   Total volume expired: 12.4 L (BTPS)
   Total breaths: 30
   This patient's V_T is approximately
   a. 0.10 L (BTPS).
   b. 0.41 L (BTPS).
   c. 1.24 L (BTPS).
   d. 4.13 L (BTPS).

2. Decreased minute ventilation might be expected in which of the following conditions?
   a. Hypercapnia with acidosis
   b. Mild hypoxemia
   c. Respiratory center depression
   d. Compensated metabolic acidosis

3. To calculate the V_D/V_T ratio, what else is needed in addition to the mixed expired CO_2 ($P_{\bar{E}CO_2}$)?
   1. V_T
   2. $\dot{V}_E$
   3. Pa_{CO_2}
   4. $P_{ET}CO_2$
   a. 1 and 2
   b. Either 1 or 2
   c. Either 3 or 4
   d. 1 and 4

4. An outpatient has her V_D/V_T ratio measured as 0.48 (48%); this finding is
   a. normal for an adult female.
   b. consistent with pulmonary hypertension.
   c. diagnostic of mild restrictive lung disease.
   d. expected after surgical removal of one lung.

5. A healthy adult subject who weighs 150 pounds has a $\dot{V}_E$ of 9.0 L/min (BTPS) and a respiratory rate of 10/min. What is his estimated $\dot{V}_A$?
   a. 7.5 L (BTPS)
   b. 6.0 L (BTPS)
   c. 4.5 L (BTPS)
   d. 3.0 L (BTPS)

Advanced

6. Questions 6 and 7 refer to the same case. The following data are recorded from a patient with suspected pulmonary embolism:
   1. $P_{\bar{E}CO_2}$: 20 mm Hg
   2. pH: 7.39
   3. Pa_{CO_2}: 40
   4. Pa_{O_2}: 72
   What is this patient's V_D/V_T ratio?
   a. 0.15
   b. 0.25
   c. 0.33
   d. 0.50

7. Based on the V_D/V_T ratio (question 6), what is the patient's alveolar ventilation ($\dot{V}_A$) if his minute ventilation ($\dot{V}_E$) is 16.0 L/min (BTPS)?
   a. 13.6 L/min
   b. 12.0 L/min
   c. 10.7 L/min
   d. 8.0 L/min

8. A patient has the following results after 4.0 minutes of a CO_2 rebreathing test:

	Time 0	4 Min
P_{ETCO_2} (mm Hg)	38	62
$\dot{V}_A / \dot{V}_E$ (L/min)	3.7	7.0

   Which of the following diagnoses is most consistent with these findings?
   a. Obesity-hypoventilation syndrome
   b. COPD
   c. Coal worker's pneumoconiosis
   d. Normal lung function

9. The purpose of a variable-speed blower in the closed-circuit rebreathing system used to measure the response to hypoxemia is to
   a. reduce the inspired F_{IO_2}.
   b. mix gas in the rebreathing circuit.
   c. maintain isocapnia.
   d. allow measurement of P_{100}.

10. A patient has the following findings during a CO_2 rebreathing test:

	Time 0	3 Min
P_{ETCO_2} (mm Hg)	41	51
$\dot{V}_A / \dot{V}_E$ (L/min)	5.7	23.0
P_{100} (cm H_2O)	2.7	7.8

   These data suggest
   a. normal ventilatory response to CO_2.
   b. decreased output of the respiratory centers.
   c. normal respiratory drive but decreased ventilatory response.
   d. abnormally increased P_{100} with hypercapnia.

11. A patient with moderate COPD wants to visit his son in Germany. During his physical exam, the physician places a pulse oximeter and records his resting SpO_2 as 95%. Based on the oximeter reading, what does the physician recommend?
   a. Perform spirometry and if the FEV_1 is less than 50%, order HAST.
   b. The patient is cleared for flight without further evaluation.
   c. Use 4 L O_2 during the flight.
   d. Perform HAST with 14% F_{IO_2}.

SELECTED BIBLIOGRAPHY

General References

Levitzky, M. G. (2003). *Pulmonary physiology* (6th ed.). Columbus, OH: McGraw-Hill.

West, J. B. (2000). *Pulmonary physiology and pathophysiology: An integrated, case-based approach*. Baltimore, MD: Lippincott Williams & Wilkins.

West, J. B. (2003). *Pulmonary pathophysiology: The essentials* (6th ed.). Baltimore, MD: Lippincott Williams & Wilkins.

Ventilation

Hardman, J. G., & Aitkenhead, A. R. (2003). Estimating alveolar dead space from the arterial to end-tidal CO_2 gradient: A modeling analysis. *Anesthesia and Analgesia, 97*, 1846–1851.

Hedenstierna, G., & Sandhagen, B. (2006). Assessing dead space. A meaningful variable? *Minerva Anestesiologica, 72*, 521–528.

Kline, J. A., Israel, E. G., Michelson, E. A., et al. (2001). Diagnostic accuracy of a bedside D-dimer assay and alveolar dead-space measurement for rapid exclusion of pulmonary embolism: A multicenter study. *JAMA, 285*, 761–768.

Koulouris, N. G., Latsi, P., Dimitroulis, J., et al. (2001). Noninvasive measurement of mean alveolar carbon dioxide tension and Bohr's dead space during tidal breathing. *European Respiratory Journal, 17*, 1167–1174.

Riley, R. L., & Cournand, A. (1949). "Ideal" alveolar air and the analysis of ventilation-perfusion relationships in the lungs. *Journal of Applied Physiology, 1*, 825.

Rodger, M. A., Jones, G., Rasuli, P., et al. (2001). Steady-state end-tidal alveolar dead space fraction and D-dimer: Bedside tests to exclude pulmonary embolism. *Chest, 120*, 115–119.

Control of Ventilation

Benlloch, E., Cordero, P., Morales, P., et al. (1995). Ventilatory pattern at rest and response to hypercapnic stimulation in patients with obstructive sleep apnea. *Respiration, 62*, 4–9.

Caruana-Montaldo, B., Gleeson, K., & Zwillich, C. W. (2000). The control of breathing in clinical practice. *Chest, 117*, 205–225.

Howard, L. S., & Robbins, P. A. (1994). Problems with determining the hypoxic response in humans using stepwise changes in end-tidal Po_2. *Respiration Physiology, 98*, 241–249.

Marin, J. M., Montes de Oca, M., Rassulo, J., et al. (1999). Ventilatory drive at rest and the perception of exertional dyspnea in severe COPD. *Chest, 115*, 1293–1300.

Misuri, G., Lanini, B., Gigliotti, F., et al. (2000). Mechanism of CO_2 retention in patients with neuromuscular disease. *Chest, 117*, 447–453.

Mohan, R. M., Amara, C. E., Cunningham, D. A., et al. (1999). Measuring central-chemoreflex sensitivity in man: Rebreathing and steady-state methods compared. *Respiration Physiology, 115*, 23–33.

Read, D. J. (1967). A clinical method for assessing the ventilatory response to carbon dioxide. *Australasian Annals of Medicine, 16*, 20–32.

Rebuck, A. S., & Campbell, E. J. M. (1974). A clinical method for assessing the ventilatory response to hypoxia. *American Review of Respiratory Disease, 109*, 345–350.

Zhang, S., & Robbins, P. A. (2000). Methodological and physiological variability within the ventilatory response to hypoxia in humans. *Journal of Applied Physiology, 88*, 1924–1932.

High-Altitude Simulation Test (or Hypoxic Inhalation Test)

Akero, A., Edvardsen, A., Christensen, C. C., et al. (2011). COPD and air travel, oxygen equipment and preflight titration of supplemental oxygen. *Chest, 140*(1), 84–90.

British Thoracic Society Standards of Care Committee. (2002). Managing passengers with respiratory disease planning air travel: British Thoracic Society recommendations. *Thorax, 57*, 289–304.

Edvardsen, A., Akero, A., Christensen, C., et al. (2012). Air travel and chronic obstructive pulmonary disease; a new algorithm for pre-flight evaluation. *Thorax, 67*, 964–969.

Federal Aviation Administration: Aircraft Cabin Pressurization Criteria ARP1270B Reaffirmed October 2015. https://www.sae.org/standards/content/arp1270b/ (assessed October 2020).

Gong, H., Tashkin, D. P., Lee, E. Y., et al. (1984). Hypoxia-altitude simulation test. *American Review of Respiratory Disease, 130*, 980–986.

Kelly, P. T., Swanney, M. P., Seccombe, L. M., et al. (2008). Air travel hypoxemia vs the hypoxia inhalation test in passengers with COPD. *Chest, 133*, 920–926.

O'Brien, M. J., Brittan, G. P., Murphy, S. P., et al. (2008). *Evaluation of high altitude simulation gas delivery methods–Pros and cons.* AARC Abstract.

Possick, S. E., & Barry, M. (2004). Evaluation and management of the cardiovascular patient embarking on air travel. *Annals of Internal Medicine, 141*, 148–154.

Robson, A. G., Hartung, T. K., & Innes, J. A. (2000). Laboratory assessment of fitness to fly in patients with lung disease: A practical approach. *European Respiratory Journal, 16*, 214–219.

Chapter 6

Blood Gases and Related Tests

CHAPTER OUTLINE

LEARNING OBJECTIVES

After studying the chapter and reviewing the figures, tables, and case studies, you should be able to do the following:

Entry-level

1. Describe how pH and P_{CO_2} are used to assess acid–base status.
2. Interpret P_{O_2} and oxygen saturation to assess oxygenation.
3. Identify the appropriate procedure for obtaining an arterial blood gas specimen.
4. List situations in which pulse oximetry can be used to evaluate a patient's oxygenation.

Advanced

1. Describe at least two limitations of pulse oximetry.
2. Describe the use of capnography to assess changes in ventilation-perfusion patterns of the lung.
3. Assess oxygenation using arterial oxygen content.
4. Calculate the shunt fraction using appropriate laboratory data.

KEY TERMS

A-a gradient	hemoximetry	pulse oximetry
a-$\bar{v}$ O_2 content difference	Henderson–Hasselbalch equation	shunt fraction
Allen test	methemoglobin	solubility
base excess (BE)	oxygen content	spectrophotometer
capnography	pH	Sp_{O_2}
cyanosis	phosphorescence	Swan–Ganz catheter
Hb affinity	polarographic	transcutaneous

Blood gas analysis is the most basic test of lung function. Evaluation of the acid–base and oxygenation status of the body provides important information about the function of the lungs themselves. Anaerobic sampling of arterial blood is required, which is an invasive procedure that carries risks involved with blood-borne pathogens. Pulse oximetry and capnography measure gas exchange parameters and have the advantage of monitoring patients noninvasively. Understanding the limitations of noninvasive techniques allows them to be used to provide appropriate patient care. The calculation of **oxygen content** and the **shunt fraction** uses blood gas measurements to assess gas exchange as it applies to oxygenation.

The chapter addresses how blood gas measurements are used in the pulmonary function laboratory. A complete description of blood gas electrodes and other measuring devices is included in Chapter 11. The use of pulse oximetry and capnography as adjuncts to traditional invasive measures is discussed. Two methods of calculating shunt fraction are detailed so that the most appropriate method may be used.

PH

The **pH** is the negative logarithm of the hydrogen ion [H^+] concentration in the blood, used as a positive number. The pH scale has no units. It is derived by converting the [H^+] to a negative exponent of 10 and calculating its logarithm. The [H^+] of water is 1×10^{-7} mol/L. The negative logarithm of 1×10^{-7} is 7. The pH of water (7) represents the midpoint of the pH scale. The physiologic range

of pH in blood in clinical practice is from approximately 6.90 to 7.80, with the normal range being 7.35 to 7.45.

CARBON DIOXIDE TENSION

P_{CO_2} is a measurement of the partial pressure exerted by CO_2 in solution in the blood. The measurement is expressed in millimeters of mercury (mm Hg) or in kilopascals (kPa) in the International System of Units (1 mm Hg × 0.133 kPa). The term *torr* is also used as a non-SI unit of pressure and is roughly equal to 1 mm Hg. It was named after Evangelista Torricelli, an Italian physicist and mathematician who discovered the principle of the barometer in 1644. The normal range for P_{CO_2} in arterial blood is 35 to 45 mm Hg (4.66–5.99 kPa). In mixed venous blood, P_{CO_2} varies from 40 to 46 mm Hg (5.32–6.12 kPa).

OXYGEN TENSION

P_{O_2} measures the partial pressure exerted by oxygen (O_2) dissolved in the blood. Like P_{CO_2}, it is recorded in millimeters of mercury or in kilopascals. The normal range for arterial P_{O_2} is 70 to 100 mm Hg (10.64–13.30 kPa) for healthy young adults breathing air at sea level. The normal range declines slightly in older adults. Mixed venous P_{O_2} averages 40 mm Hg (5.32 kPa) in healthy patients. Barometric pressure (at altitudes significantly above sea level) also influences the expected arterial P_{O_2} (see Evolve website at http://evolve.elsevier.com/Mottram/Ruppel/ for conversion and correction factors).

Techniques

pH

Blood pH is measured by exposing the specimen to a glass electrode (see Chapter 11) or by measuring light absorbance with an optical pH indicator under anaerobic conditions. pH measurements are made at 37°C. The pH of arterial blood is related to the Pa_{CO_2} by the **Henderson–Hasselbalch equation:**

$$pH = pK + \log \frac{\left[HCO_3^-\right]}{\left[CO_2\right]}$$

where:

pK = negative log of dissociation constant for carbonic acid (6.1)

$[HCO_3^-]$ = molar concentration of serum bicarbonate

$[CO_2]$ = molar concentration of CO_2

Pa_{CO_2} (measured directly by a CO_2 electrode or similar device) may be multiplied by 0.03 (the **solubility** coefficient for CO_2) to express Pa_{CO_2} in milliequivalents per liter (mEq/L). The equation then may be expressed as follows:

$$pH = pK + \log \frac{\left[HCO_3^-\right]}{\left[0.03\left(Pa_{CO_2}\right)\right]}$$

Carbon Dioxide Tension

P_{CO_2} has traditionally been measured by exposing whole blood to a modified pH electrode contained in a jacket with a Teflon membrane at its tip (see Chapter 11). The jacket contains a bicarbonate buffer. As CO_2 diffuses through the membrane, it combines with water to form carbonic acid (H_2CO_3). The H_2CO_3 dissociates into H^+ and HCO_3^-, thereby changing the pH of the bicarbonate buffer. The change in pH is measured by the electrode and is proportional to the P_{CO_2}. Newer blood gas analyzers use a **spectrophotometer** to measure the absorbance of CO_2 in the infrared portion of the spectrum. The blood must be anticoagulated and kept in an anaerobic state until analysis. P_{CO_2} may also be estimated using a **transcutaneous** electrode. Measurement of end-tidal CO_2 ($P_{ET_{CO_2}}$)

is sometimes used to track P_{CO_2} (see later section, Capnography, in this chapter).

The pH and P_{CO_2} are usually measured from the same sample, so bicarbonate can be easily calculated. Automated blood gas analyzers perform this calculation, along with others, to derive values such as total CO_2 (dissolved CO_2 plus HCO_3^-) and standard bicarbonate (i.e., HCO_3^- corrected to a Pa_{CO_2} of 40 mm Hg). If the hemoglobin (Hb) is measured or estimated, the **base excess (BE)** can be calculated. The normal buffer base at a pH of 7.40 is approximately 48 mmol/L. BE is the difference between the actual buffering capacity of the blood and the expected value. When the buffering capacity is less than the expected value, the difference is a negative value. This is sometimes referred to as a *base deficit* rather than a *negative base excess*. The main buffers that affect the BE are HCO_3^- and Hb.

Oxygen Tension

The P_{O_2} (arterial or mixed venous) has traditionally been measured by exposing whole blood, obtained anaerobically, to a platinum electrode covered with a thin polypropylene membrane. This type of electrode is called a **polarographic** electrode, or *Clark* electrode. Oxygen molecules are reduced at the platinum cathode after diffusing through the membrane (see Chapter 11). Newer blood gas analyzers use an optical system that senses the ability of O_2 to change the intensity and duration of **phosphorescence** in a phosphorescent dye. P_{O_2} may also be measured using a transcutaneous electrode (see Chapter 11).

Blood gas values (pH, P_{CO_2}, P_{O_2}) are influenced by the patient's temperature. Alteration of body temperature affects the partial pressure of dissolved CO_2, which influences pH, as described in the previous equations. Table 6.1 describes the expected blood gas changes when the patient's temperature is not 37°C. Although blood gas measurements are made at 37°C, the value reported is sometimes corrected to the patient's temperature.

Technical problems with blood gas electrodes and related measuring devices include contamination by protein or blood products. In electrode-based analyzers, depletion of buffers in the electrodes may reduce accuracy and cause unacceptable drift. Tears

TABLE 6.1			
Effects of Body Temperature on Blood Gas Values[a]			
Temperature (°C)	34°	37°	40°
pH	7.44	7.40	7.36
Pco_2	35	40	46
Po_2	79	95	114

[a]Temperature corrections based on algorithms from the Clinical and Laboratory Standards Institute. (2009). *C46-A2: Definitions of quantities and conventions related to blood pH and gas analysis; approved guideline—second edition.* https://clsi.org/media/1355/c46a2_sample.pdf

or ruptures of the membranes used to cover the electrodes are also common malfunctions. Some newer analyzers use spectrophotometric methods that can be compromised by mechanical or electronic failure of the sampling cuvette or by inadequate mixing of the specimen.

Specimen Collection for Blood Gases

Arterial samples are usually obtained from either the radial or brachial arteries via puncture or catheter in adults. Arterial specimens may also be drawn from the femoral, dorsalis pedis, posterior tibial, or umbilical arteries. The radial artery of the nondominant hand is usually the preferred site. A warmed capillary sample (arterialized) can also be obtained to approximate an arterial specimen.

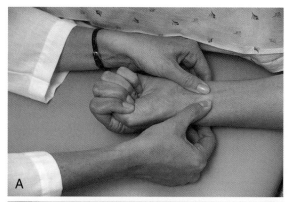
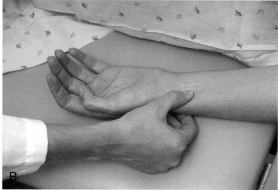

FIG. 6.1   Modified Allen test. The modified Allen test assesses collateral circulation for the hand. A "positive test" demonstrates adequate collateral circulation, and the radial artery may be used to harvest an arterial blood gas sample. (From Pagana, K. [2010]. *Mosby's manual of diagnostic and laboratory testing* (2nd ed.). St. Louis, MO: Mosby.)

PF TIP 6.1

Blood gas analyzers usually report blood gas values at 37°C. If the patient has an extreme body temperature (hypothermia or hyperthermia), correction may be useful. At low body temperatures, more gas dissolves in the blood, so Po_2 and Pco_2 show lower values when exposed to electrodes that measure their activity. At elevated temperatures, the opposite occurs; less gas dissolves, and partial pressures appear higher. The pH changes in relation to Pco_2.

Before a radial artery puncture, the adequacy of collateral circulation to the hand from the ulnar artery should be established using the modified **Allen test** (Fig. 6.1). The original Allen test was described by

Dr. Edgar Allen, a vascular surgeon at the Mayo Clinic in the 1920s, to assist in the diagnosis of thromboangiitis obliterans (e.g., Raynaud disease). A positive test in his description denoted reduced circulation; however, using the modified technique, a "positive test" demonstrates adequate collateral circulation. In performing the modified Allen test, the technologist occludes both the radial and ulnar arteries by pressing down over the wrist. The patient is instructed to make a fist and then open the hand and relax the fingers. The palm of the hand is pale and bloodless because both arteries are occluded. The ulnar artery is released while the radial remains occluded. The hand should be reperfused rapidly (5–15 seconds) if the ulnar supply is adequate. If perfusion is inadequate, an alternative site should be used.

6.1   How To ...

Perform a Modified Allen Test (See Fig. 6.1)

1. Tasks common to all procedures:
   a. Calibrate and prepare equipment.
   b. Review order.
   c. Introduce yourself and identify patient according to institutional policies.
   d. Describe and demonstrate procedure.
2. Instruct the patient to tightly close his or her hand to form a fist. Pressure is then applied at the wrist, compressing and obstructing both the radial and ulnar arteries.
3. The hand is then opened (but not fully extended), revealing a blanched palm and fingers.
4. Release pressure from the ulnar artery only while the palm and fingers, including the thumb, are observed.
5. These should become flushed within 5 to 15 seconds as the blood from the ulnar artery refills the empty capillary bed.
6. If the ulnar artery does not adequately supply the entire hand (a negative Allen test), the radial artery should not be used as a puncture site. An alternate artery should be selected.

Arterial puncture should not be performed through any type of lesion. Similarly, puncture distal to a surgical shunt (e.g., shunts used for dialysis) should be avoided. Infection or evidence of peripheral vascular disease should prompt the selection of an alternative site. Some patients may be using anticoagulant drugs such as heparin, warfarin (Coumadin), or streptokinase. High doses of these drugs or a history of prolonged clotting times may be relative contraindications to arterial puncture. Box 6.1 lists some of the potential hazards associated with arterial puncture.

Success in obtaining an arterial specimen by radial puncture requires careful positioning of the patient's wrist. The hand should be hyperextended, with good support under the wrist (Fig. 6.2, arterial puncture). A topical anesthetic may be useful for

| BOX 6.1 | COMPLICATIONS OF ARTERIAL PUNCTURE FOR BLOOD GAS TESTING |

- Pain and discomfort
- Hematoma
- Vasovagal response
- Thrombosis and embolism
- Infection or contamination
- Inadvertent needle stick
- Vascular trauma or occlusion
- Arterial spasm

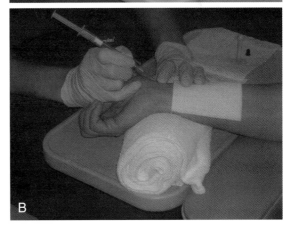

FIG. 6.2 (A) Arterial puncture with arm board. (B) Arterial puncture on towel.

some patients but is usually unnecessary. Always perform the modified Allen test to ensure adequate collateral circulation before puncturing the artery. The person drawing the sample should be in a comfortable position (i.e., sitting) to maximize control of the needle during insertion. It is recommended that the person drawing the sample use standard precautions and personal protective equipment, including gloves and eyewear. A vented syringe or similar device allows the blood to "pulse" into the syringe, ensuring that the needle is in the lumen of the artery.

Drawing a sample from a catheter-infusion system for an arterial or mixed venous sample from a pulmonary artery catheter (**Swan–Ganz catheter**) has its own nuances. Contamination of the sample with flush solution is a common problem. Withdrawing a small volume of blood into a "waste" syringe ensures that the sample is not diluted by flush solution in the catheter. Care should be taken to limit the volume of blood re-moved in this process. Significant blood loss can occur with repetitive measurements. Another problem associated specifically with mixed venous specimen collection is displacement of the Swan–Ganz catheter tip. If the catheter is advanced too far, it may "wedge" into a pulmonary arteriole. Specimens drawn from this position often reflect arterialized pulmonary capillary blood. Similarly, if the catheter tip is withdrawn or "loops back," it may be in the right ventricle or atrium rather than in the pulmonary artery. Specimens obtained from this location may not represent true mixed venous blood.

Venous samples from peripheral veins are not useful for assessing oxygenation. Venous blood reflects only the metabolism of the area drained by that particular vein. Venous samples may be used for the measurement of pH or blood lactate during exercise.

Blood is usually collected in a syringe to which an anticoagulant (e.g., heparin) has been added,

---

6.2	How To

Perform an Arterial Puncture From the Radial Artery

1. Tasks common to all procedures:
   a. Calibrate and prepare equipment.
   b. Review order.
   c. Introduce yourself and identify patient according to institutional policies.
   d. Describe and demonstrate procedure.
2. Prepare necessary equipment: self-filling heparinized syringe, needle, and personal protection equipment (e.g., gloves and eyewear).
3. Ensure the pretest conditions of the order are met (e.g., F_{IO_2}, liter flow, ventilator settings, etc.). If F_{IO_2} has been modified, wait 20 to 30 minutes before harvesting the sample. In the outpatient setting, the patient should be in a stable condition for a minimum of 5 minutes or longer once the previous criteria have been met.
4. Assess the collection site for adequate pulse and perform a modified Allen test.
5. Hyperextension of the wrist may facilitate exposure of the artery; palpate for a pulse.
6. Prepare the puncture site; clean with a laboratory-approved agent.
7. Make sure to instruct the subject to "breathe normally" and not to breath hold during the procedure.
8. Hold the syringe with the bevel up at a 30- to 45-degree angle, and advance toward the palpated artery until blood flow enters the syringe.
9. After obtaining the desired amount, place a dry gauze sponge over the puncture site and quickly remove the needle, applying pressure immediately and directly over the puncture site.
10. Immediately expel any air bubbles and mix thoroughly by rotating or inverting the sample numerous times.
11. Hold direct pressure to the site (2–5 minutes is typically adequate if the subject is not anticoagulated) until hemostasis occurs.
12. Report results and note comments related to sample quality.

CRITERIA FOR ACCEPTABILITY 6.1

Blood Gases

1. Blood should be collected anaerobically. Syringe body and plunger should be tight-fitting. Commercially available blood gas kits should be used according to manufacturers' specifications. Air bubbles should be expelled immediately.
2. The specimen must be adequately anticoagulated; sodium or lithium heparin is preferred. If liquid heparin is used, all excess should be expelled. The choice of anticoagulant should be determined by analyses to be performed (e.g., electrolytes).
3. A sample volume of 2 to 4 mL is recommended.
4. The specimen should be analyzed as soon as possible. If immediate analysis is not available, the specimen should be drawn in a glass syringe and stored in an ice-water slurry at 0°C and analyzed within 1 hour. Specimens drawn in plastic syringes should not be placed in ice water.
5. The specimen should be adequately identified, including patient name and/or number, date/time, ordering physician, and accession number. Information provided with the specimen should be the site from which it was obtained, FIO_2 (if applicable), device (e.g., nasal cannula, Oxymizer pendant), continuous flow or pulsed via a conserving device (if applicable), and ventilator or assist device (e.g., bilevel positive airway pressure [BIPAP]) settings (if applicable).
6. Analysis should be performed on an instrument that has been recently calibrated and whose function is documented by appropriate controls.

---

then sealed from the atmosphere immediately (Criteria for Acceptability 6.1). Blood gases are typically drawn using specially designed syringes containing a dry anticoagulant (i.e., a blood gas "kit"). Dry heparin is applied to the lumen of the needle and the interior of the syringe. A small heparin pellet is often placed in the syringe to provide additional anticoagulation. Care must be taken that heparin solution (sometimes used for flushing arterial catheters) does not contaminate the sample. Contamination by flush solution may affect PO_2 and PCO_2 values by dilution, but the buffering capacity of whole blood prevents large changes in pH.

After the syringe has been capped (see Chapter 12 for safe handling of blood specimens), the sample should be thoroughly mixed by rolling or gently shaking. Mixing helps prevent the sample from clotting, whether dry or liquid heparin is used. Mixing is also important for analyzers that use spectrophotometric methods for measuring blood gases. Lithium heparin or a similar preparation should be used for specimens that will also be used for electrolyte analysis.

Air contamination of arterial or mixed venous blood specimens can seriously alter blood gas values. Room air at sea level has a PO_2 of approximately 150 mm Hg and a PCO_2 near 0. If air bubbles are present in a blood gas specimen, equilibration of gases between the sample and air occurs (Table 6.2). Contamination commonly occurs during sampling when air is left in the syringe after the sample is collected. Small bubbles may also be introduced if the needle does not connect tightly to the syringe. Other sources of air contamination include poorly fitting plungers and failure to properly cap the syringe. The use of a vented syringe or one in which the pulse pressure of the blood displaces the plunger can help prevent air bubble contamination.

Sample storage depends on the type of syringe used. If a glass syringe is used, the sample may be stored in ice-water slush if the analysis is not done within a few minutes. Ice water reduces the metabolism of red and white blood cells in the sample. Specimens with O_2 tensions in the normal physiologic range (50–150 mm Hg) show minimal changes over 1 to 2 hours for glass syringes if kept in ice water. Changes in specimens held at room temperature are related to cellular metabolism in the blood, particularly in white blood cells and platelets. Specimens with PO_2 values above 150 mm

---

TABLE 6.2

Air Contamination of Blood Gas Samples

	In Vivo Values	Air Contamination[a]
pH	7.40	7.45
PCO_2	40	30
PO_2	95	110

[a]Typical values that might occur when a blood gas specimen is exposed to air, either directly or by mixing with a solution that has been exposed to air (e.g., heparinized flush solution). The change in pH occurs because of the change in PCO_2.

Hg are most susceptible to alterations resulting from gas leakage or cell metabolism. When the P_{O_2} is 150 mm Hg or more, Hb is almost completely bound with O_2. In such cases, a small change in O_2 content results in a large change in P_{O_2}.

If a plastic syringe is used, blood gas specimens should be analyzed within 30 minutes. Plastic syringes are not completely gas-tight, so room air can contaminate the sample. The influx of O_2 may be counterbalanced by the consumption of O_2 if the sample is not iced. When a blood gas specimen is placed in an ice-water bath, the solubility of O_2 increases, as does the **Hb affinity** for oxygen. This lowers the partial pressure of O_2 in the sample and increases the gradient between the sample and the environment. This gradient exaggerates the leakage of O_2 into the specimen (as occurs with plastic syringes). When the sample is introduced into the analyzer at 37°C, solubility and Hb affinity return to their normal values, the oxygen that leaked in is released, and the P_{O_2} is falsely increased. Because of these phenomena, blood gas specimens in plastic syringes should not be placed in ice water. If specimens cannot be routinely analyzed within 30 minutes, glass syringes with ice-water storage may be preferable.

Capillary samples are useful in infants when arterial puncture is impractical. The area for collection (the heel is commonly chosen) should be heated by a warm compress and lanced. Blood is then allowed to fill the required volume of heparinized glass/plastic capillary tubes. Squeezing the tissue should be avoided because predominantly venous blood will be obtained. The capillary tubes should be carefully sealed to avoid air bubbles. Guidelines for quality control of blood gas analyzers and for the safe handling of blood specimens are included in Chapter 12.

Significance and Pathophysiology

See Interpretive Strategies 6.1.

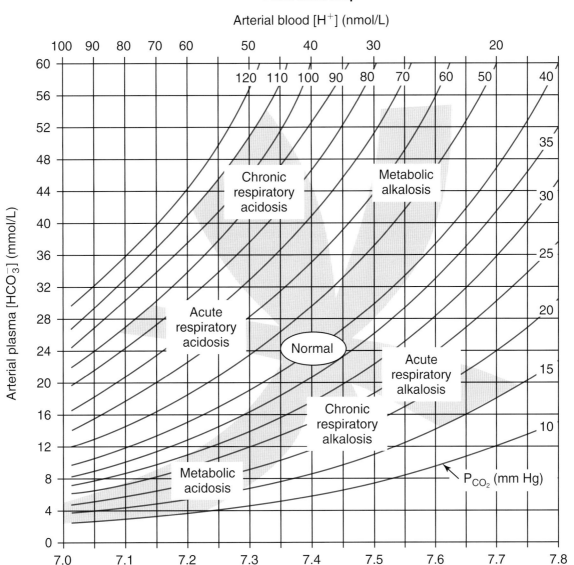

FIG. 6.3 Acid–base mapping. This tool assists the user to identify and characterize the acid–base disturbance.(From Cogan, M. G., & Rector, F. C. Jr. [1986]. Acid-base disturbances. In B. M. Brenner & F. C. Rector Jr. [Eds.], *The kidney.* Philadelphia, PA: WB Saunders.)

pH

The pH of arterial blood in healthy adults averages 7.40, with a range of 7.35 to 7.45. Arterial pH below 7.35 constitutes acidemia. A pH above 7.45 constitutes alkalemia. Because of the logarithmic scale, a change of 0.3 pH units represents a twofold change in $[H^+]$

concentration. If the pH decreases from 7.40 to 7.10 with no change in P_{CO_2}, the concentration of hydrogen ions has doubled. Conversely, if the concentration of $[H^+]$ is halved, the pH increases from 7.40 to 7.70, assuming the P_{CO_2} remains at 40 mm Hg. Changes of this magnitude represent marked abnormalities in the acid–base status of the blood and are almost always accompanied by clinical symptoms (e.g., cardiac arrhythmias; see Fig. 6.3). If a metabolic acidemia is present, examination of the anion gap (AG) needs to be assessed. The anion gap is the difference between routinely measured cations (sodium) and anions (chloride and bicarbonate) in serum, plasma, or urine. The magnitude of the difference in serum is calculated to help identify the cause of a metabolic acidemia. The anion gap also reflects unmeasured cations (e.g., proteins, organic acids, phosphates) and anions (e.g., calcium, potassium, magnesium) (Table 6.3). The anion gap is expressed in units of mEg/L or mmol/L and is calculated by subtracting the serum concentrations of chloride and bicarbonate from the concentrations of sodium and potassium. However, in routine clinical practice, the potassium is frequently ignored, which leaves the following equation:

$$AG = \left[Na^+\right] - \left[Cl^- + HCO_3^-\right]$$
$$AG = 140 - \left[105 + 24\right]$$
$$AG = 11 \, mEq/L$$

The normal range is 3 to 11 mEq/L; however, the reference range should be provided by the lab performing the tests.

Acid–base disorders arising from lung disease are often related to P_{CO_2} and its transport as carbonic acid. If the pH is outside of its normal range (i.e., acidemia or alkalemia) but P_{CO_2} is within normal limits, the condition is termed *nonrespiratory* or *metabolic* (Table 6.4). The calculated HCO_3^- is a useful indicator of the relationship between pH and P_{CO_2}. In the presence of acidemia (pH < 7.35) and normal CO_2 (P_{CO_2} of 35–45 mm Hg), HCO_3^- will be low, and a metabolic acidosis is present. A P_{CO_2} of less than 35 mm Hg in the presence of acidosis suggests that ventilatory compensation for acidemia is occurring. The acid–base status would be considered partially compensated nonrespiratory (i.e., metabolic) acidosis. Complete compensation occurs if pH returns to the normal range. This happens when ventilation reduces P_{CO_2} in proportion to the HCO_3^-.

TABLE 6.3	
Anion Gap: Metabolic Acidosis	
Wide Gap	Normal Gap
"MUDPILES"	"HARDUP"
Methanol (Osm gap high)	**H**yperventilation
Uremia	**A**cid infusion/carbonic anhydrase inhibitors/ Addison's disease
Diabetic/alcoholic ketoacidosis	**R**enal tubular acidosis (urine gap positive)
Paraldehyde	**D**iarrhea (urine gap normal; i.e., negative)
Isoniazid/Iron	**U**reterosigmoidostomy
Lactic acidosis	**P**ancreatic fistula/drainage
Ethylene glycol (Osm gap high)	
Salicylates/solvents	

TABLE 6.4			
Acid–Base Disorders			
Status	**pH**	**P_{CO_2}**	**HCO_3^-**
Simple Disorders			
Metabolic acidosis	Low	Normal	Low
Metabolic alkalosis	High	Normal	High
Respiratory acidosis	Low	High	Normal
Respiratory alkalosis	High	Low	Normal
Compensated Disorders			
Compensated respiratory acidosis or metabolic alkalosis	Normal[a]	High	High
Compensated metabolic acidosis or respiratory alkalosis	Normal[a]	Low	Low
Combined Disorders			
Metabolic/respiratory acidosis	Low	High	Low
Metabolic/respiratory alkalosis	High	Low	High

[a] Compensation cannot return values to within normal limits in severe acid–base disturbances. In addition, a normal pH may result in instances of respiratory and metabolic disturbances that occur together but are not compensatory.

In the presence of alkalemia (pH > 7.45) and normal P_{CO_2} (3–45 mm Hg), calculated bicarbonate will be increased, and metabolic alkalosis is present. If ventilatory compensation occurs, P_{CO_2} will be slightly increased. However, decreased ventilation is required so that the CO_2 can increase. Reduced minute ventilation may interfere with oxygenation. For this reason, Pa_{CO_2} seldom increases above 50 mm Hg to compensate for nonrespiratory (i.e., metabolic) alkalosis. Compensation may be incomplete if the alkalosis is severe.

Abnormal P_{CO_2} and HCO_3^- characterize combined respiratory and nonrespiratory acid–base disorders. In combined acidosis, P_{CO_2} is elevated (< 45 mm Hg), and HCO^- is low (< 22 mEq/L). In combined alkalosis, HCO^- is elevated (< 26 mEq/L), and P_{CO_2} is low (< 35 mm Hg). The pH is more severely deranged (i.e., much higher, or lower) than if just one disorder were present.

Carbon Dioxide Tension

The arterial carbon dioxide tension (Pa_{CO_2}) in a healthy adult is approximately 40 mm Hg; it may range from 35 to 45 mm Hg. The P_{CO_2} of venous or mixed venous blood is seldom used clinically. Body temperature affects Pa_{CO_2}, as described in Table 6.1.

Pa_{CO_2} is inversely proportional to alveolar ventilation ($\dot{V}_A$; see Chapter 5). When $\dot{V}_A$ decreases, CO_2 may not be removed by the lungs as fast as it is produced. This causes Pa_{CO_2} to increase. The pH falls (i.e., $[H^+]$ increases) as CO_2 is hydrated to form carbonic acid:

$$CO_2 + H_2O \leftrightarrow H_2CO_3 \leftrightarrow H^+ + HCO_3^-$$

Increasing levels of CO_2 in the blood drive this reaction to the right. The patient has respiratory acidosis resulting from hypoventilation. Conversely, when alveolar ventilation removes CO_2 more rapidly than it is produced, Pa_{CO_2} decreases. The pH increases (i.e., $[H^+]$ falls) as the patient becomes alkalotic. This condition is called *hyperventilation* or *respiratory alkalosis*.

If dead space increases, high-minute ventilation ($\dot{V}_E$) may be required to adequately ventilate alveoli and keep Pa_{CO_2} within normal limits. Respiratory dead space occurs because some lung units are ventilated but not perfused by pulmonary capillary blood. Pulmonary embolization is an example of a dead-space–producing condition. Emboli may block pulmonary arterioles, causing ventilation of the affected lung units to be "wasted." To maintain normal Pa_{CO_2}, total ventilation must be increased to compensate for wasted ventilation. Pa_{CO_2} may be normal or decreased even though significant pulmonary disease is present.

Patients who have disorders such as lobar pneumonia may increase their $\dot{V}_E$ to provide more alveolar ventilation of functional lung units. This mechanism compensates for lung units that do not participate in gas exchange. Hypoxemia is a common cause of hyperventilation (i.e., respiratory alkalosis). Hyperventilation may be seen in patients with asthma, emphysema, bronchitis, or foreign body obstruction. Anxiety, stress, or central nervous system disorders may also cause hyperventilation. Hyperventilation may also be an intentional or unintentional result of mechanical ventilation.

Increased Pa_{CO_2} (i.e., hypercapnia) commonly occurs in patients who have advanced obstructive or restrictive disease. These individuals are characterized by markedly abnormal ventilation-perfusion ($\dot{V}/\dot{Q}$) patterns. They are unable to maintain adequate alveolar ventilation. Not all patients with advanced pulmonary disease retain CO_2. Those who do become hypercapnic often have a low ventilatory response to CO_2 (see Chapter 5). Their response to the increased work of breathing caused by obstruction or restriction is to allow CO_2 to increase rather than increase ventilation. When respiratory acidosis results from increased P_{CO_2}, renal compensation usually occurs (see Table 6.4).

Increased Pa_{CO_2} may also be seen in patients who hypoventilate as a result of central nervous system or neuromuscular disorders. Whether CO_2 retention is the result of lung disease, central nervous system dysfunction, or neuromuscular disease, pH is usually maintained close to normal. The kidneys retain and produce bicarbonate (HCO_3^-) to match the increased Pa_{CO_2}. This response may completely compensate for a mildly elevated Pa_{CO_2}. However, it can seldom produce normal pH when the Pa_{CO_2}

TABLE 6.5

Causes of Hypoxia and Hypoxemia

Type	Cause
Hypoxemic hypoxia	Altitude
	Hypoventilation
	Shunt
	$\dot{V}/\dot{Q}$ mismatching
	Diffusion
Circulatory hypoxia	Hypovolemia
	Reduced cardiac output (impaired left vintricular function, outflow tract abnormalities, etc.)
Hemic hypoxia	Anemia, dyshemoglobinemias (COHb, MetHb, etc.)
Histotoxic hypoxia	Cyanide poisoning
Demand hypoxia	Seizures, exercise

is greater than 65 mm Hg. If the disorder causing the increased Pa_{CO_2} is acute (e.g., foreign body aspiration), little or no renal compensation may be observed.

Some degree of hypoxemia is always present in patients who retain CO_2 while breathing air (Table 6.5). As alveolar CO_2 increases, alveolar O_2 decreases. If the cause of hypercapnia is either obstructive or restrictive lung disease, hypoxemia may be severe because of $\dot{V}/\dot{Q}$ abnormalities (see Table 6.5). Because O_2 therapy is common in these patients, changes in P_{CO_2} while breathing supplementary O_2 must be carefully monitored. Some patients with chronic hypoxemia have a decreased ventilatory response to CO_2. O_2 administered to these patients may reduce their hypoxic stimulus for ventilation. As a result, Pa_{CO_2} may increase further. O_2 therapy is usually titrated to maintain Pa_{CO_2} values less than 60 mm Hg without hypercapnia and acidosis.

Oxygen Tension

The Pa_{O_2} of healthy young adults at sea level ranges from 85 to 100 mm Hg and decreases slightly with age. Breathing room air at sea level results in an inspired P_{O_2} of approximately 150 mm Hg:

$$\begin{aligned}
P_{IO_2} &= F_{IO_2}\left(P_B - 47\right)\\
&= 0.21(760 - 47)\\
&= 0.21(713)\\
&= 149.7
\end{aligned}$$

where:

F_{IO_2} = fractional concentration of inspired O_2
P_B = barometric pressure
47 = partial pressure of water vapor at 37°C

The partial pressure of O_2 in alveolar gas is usually close to 100 mm Hg and can be calculated using the alveolar air equation:

$$P_{AO_2} = \left(F_{IO_2} \times [P_B - 47]\right) - Pa_{CO_2}\left(F_{IO_2} + \frac{1 - F_{IO_2}}{R}\right)$$

where:

Pa_{CO_2} = arterial CO_2 tension (presumed equal to alveolar CO_2 tension)
R = respiratory exchange ratio ($\dot{V}_{CO_2}/\dot{V}_{O_2}$)

Substituting 40 mm Hg for Pa_{CO_2} and 0.8 for R gives the following:

$$\begin{aligned}
P_{AO_2} &= \left(0.21 \times [760 - 47]\right) - 40\left(0.21 + \frac{1 - 0.21}{0.8}\right)\\
&= \left(0.21 \times 713\right) - 40(1.1975)\\
&= 149.7 - 47.9\\
&= 101.8
\end{aligned}$$

In healthy lungs with good gas exchange, arterial oxygen tension can approach the value of the alveolar P_{O_2}. The difference between the alveolar and arterial oxygen tensions is described as the alveolar-arterial gradient, or **A-a gradient.** This gradient is usually less than 20 mm Hg in healthy individuals breathing air at sea level.

Hyperventilation may increase Pa_{O_2} as high as 120 mm Hg in a patient with normal lung function (see the previous alveolar air equation). Healthy subjects breathing 100% O_2 may exhibit Pa_{O_2} values higher than 600 mm Hg. The alveolar P_{O_2} (Pa_{O_2}) for a particular inspired O_2 fraction can be calculated, as previously described. Decreased Pa_{O_2} can result from hypoventilation, diffusion abnormalities, $\dot{V}/\dot{Q}$ imbalances, shunt, and inadequate atmospheric O_2 (high altitude; see Table 6.4).

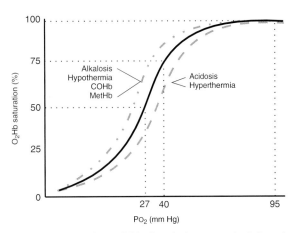

FIG. 6.4 Oxygen-hemoglobin dissociation curve. The S-shaped curve represents the relationship between partial pressure of O_2 in blood (*x*-axis) and Hb saturation (*y*-axis). "Shift to the left": ↓ 2, 3, DPG; temp; PCO_2; ↑ pH; results in an increase in oxygen affinity. "Shift to the right": ↑ 2, 3, DPG; temp; PCO_2; ↓ pH; results in a decrease in oxygen affinity.

Table 6.1 lists changes that occur in PaO_2 because of body temperatures above and below normal (37°C). Changes in PO_2 and PCO_2 reflect the solubility of the gas. The partial pressure of each gas is a measure of its activity. Hypothermia (low body temperature) is accompanied by decreased partial pressure as more gas dissolves. Hyperthermia (elevated body temperature) causes elevated gas tensions as gas comes out of solution. All blood gas analyzers perform analyses at 37°C, and most allow temperature corrections to be made. Although blood gas tensions vary with temperature, the clinical significance of correcting measurements is unclear. Blood gas values should be reported at 37°C. Care must be taken to ensure that blood gas analyzers are maintained at 37°C. Measurements made at other temperatures can significantly alter results.

PO_2 is the pressure of O_2 dissolved in blood. The amount of Hb and whether it is capable of binding O_2 have only a minimal effect on PO_2. Hypoxemia (decreased O_2 content of the blood) may occur even if PO_2 is normal or elevated by breathing O_2. Hypoxemia commonly results from inadequate or abnormal Hb (see Table 6.5). Many automated blood gas analyzers calculate oxygen saturation (SaO_2). Saturation may be calculated from the PaO_2 and pH, assuming a normal oxygen–hemoglobin reaction occurs (Fig. 6.4). Calculated SaO_2 may differ significantly from true saturation measured by a spectrophotometer (see the section on Oxygen Saturation) because a number of factors can affect the relationship of the binding capacity of hemoglobin (see Fig. 6.4).

An example of the discrepancy between calculated and measured saturation is the patient with elevated carboxyhemoglobin (COHb) resulting from smoking or smoke inhalation. The patient's PaO_2 may be normal while O_2 saturation is markedly decreased. Calculating saturation from PO_2, in this case, overestimates the O_2 content of the blood. Measured SaO_2 is preferred to a calculated value.

The severity of impaired oxygenation is indicated by the PaO_2 at rest. PaO_2 is a good index of the lungs' ability to match pulmonary capillary blood flow with adequate ventilation. If ventilation matches perfusion, pulmonary capillary blood leaves the lungs with a PO_2 close to that of the alveoli. If ventilation is adequate, pulmonary capillary blood is almost completely saturated. If either of these conditions is not met (i.e., poor ventilation or $\dot{V}/\dot{Q}$ mismatching), pulmonary capillary blood has reduced O_2 content. PaO_2 is reduced in proportion to the number of lung units contributing blood with low O_2 content. Lung units with good $\dot{V}/\dot{Q}$ cannot compensate for their poorly functioning counterparts because the pulmonary capillary blood leaving them is already almost fully oxygenated. O_2 binding to Hb is almost complete when the PaO_2 is greater than 60 mm Hg (approximately 90% saturation). As PaO_2 decreases from 60 to 40 mm Hg, saturation decreases from 90% to 75%, with increasing symptoms of hypoxia (e.g., mental confusion, shortness of breath).

Delivery of O_2 to the tissues, however, depends on Hb concentration and cardiac output, in addition to adequate gas transfer in the lungs. Arterial oxygen content (Cao_2 in mL/dL) is defined as follows:

$$Cao_2 = (1.34 \times Hb \times Sao_2) + (Pao_2 \times 0.0031)$$

where:

1.34 = O_2 binding capacity of Hb, mL/g
Hb = hemoglobin concentration, g/dL
Sao_2 = arterial oxygen saturation as a fraction
Pao_2 = arterial oxygen tension, mm Hg
0.0031 = solubility coefficient for O_2 at 37°C

Because most transported O_2 is bound to Hb, there must be an adequate supply (12–15 g/dL) of functional Hb. Adequate cardiac output (4–5 L/min) is necessary to deliver the oxygenated arterial blood to the tissues. Signs and symptoms of hypoxia may be present despite adequate Pao_2 because of severe anemia and/or reduced cardiac function (see Table 6.5).

The mixed venous oxygen tension ($P\bar{v}o_2$) in healthy patients at rest ranges from approximately 37 to 43 mm Hg, with an average of 40 mm Hg (see Fig. 6.4). Mixed venous O_2 content ($C\bar{v}o_2$) averages 15 mL/dL. In healthy individuals, arterial oxygen content (Cao_2) averages 20 mL/dL. The resulting content difference, or $C(a-\bar{v})o_2$, is thus 5 mL/dL (or 5 vol%). Although Pao_2 varies with the inspired O_2 fraction and matching of $\dot{V}/\dot{Q}$, $P\bar{v}o_2$ changes in response to alterations in cardiac output and O_2 consumption. If cardiac output increases while oxygen consumption ($\dot{V}o_2$) remains constant, the $C(a-\bar{v})o_2$ decreases. Conversely, if cardiac output decreases with no change in O_2 consumption, the $C(a-\bar{v})o_2$ increases. Increased cardiac output sometimes occurs in response to pulmonary shunting. This allows mixed venous oxygen content to increase, reducing the deleterious effect of the shunt. Critically ill patients often have low $P\bar{v}o_2$ values and increased $C(a-\bar{v})o_2$ as a result of poor cardiovascular performance. Alterations in $P\bar{v}o_2$ often occur even if Pao_2 is normal. $P\bar{v}o_2$ values of less than 28 mm Hg in critically ill patients accompanied by $C(a-\bar{v})o_2$ greater than 6 vol% suggest marked cardiovascular decompensation.

Patients who have severe obstructive or restrictive diseases may have decreased Pao_2 at rest, occasionally as low as 40 mm Hg. Mild pulmonary disease may show little decrease in Pao_2 if hyperventilation is present. Pao_2 may also be relatively normal if the disease process affects ventilation and perfusion similarly. In patients with emphysema, destruction of alveolar septa may eliminate pulmonary capillaries as well, resulting in poor ventilation and equally poor blood flow. These patients may have severe airway obstruction and markedly reduced diffusing capacity (D_{LCO}) but only a small decrease in resting Pao_2. Patients with chronic bronchitis or asthma, particularly during acute exacerbations, may have moderate or severe resting hypoxemia because of $\dot{V}/\dot{Q}$ abnormalities (see Table 6.5).

During exercise in patients with obstructive disease, Pao_2 often decreases commensurate with the extent of the disease. Pao_2 during exercise is correlated with the patient's D_{LCO} and forced expiratory volume in the first second (FEV_1), but wide variability exists. Patients with markedly decreased D_{LCO} may show low Pao_2 values at rest that decrease during exercise. Studies have demonstrated sensitivity and specificity in the range of 75% to 90% of exercise desaturation if the D_{LCO} is 50% to 60% of predicted. The degree of arterial desaturation cannot be predicted from static pulmonary function measurements.

Pao_2 may be decreased for nonpulmonary reasons, such as anatomic shunts (intracardiac) or hypoventilation because of neuromuscular disease. Tissue hypoxia can occur because of inadequate or nonfunctional Hb or because of poor cardiac output (see Table 6.5). Pao_2 should be correlated with spirometry (FEV_1), D_{LCO}, ventilation ($\dot{V}_E$, tidal volume, dead space), and lung volumes (vital capacity [VC], reserve capacity [RV], total lung capacity [TLC]) to distinguish pulmonary from nonpulmonary causes of inadequate oxygenation.

HEMOXIMETRY

Description

Hemoximetry (i.e., blood oximetry, also known as *CO-oximetry*) refers to the measurement of hemoglobin (Hb) and its derivatives by spectroscopy. Oxygen saturation is the ratio of oxygenated Hb (O_2Hb) to either total available Hb or functional Hb. Functional Hb is that portion of the total Hb capable of binding oxygen. This ratio of content to capacity is normally expressed as a percentage but is sometimes recorded as a simple fraction. The values may differ significantly, depending on the method of calculation:

Oxyhemoglobin fraction of total Hb:

$$\frac{O_2Hb}{(O_2Hb + rHb + COHb + MetHb)}$$

Oxygen saturation of available Hb:

$$\frac{O_2Hb}{O_2Hb + rHb}$$

where:

O_2Hb = oxyhemoglobin
rHb = reduced hemoglobin concentration
COHb = carboxyhemoglobin concentration
MetHb = methemoglobin concentration

The first equation is used to measure O_2 saturation with a multiple-wavelength spectrophotometer (hemoximeter); the second equation is used to measure O_2 saturation with a pulse oximeter.

Technique

O_2 saturation of Hb (O_2Hb, or SaO_2 when referring to arterial saturation) may be measured in several ways. In the first method, O_2 saturation is measured using a spectrophotometer (see Chapter 11). Whole blood is hemolyzed, and the absorbances of the various components measured. The total Hb, O_2Hb, COHb, and MetHb are usually reported. Hemoximetry is usually performed in conjunction with blood gas analysis, using a single specimen of blood.

An indirect method may be used to measure mixed venous oxygen saturation ($S\bar{v}O_2$). Saturation may be measured by a reflective spectrophotometer in a pulmonary artery catheter. In this case, absorbances are measured without hemolyzing the blood. A special catheter that includes fiberoptic bundles is used to perform in vivo measurements.

Blood specimens for hemoximetry should be prepared, as described for arterial blood gas specimens. Guidelines for quality control of blood gas analysis are included in Chapter 12. Measurement

of percent saturation allows the calculation of the O_2 content of either arterial or mixed venous blood (CaO_2 and $C\bar{v}O_2$, respectively; see the Oxygen Tension section).

Significance and Pathophysiology

See Interpretive Strategies 6.2. The SaO_2 for a healthy young adult with a PaO_2 of 95 mm Hg is approximately 97%. The O_2Hb dissociation curve is relatively flat when the PaO_2 is above 60 mm Hg (i.e., SaO_2 is 90% or more). Saturation changes only slightly when there is a marked change in PaO_2 at partial pressures above 60 mm Hg (see Fig. 6.4). Therefore PaO_2 is a more sensitive indicator of oxygenation in lungs that do not have gross abnormalities. At PaO_2 values of approximately 150 mm Hg, Hb becomes completely saturated (SaO_2 is 100%). At PaO_2 values above 150 mm Hg, further increases in O_2 content are caused by increased dissolved oxygen. Alterations in $\dot{V}/\dot{Q}$ patterns in the lungs can be monitored by allowing the patient to breathe 100% O_2 and by measuring the changes in dissolved oxygen. In practice, this is accomplished by using the clinical shunt equation (see the Shunt Calculation section).

INTERPRETIVE STRATEGIES 6.2

Oxygen Saturation

1. How was the estimate of saturation obtained? Hemoximeter? Calculated saturation? Pulse oximeter?
2. For hemoximetry or calculated saturation: Was the specimen obtained anaerobically and handled properly?
3. Is Hb within the normal limits? If low, oxygenation may be compromised; if elevated, look for clinical correlation.
4. Is O_2Hb > 90%? If so, oxygenation is probably adequate; if not, hypoxemia is likely.
5. Is O_2Hb < 85%? If so, supplementary oxygen may be indicated. Correlate with PaO_2 and a clinical history.
6. Is COHb > 3%? If so, check for a smoking history and/or environmental exposure.
7. Is MetHb > 1.5%? If so, check for environmental exposure to oxidizers or medications known to cause methemoglobin (e.g., benzocaine, dapsone, inhaled nitric oxide, etc.).

When Pa_{O_2} falls below 60 mm Hg, Sa_{O_2} decreases rapidly. Small changes in Pa_{O_2} result in large changes in saturation. As Sa_{O_2} falls below 90%, O_2 content decreases rapidly. At saturations less than 85% (i.e., $Pa_{O_2} < 55$ mm Hg), symptoms of hypoxemia increase, and supplementary O_2 may be indicated.

The ability of Hb to bind O_2 may be measured by the P_{50}. P_{50} specifies the partial pressure at which Hb is 50% saturated (see Fig. 6.4). The P_{50} of normal adult Hb is approximately 27 mm Hg. P_{50} may be determined by equilibrating blood with several gases at low oxygen tensions. An O_2Hb dissociation curve is then constructed to estimate the partial pressure at which Hb is 50% saturated. A second method of estimating P_{50} compares measured Sa_{O_2} (using a spectrophotometer) with the expected saturation. Calculated saturations presume a P_{50} of 26 to 27 mm Hg, but it may differ significantly depending on the types of Hb and interfering substances present.

Healthy individuals have small amounts of Hb that cannot carry O_2. COHb is present in blood from metabolism and from environmental exposure to carbon monoxide (CO) gas. Normal COHb, expressed as a percentage, ranges from 0.5% to 2% of the total Hb. CO comes from smoking (cigarettes, cigars, and pipes), smoke inhalation, improperly vented furnaces, automobile emissions, and other sources of combustion. In smokers, levels may increase from 3% to 15%, depending on recent smoking history. Smoke inhalation or CO poisoning from other sources also results in elevated COHb levels, sometimes as high as 50%. CO combines rapidly with Hb. Exposures of a short duration can cause a high level of COHb if high concentrations of CO are present. Because O_2Hb saturation decreases as COHb increases, COHb levels greater than 15% almost always result in hypoxemia. High levels of COHb are rapidly fatal because of the profound hypoxemia that occurs.

COHb absorbs light at wavelengths similar to O_2Hb. When COHb is elevated, arterial blood appears bright red. **Cyanosis,** which appears when there is an increased concentration of reduced Hb, is absent. In spite of elevated levels of COHb, Pa_{O_2} may be close to normal limits. Blood gas analysis that includes the calculated saturation will give erroneously high O_2 saturations. For this reason, O_2Hb and COHb should be measured by hemoximetry whenever possible.

COHb interferes with O_2 transport in two ways: it binds competitively to Hb, and it shifts the O_2Hb curve to the left (see Fig. 6.4). Increased COHb causes reduced O_2Hb with a decrease in O_2 content. The left shift of the dissociation curve causes O_2 to be bound more tightly to Hb. The combination of these two effects can seriously reduce O_2 delivery to the tissues. COHb concentrations in blood begin to decrease once the source of CO has been removed. Removal of CO from the blood depends on the minute ventilation. Breathing room air may require several hours to reduce even moderate levels to normal. Breathing 100% O_2 speeds the washout of CO. High concentrations of O_2 (often including hyperbaric therapy) are indicated whenever dangerously high levels of COHb are encountered.

Methemoglobin (MetHb) forms when iron atoms of the Hb molecule are oxidized from Fe^{++} to Fe^{+++}. The normal MetHb level is less than 1.5% of the total Hb in adults. High levels of MetHb can result from ingestion of or exposure to strong oxidizing agents. Methemoglobinemia has also been linked to high doses of medications such as benzocaine, dapsone, nitroprusside, and inhaled nitric oxide. Like COHb, MetHb reduces the O_2 carrying capacity of the blood by reducing the available Hb and shifting the O_2Hb dissociation curve to the left (see Fig. 6.4).

The saturation of mixed venous blood ($S\bar{v}_{O_2}$) in healthy patients averages 75% at a $P\bar{v}_{O_2}$ of 40 mm Hg. Healthy patients have a content difference, $C(a-\bar{v})_{O_2}$, of 5 vol%. Arterial blood in adults with normal levels of Hb typically carries approximately 20 vol% O_2, and mixed venous blood carries 15 vol% O_2. Pulmonary diseases that cause arterial hypoxemia may reduce $S\bar{v}_{O_2}$ if oxygen uptake and cardiac output remain constant. Cardiac output often increases to combat arterial hypoxemia caused by intrapulmonary shunting. Increased cardiac output increases O_2 delivery to the tissues. This results in a reduced extraction of O_2 from the blood. Mixed venous blood then returns to the lungs with normal or even increased O_2 saturation. When this blood is shunted, it has a higher O_2 content, thereby reducing the shunt effect. With or without arterial hypoxemia, $S\overline{v}O_2$ decreases if cardiac output is compromised.

$S\overline{v}O_2$ is useful in assessing cardiac function in the critical care setting and during exercise but does require the placement of a pulmonary artery catheter. Patients who have good cardiovascular reserves maintain a mixed venous saturation of 70% to 75%. Patients whose $S\overline{v}O_2$ values are in the 60% to 70% range have a limited ability to deliver more O_2 to the tissues. $S\overline{v}O_2$ values of less than 60% usually indicate cardiovascular decompensation and may be associated with tissue hypoxemia. The indwelling reflective spectrophotometer (see Chapter 11) allows continuous monitoring of this important parameter. $S\overline{v}O_2$ also decreases during exercise. Despite increased cardiac output, O_2 extraction by the exercising muscles reduces the content of blood returning to the lungs.

Estimation of SaO_2 by most pulse oximeters (**Sp**o**2**) is based on the absorption of light at two wavelengths. When only two wavelengths are analyzed, only two species of Hb can be detected. Absorption in the red and near-infrared portions of the visible spectrum allows measurement of the oxyhemoglobin and reduced Hb, providing an estimate of the oxygen saturation of available Hb (see the Pulse Oximetry section).

PULSE OXIMETRY

Description

Spo**2** estimates SaO_2 by analyzing the absorption of light passing through a capillary bed, either by transmission or reflectance. **Pulse oximetry** is noninvasive. SpO_2 is reported as percent saturation. These devices report heart rate (HR), although practitioners should be aware that this is the pulse rate derived at the probe site and may not reflect actual HR. Some pulse oximeters are also capable of measuring Hb, COHb, and MetHb.

Technique

Pulse oximeters (see Chapter 11) measure the light absorption of a mixture of two forms of Hb: O_2Hb

and reduced Hb (rHb). The relative absorptions at 660 nm (red) and 940 nm of light (near infrared) can be used to calculate the combination of the two Hb forms. Absorption at two wavelengths provides an estimate of the saturation of available Hb (see the Oxygen Saturation section). Most pulse oximeters use a stored calibration curve to estimate oxygen saturation.

Pulse oximetry may be used in any setting in which a noninvasive measure of oxygenation status is sufficient. This includes monitoring of O_2 therapy and ventilator management. Pulse oximetry is commonly used during diagnostic procedures such as bronchoscopy, sleep studies, or stress testing. It is also used for monitoring during patient transport or rehabilitation. Pulse oximetry may be used for continuous monitoring with inclusion of appropriate alarms to detect desaturation. Many pulse oximeter systems use memory (random access memory [RAM]) to record SpO_2 and HR for extended periods. This type of recorded monitoring allows pulse oximetry to be used for overnight studies of nocturnal desaturation. Alternatively, pulse oximetry can be used for discrete measurements or "spot checks."

Most pulse oximeters use a sensor that attaches to the finger, toe (nail bed), or ear. The choice of attachment site should be dictated by the type of measurement being made. The ear site may be preferred in patients undergoing exercise testing or in whom arm movement precludes the use of the finger site. Both finger and ear sites presume pulsatile blood flow. Most pulse oximeters adjust light output to compensate for tissue density or pigmentation. In some patients, impaired perfusion to one site determines which site is preferred. Low perfusion or poor vascularity can cause the oximeter to be unable to detect pulsatile blood flow. Rubbing or warming of the site often improves local blood flow and may be indicated to obtain reliable data. Some pulse oximeters use reflective sensors that detect light reflected from bone underlying the tissue bed. These sensors are usually placed on the patient's forehead and may function when finger or ear sensors do not and may be a preferred site during exercise when motion artifact can be an issue.

Some pulse oximeters display a representation of the pulse waveform derived from the absorption measurements (see Chapter 11). Such waveforms may be helpful in selecting an appropriate site or troubleshooting questionable SpO_2 values. Most pulse oximeters report HR, which is also detected from pulsatile blood flow at the sensor site. Comparison of oximeter HR with palpated pulse or with an electrocardiograph (ECG) signal can assist with the selection of an appropriate site. Inability to obtain a valid HR reading or acceptable pulse waveform suggests that SpO_2 values should be interpreted cautiously (Criteria for Acceptability 6.2).

BOX 6.2   PULSE OXIMETER LIMITATIONS

Interfering Substances

- Carboxyhemoglobin (COHb)[a,b]
- Methemoglobin (MetHb)[a]
- Intravascular dyes (indocyanine green)
- Nail polish or coverings (finger sensor)

Interfering Factors

- Motion artifact, shivering
- Bright ambient lighting
- Hypotension, low perfusion (sensor site)
- Hypothermia
- Vasoconstrictor drugs
- Dark skin pigmentation
- Artificial nails or dark nail polish

CRITERIA FOR ACCEPTABILITY 6.2

Pulse Oximetry

1. Documentation of adequate correlation with measured SaO_2 should be available. SpO_2 and SaO_2 should be within 2% from 85% to 100% saturation. Elevated COHb (> 3%) or MetHb > 2%) may invalidate SpO_2.
2. Adequate perfusion of the sensor site should be documented by agreement between the oximeter and the patient's heart rate (ECG or palpation) and reproducible pulse waveforms (if available).
3. Known interfering substances or agents should be eliminated or accounted for.
4. Pulse oximeter readings should be stable for long enough to answer the clinical question being investigated. Readings should be consistent with the patient's clinical history and presentation.

A number of factors limit the validity of SpO_2 measurements (Box 6.2). To validate pulse oximetry readings, direct measurement of arterial saturation is required. Simultaneous measurement of SpO_2 and SaO_2 can be used to confirm pulse oximeter readings. Pulse oximetry used during exercise testing has been shown to produce variable results. Hemoximetry may be necessary to validate pulse oximetry readings at peak exercise.

COHb absorbs light at wavelengths similar to oxyhemoglobin. Most pulse oximeters sense COHb as O_2Hb and overestimate the O_2 saturation; however, pulse oximeters that measure O_2Hb and COHb are available. MetHb increases absorption at each of the two wavelengths used by pulse oxime-

ters. This causes the ratio of the two Hb forms to approach 1, which is usually represented as a saturation of 85% (see Chapter 11). Other interfering substances may cause the pulse oximeter to underestimate saturation.

Significance and Pathophysiology

See Interpretive Strategies 6.3. Arterial oxygen saturation estimated by pulse oximetry (SpO_2) should approximate that measured by hemoximetry (SaO_2) in healthy nonsmoking adults. Most pulse oximeters are capable of accuracy of $\pm 2\%$ of the actual saturation when SaO_2 is above 90%. For SaO_2 values of 85% to 90%, accuracy may be slightly less. For extremely low saturations (i.e., < 80%), pulse oximeter accuracy is less of an issue because the clinical implications are the same.

Pulse oximetry is most useful when it has been shown to correlate with blood oximetry in a patient in a known circumstance. When this is the case, pulse oximetry can be used for noninvasive monitoring, either continuously or by taking discrete measurements. Uses include monitoring of O_2 therapy, ventilatory support, pulmonary or cardiac rehabilitation, bronchoscopy, surgical procedures, sleep studies, and cardiopulmonary exercise testing. In each of these applications, careful attention must be paid to minimizing known interfering agents or substances (see Box 6.2).

Because of its limitations, pulse oximetry should be used cautiously when assessing oxygen need. This is particularly true when using pulse oximetry to detect exercise desaturation. Pulse oximetry may not accurately reflect SaO_2 during exertion. For this reason, SpO_2, even if demonstrated to correlate with SaO_2 at rest, may yield false-positive or false-negative results during exercise. Blood gas analysis with hemoximetry should be used to resolve discrepancies between the SpO_2 reading and the patient's clinical presentation.

Pulse oximetry may not be appropriate in all situations. To evaluate hyperoxemia ($PaO_2 > 100$–$150\,mm\,Hg$) or acid–base status in a patient, blood gas analysis is required. Measurement of O_2 delivery, which depends on Hb concentration, cannot be adequately assessed by pulse oximetry alone.

CAPNOGRAPHY

Description

Capnography includes continuous, noninvasive monitoring of expired CO_2 and analysis of the single-breath CO_2 waveform. Continuous monitoring of expired CO_2 allows trending of changes in alveolar and dead-space ventilation. Analysis of a single breath of expired CO_2 measures the uniformity of both ventilation and pulmonary blood flow. End-tidal PCO_2 ($PETCO_2$) is reported in millimeters of mercury.

Technique

Continuous monitoring of expired CO_2 is performed by sampling gas from the proximal airway. This gas may be pumped to an infrared analyzer (see Chapter 11) or to a mass spectrometer. An alternative method inserts a "mainstream" sample window directly into the expired gas stream. The analyzer signal is then passed to either a recorder or a computer. CO_2 waveforms may be displayed either individually (Fig. 6.5) or as a series of deflections to form a trend plot. $PETCO_2$ may be read from the peaks of the waveforms. It can also be obtained by a simple peak detector and displayed digitally. Continuous CO_2 monitoring is commonly used in patients with artificial airways in the critical care setting. $PaCO_2$ can be measured at intervals to establish a gradient with $PETCO_2$. Respiratory rate may be determined from the frequency of the CO_2 waveforms. The change in CO_2 concentration

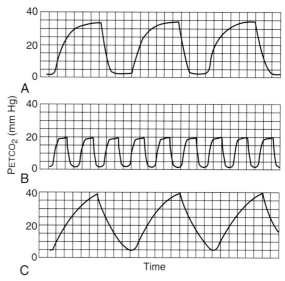

FIG. 6.5 Capnography tracings. Plots of expired CO_2 versus time for three patients are displayed. In each example, expiration is marked by a rapid increase in carbon dioxide to a peak ($PETCO_2$), followed by a return to the baseline during inspiration. (A) Normal respiratory pattern with $PETCO_2$ near $40\,mm\,Hg$ and a relatively flat alveolar phase. (B) Rapid respiratory rate and low $PETCO_2$ ($20\,mm\,Hg$), which may be found in a patient who is hyperventilating; the expiratory waveform has a normal configuration. (C) Abnormal expired CO_2 waveform is consistent with $\dot{V}/\dot{Q}$ abnormalities; no alveolar plateau is present, and the baseline does not return to zero.

during a single expiration may be analyzed to detect ventilation-perfusion abnormalities (see Fig. 6.5).

CRITERIA FOR ACCEPTABILITY 6.3

Capnography

1. The CO_2 analyzer should be calibrated at a frequency consistent with the types of measurements being made. Calibration with air and 5% CO_2 is suitable for most purposes.
2. Sample flow (except in mainstream analyzers) should be high enough to prevent damping of CO_2 waveforms. Sample flow should not be changed after calibration. The sample chamber and tubing should be free of secretions or condensation that may affect the accuracy of the results.
3. $Paco_2$ should be obtained to establish the gradient with $Petco_2$.
4. CO_2 waveforms (if displayed) should be consistent with the patient's clinical condition.
5. CO_2 waveforms (if displayed) should return to baseline during inspiration, indicating appropriate washout of dead space.

Technical problems involved in capnography include the necessity of accurate calibration and management of the gas sampling system (Criteria for Acceptability 6.3). Calibration using known gases (preferably two gas concentrations) is required if the system will be used to monitor $Paco_2$. Many systems use ambient air containing minimal CO_2 and a 5% CO_2 mixture for calibration (see Chapter 12). Condensation of water in sample tubing, connectors, or the sample chamber can affect accuracy. Some infrared analyzers may be affected if sample flow changes after calibration. Saturation of a desiccator column, if used, can also lead to inaccurate readings. Long sample lines or low sample flows can cause damping of the CO_2 waveform, invalidating analysis of the shape of the expired gas curve.

Significance and Pathophysiology

See Interpretive Strategies 6.4. In healthy patients, CO_2 rises to a plateau as alveolar gas is expired (see Fig. 6.5). If all lung units empty CO_2 evenly, the plateau appears flat. However, even healthy lungs have ventilation and blood flow imbalances. Healthy lung units empty CO_2 at varying rates. Alveolar CO_2 concentration increases slightly as the exhalation

continues. $Petco_2$ theoretically should not exceed $Paco_2$. In healthy patients at rest, the $Petco_2$ is usually close to the arterial value. During maximal exercise $Petco_2$ may exceed $Paco_2$. When ventilation and perfusion become grossly mismatched (e.g., in severe obstruction), end-tidal CO_2 may exceed the $Paco_2$ as well. $Paco_2$ reflects the gas exchange characteristics of the entire lung. Thus $Petco_2$ may differ significantly if some lung units are poorly ventilated.

Continuous CO_2 analysis provides useful data for monitoring critically ill patients, particularly those requiring ventilatory support. $Petco_2$ measurements allow trending of changes in $Paco_2$, provided there is little or no change in the shape of the CO_2 waveform (indicating $\dot{V}/\dot{Q}$ abnormalities). When a reference blood gas sample is obtained, $Petco_2$ can be used as a continuous noninvasive monitor. Respiratory rate can be measured from the frequency of expired CO_2 waveforms. Marked changes in breathing rate (e.g., hyperpnea or apnea) can be detected quickly. Analysis of the individual CO_2 waveforms along with $Paco_2$ may help identify abrupt changes in dead space. This can be useful in detecting pulmonary embolization or reduced cardiac output.

Problems related to ventilatory support devices can also be detected. Disconnection or leaks in breathing circuits can be quickly recognized by the loss of the CO_2 signal. Increased mechanical dead space (i.e., gas rebreathed in the ventilator circuit) can be identified by a baseline CO_2 concentration of greater than zero. Irregularities in the CO_2 waveform often signal that the patient is "out of phase" with the ventilator.

INTERPRETIVE STRATEGIES 6.4

Capnography

1. Was there an appropriate calibration of the CO_2 analyzer? If not, arterial–to–end-tidal CO_2 gradients may be inaccurate.
2. Are CO_2 waveforms (if available) consistent with the patient's clinical condition? Do waveforms show an obvious alveolar plateau?
3. Was the $Paco_2$ measured? If so, what is the $Paco_2$-to-$Petco_2$ gradient? If greater than 5 mm Hg, consider marked ventilation-perfusion abnormalities.
4. Has the $Petco_2$ changed (serial measurements)? Consider acute changes in dead space or cardiac output.

The shape of the expired CO_2 curve is determined by ventilation-perfusion matching. Only lung units that are ventilated and perfused contribute CO_2 to expired gas. In patients without lung disease, the CO_2 waveform shows a flat initial segment of anatomic dead-space gas containing little or no CO_2. This phase is followed by a rapid increase in CO_2 concentration, reflecting a mixture of dead space and alveolar gas. Finally, an "alveolar" plateau occurs in which gas composition changes only slightly. This slight change is caused by different emptying rates of various lung units. The absolute concentration of CO_2 at the alveolar plateau depends on factors such as minute ventilation and CO_2 production. Dead-space–producing disease (e.g., pulmonary embolization or marked decrease in cardiac output) may show a profound decrease in expired CO_2 concentration. Patients who have pulmonary disease, especially obstruction, show poorly delineated phases of the CO_2 washout curve. The alveolar plateau may actually be a continuous slope throughout expiration, causing the measurement of P_{ETCO_2} to be misleading.

SHUNT CALCULATION

Description

A shunt is that portion of the cardiac output that passes from one side of the heart to the other side without participating in gas exchange. This most commonly occurs from the right side to the left side. When the defect is in the lungs, it is a pulmonary shunt. If it occurs in the heart (e.g., atrial or ventricular septal defects), it is referred to as an *intracardiac shunt*. The shunt calculation determines the ratio of shunted blood ($\dot{Q}s$) to total perfusion ($\dot{Q}t$). Shunt is reported as a percentage of total cardiac output or sometimes as a simple fraction. Left-to-right shunting can occur when cardiac physiology is abnormal, such as in patent ductus arteriosus (PDA). These types of shunts are usually detected by Doppler echocardiography rather than by the shunt measurement, as described here.

Technique

Two methods for measuring the shunt fraction are available. The first uses O_2 content differences between arterial and mixed venous blood. The first method is called the *physiologic shunt equation:*

Equation 1

$$\frac{\dot{Q}s}{\dot{Q}t} = \frac{Cc_{O_2} - Ca_{O_2}}{Cc_{O_2} - C\bar{v}_{O_2}}$$

where:

Cc_{O_2} = O_2 content of end-capillary blood, estimated from saturation associated with calculated P_{AO_2}
Ca_{O_2} = arterial O_2 content, measured from an arterial sample
$C\bar{v}_{O_2}$ = mixed venous O_2 content, measured from a sample obtained from a pulmonary artery catheter

The term in the denominator of this equation reflects potential arterialization of mixed venous blood. The term in the numerator reflects the actual arterialization.

The second method is more commonly used in clinical practice. The patient breathes 100% O_2 in a unidirectional valved system until the Hb is completely saturated (Fig. 6.6). Twenty minutes of O_2 breathing is usually sufficient. Percent shunt is then calculated from differences in dissolved O_2. The second method is called the *clinical shunt equation:*

Equation 2

$$\frac{\dot{Q}s}{\dot{Q}t} = \frac{(P_{AO_2} - Pa_{O_2}) \times 0.0031}{C(a-\bar{v})o_2 + \left[(P_{AO_2} - Pa_{O_2}) \times 0.0031\right]}$$

where:

P_{AO_2} = alveolar O_2 tension
Pa_{O_2} = arterial O_2 tension
$C(a-\bar{v})o_2$ = arteriovenous O_2 content difference
0.0031 = solubility factor for O_2 at 37°C

When the patient is breathing 100% O_2, P_{AO_2} can be estimated from an abbreviated form of the alveolar gas equation, as follows:

$$P_{AO_2} = P_B - P_{H_2O} - \left(\frac{Pa_{CO_2}}{0.8}\right)$$

where:

P_B = barometric pressure
P_{H_2O} = partial pressure of water vapor at body temperature (47 mm Hg)
Pa_{CO_2} = arterial CO_2 tension (as an estimate of alveolar P_{CO_2})
0.8 = normal (assumed) respiratory exchange ratio

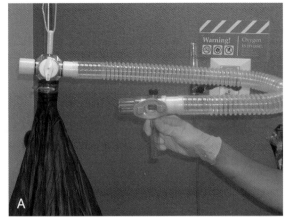

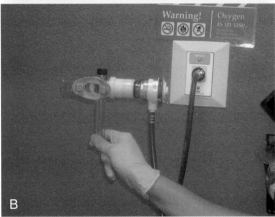

FIG. 6.6 Equipment used for clinical shunt measurement. (A) Shunt performed using a unidirectional breathing valve attached to a reservoir bag filled with 100% oxygen. (B) Shunt performed using a unidirectional breathing valve attached to a demand valve driven with oxygen.

This calculation of alveolar P_{O_2} assumes that the inspired gas is 100% O_2. If the F_{IO_2} is measured and found to be less than 1, the standard alveolar air equation can be used (see Evolve website, http://evolve.elsevier.com/Mottram/Ruppel/).

The clinical shunt calculation is accurate only when Hb is completely saturated. This normally requires a Pa_{O_2} greater than 150 mm Hg. A saturation of 100% is usually easily accomplished if O_2 is breathed long enough. If breathing 100% O_2 does not increase the Pa_{O_2} high enough to completely saturate Hb, the content difference method (physiologic method) should be used. With either method, the shunt fraction may be multiplied by

100 and reported as a percentage (e.g., 0.20 ratio × 100 equals a 20% shunt).

Several technical considerations should be noted regarding shunt measurement (Criteria for Acceptability 6.4). Using O_2 content differences (Equation 1) requires a pulmonary artery catheter to obtain mixed venous O_2 content. Using dissolved O_2 differences (Equation 2) also relies on measured $C(a-\bar{v})_{O_2}$. If the placement of a pulmonary artery catheter is not practical, the clinical shunt equation may be used with an assumed a-$\bar{v}$ content difference or a presentation of the calculated data with several a-$\bar{v}$ content differences (Table 6.6; see the Significance and Pathophysiology subsection in this section). The estimated technique assumes the subject is breathing 100% oxygen, so a closed circuit with directional value is required. This can be accomplished with a demand valve driven with a 50-psig 100% oxygen gas source or reservoir bag (e.g., Douglas bag) filled with 100% oxygen connected to a directional valve. The subject needs to be monitored for leaks around the mouthpiece or nose clips. The sample should be collected in a glass syringe or analyzed immediately to reduce the decrease in Pa_{O_2} secondary to environmental exposure (How To ... Box 6.3).

CRITERIA FOR ACCEPTABILITY 6.4

Shunt Calculation

1. For physiologic shunt, the patient must have simultaneous arterial and mixed venous blood specimens drawn over a 30-second interval.
2. For clinical shunt, patient should breathe 100% O_2 for at least 20 minutes or until Hb is completely saturated ($Pa_{O_2} > 150$ mm Hg). If $Pa_{O_2} > 150$ mm Hg cannot be achieved, clinical shunt calculation may underestimate true shunt.

   Ca_{O_2} and $C\bar{v}_{O_2}$ must be measured for physiologic shunt. Measured contents should be used for clinical shunt if available; otherwise, the estimated a-$\bar{v}$ content difference should be based on clinical status.
3. F_{IO_2} should be accurately determined; this is required to calculate capillary content for physiologic shunt. An F_{IO_2} of 1.00 can be assumed for clinical shunt calculation, but a measured value improves accuracy.

TABLE 6.6

Shunt Study

Male, Age 48, Barometer: 719, Time: 10:00

Sample No.	Position	Activity	Pa_{O_2} (mm Hg)	Pa_{CO_2} (mm Hg)	$P(A\text{-}a)_{O_2}$ (mm Hg)	$C(a\text{-}\bar{v})_{O_2}$ (cc/100 mL)	$\dot{Q}sp/\dot{Q}tot$ (%)
3	Supine	Rest	228.0	38-6	405-4	4	23.9
						5	20.1
						6	17.3
						8	13.6
4	Stand	Rest	355.0	36	281.0	4	17.9
						5	14.8
						6	12.7
						8	9.8

The shunt fraction ($\dot{Q}sp/\dot{Q}tot$) is estimated from arterial blood gas while breathing at 100% oxygen. Mixed venous blood is not sampled. ($\dot{Q}sp/\dot{Q}tot$) is reported assuming a 4-, 5-, 6-, and 8-C_{cO_2}/100-mL difference between arterials and mixed venous blood. Clinical evaluation should dictate which value is appropriate.

6.3   How To...

Perform an Estimated Shunt Study

1. Tasks common to all procedures:
   a. Calibrate and prepare equipment.
   b. Review order.
   c. Introduce yourself and identify patient according to institutional policies.
   d. Describe and demonstrate procedure.
2. Prepare necessary equipment: self-filling heparinized syringe, needle, personal protective equipment (e.g., gloves and eyewear), and oxygen delivery apparatus.
3. Place the subject on the 100% breathing apparatus, apply nose clips, and instruct him or her on the importance of maintaining a tight seal on the mouthpiece throughout the procedure (unless using a mask).
4. After 20 minutes, obtain an arterial blood gas according to the laboratory procedure, making sure an analysis can occur immediately after drawing the sample (<5 minutes).
5. Oftentimes, a clinician is interested in performing the estimated shunt in various positions (e.g., sitting, standing, supine). The patient should be placed in the specified position for a minimum of 10 additional minutes before sampling. (See Criteria for Acceptability Box 6.4.)
6. Calculate the estimated shunt.

The physiologic shunt equation may be used for patients on any known F_{IO_2}. The clinical shunt measurement requires O_2 breathing for 20 minutes or longer. Prolonged O_2 breathing may be contraindicated in patients whose respiration is driven by hypoxemia. Breathing 100% O_2 washes nitrogen (N_2) out of the lungs. Washout of N_2 combined with O_2 uptake by perfusing blood flow can reduce the size of alveoli to their critical limit. In poorly ventilated lung units, this may cause alveolar collapse. The effect of this "nitrogen shunting" may be shunt values that are falsely high because some shunting was induced by the test itself.

INTERPRETIVE STRATEGIES 6.5

Blood Gases

Shunt Calculations

1. For a physiologic shunt: Were arterial and mixed venous samples obtained correctly? Analyzed promptly? FiO_2 accurately determined?
2. For a clinical shunt: Did the patient breathe O_2 long enough to maximally saturate Hb? Was an estimated or measured content difference used? Was blood gas analysis performed promptly?
3. Was the calculated shunt ≤ 5%? If so, no significant shunting is present.
4. Was the calculated shunt > 5% but < 10%? If so, some shunting is likely. Consider technical causes (assumed content difference, assumed FiO_2).
5. Was the calculated shunt > 10% but < 30%? If so, significant shunting is present. Consider a clinical correlation.
6. Was the calculated shunt > 30%? If so, severe shunting is present. Further testing is indicated to determine the site and physiologic basis for the shunt.

Significance and Pathophysiology

See Interpretive Strategies 6.5. In healthy individuals, approximately 5% of the cardiac output is shunted past the pulmonary system. An increased pulmonary shunt fraction indicates that some lung units have little ventilation in relation to their blood flow. These patterns may be found in both obstructive and restrictive diseases. However, even in severe obstruction or restriction, blood flow to areas of poor ventilation may be reduced by the lesions themselves. In emphysema, destruction of the alveolar septa obliterates pulmonary capillaries. As the terminal airways lose their support, they also have reduced blood flow. In poorly ventilated lung units, vasoconstriction of pulmonary arterioles redirects blood flow away from the affected area. In these cases, there may be minimal shunting even though severe ventilatory impairment exists.

Intrapulmonary shunting is common in acute disease patterns such as atelectasis or foreign body aspiration. Diseases such as pneumonia or adult respiratory distress syndrome (ARDS; in some references, this has been broadened to *acute respiratory distress syndrome*) often result in a "shunt-like effect." This is caused by reduced ventilation in relation to blood flow in many lung units. Foreign body aspiration may cause shunting by blocking an airway and depriving all distal lung units of ventilation. Blood flow to the affected units cannot participate in gas exchange. The degree of shunting is directly related to the number of lung units with $\dot{V}/\dot{Q}$ ratios close to zero.

Intrapulmonary shunting may also occur when the pulmonary vascular system is involved, as is the case in hepatopulmonary syndrome. Patients who have liver disease with portal hypertension commonly have arteriovenous malformations that allow significant volumes of blood to pass through the lungs without participating in gas exchange. These malformations are prominent at the lung bases and result in increased shunting when the patient is upright.

Intracardiac shunting occurs when defects in the atrial or ventricular septa allow mixed venous blood to pass from the right side of the heart to the left side of the heart without traversing the pulmonary capillaries. In the ventricles, shunting usually requires an elevated right-heart pressure to overcome the normal pressure difference between the systemic and pulmonary systems. Atrial septal defects, such as patent foramen ovale (PFO), allow blood to pass from the right atrium to the left atrium during systole.

PF TIP 6.4

There are several key values to remember when assessing oxygen saturation. When SaO_2 is above 90%, PaO_2 is usually greater than 60 mm Hg. At a PaO_2 of 60, the saturation is 90%, and O_2 therapy may be needed. At a PaO_2 of 55, the saturation is 85%, and O_2 therapy is indicated. At a PaO_2 of 40, the saturation is approximately 75% (the same as mixed venous blood).

Very large shunt values (>30%) suggest that a significant volume of blood is moving from the right side of the heart to the left side of the heart without participating in gas exchange. Further testing may be required to determine whether the shunt is occurring in the lungs or in the heart. Echocardiography with contrast media or cardiac catheterization may be necessary to identify intracardiac shunts.

The accuracy of clinical shunt measurement (i.e., dissolved O_2 differences) depends on the accuracy of Po_2 determinations. In small shunts, Hb becomes 100% saturated. The difference between alveolar and arterial Po_2 values results simply from the amount of O_2 dissolved. The difference between the actual content of dissolved oxygen and the content that can potentially dissolve is the basis for the calculation. Measurements of Po_2 used for shunt calculations (200–600 mm Hg) are much higher than the normal physiologic range. Additional calibration and quality control of the Po_2 electrode may be necessary to provide accurate values for oxygen tension. Blood gases drawn for shunt studies should be analyzed immediately to avoid large changes in Pao_2 values caused by cell metabolism in the specimen and the effect of diffusion across a plastic syringe if used. Glass syringes should be used if any delay in sampling greater than a few minutes is expected.

The calculated shunt fraction also depends on the O_2 content difference between arterial and mixed venous blood. $C(a-\bar{v})o_2$ is a component of the denominator in the clinical shunt equation. The **a-$\bar{v}O_2$ content difference** is determined not only by the lungs but also by cardiac output and the perfusion status of the tissues. Ideally, the value used in the equation should be measured rather than estimated. Arterial content can be determined easily from a sample taken from a peripheral artery. However, mixed venous content can only be measured accurately from a pulmonary artery sample. In patients who do not have a pulmonary artery catheter in place, an estimated value

must be used. $C(a-\bar{v})o_2$ values from 4.5 to 5.0 vol% are reasonable content differences in patients who have good cardiac output and perfusion status. Values of 3.5 vol% may be more realistic in patients who are critically ill.

In some instances, the a-$\bar{v}$ content difference cannot be reliably estimated or Hb cannot be maximally saturated by breathing 100% oxygen. In such cases, the alveolar-arterial oxygen gradient $P(A-a)o_2$ may be useful as an index of ventilation to blood flow. In healthy patients breathing 100% O_2 at sea level, arterial Pao_2 should increase to approximately 600 mm Hg. $\dot{Q}s/\dot{Q}t$ does not directly provide absolute values for $\dot{Q}s$, but if the cardiac output ($\dot{Q}t$) is known, $\dot{Q}s$ can be determined simply. Measurement of the shunt fraction is sometimes performed in conjunction with the determination of the V_D/V_T ratio (see Chapter 5) to assess both types of gas exchange abnormalities together.

SUMMARY

· The chapter describes the measurement of pH, Pco_2, Po_2, and blood oximetry used as part of pulmonary function testing. Technical aspects of obtaining samples are discussed in detail because accurate interpretation makes numerous assumptions regarding proper specimen handling.

· Two noninvasive methods of assessing gas exchange are commonly used: pulse oximetry and capnography. Pulse oximetry offers a simple means of assessing oxyhemoglobin saturation. Capnography is useful for monitoring changes in $Petco_2$, particularly for patients in critical care settings.

· Shunt measurements allow estimates of severe ventilation-perfusion imbalances in the lungs. Two methods are described: the clinical and physiologic equations. The advantages and disadvantages of each are also discussed.

CASE STUDIES

CASE 6.1

HISTORY

A 57-year-old man is referred to the pulmonary function laboratory for increasing shortness of breath. He admits having a chronic cough with a production of thick, white sputum, mainly upon awakening. The subject reports that he quit smoking 3 months ago. He averaged approximately two packs of cigarettes per day for 30 years (60 pack-years) before quitting. His referring physician performed pulse oximetry in the outpatient clinic and obtained readings of 90% to 91%. Complete pulmonary function studies with arterial blood gases were requested.

PULMONARY FUNCTION TESTS

Personal Data

Sex:	Male, Caucasian
Age:	57 yr
Height:	66 in. (168 cm)
Weight:	197 lb (89.5 kg)

Spirometry

	Before Drug	LLN	Predicted	%	After Drug	%	% Change
FVC (L)	3.97	3.51	4.10	97	4.04	99	2
FEV$_1$ (L)	2.31	2.35	2.99	77	2.50	84	8
FEV$_{1\%}$ (%)	58	64	73	—	62	—	7
MVV (L)	83	116	72	92	79	11	

FVC, Forced vital capacity; *LLN,* lower limit of normal; *MVV,* maximal voluntary ventilation.

Lung Volumes

	Before Drug	LLN	Predicted	%
VC (L)	3.97	3.20	4.10	97
IC (L)	2.66	2.76		96
ERV (L)	1.31	1.35		97
FRC (L)	3.65	3.42		107
RV (L)	2.34	2.07		113
TLC (L)	6.31	4.64	6.18	102
RV/TLC (%)	37		34	—

ERV, Expiratory reserve volume; *IC,* inspiratory capacity; *RV,* residual volume.

D$_{LCO}$

	Before Drug	LLN	Predicted	%
D$_{LCO}$ (mL/min/mm Hg)	16.7	19.5	26.3	63
D$_{LCO}$ (corrected)	16.7	26.3	63	
D$_L$/V$_A$	5.09	4.38	86	

Blood Gases

pH	7.37
P$_{CO_2}$ (mm Hg)	44
P$_{O_2}$ (mm Hg)	57
HCO$_3^-$ (mEq/L)	26.4
BE (mEq/L)	~ 1.7
Hb (g/dL)	16.2
O$_2$Hb (%)	80.1
COHb (%)	5.9
MetHb (%)	0.2

Technologist's Comments

All spirometry maneuvers were performed acceptably. Lung volumes by helium (He) dilution were also performed acceptably. D$_{LCO}$ was performed acceptably; predicted D$_{LCO}$ was corrected for an Hb of 16.2 and a COHb of 5.9.

QUESTIONS

1. What is the interpretation of the following?
   a. Prebronchodilator and postbronchodilator spirometry
   b. Lung volumes

c. D$_{LCO}$
d. Blood gases
2. What is the most likely cause of the subject's symptoms?
3. What other treatment or tests might be indicated?

DISCUSSION
Interpretation

All spirometry, lung volumes, and diffusing capacity maneuvers were performed acceptably. Spirometry reveals moderate airway obstruction with minimal response to inhaled bronchodilators. Lung volumes by He dilution show a normal TLC but with a slightly increased FRC, RV, and RV/TLC ratio. These changes are suggestive of air trapping. D$_{LCO}$ is moderately decreased even after a correction for increased Hb and elevated COHb. Arterial blood gas results reveal normal acid–base status with a P$_{CO_2}$ of 44. There is moderate to severe hypoxemia, as indicated by a P$_{O_2}$ of 57 and an oxyhemoglobin saturation of 80%. The hypoxemia is further aggravated by an increased COHb, consistent with cigarette smoking or environmental exposure.

Impression: Moderate obstructive airway disease with no significant improvement after inhaled bronchodilator. There is a moderate loss of diffusing capacity. There is significant hypoxemia on room air, which is further increased by an elevation of COHb. Recommend further investigation of source of CO and clinical evaluation of O$_2$ supplementation.

Cause of Symptoms

This case demonstrates the importance of arterial blood gas analysis in the diagnosis of pulmonary disorders. The subject's complaint of increased shortness of breath was not explained by the borderline value of pulse oximetry (SpO$_2$) performed in the referring physician's office. The referring physician correctly suspected a pulmonary problem resulting from the subject's previous smoking history.

The spirometric measurement shows obstruction as evidenced by the FEV$_{1\%}$ of 58%, well below the LLN (64% for this subject). The subject's FEV$_1$ is also below its LLN. The response of FEV$_1$ to the inhaled bronchodilator is slightly less than 200 mL and represents only an 8% improvement over prebronchodilator values. Lung volumes are also consistent with an obstructive pattern, suggesting the beginnings of air trapping.

Diffusing capacity is also reduced in a pattern consistent with mild to moderate airway obstruction. The predicted D$_{LCO}$ has been corrected for an elevated Hb and COHb. The combination of these two corrections results in a predicted D$_{LCO}$ that is identical to the uncorrected predicted value (see Chapter 3).

Of the pulmonary function variables measured, the arterial blood gas values are most abnormal. Although pH and P$_{CO_2}$ are within normal limits, P$_{O_2}$ is markedly decreased. As a result, oxygen saturation is low. Elevated COHb further complicates oxygenation. This level is characteristic of individuals who currently smoke or who are chronically exposed to low levels of CO in their environment. The subject's spouse reported that he was still smoking 5 to 10 cigarettes per day.

Treatment and Other Tests

The subject was referred to a smoking cessation program and prescribed a nicotine replacement medication. He was able to stop smoking. Blood gas analysis 2 weeks later confirmed his smoking cessation (i.e., COHb was 1.7%). However, his P$_{O_2}$ improved only slightly to 61 mm Hg (SaO$_2$ was 87%). He was referred for evaluation of possible exercise desaturation. His arterial oxygenation was shown to actually increase with exercise, so O$_2$ supplementation was unnecessary. His lung function continued to improve over several months, presumably because of his smoking cessation.

CASE 6.2

HISTORY

A 31-year-old woman is referred to the pulmonary function laboratory for a shunt study. Her chief complaint is shortness of breath with exertion and at other times. Her referring physician suspected a shunt and requested a shunt study. The subject was in no apparent distress on arrival at the laboratory. She never smoked and had no significant environmental exposure to respiratory irritants. Her mother died of a stroke at age 50 years, but there is no heart or lung disease in her immediate family.

SHUNT STUDY
Personal Data
Age:	31 yr
Height:	69 in. (175 cm)
Weight:	200 lb (91 kg)
Race:	Caucasian

Blood Gases (Drawn After 20 Minutes of O_2 Breathing)

F_{IO_2}	1.00
P_B	752
pH	7.43
P_{CO_2}	38
P_{O_2}	557
HCO_3^-	24.1
BE	0.1
Hb	7.4
O_2Hb	99.6
COHb	0.3
MetHb	0.1

QUESTIONS
1. What is the subject's calculated shunt?
2. What is the interpretation of the following?
   a. Blood gases
   b. Shunt
3. What is the cause of the subject's symptoms?
4. What other treatment or tests might be indicated?

DISCUSSION
Calculations
The P_{AO_2} is calculated as follows:

$$P_{AO_2} = P_a - P_{H_2O} - \left(\frac{P_{aCO_2}}{0.8}\right)$$

$$= 752 - 47 - \left(\frac{38}{0.8}\right)$$

$$= 705 - 48$$

$$P_{AO_2} = 657$$

Substituting this value in the clinical shunt equation and assuming an $a - \bar{v}$ content difference of 4.5 gives the following:

$$\frac{\dot{Q}s}{\dot{Q}t} = \frac{\left(P_{AO_2} - P_{aO_2}\right) \times 0.0031}{C(a-\bar{v})o_2 + \left[\left(P_{AO_2}\right) \times 0.0031\right]}$$

$$= \frac{(657 - 557) \times 0.0031}{4.5 + \left[(657 - 557) \times 0.0031\right]}$$

$$= \frac{0.31}{45 + (031)}$$

$$\frac{\dot{Q}s}{\dot{Q}t} = 0.06$$

Interpretation
The subject's blood gas results show a normal acid–base status. The P_{aO_2} reflects an appropriate increase after breathing 100% O_2 for 20 minutes. The Hb as measured by hemoximetry (7.4 mg/dL) is markedly decreased. The subject's shunt is 6% (0.06 as a fraction). This is within normal limits.

Impression: Normal arterial blood gas results and normal shunt with markedly reduced Hb. Recommend clinical correlation.

Cause of Symptoms
The subject's primary symptom of dyspnea does not appear to be caused by any significant shunting. In a shunt, blood passes from the right side of the heart to the left side without coming into contact with alveolar gas. The shunt may be in the heart or in the lungs themselves. Breathing high concentrations of oxygen will not relieve this problem. This subject increased her P_{aO_2} appropriately, which rules out a large shunt.

A more likely cause of the symptoms described is the subject's low Hb level. Severe anemia reduces the arterial oxygen content dramatically. Oxygen delivery to the tissues is reduced. Dyspnea can result during exertion or times of increased metabolic demand. The subject's arterial content (mL/dL) can be calculated as follows:

$$CaO_2 = (13.4 \times Hb \times O_2Hb) + \left(P_{aO_2} \times 0.0031\right)$$

$$= (13.4 \times 7.4 \times 0.996) + (557 \times 0.0031)$$

$$= (9.9) + (1.7)$$

$$CaO_2 = 11.6$$

This value is much lower than the normal arterial content of about 20 mL/dL. It should be noted that the term in the second parentheses represents dissolved O_2 and would be much lower if the subject were breathing room air.

Treatment and Other Tests

The subject's anemia could have been diagnosed by any test that measures total Hb. Hemoximetry, in addition to providing accurate saturation data, also provides a measurement of total Hb. The shunt study could have been performed using calculated Hb saturation, but the low arterial content would have been missed.

No treatment is indicated until the cause of anemia can be identified. The subject was referred to a hematologist for further evaluation. Additional testing revealed a hemolytic form of anemia, which was successfully treated.

SELF-ASSESSMENT QUESTIONS

Entry-Level

1. A patient referred for a pulmonary function test has blood gases drawn, and the following data are reported:

pH	7.43
Pa_{CO_2} (mm Hg)	38
Hco_3^- (mEq/L)	25.1

These values are consistent with
a. normal acid–base status.
b. respiratory alkalosis.
c. metabolic acidosis.
d. compensated respiratory acidosis.

2. A patient with chronic obstructive pulmonary disease (COPD) has blood gases drawn, and the following values are reported:

pH	7.37
P_{CO_2}	47 mm Hg
P_{O_2}	52 mm Hg
HCO_3^-	27.1 mEq/L
Hb	15.8 g/dL
O_2Hb	82%

Which of the following best describes these results?
a. Normal blood gases
b. Compensated metabolic alkalosis
c. Moderate hypoxemia with compensated respiratory acidosis
d. Erroneous blood gas results

3. A patient being monitored by ECG has an HR of 120/min. A pulse oximeter on this patient displays a saturation of 84% with an HR of 118. Which of the following should the pulmonary function technologist conclude based on these findings?

a. The patient's COHb level is likely elevated.
b. The pulse oximeter's sensor should be moved to an alternate site.
c. The patient needs supplementary O_2.
d. The pulse oximeter is malfunctioning.

4. An outpatient is referred for arterial blood gas analysis. While performing the modified Allen test, the pulmonary function technologist notes that the patient's hand reperfuses after 30 seconds. The technologist should take which action?
a. Use a 23-gauge or smaller needle for the puncture.
b. Proceed to obtain the specimen.
c. Draw blood from an alternate site.
d. Check the patient's blood pressure before proceeding.

5. A patient with interstitial lung disease has an arterial oxygen tension (Pa_{O_2}) of 60 mm Hg, but hemoximetry is not performed. What calculated Sa_{O_2} should the pulmonary function technologist report?
a. 95%
b. 90%
c. 85%
d. 75%

Advanced

6. A patient with chronic bronchitis has a resting Sp_{O_2} of 80%, but an arterial blood gas reveals an Sa_{O_2} of 90%. Which of the following should the pulmonary function technologist conclude?
a. The patient has an elevated COHb.
b. The patient has compensated respiratory acidosis.
c. The pulse oximeter reading is erroneous.
d. These results are expected in patients with polycythemia.

7. A patient who has COPD performs a maximal exercise test. At peak exercise, his SpO_2 is 94%, and a blood gas shows an SaO_2 of 87%. Which of the following might explain these results?
   1. Carboxyhemoglobinemia
   2. Methemoglobinemia
   3. Motion artifact
   4. Metabolic acidosis
      a. 1 and 2 only
      b. 1 and 3 only
      c. 2 and 4 only
      d. 3 and 4 only

8. A patient being monitored by capnography shows the following data:

Time	8:35	8:40	8:45	8:50	8:55	9:00
$PETCO_2$	38	39	39	29	25	26

Which of the following best explains the change occurring at 8:50?
   a. Hypoventilation
   b. Respiratory acidosis
   c. Acute bronchospasm
   d. Decreased cardiac output

9. A patient with dyspnea on exertion has arterial blood gases drawn at rest before beginning an exercise test, and the following data are obtained:

pH	7.44
$PaCO_2$	36 mm Hg
HCO_3^-	24.4 mEq/L
PaO_2	64 mm Hg
SaO_2	91%
Hb	6.9 mg/dL
COHb	1.2%

What is the subject's arterial oxygen content (CaO_2)?
   a. 10.0 mL/dL
   b. 9.3 mL/dL
   c. 8.6 mL/dL
   d. 8.4 mL/dL

10. A patient with dyspnea at rest has a clinical shunt study performed. The following data are obtained:

P_B	761 mm Hg
FIO_2	1.00
PaO_2	597 mm Hg
$PaCO_2$	38 mm Hg
SaO_2	100%
Hb	15.1 mg/dL

On the basis of these results, the patient's $\dot{Q}s/\dot{Q}t$ is approximately
   a. 5%.
   b. 9%.
   c. 12%.
   d. 15%.

SELECTED BIBLIOGRAPHY

General References

Shapiro, B. A., Kozlowski-Templin, R., & Peruzzi, W. T. (1994). *Clinical application of blood gases* (5th ed.). St. Louis, MO: Mosby.

West, J. B. (2003). *Pulmonary pathophysiology: The essentials* (6th ed.). Baltimore, MD: Lippincott Williams & Wilkins.

Blood Gases

Breen, P. H. (2001). Arterial blood gas and pH analysis: Clinical approach and interpretation. *Anesthesiology Clinics of North America, 19*, 885–906.

Hadeli, K., Siegel, E., Sherrill, D., et al. (2001). Predictors of oxygen desaturation during submaximal exercise in 8,000 patients. *Chest, 120*, 88–92.

Hess, D. (2000). Detection and monitoring of hypoxemia and oxygen therapy. *Respiratory Care, 45*, 65–80.

Knowles, T. P., Mullin, R. A., Hunter, J. A., et al. (2006). Effects of syringe material, sample storage time, and temperature on blood gases and oxygen saturation in arterialized human blood samples. *Respiratory Care, 51*, 732–736.

Mahoney, J. J., Harvey, J. A., Wong, R. J., et al. (1991). Changes in oxygen measurements when whole blood is stored in iced plastic or glass syringes. *Clinical Chemistry, 37*, 1244–1248.

Siggard-Anderson, O. (1968). Acid-base and blood gas parameters: Arterial or capillary blood? *Scandinavian Journal of Clinical and Laboratory Investigation, 21*, 289–292.

Swenson, E. R. (2001). Metabolic acidosis. *Respiratory Care, 46*, 342–353.

Pulse Oximetry

Barker, S. J. (2002). Motion-resistant pulse oximetry: A comparison of new and old models. *Anesthesia and Analgesia*, *95*(4), 967–972.

Fussell, K. M., Ayo, D. S., Branca, P., et al. (2003). Assessing need for long-term oxygen therapy: A comparison of conventional evaluation and measures of ambulatory oximetry monitoring. *Respiratory Care*, *48*, 115–119.

Gehring, H., Hornberger, C., Matz, H., et al. (2002). The effects of motion artifact and low perfusion on the performance of a new generation of pulse oximeters in volunteers undergoing hypoxemia. *Respiratory Care*, *47*, 48–60.

Giuliano, K. K., & Higgins, T. L. (2005). New-generation pulse oximetry in the care of critically ill patients. *American Journal of Critical Care*, *14*, 26–37.

McMorrow, R. C., & Mythen, M. G. (2006). Pulse oximetry. *Current Opinion in Critical Care*, *12*, 269–271.

Netzer, N., Eliasson, A. H., Netzer, C., et al. (2001). Overnight pulse oximetry for sleep-disordered breathing in adults: A review. *Chest*, *120*, 625–633.

Roth, D., Herkner, H., Schreiber, W., & Hubmann, N. (2011). Accuracy of noninvasive multiwave pulse oximetry compared with carboxyhemoglobin from blood gas analysis in unselected emergency department patients. *Annals of Emergency Medicine*, *58*(1), 74–79.

Sinex, J. E. (1999). Pulse oximetry: Principles and limitations. *American Journal of Emergency Medicine*, *17*, 59–67.

Capnography

Anderson, C. T., & Breen, P. H. (2000). Carbon dioxide kinetics and capnography during critical care. *Critical Care*, *4*, 207–215.

Blanch, L., Romero, P. V., & Lucangelo, U. (2006). Volumetric capnography in the mechanically ventilated patient. *Minerva Anestesiologica*, *72*, 577–585.

Koulouris, N. G., Latsi, P., Dimitroulis, J., et al. (2001). Noninvasive measurement of mean alveolar carbon dioxide tension and Bohr's dead space during tidal breathing. *European Respiratory Journal*, *17*, 1167–1174.

St. John, R. E. (1999). Thomson PD. Noninvasive respiratory monitoring. *Critical Care Nursing Clinics of North America*, *11*, 423–435.

Walsh, B. K., Crotwell, D. N., & Restrepo, R. D. (2011). Capnography/capnometry in the mechanically ventilated patient: 2011. *Respiratory Care*, *56*(4), 503–509.

Shunt Calculation

Cane, R. D., Shapiro, B. A., Harrison, R. A., et al. (1980). Minimizing errors in intrapulmonary shunt calculations. *Critical Care Medicine*, *8*, 294.

Cane, R. D., Shapiro, B. A., Templin, R., et al. (1988). Unreliability of oxygen tension-based indices in reflecting intrapulmonary shunting in critically ill patients. *Critical Care Medicine*, *16*, 1243–1245.

Harrison, R. A., Davison, R., Shapiro, B. A., et al. (1975). Reassessment of the assumed A-V oxygen content difference in the shunt calculation. *Anesthesia and Analgesia*, *54*, 198.

Henig, N. R., & Pierson, D. J. (2000). Mechanisms of hypoxemia. *Respiratory Care Clinics of North America*, *6*, 501–521.

McCarthy, K., & Stoller, J. K. (1999). Possible underestimation of shunt fraction in the hepatopulmonary syndrome. *Respiratory Care*, *44*, 1486–1488.

Moller, S., Krag, A., & Madsen, J. L. (2009). Pulmonary dysfunction and hepatopulmonary syndrome in cirrhosis and portal hypertension. *Liver International*, *29*(10), 1528–1537.

Smeenk, F. W., Janssen, J. D., Arends, B. J., et al. (1997). Effects of four different methods of sampling arterial blood and storage time on gas tensions and shunt calculations in the 100% oxygen test. *European Respiratory Journal*, *10*, 910–913.

Standards and Guidelines

Clinical Practice Guideline, A. A. R. C. (2003). Capnography/capnometry during mechanical ventilation–2003 revision & update. *Respiratory Care*, *48*, 534–539.

Clinical Practice Guideline, A. A. R. C. (2013). Blood gas analysis and hemoximetry 2013. *Respiratory Care*, *58*, 1694–1703.

CLSI. (2008). *Procedures and devices for the collection of diagnostic capillary blood specimens: Approved standard. CLSI document H04-A6* (6th ed.). Wayne, PA: Clinical and Laboratory Standards Institute.

CLSI. (2004). *Procedures for the collection of arterial blood specimens: Approved standard. CLSI document H11-A4* (4th ed.). Wayne, PA: Clinical and Laboratory Standards Institute.

CLSI. (2005). *Protection of laboratory workers from occupationally acquired infections: Approved guideline. CLSI document M29-A3* (3rd ed.). Wayne, PA: Clinical and Laboratory Standards Institute.

CLSI. (2009). *Blood gas and pH analysis and related measurements: Approved guideline. CLSI document C46-A2* (2nd ed.). Wayne, PA: Clinical and Laboratory Standards Institute.

CLSI. (2010). *Pulse oximetry. CLSI document p OCT11–A2*. Wayne, PA: Clinical and Laboratory Standards Institute.

Guideline for isolation precautions: Preventing transmission of infectious agents in healthcare settings. (2007; Updated July 2019) Accessed October 2020. http://www.cdc.gov/ncidod/dhqp/gl_isolation.html.

Chapter 7

Cardiopulmonary Exercise Testing and Field Tests

CHAPTER OUTLINE

LEARNING OBJECTIVES

After studying the chapter and reviewing the figures, tables, and case studies, you should be able to do the following:

Entry-level

1. Understand and select an appropriate exercise protocol based on the reason for performing the test.
2. Describe and understand the performance of field tests.
3. Identify the ventilatory/anaerobic threshold.
4. Describe two methods for measuring ventilation, oxygen consumption, and carbon dioxide production during exercise.
5. Identify indications for terminating a cardiopulmonary stress test.

Advanced

6. Describe the normal physiologic changes that occur during exercise when workload is increased.
7. Classify exercise limitation as caused by cardiovascular, ventilatory, gas exchange, or blood gas abnormalities or deconditioning.
8. Understand the importance of evaluating breathing kinetics during exercise.
9. Evaluate exercise flow-volume loop data.

KEY TERMS

anaerobic threshold (AT)
Borg scale
breathing strategy
carbon dioxide production $(\dot{V}co_2)$
Endurance Shuttle Walk Test
field test
Incremental Shuttle Walk Test
lactic acid
metabolic equivalents (METs)

minute ventilation $(\dot{V}_E)$
oxygen consumption $(\dot{V}o_2)$
O_2 prescription
O_2 pulse
progressive multistage exercise tests
ramp test
ratings of perceived exertion (RPE)
6-Minute Walk Test (6MWT)

steady-state tests
ventilatory equivalent for CO_2 $(\dot{V}_E / \dot{V}co_2)$
ventilatory equivalent for oxygen $(\dot{V}_E / \dot{V}o_2)$
ventilatory threshold
V-slope method
watts
work
workload

The efficiency of the cardiopulmonary system may be different during increased metabolic demand than at rest. Tests designed to assess exercise capacity, ventilatory response, gas exchange, and cardiovascular function during exercise can provide information not obtainable with the patient at rest. **Field tests** assess functional capacity in patients with chronic disease, do not require any sophisticated testing equipment, and would fit into the category of simple pulmonary stress tests. Cardiopulmonary exercise tests, which are characterized as complex pulmonary stress tests, allow for the evaluation of the heart and lungs under conditions of increased metabolic demand. Limitations to work are not entirely predictable from any single resting measurement of pulmonary function. To define work limitations, a cardiopulmonary exercise test is necessary. In most exercise tests, cardiopulmonary variables are assessed in relation to the **workload** (i.e., the level of exercise). The patterns of change in any particular variable (e.g., heart rate [HR]) are then compared with the expected normal response.

The primary indications for performing exercise tests are dyspnea on exertion, pain (especially angina), and fatigue. Other indications include exercise-induced bronchospasm, assessing functional capacity, and arterial desaturation. Exercise testing can detect the following:

1. Presence and nature of ventilatory limitations to work
2. Presence and nature of cardiovascular limitations to work
3. Extent of conditioning or deconditioning
4. Maximum tolerable workload and safe levels of daily exercise
5. Extent of disability for rehabilitation purposes
6. Oxygen (O_2) desaturation and appropriate levels of supplemental O_2 therapy
7. Outcome measurement after a treatment plan (e.g., surgery or medical)

Exercise testing may be indicated in apparently healthy individuals, particularly in adults older than 40 years. Cardiopulmonary exercise testing is indicated to assess fitness before engaging in vigorous physical activities (e.g., running). Cardiopulmonary exercise testing may be useful in assessing the risk of postoperative complications, particularly in patients undergoing thoracotomy.

Exercise testing and the protocols used can be diverse in purpose and complexity. The chapter deals primarily with cardiopulmonary measurements during exercise and field tests. This does not include simple cardiac stress testing during which only the electrocardiogram (ECG) and blood pressure (BP) are monitored, or more sophisticated tests involving injection of radioisotopes.

FIELD TESTS

Six-Minute Walk Test

The **6-Minute Walk Test (6MWT)** is a simple test that does not require any sophisticated equipment. It is typically performed to assess the response of functional capacity to a medical or surgical intervention, as well as to estimate morbidity and mortality. Absolute and relative contraindications are the same as for a maximal exercise test (Box 7.1). A 30-m (100-ft) hallway free of obstructions is needed

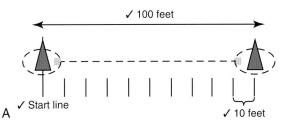

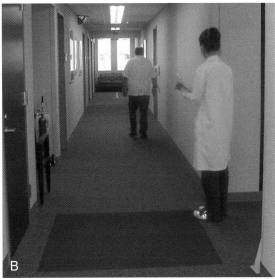

FIG. 7.1   Six-Minute Walk Test. (A) and (B) The corridor should be a minimum of 100 ft (30 m), with the ends of the course marked with small traffic cones. The technologist should remain in the center of the course when feasible and give standardized statements of encouragement to decrease intratester variability. Monitoring of oxygenation using pulse oximetry can be facilitated by using telemetry–pulse oximetry. Standard phases of encouragement: "You are doing well—you have 5 minutes to go." "You are doing well—you have 4 minutes to go." "You're halfway done."

> **BOX 7.1   CONTRAINDICATIONS TO EXERCISE TESTING[a]**
>
> Absolute Contraindications
>
> - Acute myocardial infarction within 2 days
> - Ongoing unstable angina
> - Uncontrolled cardiac arrhythmia with hemodynamic compromise
> - Active endocarditis
> - Severe aortic stenosis
> - Decompensated heart failure
> - Acute aortic dissection
> - Acute myocarditis or pericarditis
> - Pao_2 less than 40 mm Hg on room air (unless an oxygen environment is provided)
> - Pao_2 greater than 70 mm Hg
> - Physical disability that precludes safe testing
>
> Relative Contraindications
>
> - Known obstructive left main coronary artery stenosis
> - Moderate to severe aortic stenosis
> - Tachyarrhythmia's with uncontrolled ventricular rates
> - Complete heart block
> - Hypertrophic cardiomyopathy
> - Recent stroke or transient ischemic attack
> - Mental impairment
> - Resting hypertension > 200/110 mm Hg
> - Uncorrected medical condition (e.g., anemia, electrolyte imbalance)
>
> ---
> [a]These conditions represent relative contraindications to exercise testing; the risk to the patient must be evaluated on a case-by-case basis.
> Adapted from the 2013 American Heart Association (AHA) exercise standards for testing and training.

to perform the test (Fig. 7.1A). Equipment needed includes the following:

- At least one chair positioned at one end of the walking course
- Countdown timer (stopwatch)
- Mechanical lap counter
- A method to mark the endpoints of the course (small traffic cones)
- A method to measure distance covered less than a complete lap (e.g., premeasured marks on floor or measuring wheel)
- Sphygmomanometer and appropriately sized cuff

- A validated scale to measure dyspnea and subjective fatigue (e.g., rating of perceived exertion scale, such as **Borg scale**)
- Clipboard with reporting sheet and list of standard statements
- Pulse oximeter
- Access to oxygen and easy access to the emergency response team (e.g., telephone, nurse call light)
- Portable supplemental oxygen if required to perform exercise test by patient
- An emergency plan

Patient assessment and preparation would include a review of the medical history to identify any absolute or relative contraindications. The patient should wear comfortable clothing and appropriate shoes for walking and be instructed to use their usual medications. Any other scheduled pulmonary function tests should be performed before testing, and the subject should rest for at least 15 minutes before starting the test. Resting measurements obtained before testing with the subject seated include Sp_{O_2}, HR, **ratings of perceived exertion (RPE),** and BP. The technologist should provide the subject with standardized instructions.

The objective of the test is to have the patient walk as far as possible in 6 minutes. The patient should be encouraged throughout the test, and it is recommended that standard phrases be used to reduce intratester and test-to-test variability (How To ... 7.1). The use of supplemental oxygen and wheeled walkers can affect the results and must be kept constant in repeat testing. Resting during the tests is permitted, with encouragement to continue walking as soon as possible. Pulse oximetry (Sp_{O_2}) monitoring is required. The testing personnel should not influence the walking pace if a cabled pulse oximeter is used. Telemetry or Bluetooth technology would be advantageous for continual Sp_{O_2} monitoring during field testing. If the subject desaturates less than 80%, the tester should pause the test until the Sp_{O_2} returns to greater than 85%, upon which the subject may continue the test. It should be emphasized that the timer continues to run during any pause during the test. The primary outcome measurement is the 6-Minute Walk Distance (6MWD). Reporting documentation should include the 6MWD, the lowest Sp_{O_2}, the end-exercise HR, oxygen flow and delivery device if used, the mode of oxygen transport (e.g., pulling an O_2 cart has a different effect on work than carrying a unit), and the RPE. See Table 7.1 for an example of a data record used to record 6-minute walk data from a patient. It is recommended that the test be repeated at the initial visit secondary to a training effect, which is the same as the minimally important distance.

7.1   How To ...
Perform a 6-Minute Walk Test

1. Tasks common to all procedures:
   a. Prepare equipment.
   b. Review order.
   c. Introduce yourself and identify patient according to institutional policies.
2. Describe the procedure: "The aim of this test is to walk as far as possible for 6 minutes. You will walk along this hallway between the markers as many times as you can in 6 minutes."
3. Explain to the patient: "I will let you know as each minute goes past, and then at 6 minutes, I will ask you to stop where you are. Six minutes is a long time to walk, so you will be exerting yourself."
4. Encourage the patient throughout the test using standardized phrases noted in the technical statement.
5. Permit the patient to slow down, stop, and rest if necessary, but encourage the patient to resume walking as soon possible.
6. Remind the patient that the objective is to walk as far as possible for 6 minutes, not to run or jog.
7. If at any time the patient feels chest discomfort or lightheadedness, the tester should be told.
8. If the subject is oxygen dependent, titrate the oxygen before the 6MWT using an independent test. Do not use the 6MWT as a titration test.
9. Pulse oximetry: do not influence the subject's walking pace to monitor. Telemetry or Bluetooth oximetry would be preferred. Pause the test if the Sp_{O_2} is <80%. The subject can restart once the Sp_{O_2} reaches >85%.
10. Record the 6MWD, nadir Sp_{O_2}, end-exercise HR, and RPE.
11. Report results and note comments related to test performance or quality.

TABLE 7.1							
Six-Minute Walk Report							
Date	Distance (ft/meters)	Inspired Gas	Mode of O_2 Transport	SpO_2 Nadir	SpO_2 (End Exercise)	HR (End Exercise)	RPE (6–20)
8/12/2019	1173/486	4.0 L/min NC	Patient carried unit	93	94	112	17
12/09/2019	1569/478	4.0 L/min NC	Patient carried unit	94	95	115	18
3/18/2019	1506/451	4.0 L/min	Patient carried unit	91	92	118	17

RPE, ratings of perceived exertion.

Six-Minute Walk Test Reference Set

Enright and Sherrill suggested the following 6MWD formulas based on a study in 117 healthy men and 173 healthy females with an age range of 40 to 80 years. The median 6MWD was 576 m (1889 ft) for men and 494 m (1620 ft) for women.

$$Men = (7.57 \times ht[cm]) - (5.02 \times age)$$
$$-1.76 \times (wt[kg]) - 309\,m$$
$$Women = (2.11 \times ht[cm]) - (2.29 \times wt[kg])$$
$$-(5.78 \times age) - 667\,m$$

Casanova et al. published their results from the Six-Minute Walk Distance Project. They studied 444 subjects (238 males) from ages 40 to 80 and found that the best predictive equation for the 6MWD included age, height, weight, sex, and HRmax/HRmax% predicted.

$$Predicted\ 6MWD = 361 - (age\ in\ yr \times 4) + (ht[cm] \times 2)$$
$$+ (HRmax / HRmax\%pred \times 3)$$
$$(wt[kg] \times 1.5) - 30\,(if\ female)$$

The 2014 American Thoracic Society–European Respiratory Society (ATS-ERS) standard does not identify a preferred predicted set for the 6MWT.

The minimal important difference (MID) for the 6MWT is 30 m based on the current evidence. The 2014 ATS-ERS field-testing standard subdivided the threshold to predict survival into four categories: chronic obstructive pulmonary disease (COPD; 317 m), interstitial lung disease (254 m), pulmonary hypertension (337 m), and other (294 m).

Shuttle Walk Tests

The **Incremental Shuttle Walk Test** (ISWT) is another simple field test used to define functional exercise capacity. The pretest instructions, equipment used, required patient assessment, and absolute and related contraindications (see Box 7.1) are all the same as for the 6MWT. The test is a 10-m course with the traffic cones inset 0.5 m on each end. The test is an externally paced maximal exercise test where speed is controlled by a series of prerecorded signals. The walking speed increases until the participant can no longer continue. At the beginning of the test, play the pretest instructions from the audio recording, and confirm the subject understands the expectations of the test. There is a triple beep from the audio recording to indicate the start of the test, and the timer is activated. The walking speed is increased every minute, indicated by a triple beep; instruct the patient, "You need to increase your speed of walking." Only one statement of encouragement can be used if the subject is falling behind, "You need to increase your speed to keep up with the test." The test is terminated if the patient is unable to continue, if the technologist determines the patient is not fit to continue, or if the technologist determines the patient is unable to sustain the speed or cover the distance to the cone before the next beep. The latter is determined as the patient being more than 0.5 m from the cone when the beep sounds on a second successive 10-m length. The test should also be discontinued if the $SpO_2 < 80\%$. The MID for the ISWT is 47.5 m or five shuttles. Report the number of lengths walked in meters (to the last 10 completed).

The ATS-ERS field-testing standard cites there are not enough studies to recommend a predicted reference set.

The **Endurance Shuttle Walk Test** (ESWT) is conducted along the course as described for the ISWT. The pretest instructions, equipment used, required patient assessment, and absolute and related contraindications (see Box 7.1) are all the same as for the 6MWT. The ESWT is a constant walking speed after a 1.5-minute warm-up period. There are standardized audio instructions and an audio beep that assists in determining the walking pace. The pace is calculated from the ISWT as a predefined percentage of the peak performance of the ISWT (70%–85% estimated peak $\dot{V}o_2$) or as a percentage of the peak speed achieved. After the instructions are given, a triple beep indicates the test has started. The timer is activated after the warm-up period. The subjects are paced for the first two shuttles. During the test, only one statement of encouragement can be given, "You need to increase your speed to keep up with the test." Termination of the test is the same as for the ISWT. The reporting of the test is in time (seconds). It is also important that the walking speed is recorded.

EXERCISE PROTOCOLS AND REFERENCE SETS

Cardiopulmonary exercise tests can be divided into two general categories depending on the protocols used to perform the test: progressive multistage tests and steady-state tests. The 6MWT contains elements of each of these general categories.

Progressive multistage exercise tests examine the effects of increasing workloads on various cardiopulmonary variables without necessarily allowing a steady state to be achieved. These protocols are often used to determine the workload at which the patient reaches a maximum oxygen uptake ($\dot{V}o_2$max). Multistage protocols can determine maximal ventilation, maximal HR, or a symptom limitation (e.g., chest pain) to exercise. Progressive multistage protocols (also called *incremental tests*) allow cardiopulmonary variables to be compared with expected patterns as workload increases.

In a typical incremental test, the patient's workload increases at predetermined intervals (Table 7.2). The workload may be increased at intervals of 1 to 5 minutes. Measurements (e.g., ECG, BP, or blood gases) are usually made during the last 20 to 30 seconds of each or alternating intervals. Computerized systems that continuously measure ventilation, gas exchange, and cardiopulmonary variables permit shorter intervals to be used. The combination of intervals and work increments should allow the patient to reach exhaustion or symptom limitation within a reasonable period. An incremental test lasting 8 to 10 minutes after a warm-up is typically used as the target. If a computerized cycle ergometer is used, a "ramp" test may be performed. In a ramp protocol, the ergometer's resistance is increased continuously at a predetermined rate (usually measured in watts per minute).

During incremental tests with short intervals (1–3 minutes or a ramp protocol), a steady state of gas exchange, ventilation, and cardiovascular response may not be attained. Healthy patients may reach a steady state in 2 to 3 minutes at low and moderate workloads. Attainment of a steady state, however, is unnecessary if the primary objective of the evaluation is to determine the maximum values (oxygen uptake, HR, or ventilation). Short exercise intervals also lessen the muscle fatigue that may occur with prolonged tests. Short-interval or ramp protocols may allow better delineation of gas exchange ($\dot{V}o_2$, $\dot{V}co_2$) kinetics. Progressive multistage tests using intervals of 4 to 6 minutes may result in a steady state.

Steady-state tests are designed to assess cardiopulmonary function under conditions of constant metabolic demand. Steady-state conditions are usually defined in terms of HR, oxygen consumption ($\dot{V}o_2$), or ventilation ($\dot{V}_E$). If the HR remains unchanged for 1 minute at a given workload, a steady state may be assumed. Steady-state tests are useful for assessing responses to a known workload. Steady-state protocols may be used to evaluate the effectiveness of various therapies or pharmacologic agents on exercise ability. For example, an incremental test may be performed initially to determine a patient's maximum tolerable

TABLE 7.2

Exercise Protocols

Treadmill	Speed (mph)/Grade (%)	Interval (min)	Comment
Bruce	1.7/10 2.5/12 3.4/14 4.2/16 5.0/18 5.5/20 6.0/22	3	Large workload increments 1.7/0 and 1.7/5 may be used as preliminary stages for deconditioned patients
Balke	3.3–3.4/0 increasing grade by 2.5% to exhaustion	1	Small workload increments: may use 3 mph and 2-minute intervals for deconditioned subjects, or reduce slope changes to 1%
Jones	1.0/0 2.0/0 2–3.5/2.5 increasing grade by 2.5% to exhaustion	1	Small workload increments and low starting workload

Cycle Ergometer	Workload	Interval (min)	Comment
Astrand	50 W/min (300 kpm) to exhaustion	4	Large workload increments and long intervals; 33 W (200 kpm) may be used for women
Incremental	Variable (5-, 10-, 15-, up to 50-watt increments)	Warm-up followed by 1-minute increments in work	Workload increments are based on subject conditions.
"RAMP"	Variable (e.g., 5, 10, 15) W/min to exhaustion	Continuous	Requires electronically braked ergometer; different work rates may be used to alter ramp slope
Jones	16 W/min (100 kpm) to exhaustion	1	Smaller increments (50 kpm) may be used for deconditioned subjects

Other	Description	Interval (min)	Comment
Master step test	Either constant or variable step height combined with increasing step rates	Variable	Simple to perform; workload may be difficult to qualify

workload. Then, a steady-state test may be used to evaluate specific variables at a submaximal level, such as 50% and 75% of the highest $\dot{V}o_2$ achieved. The patient exercises for 5 to 8 minutes at a predetermined level to allow a steady state to develop. Measurements are performed during the last 1 or 2 minutes of the period. Successive steady-state determinations at higher power outputs may be made continuously or spaced with short periods of light exercise or rest. A similar protocol may be used for evaluation of exercise-induced bronchospasm (see Chapter 9).

Reference Sets

Numerous reference equations for predicting $\dot{V}o_2$ max have been published in the literature (see Table 7.3). As with all reference equations, it is important for the laboratory management team to select a set or multiple sets that match their patient population. Recently, the Fitness Registry and Importance of Exercise National Database (FRIEND) published reference equations for normal standards for $\dot{V}o_2$max. Their published data have separate equations for both treadmill and cycle ergometer performed tests.

TABLE 7.3				
Common Predicted $\dot{V}o_2$max Reference Sets				
Author/Name	Sample size	Age range	Year published	Comments
Pediatric				
Cooper	109 (M-58, F-51	6–17	1984	Ramp protocol cycle
James	149 (M-90, F-59)	5–33	1980	Steady-state cycle
Adult				
Blackie	170 (M-47, F-81)	55–80	1991	Increment cycle
Friend Cycle	5100 (M-3378, F-1722	18->70	2018	Grouped in < 40, 40–50, 50–70 and > 70 years
Friend treadmill	7759 (M-4601, F-3158)	20–80	2017	Grouped in 6 decade ranges (e.g., 20–29, 30–39, etc.)
Hanson, Sue, Wasserman	400 (NK)	Mean 54	1984	Ramp protocol (shipyard workers)
Jones	100 (M-50, F-50)	15–71	1984	Incremental cycle
SHIP	534 (M-253, F-281)	20–79	2009	Incremental cycle (German population study)
Whipp	120 (M-60, F-60)	20–80	2001	Incremental cycle

M, Male; *F*, female.

EXERCISE WORKLOAD

Two methods of varying exercise workload are commonly used: the treadmill and the cycle ergometer (Figs. 7.2 and 7.3). Each device has advantages and disadvantages (Table 7.4). Other methods sometimes used include arm ergometers and steps.

Workload on a treadmill is adjusted by changing the speed and/or slope of the walking surface. The speed of the treadmill may be calibrated either in miles per hour or in kilometers per hour. Treadmill slope is registered as "percent grade." *Percent grade* refers to the relationship between the length of the walking surface and the elevation of one end above level. A treadmill with a 6-foot surface and one end elevated 1 foot above level would have an elevation of $1/6 \times 100$ or approximately 17%. The primary advantage of a treadmill is that it elicits walking, jogging, and running, which are familiar forms of exercise. An additional advantage is that maximal levels of exercise can be easily attained even in conditioned, healthy patients. However, the actual work performed during treadmill walking is a function of the weight of the patient. Patients of different weight walking at the same speed and slope perform different work. Different walking patterns or stride length may also affect the actual amount of work being done. Patients who grip the handrails of the treadmill may use their arms to reduce the amount of work being performed. For these reasons, estimating $\dot{V}o_2$ from a patient's weight and the speed and slope of the treadmill may produce erroneous results. $\dot{V}o_2$ max has been shown to be measured slightly higher (approximately 7%–10%) on a treadmill compared with a cycle ergometer.

The cycle ergometer allows workload to be varied by adjustment of the resistance to pedaling and by the pedaling frequency, usually specified in revolutions per minute (rpm). The flywheel of a *mechanical* ergometer turns against a belt or strap, both ends of which are connected to a weighted physical balance. The diameter of the wheel is known, and the resistance can be easily measured. When pedaling speed (usually 50–90 rpm) is determined, the amount of work performed can be accurately calculated. One of the chief advantages of the cycle ergometer is that the workload is independent of the weight of the patient. Unlike the treadmill, $\dot{V}o_2$ can be reasonably

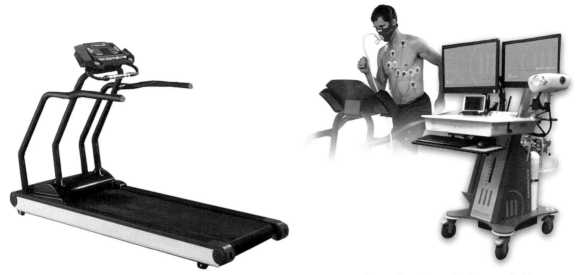

FIG. 7.2 Treadmill with computerized electrocardiogram (ECG) and controller. The treadmill is controlled by a programmable interface so that different protocols (e.g., speeds and percent grade) can be selected. Manual control is also provided. Cardiac monitoring and exhaled gas analysis are integrated in a single computer system. The 12-lead ECG recordings or rhythm strips can be taken automatically at each exercise level. Most automated systems provide "freeze-frame" technology that allows for close review during the test and storage of data for retrieval and analysis for significant arrhythmia and ST abnormalities after the test. The same system can be interfaced with a cycle ergometer (see Fig. 7.3). (Courtesy MGC Diagnostics., St. Paul, MN.)

TABLE 7.4		
Ergometers		
	Advantages	Disadvantages
Treadmill	Natural form of exercise, easy to verify calibration, higher $\dot{V}o_2$max	Risk of accidents Patient anxiety Motion artifact Difficult to obtain blood Difficult to quantify work
Cycle ergometer	Lower cost and smaller footprint Safer than treadmill Easy to monitor Easy to quantify work Easier to obtain blood samples	Difficult to verify calibration, leg fatigue more of an issue, Lower $\dot{V}o_2$max

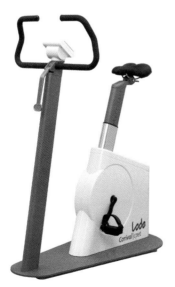

FIG. 7.3 Electronically braked cycle ergometer. Workload (i.e., resistance) is usually managed by interfacing the ergometer with a computer. (Courtesy MGC Diagnostics., St. Paul, MN.)

estimated if the pedaling speed and resistance are carefully measured. The normal relationship of workload in watts to oxygen consumption is 10 mL/watt (range 8–13 mL/watt, with some suggesting 10.8 mL/watt). Another advantage of ergometers is better stability of the patient for gas collection, blood sampling, and BP monitoring. *Electronically braked cycle ergometers* (see Fig. 7.3) provide a smooth, rapid, and more reproducible means of changing exercise workload than mechanical ergometers. Electronically braked ergometers allow continuous adjustment of workload independent of pedaling speed. However, the accuracy of the ergometer output may be dependent on a manufacturer's specified pedal cadence range (e.g., 40–100 rpm). This feature permits the exercise level to be ramped (i.e., the workload increases continuously rather than in increments). The **ramp test** allows the patient to advance from low to high workloads quickly and provides all of the information normally sought during a progressive maximal exercise test. A ramp protocol typically requires electronic control (usually by a computer) for adjustment of the workload and rapid collection of physiologic data. Box 7.2 provides a systematic method for determining the desired workload increments using a cycle ergometer.

Some differences in maximal performance exist between the treadmill and the cycle ergometer. These differences primarily result from the muscle groups used. In most patients, cycling does not produce as high of a maximum O_2 consumption as walking on the treadmill (approximately 7%–10% less). Ventilation and lactate production may be slightly greater on the cycle ergometer because of the different muscle groups used. Differences between the treadmill and cycle ergometer are not significant in most clinical situations. The choice of device may be dictated by the patient's clinical condition (e.g., orthopedic impairments or chief complaint occurs with running only), the types of measurements to be made, or the space and availability of equipment in the laboratory.

PF TIP 7.1

MET is a commonly used term to describe the level of work performed during an exercise evaluation or in relation to activities of daily living. One MET equals the O_2 uptake at rest. For clinical purposes, 1 MET is equivalent to an O_2 uptake of 3.5 mL O_2/min/kg. If O_2 consumption is measured during a cardiopulmonary exercise test, the MET level achieved can be calculated easily. For example, if a patient reaches a peak $\dot{V}O_2$ of 15 mL O_2/min/kg, the MET equivalent would be 15/3.5, or approximately 4.3 METs. Healthy sedentary patients should be able to exercise up to approximately 7 METs.

Workload may be expressed quantitatively in several ways:

- **Work** is normally expressed in kilopond-meters (kpm). One kilopond-meter equals the work of moving a 1-kg mass a vertical distance of 1 m against the force of gravity.
- Power is expressed in kilopond-meters per minute (i.e., work per unit of time) or in **watts**. One watt equals 6.12 kpm/min (100 watts = ~600 kpm/min). The normal relationship of work, in watts, to oxygen consumption is 10 mL/watt.

Energy is expressed by oxygen consumption ($\dot{V}O_2$) in liters or milliliters per minute (standard temperature, pressure, dry [STPD]) or in terms of **metabolic equivalents (METs)**. Resting or baseline $\dot{V}O_2$ can be measured as described in the following paragraphs or estimated. For purposes of standardization, 1 MET is considered equal to 3.5 mL O_2/min/kg.

For cardiopulmonary exercise evaluation, it is particularly useful to relate the ventilatory, blood gas, and hemodynamic measurements to the $\dot{V}O_2$ as the independent variable. This requires measurement of ventilation and analysis of expired gas during exercise.

BOX 7.2   METHOD FOR PREDICTING INCREMENT OR RAMP PROTOCOL

($\dot{V}O_2$max predicted – $\dot{V}O_2$ rest)/100 = predicted max power output (watts) to achieve in 10 minutes.

- Reduce the predicted max workload for subjects with reduced exercise tolerance.
- Increase the estimated maximal power output for very fit subjects.
  Example: Predicted $\dot{V}O_2$ max 2300 mL, resting $\dot{V}O_2$ max 300 mL (2300 – 300)/100 = 20 watts/min incremental or ramp protocol
- A method to determine workload in subjects with lung disease can be derived from the maximal voluntary ventilation (MVV): >80 L/min, use previous method; <80 L/min, use a 10-watt increment; <40 L/min, use a 5-watt increment.

A number of cardiopulmonary exercise variables may be used, depending on the clinical questions to be answered. Schemes for measuring these variables are described in Table 7.5. Graded exercise with monitoring of only BP and ECG may be limited to the evaluation of patients with suspected or known coronary artery disease.

Measurement of ventilation, oxygen consumption, carbon dioxide production, and related variables permits a comprehensive evaluation of the cardiovascular system. The addition of these measurements to ECG, BP, and pulse oximetry makes it possible to grade the adequacy of cardiopulmonary function. In addition, analysis of exhaled gas allows the relative contributions of cardiovascular, pulmonary, or conditioning limitations to work to be determined. All of these variables can be measured noninvasively. When using pulse oximetry to assess gas exchange, the practitioner needs to be aware of the limitations of the device that may lead to a false-positive result (e.g., motion artifact, peripheral vasoconstriction).

Adding arterial blood gases (ABGs) to the exercise protocol enables detailed analysis of the pulmonary limitations to exercise. Placement of an arterial catheter is preferable to a single sample obtained at peak exercise, although this is subject to the laboratory having the skilled personnel available to place an arterial line. Multiple specimens permit comparison of blood gases at each workload. A single sample at peak exercise may be difficult to obtain and may not adequately describe the pattern of gas exchange abnormality. However, if this technique is used, the sample should be harvested within 30 seconds of achieving the maximal workload because variables of gas exchange return rapidly to baseline in some individuals. In some patients, measurement of CO using either noninvasive or invasive techniques such as a pulmonary artery (Swan–Ganz) catheter may be indicated. Noninvasive CO determination depends on the availability of the technology and the underlying cause of the patient's condition (e.g., may not work well in patients with COPD). Invasive techniques require the placement of a catheter that allows measurement of mixed venous blood gases, CO via the Fick method, and many other derived variables. Thermal dilution CO is also available with most pulmonary artery catheters.

TABLE 7.5

Cardiopulmonary Exercise Variables

Variables Measured	Uses
ECG, blood pressure, Sp_{O_2}	Limited to suspected or known coronary artery disease; pulse oximetry may be misleading if used without blood gases
All of the above plus ventilation $\dot{V}_{O_2}$, $\dot{V}_{CO_2}$, and derived measurements	Noninvasive estimate of ventilatory/anaerobic threshold (AT), quantify workload; discriminate between cardiovascular and pulmonary limitation to work
All of the above plus arterial blood gases	Detailed assessment of gas exchange abnormalities; calculation of V_D/V_T; titration of O_2 in exercise desaturation; measurement of pH and lactate possible
All of the above plus mixed venous blood gases	Cardiac output by Fick method, noninvasive techniques, calculation of shunt, thermodilution cardiac output, pulmonary artery pressures, calculation of pulmonary and systemic vascular resistances

ECG, Electrocardiogram.

CARDIOVASCULAR MONITORS DURING EXERCISE

Continuous monitoring of HR and ECG during exercise is essential to the safe performance of the test. Intermittent or continuous monitoring of BP is equally important to ensure that exercise testing is safe. Recording of HR, ECG, and BP allows work limitations caused by cardiac or vascular disease to be identified and quantified. The level of fitness or conditioning can be gauged from the HR response in relation to the maximal work rate achieved during exercise.

Heart Rate and Electrocardiogram

HR and rhythm should be monitored continuously using one or more modified chest leads. Standard precordial chest lead configurations (V_1–V_6) allow comparison with resting 12-lead tracings (Criteria for Acceptability 7.1). Twelve-lead monitoring during exercise is practical with electrocardiographs designed for exercise testing. These instruments incorporate filters (digital or analog) that eliminate movement artifact and provide ST-segment monitoring. Limb leads normally must be moved to the torso for ergometer or treadmill testing (modified leads). A resting ECG should be performed to record both the standard and modified leads. Single-lead monitoring allows only for gross arrhythmia detection and HR determination. It may not be adequate for testing patients with known or suspected cardiac disease.

CRITERIA FOR ACCEPTABILITY 7.1

Cardiovascular Monitors During Exercise

1. Heart rate and rhythm (ECG) should be monitored continuously. At least one precordial lead is required; full 12-lead monitoring using modified limb leads is recommended.
2. A resting 12-lead ECG should be available for comparison with exercise tracings.
3. All exercise tracings should be free from artifact caused by motion or electrical interference.
4. ECG monitoring devices should allow manual or automated storage of arrhythmia events for later review.
5. "Raw" ECG tracings should be available for comparison with computer-averaged complexes.
6. Heart rates should be checked by visual inspection of the ECG tracing.
7. Systemic BP should be monitored at appropriate intervals.
8. BP may be monitored using an appropriate-sized cuff or by automated noninvasive blood pressure (NIBP) monitor. A cuff/stethoscope should be available as backup for the NIBP.
9. If BP is monitored by an indwelling arterial catheter, the pressure transducer must be zeroed and calibrated appropriately. The catheter should be secured to minimize movement artifact.

The ECG monitor should allow the assessment of intervals and segments up to the patient's maximal HR (HRmax). Computerized arrhythmia recording or manual "freeze-frame" storage allows the sub-

sequent evaluation of conduction abnormalities while the testing protocol continues (see Fig. 7.4A). Some digital ECG systems generate computerized "median" complexes averaged from a series of beats. These may be helpful in analyzing ST-segment depression. The "raw," or nondigitized, ECG should also be available. Significant ST-segment changes should be easily identifiable from the tracing up to the predicted HRmax.

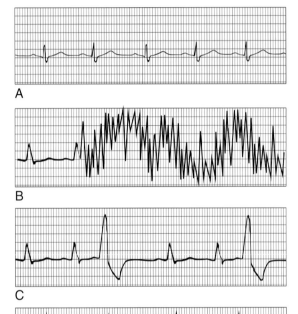

A

B

C

D

FIG. 7.4 Electrocardiographic (ECG) monitoring during exercise. (A) Standard rhythm lead showing normal sinus rhythm. (B) Motion artifact. The most common monitoring problem during exercise is poor ECG signals because of motion. (C) Premature ventricular contractions (PVCs). PVCs are a common occurrence during exercise in patients with underlying cardiac disease. Increased rate of PVCs, couplets (two in a row), or triplets (three in a row) may be indications for limiting the exercise test. (D) ST-segment changes. Depression (and sometimes elevation) of the ST segment of the ECG is usually considered evidence of cardiac ischemia. Depression (or elevation) of the ST segment greater than 1 to 2 mm for 0.08 seconds or longer is consistent with significant ischemia.

PF TIP 7.2

Exercise tests are often performed to determine a patient's maximal exercise capacity. An endpoint commonly used is the patient's predicted maximal HR. Maximal HR is easily computed using formulas such as 220 – age or 210 – 0.65 (age). A subject who is 40 years old would have a predicted maximal HR of 220 – 40, or 180 beats/min. If the subject achieves at least 85% of the predicted value (153 beats/min in this case), he or she is considered to have made a maximal effort. Because maximal HR varies among individuals, some patients may reach or exceed their predicted maximum. Many patients will reach a "symptom-limited" endpoint before reaching 85% of the predicted maximal HR. In these cases, the patient becomes exhausted, is dyspneic, or has chest pain. The technologist should always record what symptoms caused the patient's inability to continue.

HR should be analyzed by visual inspection of the ECG with manual measurement of the rate rather than by an automatic sensor. Most HR meters average RR intervals over multiple beats. Inaccurate HR measurements may occur with nodal or ventricular arrhythmias or because of motion artifact. Tall P or T waves may be falsely identified as R waves, causing automatic calculation of HR to be incorrect. Accurate measurement of HR is necessary to determine the patient's maximal HR in comparison with the age-related predicted value.

Motion artifact is the most common cause of unacceptable ECG recordings during exercise (Fig. 7.4B). Allowing the patient to practice pedaling on the ergometer or walking on the treadmill permits the adequacy of the ECG signal to be checked. Carefully applied electrodes, proper skin preparation, and secured lead wires greatly minimize movement artifact (see Criteria for Acceptability 7.1). Electrodes specifically designed for exercise testing are helpful. Most use extra adhesive to ensure electrical contact even when the patient begins perspiring. The skin sites should be carefully prepared. Removal of surface skin cells by gentle abrasion is recommended. Patients with excessive body hair may require shaving of the electrode site to ensure good electrical contact. Lead wires must be securely attached to the electrodes. Devices that limit the movement of the lead wires can greatly reduce motion artifact. Spare electrodes and lead wires should be available to avoid test interruption in the event of an electrode failure.

HR increases linearly with increasing workload, up to an age-related maximum. Several formulas are available for predicting HRmax. For most predicted HRmax values, a variability of ± 10 to 15 beats/min exists in healthy adult patients. Two commonly used equations for predicting HRmax are as follows:

(1)
$$HRmax = 220 - Age(years)$$

(2)
$$HRmax = 210 - (0.65 \times Age[years])$$

Equation 1 yields slightly higher predicted values in young adults. Equation 2 produces higher values in older adults. Other methods of predicting HRmax vary, depending on the type of exercise protocol used in deriving the regression data. Specific criteria for terminating an exercise test should include factors based on symptom limitation, as well as HR and BP changes (see the Safety section).

HR increases almost linearly with increasing $\dot{V}o_2$. The increase in CO depends on both HR and stroke volume (SV), according to the following equation:

$$CO = HR \times SV$$

Increases in SV account for a smaller portion of the increase in CO, primarily at low and moderate workloads (Fig. 7.5). While HR increases from 70 beats/min up to 200 beats/min in young, healthy, upright patients, SV increases from 80 mL to approximately 110 mL. At low workloads, an increase in CO depends on the patient's ability to increase both HR and SV. At high workloads, further increases in CO result almost entirely from the increase in HR.

Deconditioned patients usually have a limited SV. High HR values occur with moderate workloads in deconditioned individuals because it is the primary mechanism for increasing CO. Training (e.g., endurance or aerobic) typically improves SV response. This allows the same CO to be achieved at

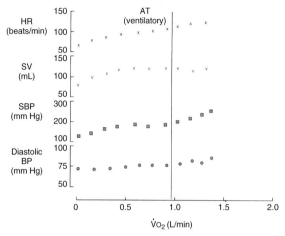

FIG. 7.5 Normal cardiovascular responses during exercise. Four cardiovascular parameters are plotted against $\dot{V}O_2$ as a measure of work rate, as they might appear in a normal, healthy adult. Heart rate (HR) increases linearly with work. Maximal HR is predicted by the age of the patient. Stroke volume (SV) increases initially at low to moderate workloads but then becomes relatively constant. Cardiac output (HR × SV) increases at low and moderate workloads because of increases in both HR and SV (see text). At higher levels of work, increases in HR are responsible for increasing cardiac output. Systolic blood pressure (BP) increases by approximately 100 mm Hg in a linear fashion, whereas diastolic BP increases only slightly.

a lower HR. Training usually results in a lower resting HR and a higher tolerable maximum workload. Except in highly trained patients, maximal exercise in healthy individuals is limited by the inability to further increase the CO. Reductions in SV are usually related to the preload or afterload of the left ventricle. Increased HR response, in relation to the workload, implies that SV is compromised.

Reduced HR response may occur in patients who have ischemic heart disease or complete heart block (Interpretive Strategies 7.1). Low HR is also common in patients who have been treated with drugs that block the effects of the sympathetic nervous system (beta-blockers, calcium channel blockers). HR response may also be reduced if the autonomic nervous system is impaired or the heart is denervated, as occurs after cardiac transplantation (e.g., chronotropic insufficiency).

In patients who have heart disease (e.g., coronary artery disease, cardiomyopathy), increased HR is typically accompanied by ECG changes such as arrhythmias or ST-segment depression. Deconditioned patients without heart disease show

a high HR at lower-than-maximal workloads but usually without ECG abnormalities. Horizontal or down-sloping ST-segment depression greater than 1 mm (from the resting baseline) for a duration of 0.08 seconds is usually considered evidence of ischemia (Fig. 7.4D). ST-segment depression at low workloads that increases with HR and continues into the postexercise period is usually indicative of multivessel coronary artery disease. ST-segment depression accompanied by exertional hypotension or a marked increase in diastolic pressure is usually associated with significant coronary disease. The predictive value of ST-segment changes during exercise must be related to the patient's clinical history and risk factors for heart disease.

INTERPRETIVE STRATEGIES 7.1

Cardiovascular Monitors During Exercise

1. Is ECG recording acceptable? Free from motion and other artifact?
2. Is resting tracing consistent with previous 12-lead ECGs? If not, are differences caused by lead placement?
3. What is the rate and rhythm at rest? Is there evidence of heart block at rest? Is there evidence of ischemia (ST-segment changes) at rest?
4. Was maximal heart rate greater than 85% of predicted? If so, patient probably exerted maximal effort. If not, what factors limited exercise? Ventilation? Pain? Fatigue? Other?
5. Did the rhythm change with exercise? Increased or decreased PVCs? Was there evidence of ischemia (ST- or T-wave changes)?
6. Was BP normal at rest? If not, consider clinical correlation.
7. Did systolic BP increase appropriately? Did it exceed 250 mm Hg at maximal exercise?
8. Did diastolic BP remain constant or increase slightly? If not, consider clinical correlation.

The most common arrhythmia that occurs during exercise testing is premature ventricular contractions (PVCs; see Fig. 7.4C). Exercise-induced PVCs occurring at a rate of more than 10 per minute are often found in ischemic heart disease. Increased PVCs during exercise may also be seen in mitral valve prolapse. Coupled PVCs (couplets) often precede ventricular tachycardia or ventricular fibrillation. Occurrence of couplets or frequent PVCs may be an indication for terminating the

TABLE 7.6				
Exercise Variables and Dyspnea[a]				
	Cardiac	**Ventilatory**	**Deconditioned**	**Poor Effort**
$\dot{V}_{O_2}$max	Less than 80% of predicted	Less than 80% of predicted	Less than 80% of predicted	Less than 80% of predicted
$\dot{V}_E$max	Less than 70% of MVV	Greater than 90% of MVV; MVV –$V_E$max < 15 L	Less than 70% of MVV	Variable
Anaerobic threshold	Achieved at low $\dot{V}_{O_2}$	Usually not achieved	Achieved at low $\dot{V}_{O_2}$	Not achieved
HR	Greater than 85% of predicted	Less than 85% of predicted	Greater than 85% of predicted	Less than 85% of predicted
ECG/signs of ischemia	ST changes, arrhythmias, chest pain	Usually normal	Normal	Normal
Sa_{O_2}	Greater than 90%	Often less than 90%, hypoxemia	Greater than 90%	Greater than 90%

[a]This table compares the usual findings for the exercise variables listed in subjects with dyspnea caused by cardiac disease, pulmonary disease, or deconditioning. Some subjects may have dyspnea because of a combination of causes. Poor effort during exercise may result from improper instruction, lack of understanding by the subject, or lack of motivation by the subject.
ECG, Electrocardiogram; *HR,* heart rate; *MVV,* maximal voluntary ventilation; Sa_{O_2}, arterial oxygen saturation.

exercise evaluation. Some patients with PVCs at rest or at low workloads may have these ectopic beats suppressed as exercise intensity increases. The most serious ventricular arrhythmias are sometimes seen in the immediate postexercise phase.

Shortness of breath (SOB) brought on by exertion is perhaps the most widespread indication for cardiopulmonary exercise evaluation. The combination of cardiovascular parameters (e.g., HR, SV) with data obtained from the analysis of exhaled gas (i.e., $\dot{V}_{O_2}$) permits the assessment of dyspnea on exertion. Table 7.6 generalizes some of the basic relationships between cardiovascular and pulmonary exercise responses. These relationships help delineate whether exertional dyspnea is a result of cardiac or pulmonary disease or whether the patient is simply deconditioned. In some instances, poor effort may mimic exertional dyspnea. Comparison of data from cardiovascular and exhaled gas variables can confirm inadequate patient effort.

Blood Pressure

Systemic BP may be monitored intermittently with the standard cuff method. Automated noninvasive cuff devices for monitoring BP are also available. Although these methods work well at rest and at low workloads, they may be difficult to implement during high levels of exercise. However, recent advances in automated systems that pair sophisticated Korotkoff sound detection with QRS complex activation have improved the ability to measure exercise BP more accurately with these devices. BP sounds may be difficult to detect because of treadmill noise or patient movement. It is important to monitor the pattern of BP response at low and moderate workloads to establish that both systolic and diastolic pressures respond as anticipated.

Continuous monitoring of the BP may be accomplished by the connection of a pressure transducer to an indwelling arterial catheter (Fig. 7.6). An indwelling line allows the continuous display and recording of systolic, diastolic, and mean arterial pressures. In addition, the catheter provides ready access for arterial blood sampling. Arterial catheterization may be easily accomplished using either the radial or the brachial site. The catheter must be adequately secured to prevent loss of patency during vigorous exercise. The insertion of arterial catheters presents some risk of blood splashing or spills. Adequate protection for the individual inserting the catheter and for those withdrawing specimens is essential. See Chapter 6 for specific recommendations regarding arterial sampling via catheters.

Systolic BP increases in healthy patients during exercise from 120 mm Hg up to approximately 200 to 250 mm Hg (see Fig. 7.5). Diastolic pressure

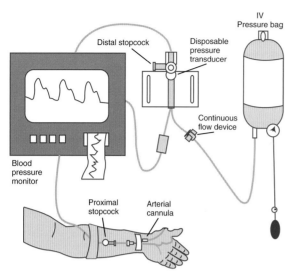

FIG. 7.6 Pressure transducer setup for continuous arterial monitoring. A catheter is inserted into the radial or brachial artery. Pressure tubing connects the catheter to a continuous flow device that maintains a constant pressure (and a small flow of solution) against the arterial line to prevent backflow of blood into the system. The continuous flow device also allows flushing of the system. A pressure transducer assembly is connected in line with the tubing. Pressure changes in the system are transmitted via a thin membrane to the transducer. Blood samples may be drawn by inserting a heparinized syringe at a stopcock located near the indwelling catheter (blood pressure signal is temporarily lost during sampling). A similar assembly can be used for connection to a Swan-Ganz catheter for pulmonary artery monitoring during exercise.

normally rises only slightly (10–15 mm Hg) or not at all. The mean arterial pressure rises from approximately 90 mm Hg to approximately 110 mm Hg, depending on the changes in systolic and diastolic pressures. The increase in systolic pressure is caused almost completely by increased CO and mostly by the SV. Even though CO may increase fivefold (e.g., from 5–25 L/min), the systolic pressure only increases twofold. Systolic pressure only doubles because of the tremendous decrease in peripheral vascular resistance. Most of this decrease in resistance results from vasodilatation in exercising muscles. Increased systolic pressure (> 250–300 mm Hg) should be considered an indication for terminating the exercise evaluation (Box 7.3). Similarly, if the systolic pressure fails to rise with increasing workload, the exercise test should be terminated and the patient's condition stabilized. Variations in BP during exercise are often caused by the patient's respiratory effort. Phasic changes with respiration are particularly common in patients who have large transpulmonary pressures because of lung disease (e.g., pulsus paradoxus). Differences of as much as 30 mm Hg between inspiration and expiration may be seen during the continuous monitoring of arterial pressure.

In maximal tests (e.g., the patient reaches HRmax), it may be impossible to obtain a reliable BP at peak exercise. Even with an arterial catheter, motion artifact may prevent the recording of a usable tracing. Systolic pressure may transiently drop, and diastolic pressure may drop to zero at the termination of exercise. To minimize the degree of hypotension resulting from abrupt cessation of heavy exercise, the patient should "cool down." This is accomplished easily by having the patient continue exercising at a low work rate until BP and HR have stabilized at or slightly above baseline levels.

Safety

Safe and effective exercise testing for cardiopulmonary disorders requires careful pretest evaluation to identify contraindications to the test procedure (see Box 7.1). A preliminary workup should include a complete history and physical examination by the referring physician or the physician performing the stress test. Preliminary laboratory tests should include a 12-lead ECG, chest x-ray study, baseline pulmonary function studies before and after bronchodilator therapy, and routine laboratory examinations such as complete blood count and serum electrolytes.

The risks and benefits of the entire exercise procedure should be explained to the patient. Appropriate informed consent should be obtained. This includes an explanation of any alternative tests that might be done and what the consequences of not performing the stress test might be. A physician experienced in exercise testing should supervise the test. Tests may be performed by qualified practitioners on patients younger than 40 years with no known risk factors provided a physician is immediately available. Criteria for terminating the exercise evaluation before the specified endpoint or symptom limitation occurs are listed in Box 7.3.

After termination of the exercise evaluation for whatever reason, the patient should be monitored until HR, BP, and ECG return to pretest levels. ECG monitoring should continue for at least 5 minutes (as recommended by the American College of Sports Medicine). Tracings should be made at frequent intervals immediately after exercise.

Personnel conducting exercise tests should be trained in handling cardiovascular emergencies and all aspects of cardiopulmonary resuscitation (e.g., advanced cardiac life support [ACLS]). The laboratory should have available resuscitation equipment, including the following:

1. Standard intravenous (IV) medications (e.g., epinephrine, atropine, lidocaine)
2. Syringes, needles, IV infusion apparatus
3. Portable O_2 and suction equipment
4. Airway equipment, endotracheal tubes, and laryngoscope
5. Direct current (DC) defibrillator and appropriate monitor

All emergency equipment should be checked daily or immediately before any cardiopulmonary exercise evaluation. Equipment such as defibrillators, laryngoscopes, and suction apparatus should be routinely evaluated for proper function according to institutional policies.

VENTILATION DURING EXERCISE

Collection and analysis of expired gas during cardiopulmonary exercise testing provide a noninvasive means of obtaining the following variables:
- Minute ventilation $\left(\dot{V}_E\right)$
- Tidal volume (V_T)
- Frequency of breathing; respiratory rate (f_b)
- Oxygen consumption; oxygen uptake $\left(\dot{V}o_2\right)$
- Carbon dioxide production $\left(\dot{V}co_2\right)$
- Respiratory exchange ratio (RER)
- Ventilatory equivalent for oxygen $\left(\dot{V}_E / \dot{V}o_2\right)$
- Ventilatory equivalent for carbon dioxide $\left(\dot{V}_E / \dot{V}co_2\right)$

Equipment Selection and Calibration

The two common methods of exhaled gas analysis use either a mixing chamber (Fig. 7.7) or computerized breath-by-breath measurements (Fig. 7.8). Pneumotachometers are used in both mixing chamber and breath-by-breath systems and should be calibrated with a known volume (3-L syringe) or flow signal (Criteria for Acceptability 7.2). The flow sensor's accuracy should comply with the

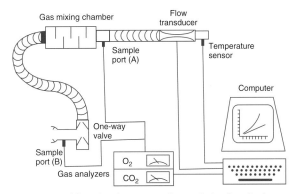

FIG. 7.7 Mixing chamber system for analysis of expired gas. The patient inspires room air through a one-way valve and expires through large-bore tubing into a mixing chamber with a volume of approximately 5 L. Baffles in the chamber cause the gas to be thoroughly mixed so that it is representative of mixed expired gas. A small volume is extracted at *sample port A* and directed to the O_2 and CO_2 analyzers for determination of F_{EO_2} and F_{ECO_2}. Expired gas then passes through a flow-sensing device (pneumotachometer) from which volume can be obtained by integration. The mixing chamber system can be used for exercise protocols and for resting metabolic measurements.

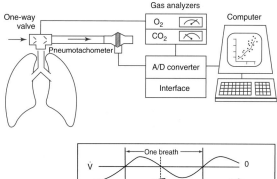

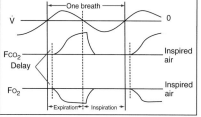

FIG. 7.8 Breath-by-breath system for determination of $\dot{V}_{O_2}$, $\dot{V}_{CO_2}$, and ventilation. The patient inspires and expires through a pneumotachometer or similar flow-sensing device, which may or may not require the use of a unidirectional valve. Gas is continuously sampled at the patient's mouth to determine fractional concentrations of O_2 and CO_2. The flow signal and signals from the gas analyzers are integrated to measure volume, F_{EO_2}, and F_{ECO_2} and to calculate $\dot{V}_E$, $\dot{V}_{O_2}$, $\dot{V}_{CO_2}$, rate, and V_T. Simultaneous recording of flow $\left(\dot{V} \right)$ and fractional concentrations of O_2 and CO_2 are shown *(insert)*. During expiration, F_{CO_2} increases and F_{O_2} decreases. Gas concentrations and flow are out of phase because of the time required to transport gas from the mouthpiece to the analyzers and the response time of the analyzers themselves. Storing appropriate phase-delay corrections (determined during calibration) in the computer can align signals. For exercise tests or metabolic measurements, breath-by-breath data are averaged over a short interval (10–60 seconds) or specific number of breaths.

criteria set by the ATS-ERS for flow-measuring devices (e.g., $\pm 3.0\%$ at three flow rates). Validation of a flow-measuring device can be performed by connecting it in series with a volume-based spirometer of known accuracy. Gas analyzers should also be calibrated and checked before each test procedure. Two-point calibration with gases that approximate the physiologic range to be tested provide the most appropriate means of ensuring accuracy. Three-point calibration is necessary to check the linearity of the analyzers. Table 7.7 lists some recommended gas concentrations for calibration of analyzers to be used for exercise tests.

TABLE 7.7

Recommended Calibration Gases for Exercise Systems

Type of Exercise Test	Suggested Calibration Gases
Maximal or submaximal with subject breathing room air	Reference tank: 20.9% O_2, 0% CO_2, Bal N_2 Cal tank: 12% O_2, 5% CO_2, Bal N_2
Maximal or submaximal with subject breathing supplementary O_2 (may also be used to check linearly)	Reference tank: 20.9% O_2, 0% CO_2, Bal N_2 Cal tank: 12% O_2, 5% CO_2, Bal N_2 O_2 tank: 30% O_2, 0% CO_2, Bal N_2

If a gas collection valve (see Chapter 11) is used in the breathing circuit, it should have a low resistance (1–2 cm H_2O at 100 L/min) and a small dead space. In healthy adults, a valve dead space of 100 mL is acceptable. A valve with reduced dead space (25–50 mL) may be more appropriate for children or for patients who have dead-space–producing disease or small tidal volumes. Some breath-by-breath systems can be programmed to reject small breaths (<100 mL). If this feature is used, the volume of rejected breaths should be matched to valve dead space. Breaths that do not clear valve dead space should be discarded. If valve dead space is too large for the patient, significant rebreathing may occur. In breath-by-breath exercise systems, this may show up as an expired CO_2 level that does not decrease to zero during inspiration. Many modern exercise systems have small flow sensors that do not require a valve system, so dead space and valve resistance become less critical.

If a mixing chamber is used, the patient should be allowed to breathe through the circuit with a nose clip in place long enough to wash out room air with expired gas. The exact washout volume, or time, depends on the volume of the mixing chamber. Breath-by-breath systems (see Fig. 7.8) normally require minimal washout because fractional gas concentrations are sampled directly at the mouthpiece. If supplemental O_2 is breathed, the inspiratory portion of the breathing circuit and the patient's lungs should be in equilibrium before gas sampling starts.

Depending on the protocol and equipment used, gas collection and analysis are performed over a specified interval during each exercise level. For steady-state protocols, gas collection is usually performed after 3 to 6 minutes at a constant workload. For incremental protocols, sampling may be averaged during the last minute of each stage. In breath-by-breath systems, sampling is done continuously with data being displayed for each breath.

Breath-by-breath data may also be averaged over several breaths.

In gas collection or mixing chamber systems, raw data collected include the following:
- Volume expired, in liters
- Temperature of gas at the measuring device (Celsius)
- Time of collection, seconds or minutes
- Respiratory rate during the collection interval
- Fraction of mixed expired O_2 (F_{EO_2})

Fraction of Mixed Expired CO_2 (F_{ECO_2})

In most modern systems, the data are gathered into a computer by means of an analog-to-digital (A/D) converter (see Chapter 11). Computerized data reduction offers the advantage of immediate feedback for all measurements. Automated data collection also offers greater flexibility for using different exercise protocols (see Table 7.2). Breath-by-breath gas analysis requires that signals from the flow sensor be integrated with the gas analyzer signals for F_{EO_2} and F_{ECO_2}. The phase delay between volume and gas concentration signals must be considered (see Fig. 7.8). This is done by measuring phase delay time (for each gas analyzer) during calibration. The phase delay is then stored, and subsequent measurements use this factor to align the volume and gas signals. Sampling flow or sample lines should not be altered after calibration because phase-delay values may change. Water or particulate contamination of the gas analyzer sample line or damage to the sample line can also affect phase delay. Alterations of the phase delay can have a profound effect on the accuracy of the data (up to $\pm 30\%$ error in the calculated $\dot{V}_{O_2}$), especially at higher respiratory rates.

Minute Ventilation

Minute ventilation ($\dot{V}_E$) is the volume of gas expired per minute by the exercising patient, expressed in liters, body temperature, pressure, and saturation (BTPS). For an exercise system in which gas is collected, $\dot{V}_E$ may be calculated as follows:

$$\dot{V}_E = \frac{\text{Volume expired} \times 60}{\text{Collection time(sec)}} \times \text{BTPS factor}$$

Ventilatory Measurements During Exercise

< Box Type E >

1. Were data collected over an interval appropriate to the type of exercise test?
2. Was resting ventilation within normal limits (≈ 5 to $10\,L/min$)? If not, why?
3. Did minute ventilation increase appropriately with workload?
   Was $\dot{V}_E$max less than 70% of MVV or $FEV_1 \times 35$–40? Was the absolute difference greater than 10 to $15\,L/min$? If so, some ventilatory reserve is present. If not, ventilatory limitation to exercise is likely.
   Was breathing kinetics appropriate? Did V_T increase to approximately 50% to 60% of VC? If not, why? Was increased respiratory rate primarily responsible for increased $\dot{V}_E$? If so, suspect a restrictive ventilatory pattern or inappropriate breathing kinetics.
4. Was there flow limitation evidenced by the tidal breathing superimposed on the maximal flow-volume curve? If so, to what extent?
5. Were changes in V_T consistent with an appropriate breathing strategy?
6. What reason did the patient offer for stopping exercise (if applicable)? Was this finding consistent with the pattern of ventilation observed?

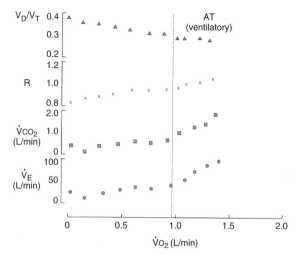

FIG. 7.9 Normal ventilation/gas exchange responses during exercise. Four variables as they might appear in a healthy young adult are plotted against $\dot{V}_{O_2}$. The *dotted vertical line* represents ventilatory/anerobic threshold (AT). $\dot{V}_E$ increases linearly with work rate at low and moderate workloads up to the AT, as does $\dot{V}_{CO_2}$. At higher levels, $\dot{V}_E$ and $\dot{V}_{CO_2}$ increase at a faster rate as HCO_3^- buffers lactic acid and as CO_2 is produced. The ratio of $\dot{V}_{CO_2}$ to $\dot{V}_{O_2}$ (RER) follows a similar pattern as RER approaches and then exceeds 1. V_D/V_T initially decreases rapidly as V_T increases; it then continues to decrease but at a slower rate (see text).

Sample calculations and BTPS factors are on the Evolve website at http://evolve.elsevier.com/Mottram/Ruppel/. Modern breath-by-breath systems measure the volume of each breath and continuously compute the minute ventilation.

Healthy adults at rest breathe 5 to $10\,L/min$. During exercise, this value may increase to more than $200\,L/min$ in trained patients. It commonly exceeds $100\,L/min$ in healthy adults (Figs. 7.9 and 7.10). The increase in ventilation removes CO_2, the primary product of exercising muscles, as workload increases. Ventilation increases linearly with an increasing workload (i.e., $\dot{V}_{O_2}$) at low and moderate levels of exercise. In healthy patients, this increase in ventilation during exercise follows the rise in $\dot{V}_{CO_2}$. Relating the $\dot{V}_E$max to resting ventilatory function provides an index of ventilatory limitations to exercise. MVV (see Chapter 2) can be related to the $\dot{V}_E$ achieved at the highest workload attained ($\dot{V}_E$max). Ventilatory capacity (sometimes called *ventilatory ceiling*) is defined by the measured MVV or the

FEV_1 (forced expiratory volume in 1 second) $\times 35$ (some clinicians prefer $FEV_1 \times 40$). The difference between $\dot{V}_E$max and ventilatory capacity is often called the *ventilatory* (or *breathing*) *reserve* (Fig. 7.11). Ventilatory reserve is calculated as follows:

$$\text{Ventilatory reserve} = \left[1 - \left(\frac{\dot{V}_E\max}{MVV}\right)\right] \times 100$$

where:

$\dot{V}_E$max = ventilation at highest exercise level reached, liters/minute

MVV = maximal voluntary ventilation, liters/minute (measured or estimated)

The ventilatory reserve is usually expressed as a percentage but can also be denoted as the actual difference. In healthy patients, the ventilatory reserve is typically 20% to 40%. In patients with pulmonary disease, the reserve is less than 20%, or the absolute difference between MVV and $\dot{V}_E$max is less than 10 to $15\,L$. The latter relationship is important in individuals with a disease process that affects the ability to

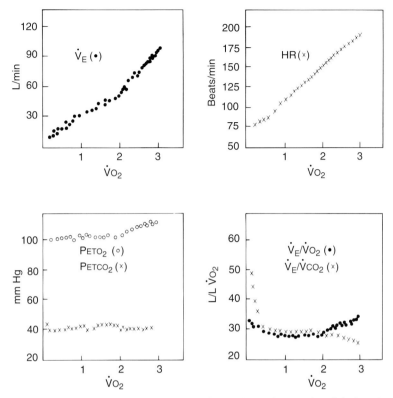

FIG. 7.10 Breath-by-breath exercise data. Four plots of data obtained using a breath-by-breath technique, as in Fig. 7.8. Although data are recorded for each breath, the plots represent 30-second averages. All parameters are plotted against $\dot{V}O_2$ as the measure of work being performed. $\dot{V}_E$ increases linearly up to approximately 2 L/min $\dot{V}O_2$; HR increases linearly throughout the test. $PETO_2$ and $PETCO_2$ (end-tidal partial pressures of O_2 and CO_2, respectively) remain relatively constant up to approximately 2 L/min $\dot{V}O_2$. At this point, end-tidal O_2 begins to increase, and end-tidal CO_2 begins to decrease. A similar pattern is seen on the plot of ventilatory equivalents for oxygen and carbon dioxide ($\dot{V}_E/\dot{V}O_2$ and $\dot{V}_E/\dot{V}CO_2$, respectively). A primary advantage of breath-by-breath analysis is that plots may be viewed in "real time," thus allowing modification of the testing protocol as required. Data in this example indicate the occurrence of ventilatory/anaerobic threshold at approximately 2 L/min of $\dot{V}O_2$.

perform an MVV (i.e., those who have a low or abnormal MVV). In some cases, the abnormally low MVV can yield a $\dot{V}_E$max/MVV ratio in the normal range, but the actual difference is reduced (see Table 7.6). A valid MVV maneuver is essential to compare exercise ventilation with MVV. Patients who have airway obstruction may actually achieve $\dot{V}_E$ during exercise that equals or exceeds their ventilatory capacity. In both scenarios, exercise is limited by their inability to further increase ventilation, and they are therefore identified as being "ventilatory limited."

At high levels of ventilation in healthy patients (> 120 L/min), increases in O_2 uptake gained by increased ventilation serve mainly to supply O_2 to the respiratory muscles. The same phenomenon may occur at much lower levels of ventilation in patients with severe lung disease because of the increased work of breathing. Because of the ventilatory reserve in healthy patients, exercise is seldom limited by ventilation. Maximal exercise is normally limited by the inability to further increase CO or the inability to extract more O_2 at the tissue level in exercising muscles. Some highly trained athletes may achieve ventilatory limitation. Aerobic training can improve cardiovascular function so that ventilation, not CO, limits maximal work.

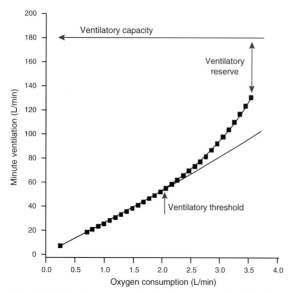

FIG. 7.11 Ventilatory capacity. *Ventilatory capacity* is defined as the measured maximal voluntary ventilation (MVV) or MVV calculated from FEV$_1$ × 35 or 40. The difference between the $\dot{V}_E$max (highest level of ventilation achieved during exercise) and the ventilatory capacity is termed the *ventilatory reserve* or *breathing reserve*.

Tidal Volume and Respiratory Rate

V_T during exercise may be calculated by dividing $\dot{V}_E$ by f_b. Breath-by-breath systems record individual breaths and then report an average V_T over a short interval or after a fixed number of breaths has been analyzed. Observation of the breathing kinetics

or **breathing strategy** of a patient during exercise can be an important adjunct in the interpretation of the exercise results. The normal response to exercise is to increase the V_T at low and moderate workloads. Increased V_T accounts for most of the rise in ventilation at these workloads; only a small amount results from increased f_b. This pattern continues until the V_T approaches approximately 50% to 60% of vital capacity (VC). Further increases in total ventilation are accomplished by increasing f_b. These kinetic changes can be important in a patient complaining of SOB with normal lung function. A high-frequency low–tidal volume breathing strategy will result in an increased V_D/V_T. More important, however, it may be the only physiologic reason for the patient's perceived SOB. Likewise, a patient using a large V_T and low f_b may also complain of SOB without a physiologic abnormality.

In healthy individuals, the increase in V_T is accomplished both by using the inspiratory reserve volume (IRV) and by reducing the end-expiratory lung volume (EELV; Fig. 7.12A). This allows efficient use of the respiratory muscles and chest wall pump. In patients with chronic airflow limitation, the inability to increase ventilation may be related to dynamic compression of the airways and dynamic hyperinflation (i.e., increased lung volume) that can occur during exertion. These patients have large resting lung volumes (hyperinflation). During

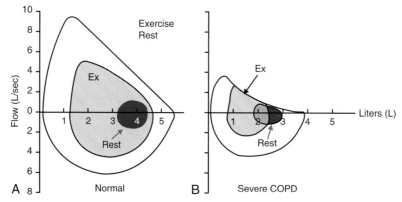

FIG. 7.12 Flow-volume (F-V) loop kinetics. (A) Normal F-V loop kinetics are shown with recruitment of exercise tidal breathing from both the inspiratory reserve volume (IRV) and the expiratory reserve volume (ERV) and not touching the resting maximal F-V curve (MFVC). (B) The breathing kinetics of a patient with severe chronic obstructive pulmonary disease (COPD) are also shown. The patient has to move up in absolute lung volumes to recruit tidal volume. This, along with the fact that they are flow limited throughout much of the tidal breath, increases the work of breathing. Tracking changes in inspiratory capacity (IC) can characterize the degree of exercise-induced hyperinflation.

exercise, EELV tends to increase even more as the patient attempts to optimize expiratory flow to meet ventilatory demand. The dynamic shift in lung volume places the respiratory muscles at an even greater disadvantage. The sensation of dyspnea increases tremendously, and the patient is unable to continue exercise. The consequence for these patients is an increase in the work of breathing from both flow limitation and breathing at higher lung volumes (see Fig. 7.12B). Patients who have airway obstruction may also be able to increase their $\dot{V}_E$ but cannot attain predicted values (see Interpretive Strategies 7.1). If VC is markedly reduced by the obstructive process, there may be little reserve to accommodate an increased V_T. Obstructed patients who have a normal VC but increased resistance to flow may increase their V_T at a low f_b during exercise in an effort to minimize the work of breathing. This pattern continues until the V_T reaches a plateau, as described previously. Then the f_b must be augmented to further increase $\dot{V}_E$. Because of flow limitation, particularly during the expiratory phase, increases in f_b must be accomplished by shortening the inspiratory portion of each breath. Reduction of the inspiratory time in relation to the total breath time (T_I/T_{tot}) requires the inspiratory muscles to generate increasingly greater flows. The increased load placed on the muscles of inspiration typically results in dyspnea.

Unlike the pattern in obstruction, in restrictive disease, V_T may remain relatively fixed. Increases in $\dot{V}_E$ during exercise are accomplished primarily by increasing breathing frequency. It is usually more efficient for patients who have "stiff" lungs to move small tidal volumes at fast rates to increase ventilation. However, these tidal volumes may still comprise a relatively large portion of their VC (60%–70%). F-V loop profiles may be close to normal, whereas the work of distending the lung is increased in restrictive patterns. The mechanism of increasing ventilation primarily by increasing respiratory rate places a load on the respiratory muscles. In combination with hypoxemia, this increased load often results in extreme SOB.

7.2   **How To ...**

Perform a Cardiopulmonary Exercise Test

1. Tasks common to all procedures:
   a. Calibrate and prepare equipment.
   b. Review order.
   c. Introduce yourself and identify patient according to institutional policies.
   d. Describe and demonstrate procedure.
2. Review the patient's medical record to determine absolute or relative contraindications to exercise. Review may include physical limitations that would preclude or affect the testing device selected.
3. Explain to the patient, "You will be asked to rate your perceived exertion throughout the procedure using this chart (review the Ratings of Perceived Exertion [Borg] or modified RPE scale). We will also ask you to rate any chest discomfort (or lightheadedness, chest tightness, etc.) using a 0 to 4 scale, zero being nothing at all and 4 very severe."
4. Communicate, communicate, communicate! Use words of encouragement, such as, "You are doing a great job"; "Everything looks good"; "Your heart rate is 120, and we expect to reach 165"; and "Keep pushing!" Communication will go a long way in making the patient feel safe and thus give you their best effort.
5. Check blood pressure every 1 to 2 minutes. Monitor heart rate (ECG) continuously and perform other adjunct procedures as previously determined (e.g., FV loops, ABGs).
6. Monitor subject for early termination criteria or predetermined endpoints (e.g., maximal or submaximal heart rate or workload).
7. Reduce workload for a cool-down period of 3 to 5 minutes. Postexercise syncope is very common, which can be reduced with a cool-down workload. However, warn the patient in advance that it does happen, and, once again, communicate and monitor closely.
8. Ask the subject the reason he or she stopped (e.g., shortness of breath, leg fatigue, or both), unless terminated by the examiner.
9. Monitor in recovery for 5 to 10 minutes or until ECG variables return close to baseline.
10. Select average data, enter variables such as ABGs and BPs, and process the report. Note comments related to test quality.

Flow-Volume Loop Analysis

Another method of determining the degree of ventilatory limitation is by monitoring F-V loop dynamics during exercise. Exercise tidal-volume loops may be plotted against the resting maximal F-V loop. This technique quantifies the amount of time the patient spends on the maximal flow-volume envelope and allows the clinician to identify the percent of flow limitation (Fig. 7.13). This method may better define the increased work of breathing in individuals who do not reach a classic definition of ventilatory limitation but have a substantial component of flow limitation during exercise. Monitoring the tidal F-V loop during exercise can also show dynamic changes in the flow pattern. These changes can alert the clinician to intrathoracic, extrathoracic, or fixed-airway abnormalities that are demonstrated during exercise

only. This technique may also be useful in monitoring breathing kinetics during exercise. As discussed previously, the normal method of increasing tidal volume during exercise is to use both inspiratory and expiratory reserve volumes. Patients with obstructive lung disease have to "move up" in their lung volumes (see Fig. 7.12) to recruit tidal volume. In some cases, individuals with normal lung function can use an inappropriate breathing strategy by moving up in their lung volumes to recruit tidal volume without evidence of flow limitation. Using these inappropriate breathing strategies may cause a concomitant sensation of dyspnea. Some patients may breathe at low lung volumes, which approach residual volume. Breathing at these low lung volumes can cause flow limitation resulting from the position of tidal breathing along the absolute lung volume scale. This breathing strategy can elicit

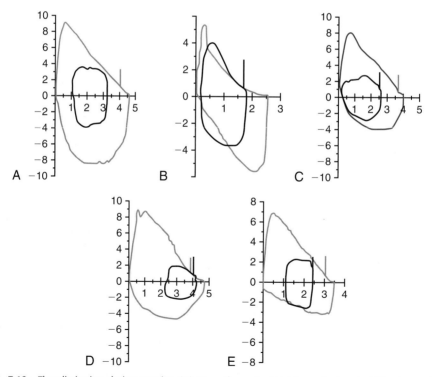

FIG. 7.13   Flow limitation during exercise. (A) Normal exercise tidal loop displayed within the maximal flow-volume (F-V) loop. (B) Flow limitation with tidal loop shifting toward total lung capacity (TLC). (C) Inappropriate breathing strategy with upward shift without flow limitation. (D) Inappropriate breathing strategy with shift toward residual volume (RV; reduced end-expiratory lung volume [EELV]). (E) Reduced inspiratory flows consistent with variable extrathoracic obstruction (e.g., vocal cord dysfunction [VCD]) in both maximal flow-volume and tidal-volume loops.

wheezing and SOB that can mimic asthma and has been coined a type of "pseudo-asthma." This phenomenon is often seen in morbidly obese subjects secondary to the weight on their thoracic cage that facilitates a reduction in their functional residual capacity (FRC).

OXYGEN CONSUMPTION, CARBON DIOXIDE PRODUCTION, AND RESPIRATORY EXCHANGE RATIO DURING EXERCISE

Oxygen Consumption

Oxygen consumption $(\dot{V}_{O_2})$ is the volume of O_2 taken up by the exercising (or resting) patient in liters or milliliters/minute, STPD. Oxygen consumption is also commonly reported in milliliters/kilogram (mL/kg) of body weight. $\dot{V}_{O_2}$ is the product of ventilation minute and the rate of extraction from the gas breathed (i.e., the difference between the F_{IO_2} and the F_{EO_2}; see the following paragraph). Healthy patients at rest have a $\dot{V}_{O_2}$ of approximately 0.25 L/min (STPD) or approximately 3.5 mL O_2/min/kg (1 MET). During exercise, $\dot{V}_{O_2}$ may increase to over 5.0 L/min (STPD) in trained patients. $\dot{V}_{O_2}$ is the best single measure of external work being performed. Exercise limitation caused by ventilatory, gas exchange, or cardiovascular abnormalities may be quantified by relating exercise variables to $\dot{V}_{O_2}$. Figs. 7.5 and 7.9 provide examples of ventilatory and cardiovascular variables related to $\dot{V}_{O_2}$ in healthy patients. The causes of work limitation may be defined by comparing these patterns in the exercising patient. Exercise limitation may be a result of pulmonary disease, cardiovascular disease, muscular abnormalities, deconditioning, poor effort, or a combination of these factors.

To calculate $\dot{V}_{O_2}$ and $\dot{V}_{CO_2}$, the fractional concentrations of O_2 and CO_2 in expired gas must be analyzed (Criteria for Acceptability 7.3). Exhaled gas is sampled from a mixing chamber (see Fig. 7.7) or a breath-by-breath system (see Fig. 7.8). In systems that accumulate gas (e.g., mixing chamber), a pump is used to draw the sample through the O_2 and CO_2 analyzers. Water vapor is removed from the mixed expired sample by passing the gas through a drying tube (usually containing calcium chloride). In

breath-by-breath systems, fractional gas concentrations are sampled at the mouth using rapid gas analyzers. Most systems use sample tubing permeable to water vapor so that the effects of humidity can be accommodated (see Chapter 11). Gas concentration signals from the analyzers are integrated with the expiratory flow signal to measure the volumes of O_2 and CO_2 exchanged for each breath (see Fig. 7.8).

$\dot{V}_{O_2}$ is calculated from an accumulated gas volume using the following equation:

$$\dot{V}_{O_2} = \left(\left[\frac{1 - FEO_2 - FECO_2}{1 - FIO_2} \times FIO_2 \right] - FEO_2 \right) \times \dot{V}_E \, (\text{STPD})$$

where:

FEO_2 = fraction of O_2 in the expired sample
$FECO_2$ = fraction of CO_2 in the expired sample
FIO_2 = fraction of O_2 in inspired gas (room air = 0.2093)

The term

$$\left(\frac{1 - FEO_2 - FECO_2}{1 - FIO_2} \right)$$

CRITERIA FOR ACCEPTABILITY 7.3

Oxygen Consumption and Carbon Dioxide Uptake per Minute

1. There should be documentation of appropriate gas analyzer calibrations; two-point calibration recommended for room air exercise, three-point for exercise with supplemental oxygen.
2. Phase delay calibration (breath-by-breath systems) should be documented within manufacturer's specifications.
3. Volume transducer should be calibrated before testing.
4. Breathing valve (if used) should have appropriate resistance and dead space volume for patient tested.
5. There should be evidence of appropriate washout of collection device or mixing chamber (if used).
6. RER at rest should be within the physiologic range of 0.70 to 1.10; RER values greater than 1.0 may be present because of hyperventilation. $\dot{V}_{O_2}$ and $\dot{V}_{CO_2}$ should be within normal limits with the patient at rest; each should increase with increasing workloads.

is a factor to correct for the small differences between inspired and expired volumes when only expired volumes are measured. Ventilation is corrected to STPD as follows:

$$\dot{V}_E(STPD) = \dot{V}_E(BTPS) \times \left(\frac{P_B - 47}{760}\right) \times 0.881$$

O_2 consumption at the highest level of work attainable by normal patients is termed the $\dot{V}o_2max$. $\dot{V}o_2$ max is characterized by a plateau of the oxygen uptake despite increasing external workloads. $\dot{V}o_2$ max is useful for comparing exercise capacity among patients. $\dot{V}o_2$ max may also be used to compare a patient with his or her age-related predicted value of $\dot{V}o_2$ max. Equations for deriving predicted $\dot{V}o_2$ max are included on the Evolve website at http://evolve.elsevier.com/Mottram/Ruppel/.

One measure of impairment is the percentage of expected $\dot{V}o_2$ max attained by the exercising patient. Height, sex, age, and fitness level all affect the "normal" maximal oxygen consumption. Because of these factors, most reference equations show a large variability ($\pm 20\%$). Patients who have a 20% to 40% reduction in their $\dot{V}o_2$ max have mild to moderate impairment. Those who have $\dot{V}o_2$ max values less than 50% of their predicted values have severe exercise impairment. Some studies have attempted to estimate $\dot{V}o_2$ based on the height and weight of the patient and the speed and slope of a treadmill. O_2 consumption estimated from treadmill walking is sufficiently variable, so its use is limited. Power output from a calibrated cycle ergometer may be used to estimate $\dot{V}o_2$ more accurately than from treadmill exercise. Workload estimated from cycle ergometry is not influenced by weight or stride. Actual $\dot{V}o_2$ may differ significantly from the estimated value even with an ergometer. Cycle ergometry usually produces slightly lower maximal $\dot{V}o_2$ values than treadmill walking in healthy patients (see the Exercise Protocols section).

Carbon Dioxide Production

Carbon dioxide production ($\dot{V}co_2$) is a direct reflection of metabolism. It is expressed in liters or milliliters per minute, STPD. $\dot{V}co_2$ may be calculated using the following equation:

$$\dot{V}_Eco_2 = (FECO_2 - 0.0003) \times \dot{V}_E(STPD)$$

where:

$FECO_2$ = fraction of CO_2 in expired gas
0.0003 = fraction of CO_2 in room air (may vary)
$\dot{V}_E(STPD)$ = calculated as in the equation for $\dot{V}o_2$

Pulmonary ventilation, consisting of alveolar ventilation ($\dot{V}_A$) and dead-space ventilation ($\dot{V}_D$), may be related in terms of the $\dot{V}co_2$. The fraction of alveolar carbon dioxide (F_ACO_2) is directly proportional to $\dot{V}co_2$ and inversely proportional to $\dot{V}_A$. The concentration of CO_2 in the lung is determined by CO_2 production and the rate of removal from the lung by ventilation. This relationship may be expressed as follows:

$$F_Aco_2 = \frac{\dot{V}co_2}{\dot{V}_A}$$

$\dot{V}co_2$ in a healthy patient at rest is approximately 0.20 L/min (STPD). It may increase to more than 5 L/min (STPD) during maximal exercise in trained individuals. The adequacy of $\dot{V}_A$ in response to the increase in $\dot{V}co_2$ is indicated by how well $Paco_2$ is maintained near normal levels. Alveolar ventilation keeps $Paco_2$ in equilibrium with alveolar gas at low and moderate workloads. At high workloads, $\dot{V}_A$ increases dramatically to reduce $Paco_2$ when buffering of lactic acid takes place. At maximal workloads, even high levels of ventilation cannot keep pace with CO_2 produced metabolically and from lactate buffering. As a result, acidosis develops.

Respiratory Exchange Ratio

The RER is defined as the ratio of $\dot{V}co_2$ to $\dot{V}o_2$ at the mouth. RER is calculated by dividing $\dot{V}co_2$ by $\dot{V}o_2$; it is expressed as a fraction. In some circumstances, RER at rest is assumed to be equal to 0.8. For exercise evaluation or metabolic studies, however, the actual value is calculated. RER normally varies between 0.70 and 1.00 in resting patients, depending on the nutritional substrate being metabolized (see Chapter 10). RER reflects the respiratory quotient (RQ) at the cellular level only when the patient is in a true steady state. RER may differ significantly from RQ, depending on the patient's ventilation.

RER typically increases from a resting level of between 0.75 and 0.85 as work increases. When anaerobic metabolism (see next paragraph) begins to produce CO_2 from the buffering of lactate, $\dot{V}_{CO_2}$ approaches $\dot{V}_{O_2}$. As exercise continues, $\dot{V}_{CO_2}$ exceeds $\dot{V}_{O_2}$ and the RER becomes greater than 1. RER is commonly elevated at rest because many patients hyperventilate during exhaled gas analysis before exercise begins (see Criteria for Acceptability 7.3). In steady-state exercise tests (i.e., 4–6 minutes at a constant workload), RER may equal RQ, and it then reflects the ratio of $\dot{V}_{CO_2}/\dot{V}_{O_2}$ at the cellular level. Under steady-state conditions, $\dot{V}_{CO_2}$ reflects the CO_2 produced metabolically at the cellular level.

PF TIP 7.4

The RER is a good indicator of maximal effort during a cardiopulmonary exercise test. Patients who exert maximal effort are usually able to exceed their **anaerobic threshold (AT)**. During exercise, the RER increases; at the highest workloads, it exceeds 1.00. An RER value greater than 1.15 is usually consistent with a maximal effort. Patients with pulmonary disease are often limited by ventilation and may not reach an RER greater than 1.

Anaerobic or Ventilatory Threshold

Measurement of and the analysis of exhaled gases during exercise allow a noninvasive estimate of the AT. This threshold is also termed the **ventilatory threshold** when it is denoted by a change in ventilation and CO_2 production. The AT occurs when the energy demands of the exercising muscles exceed the body's ability to produce energy by aerobic metabolism. The workload at which AT occurs is considered an index of fitness in healthy patients. The AT is also used to assess cardiac performance in patients with heart disease.

Historically, anaerobic metabolism was detected by noting an increase in the blood lactate level of an exercising patient. Analysis of $\dot{V}_E$ and $\dot{V}_{CO_2}$ in relation to workload ($\dot{V}_{O_2}$) can be used to detect the onset of anaerobic metabolism without drawing blood. This threshold is commonly referred to as the *ventilatory threshold*.

At low and moderate workloads, $\dot{V}_E$ increases linearly with increases in $\dot{V}_{CO_2}$. When the body's energy demands exceed the capacity of aerobic pathways, further increases in energy are produced anaerobically. The primary product of anaerobic metabolism is lactate. The increased **lactic acid** (from lactate) is buffered by HCO_3^-, resulting in an increase in CO_2 in the blood. $\dot{V}_{CO_2}$ measured from exhaled gas increases because CO_2 is being produced by both the exercising muscles and the buffering of lactate. To maintain the pH near normal, $\dot{V}_E$ increases to match the increased $\dot{V}_{CO_2}$. This pattern of increasing ventilation and CO_2 production can be detected when these parameters are plotted against $\dot{V}_{O_2}$ (see Fig. 7.9). Determination of the ventilatory-anaerobic threshold may be accomplished by visual inspection of an appropriate plot. Statistical analysis can also be used to determine the inflection point as displayed by the graph in Fig. 7.14. Several different algorithms may be used to identify the AT. One of the most common techniques uses regression analysis to determine the "breakpoint" at which $\dot{V}_{O_2}$ and $\dot{V}_{CO_2}$ change abruptly (**V-slope method**).

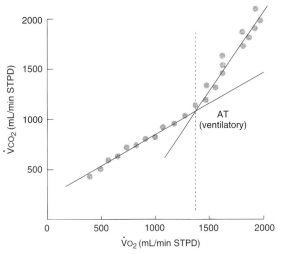

FIG. 7.14 V-slope determination of ventilatory/anaerobic threshold (AT). By plotting $\dot{V}_{CO_2}$ against $\dot{V}_{O_2}$, an inflection point can typically be identified, indicating an abrupt increase in CO_2 production. A more precise method fits two regression lines to the data gathered. One line is a best-fit line through the low- and moderate-workload portion of the data; the second is fit through the high-workload points. These lines are recalculated repeatedly until the best statistical "fit" is obtained. The point at which the two lines intersect represents the onset of lactate production (anaerobic threshold).

Noninvasive AT determination may be useful in assessing cardiovascular or pulmonary diseases (Interpretive Strategies 7.3). In healthy patients, AT occurs at 60% to 70% of the $\dot{V}_{O_2}$ max. Patients who have cardiac disease often reach their AT at a lower workload ($\dot{V}_{O_2}$). Early onset of anaerobic metabolism occurs when the demands of exercising muscles exceed the capacity of the heart to supply O_2. Occurrence of the anaerobic threshold at less than 40% of the $\dot{V}_{O_2}$ max is considered abnormally low. Patients who have a ventilatory limitation to exercise (i.e., pulmonary disease) may be unable to exercise at a high enough workload to reach their anaerobic threshold. In these patients, O_2 delivery is limited by the lungs rather than by CO or extraction by the exercising muscle.

Aerobic training improves cardiac performance, specifically the SV. Training allows more O_2 to be delivered to the tissues and increased utilization at the cellular level (e.g., more mitochondria), resulting in a delay in the AT until higher workloads are reached. Measurement of the AT is often used to select a training level (e.g., exercise prescription). Maximum training effects seem to occur when the patient exercises at a workload slightly below the AT. In sedentary patients, deconditioning may occur. Deconditioning is characterized by reduced SV and poor O_2 extraction by the muscles from a lack of use. Deconditioning may be present when the AT occurs at a lower-than-expected workload and there is no evidence of cardiovascular disease.

The AT may also be determined by inspecting graphs of the ventilatory equivalents for O_2 and CO_2 (see the next section) plotted against workload ($\dot{V}_{O_2}$). When $\dot{V}_E/\dot{V}_{CO_2}$ increases without an increase in $\dot{V}_E/\dot{V}_{CO_2}$, the AT has been reached. A similar pattern can be seen when the end-tidal O_2 and CO_2 gas tensions are plotted (see Fig. 7.10). Sample calculations of $\dot{V}_E, \dot{V}_{O_2}, \dot{V}_{CO_2}$, and RER, as used with one of the gas collection methods, are included on the Evolve website at http://evolve.elsevier.com/Mottram/Ruppel/.

Ventilatory Equivalent for Oxygen

Minute ventilation during exercise may be related to the work being performed (expressed as $\dot{V}_{O_2}$). This ratio is termed the **ventilatory equivalent for oxygen** or $\dot{V}_E / \dot{V}_{O_2}$. It is calculated by dividing $\dot{V}_E$ (BTPS) by $\dot{V}_{O_2}$ (STPD) and expressing the ratio in liters of ventilation/liters of O_2 consumed per minute. The $\dot{V}_E/\dot{V}_{O_2}$ is a measure of the efficiency of the ventilatory pump at various workloads.

During resting data collection in healthy patients, the ratio is in the range of 30 to 40 L depending on the degree of ventilation, including anticipatory hyperventilation. As the patient begins to exercise, this ratio decreases to about 25 ± 4 (Fig. 7.15). This initial kinetic change is assumed to be related to an improvement in $\dot{V}/\dot{Q}$ matching with increased CO during exercise. At low and moderate workloads, ventilation increases linearly with increasing $\dot{V}_{O_2}$ and $\dot{V}_{CO_2}$. The absolute level of ventilation depends on the response to CO_2, the adequacy of $\dot{V}_A$, and the V_D/V_T ratio. At workloads above 60% to 75% of the $\dot{V}_{O_2}$ max, $\dot{V}_E$ is more closely related to $\dot{V}_{CO_2}$. As ventilation increases to match the $\dot{V}_{CO_2}$ above the AT, the ventilatory equivalent for O_2 also increases.

INTERPRETIVE STRATEGIES 7.3

Oxygen Consumption and Carbon Dioxide Uptake per Minute

1. Were the data obtained acceptably? Were all calibrations appropriate? Gas analyzers? Volume transducer? Phase delay?
2. Were appropriate reference values selected? Age? Sex? Height? Weight?
   Was $\dot{V}_{O_2}$ max (mL/kg) achieved? If so, there is no aerobic impairment.
   Was $\dot{V}_{O_2}$ max (mL/kg) less than 80% of predicted? If so, some aerobic impairment is present. Was $\dot{V}_{O_2}$ max (mL/kg) less than 60% of predicted? If so, there is moderate to severe exercise limitation.
   Was ventilatory AT reached? If so, at what % $\dot{V}_{O_2}$ max? If less than 50% to 60%, early onset of anaerobic metabolism is likely. Consider clinical correlation.
   What factors contributed to the reduced $\dot{V}_{O_2}$ max? Cardiac (arrhythmias, ischemic changes)? Vascular (BP response)? Pulmonary (ventilation, hypoxemia, V_D/V_T)? Other (poor effort, deconditioning, pain, orthopedic problems)?
3. What reason did the patient cite for stopping exercise (incremental tests)? Is it consistent with physiologic patterns observed?

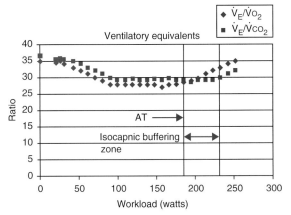

FIG. 7.15 Determination of ventilatory/anaerobic threshold (AT) using ventilatory equivalents data. The *ventilatory threshold* is defined as the point where the $\dot{V}_E/\dot{V}o_2$ begins to increase while the $\dot{V}_E/\dot{V}co_2$ remains constant or begins to decrease. The period from the onset of AT until $\dot{V}_E/\dot{V}co_2$ increases is the isocapnic buffering zone. Minute ventilation is appropriate for $\dot{V}co_2$, which now exceeds $\dot{V}o_2$ because of acid buffering created by anaerobic metabolism ($H^+ + HCO_3^- \leftrightarrow H_2CO_3^- \leftrightarrow H_2O + CO_2$).

Ventilation helps determine how much O_2 can be transported per minute. Therefore it is often useful to evaluate the level of total ventilation required for a particular workload to assess the role of the lungs in exercise limitations. In some pulmonary disease patterns, the $\dot{V}_E/\dot{V}o_2$ may be close to normal at rest but increases with exercise out of proportion to increases in either $\dot{V}o_2$ or $\dot{V}co_2$. This usually occurs in individuals who have abnormalities that worsen as CO increases during exercise. Some patients who have pulmonary disease may have an elevated $\dot{V}_E/\dot{V}o_2$ at rest (i.e., $> 40\,L\ \dot{V}o_2$) that decreases during exercise but does not return to the normal range. Many patients hyperventilate during the resting phase at the beginning of an exercise evaluation. The result is an increased $\dot{V}_E/\dot{V}o_2$ that usually returns to the normal range during exercise. This pretest hyperventilation is usually denoted by an RER of greater than 1 that returns to a normal level when the patient begins to exercise.

Ventilatory Equivalent for Carbon Dioxide

The **ventilatory equivalent for CO_2 ($\dot{V}_E / \dot{V}co_2$)** is calculated in a manner similar to that used for the $\dot{V}_E/\dot{V}o_2$. Minute ventilation (BTPS) is divided by

CO_2 production (STPD). The $\dot{V}_E/\dot{V}co_2$ mimics the initial $\dot{V}_E/\dot{V}o_2$ kinetic change, decreasing to a normal range of 25 to 35 $L\ \dot{V}co_2$. $\dot{V}_E$ tends to match $\dot{V}co_2$ from low up to high workloads. Thus the $\dot{V}_E/\dot{V}co_2$ remains constant in healthy patients until the highest workloads are reached. The $\dot{V}_E/\dot{V}co_2$ may be useful for estimating the maximum tolerable workload in patients who have moderate or severe ventilatory limitations. The ventilatory equivalents for O_2 and CO_2, measured with a breath-by-breath technique, may be useful in identifying the onset of the AT. Anaerobic metabolism is usually accompanied by a steady increase in the $\dot{V}_E/\dot{V}o_2$ while the $\dot{V}_E/\dot{V}co_2$ remains constant or decreases slightly. The period in which $\dot{V}_E/\dot{V}o_2$ is increasing yet $\dot{V}_E/\dot{V}co_2$ is constant is called the *isocapnic buffering zone* (see Fig. 7.15). This zone indicates the onset of metabolic acidosis where $\dot{V}_E$ is no longer proportional to $\dot{V}o_2$ but is appropriate for $\dot{V}co_2$. The occurrence of this pattern coincides with the buffering of the lactate (AT). Eventually, the buffering system cannot keep pace with the metabolic acidemia, and the $\dot{V}_E/\dot{V}co_2$ increases as attempts to maintain pH. This same pattern may also be seen on a breath-by-breath display of P_{ETO_2} and P_{ETCO_2} (see Fig. 7.10). A markedly elevated $\dot{V}_E/\dot{V}co_2$ (> 50) may also be observed in pulmonary hypertensive disease.

Oxygen Pulse

The efficiency of the circulatory pump may be related to the workload (i.e., $\dot{V}o_2$) during exercise by the O_2 pulse. **O_2 pulse** is defined as the volume of O_2 consumed per heartbeat and is derived from the Fick equation:

$$\text{Cardiac output} = \frac{\dot{V}o_2}{C_aO_2 - C_{\bar{v}}O_2}$$

$$HR \times SV = \frac{\dot{V}o_2}{C_aO_2 - C_{\bar{v}}O_2}$$

$$\frac{\dot{V}o_2}{HR}(O_2\ \text{pulse}) = SV \times (C_aO_2 - C_{\bar{v}}O_2)$$

O_2 pulse is sometimes called the "poor man's" estimate of SV because of the relatively "consistent" change in the $CaO_2 - C\bar{v}o_2$ difference with exercise. The ratio is expressed as milliliters of O_2 per heartbeat. In healthy patients, O_2 pulse varies between

2.5 and 4.0 mL O_2/beats at rest. It increases to 10 to 15 mL O_2/beats during strenuous exercise.

In patients with cardiac disease, the O_2 pulse may be normal or even low at rest but does not increase to expected levels during exercise. This pattern is consistent with an inappropriately high HR for a particular level of work. CO normally increases linearly with increasing exercise (see Fig. 7.5). A low O_2 pulse is consistent with an inability to increase the SV because of the relationship noted in the preceding paragraphs. O_2 pulse may even decrease in patients with poor left ventricular function. The pattern of low O_2 pulse with increasing work rate may be seen in patients with coronary artery disease or valvular insufficiency, but it is most pronounced in cardiomyopathy. Tachycardia or tachyarrhythmias tend to lower the O_2 pulse because of the abnormally elevated HR. Conversely, beta-blocking agents, which tend to reduce HR, may elevate the O_2 pulse.

O_2 pulse is often used as an index of fitness. At similar power outputs, a fit patient will have a higher O_2 pulse than one who is deconditioned. Fitness is generally accompanied by a lower HR, both at rest and at maximal workloads. Lower HR occurs because conditioning exercises (e.g., aerobic training) tend to increase SV. As a result, the heart beats less frequently but produces the same CO. Trained patients can thus achieve higher work rates before reaching their limiting cardiac frequency (i.e., attain a higher O_2 pulse).

EXERCISE BLOOD GASES

Arterial Catheterization

Although invasive, blood gas sampling during exercise testing is often indicated in patients with primary pulmonary disorders. An indwelling arterial catheter permits the analysis of blood gas tensions (PaO_2, $PaCO_2$), arterial saturation (SaO_2), O_2 content (CaO_2), pH, and lactate levels at various workloads. Box 7.4 lists some of the indications for arterial catheterization for exercise testing.

Arterial catheterization, at either the radial or the brachial site, has been demonstrated to be relatively safe. The modified Allen's test is performed to ascer-

> **BOX 7.4   INDICATIONS FOR ARTERIAL CATHETERIZATION WITH EXERCISE TESTING**
>
> - Moderate or severe pulmonary disease
> - Clinical suspicion of a gas exchange abnormality
> - Low diffusion capacity for carbon monoxide (<50% predicted)
> - Low or borderline PaO_2 at rest (55–60 mm Hg)
> - Multiple blood specimens required (blood gases, lactate)

tain adequate collateral circulation (see Chapter 6). The site is cleaned with a skin preparation antiseptic, typically applied with a sterile applicator. Local anesthetic (1%–2% lidocaine [Xylocaine]) is injected subcutaneously. An appropriately sized catheter is inserted percutaneously. The catheter needs to be secured to prevent being dislodged during the exercise study. The catheter is then connected to a high-pressure flush system to maintain patency. Care must be taken when drawing blood samples from the catheter not to contaminate the specimen with flush solution (Criteria for Acceptability 7.4). If flush solution mixes with the specimen, dilution occurs and can affect pH, PCO_2, PO_2, and hemoglobin (Hb) values.

The catheter may also be connected to a suitable pressure transducer (see Fig. 7.6) for continuous monitoring of systemic BP. The BP transducer should be balanced ("zeroed") at the level of the left ventricle during exercise. See Chapter 6 for precautions concerning the insertion of arterial catheters.

Arterial Puncture

An alternate technique is to obtain a specimen by a simple arterial puncture at peak exercise. Use of a cycle ergometer for testing allows better stabilization of the radial or brachial artery sites. The site should be identified and the modified Allen's test performed before beginning exercise. The sample should be obtained within 15 seconds of peak exercise. Blood gas tensions, particularly PaO_2, may change rapidly as blood recirculates. A serious disadvantage of the single puncture is that if the specimen cannot be obtained within 15 seconds, the procedure must be repeated. If any of the conditions listed in Box 7.4 are present, arterial catheterization should be considered.

CRITERIA FOR ACCEPTABILITY 7.4

Exercise Blood Gases

1. Blood gases should be drawn from either a radial or a brachial catheter. Care should be taken that specimens are not contaminated with flush solution.
2. Exercise blood gas specimens should be handled like any other sample for blood gas analysis, according to the Clinical and Laboratory Standards Institute (CLSI) publication C46-A2, *Blood Gas and pH Analysis and Related Measurements*.
3. Specimens from multiple exercise levels should be labeled to indicate the exercise workload and related conditions.
4. Blood obtained by a single arterial puncture at peak exercise should be obtained within 30 seconds of the observed maximal workload.
5. If pulse oximetry is used to evaluate exercise desaturation, it should be validated by correlation with co-oximetry, preferably at rest and peak exercise.

If pulse oximetry is used to titrate supplemental O_2 administration and Spo_2 does not increase, an arterial blood specimen may be required.

Pulse Oximetry

Oxygen saturation during exercise may be monitored with a pulse oximeter (Spo_2) using the ear, finger, or forehead sites (see Chapter 11). Wherever the pulse oximeter is attached, the probe should be adequately secured. Motion artifact is a common problem, particularly with treadmill exercise.

An advantage of pulse oximetry is that it provides continuous measurements of saturation, compared with discrete measurements of arterial sampling. Continuous measurements can be helpful in evaluating patients who have pulmonary disease. These patients often display rapid changes in Pao_2 and Sao_2 during exercise. A decrease of 4% to 5% in Sao_2 is indicative of exercise desaturation even if some other factor (e.g., ventilation, arrhythmia) limits exercise.

Pulse oximetry may overestimate the true saturation if a significant concentration of carboxyhemoglobin (COHb) is present (see Criteria for Acceptability 7.4). A low total Hb level (i.e., anemia) sometimes contributes to exercise limitation. This condition may not be detected by pulse oximetry alone. Inadequate perfusion at the site of the probe (e.g., ear or finger) may also cause erroneous readings (false positive) during exercise testing. Motion artifact, light scattering within the tissue at the probe site, and dark skin pigmentation may all cause discrepancies between Spo_2 and actual Sao_2 (see Chapter 6). A single arterial sample, preferably at peak exercise, may be used to correlate the Spo_2 reading with true saturation if the specimen is analyzed with a multiwavelength blood oximeter (see Chapter 11). If adequate correlation between Sao_2 and Spo_2 during exercise is established, further blood sampling may be unnecessary.

Arterial Oxygen Tension During Exercise

In healthy patients, Pao_2 remains relatively constant even at high workloads (Interpretive Strategies 7.4). Alveolar Po_2 increases at maximal exercise from the increased ventilation accompanying the increase in $\dot{V}co_2$. The alveolar-arterial (A-a) gradient (normally approximately 10 mm Hg) widens as a result of the increase in alveolar oxygen tension. The A-a gradient also increases somewhat because of a lower mixed venous O_2 content during exercise. The A-a gradient may increase to 20 to 30 mm Hg in healthy patients during heavy exercise because of these mechanisms.

PF TIP 7.5

The V_D/V_T ratio is often measured during cardiopulmonary exercise testing. This ratio is usually about 0.3 at rest and should decrease with exercise in healthy subjects. V_D/V_T can be estimated noninvasively with a breath-by-breath metabolic measurement system. These systems use the end-tidal Pco_2 ($Petco_2$) along with the mixed expired CO_2 to calculate the ratio. In patients with pulmonary disease, $Petco_2$ may not accurately reflect the arterial Pco_2 ($Paco_2$). For such patients, arterial blood gases drawn during exercise may be required to accurately assess the V_D/V_T ratio.

A decrease in Pao_2 with increasing exercise can result from increased right-to-left shunting. Similarly, inequality of $\dot{V}_A$ in relation to pulmonary capillary perfusion may result in a reduced Pa_{O_2}. Diffusion limitation at the alveolocapillary interface can also affect Pa_{O_2}. Because exercise reduces the mixed venous oxygen tension ($P\bar{v}_{O_2}$), a shunt or ventilation/perfusion inequality may result in a decrease in the Pa_{O_2} or widening of the A-a gradient. This change in Pa_{O_2} may occur without an absolute change in the magnitude of the shunt. Mixed venous blood with a lowered O_2 content (from extraction by the exercising muscles) passes through abnormal lung units and then mixes with normally arterialized blood.

INTERPRETIVE STRATEGIES 7.4

Exercise Blood Gases

1. Were blood gas samples obtained acceptably? Was there dilution or contamination with flush solution or air?
2. Were blood gas samples obtained at each exercise level or just at peak exercise? If drawn by arterial puncture at peak exercise only, were they obtained within 15 seconds?
3. Did Pa_{O_2} decrease with increasing workloads? Did the A-a gradient increase to greater than 30 mm Hg? If so, exercise desaturation is likely.
4. Did Pa_{O_2} decrease to less than 55 mm Hg or Sa_{O_2} decrease to less than 85%? If so, supplemental O_2 is indicated. Retesting on O_2 may be indicated.
5. Did Pa_{CO_2} remain constant or decrease slightly with increasing workloads? If not, respiratory acidosis may be contributing to work limitation.
6. Did pH decrease to the range of 7.20 to 7.35 (or lower) at the highest workload? If so, metabolic acidosis is present; the patient made a good effort. If not, did ventilation limit work below the anaerobic threshold?
7. Was V_D/V_T normal at rest? Did it decrease with increasing workloads? If not, suspect pulmonary hypertension, pulmonary vascular disease, or inappropriate breathing strategy.
8. Are blood gas test results consistent with observed changes in ventilatory and cardiovascular variables during exercise?

In some patients who have decreased Pa_{O_2} and increased $P(A\text{-}a)_{O_2}$ at rest, oxygenation may improve with exercise. Increased CO or redistribution of ventilation during exercise may actually cause an increase in Pa_{O_2}. Some improvement of Pa_{O_2} may

occur as a result of an increased Pa_{O_2} caused by a reduction of Pa_{CO_2} at moderate to high work rates. Improved $\dot{V}/\dot{Q}$ relationships resulting directly from the changes in ventilation or CO may also improve Pa_{O_2}. Because Pa_{O_2} may either increase or decrease during exercise, measuring Pa_{O_2} during exercise may be particularly valuable in patients with pulmonary disorders.

When Pa_{O_2} decreases to less than 55 mm Hg or Sa_{O_2} decreases to less than 85%, the exercise evaluation should be terminated. Patients with hypoxemia at rest or who desaturate at low work rates should be tested with supplemental O_2 (e.g., a nasal cannula) to determine an appropriate exercise **O_2 prescription**. Different flows of supplemental O_2 may be required at rest and for various levels of exertion. The correlation of Pa_{O_2} while breathing supplemental O_2 at different exercise workloads allows precise titration of therapy to the patient's needs. Measurement of $\dot{V}_{O_2}$ while the patient breathes supplemental O_2 presents special problems. A closed system in which the patient breathes from a reservoir containing blended gas, typically F_{IO_2} 0.30, is usually required.

Reported in some elite athletes at high levels of work (e.g., 400–500 watts or 9 mph/18% grade) is a widening of the A-a gradient with $Pa\dot{v}_{O_2}$ values falling into the range of 50 to 60 mm Hg. This phenomenon is thought to be related to the time constants of blood in the lung with very high CO and high oxygen extraction at the cellular level.

Arterial Carbon Dioxide Tension During Exercise

In healthy patients, Pa_{CO_2} remains relatively constant at low and moderate work rates (see Interpretive Strategies 7.4). $\dot{V}_A$ increases to match the increase in $\dot{V}_{CO_2}$. End-tidal CO_2 increases at submaximal workloads, indicating that less ventilation is "wasted" (V_D/V_T decreases). At workloads in excess of 50% to 60% of the $\dot{V}_{O_2}$ max, metabolic acidosis from anaerobic metabolism stimulates an increase in $\dot{V}_E$. This occurs in response to the augmented $\dot{V}_{CO_2}$ from the buffering of lactic acid, as noted previously. Ventilation thus increases in excess of that required to keep Pa_{CO_2} constant. A progressive decrease in Pa_{CO_2} results, which causes respiratory compensation for the acidosis associated with anaerobic metabolism (see Figs. 7.9 and 7.10). P_{ETCO_2} decreases along with Pa_{CO_2} at high work rates.

Some individuals who have airway obstruction can increase $\dot{V}_A$ to maintain a normal Pa_{CO_2} at low workloads. At higher workloads, however, they may be unable to reduce Pa_{CO_2} to compensate for the metabolic acidosis. In many patients with airway obstruction, maximal exercise is limited by a lack of ventilatory reserve. These individuals typically do not reach the AT. Ventilatory limitation prevents them from attaining a workload high enough to induce anaerobic metabolism. In patients with severe airflow obstruction, $\dot{V}_A$ may be unable to match any increment in $\dot{V}_{CO_2}$, resulting in hypercapnia and respiratory acidosis. Increased work of breathing and reduced sensitivity to CO_2, combined with the increased $\dot{V}_{CO_2}$ of exercise, allow Pa_{CO_2} to increase.

Acid–Base Status During Exercise

The pH, like Pa_{CO_2}, is regulated by the $\dot{V}_A$ at low work rates. $\dot{V}_A$ increases in proportion to $\dot{V}_{CO_2}$ up to the ventilatory AT. At work rates above AT, proportional increases in ventilation maintain the pH at near-normal levels. Most of the buffering of lactic acid is provided by HCO_3^- and a decrease in Pa_{CO_2}. At the highest work rates (above 80% of the $\dot{V}_{O_2}$ max), pH decreases despite hyperventilation because compensation for lactic acidosis becomes incomplete. In the presence of airway obstruction, ventilatory limitations may prevent compensation above the anaerobic threshold, with the development of significant respiratory acidosis. However, patients who have moderate or severe obstruction generally cannot exercise up to a level that elicits anaerobic metabolism. Increased Pa_{CO_2} (respiratory acidosis) may be the primary cause of acidosis in these patients.

Exercise Variables Calculated from Blood Gases

Arterial blood gases drawn during exercise allow several other parameters of gas exchange to be determined (see Interpretive Strategies 7.4). These include physiologic dead space, alveolar ventilation, and the V_D/V_T ratio.

Calculation of V_D, $\dot{V}_A$, and V_D/V_T requires measurement of Pa_{CO_2}. V_D may be calculated with the following equation:

$$V_D = \left(V_T \times \left[1 - \frac{F_{ECO_2} \times (P_B - 47)}{Pa_{CO_2}} \right] \right) - V_{Dsys}$$

where:

V_T = tidal volume, liters (BTPS)
F_{ECO_2} = fraction of expired CO_2
$P_B - 47$ = dry barometric pressure
Pa_{CO_2} = arterial CO_2 tension
V_{Dsys} = dead space of one-way breathing valve, liters

When V_D has been determined, $\dot{V}_A$ can be calculated with the following equation:

$$\dot{V}_A = \dot{V}_E - (f_b \times V_D)$$

where:

$\dot{V}_E$ = minute ventilation (BTPS)
f_b = respiratory rate (breaths/minute)
V_D = respiratory dead space (BTPS)

The V_D/V_T ratio may be calculated as the quotient of the V_D (as just determined) and the V_T, averaged from the $\dot{V}_E$ divided by f_b. Alternatively, V_D/V_T may be derived simply from the difference between arterial and mixed expired CO_2 at each exercise level:

$$V_D/V_T = \frac{\left(Pa_{CO_2} - P_{\bar{E}}CO_2 \right)}{Pa_{CO_2}}$$

where:
$P_{\bar{E}}CO_2$ = partial pressure of CO_2 in expired gas

Most breath-by-breath systems calculate V_D/V_T noninvasively by substituting end-tidal CO_2 for Pa_{CO_2}. This method assumes that P_{ETCO_2} and Pa_{CO_2} are equal. This may not be the case at higher workloads and in patients who have pulmonary disease.

V_D, which is composed of anatomic and alveolar dead space, is the part of $\dot{V}_E$ that does not participate in gas exchange. V_D/V_T expresses the relationship between "wasted" and tidal ventilation for the average breath. The healthy adult at rest has a $\dot{V}_A$ of 4–7 L/min (BTPS) and a V_D/V_T ratio of approximately 0.20 to 0.35. The absolute volume of dead space increases during exercise in conjunction with increased $\dot{V}_E$. Because of increases in V_T and increased perfusion of well-ventilated lung units (e.g., at the apices), the V_D/V_T ratio decreases. This pattern is expected in healthy patients (see Fig. 7.9). V_D/V_T increases with age, but the kinetic change with exercise remains the same. V_D/V_T may decrease in mild or moderate pulmonary disease states as well. In severe airway obstruction or in pulmonary vascular disease, V_D/V_T remains fixed or may even increase. An increase in V_D/V_T with exertion indicates ventilation increasing in excess of perfusion. This pattern is often associated with pulmonary hypertension. The vascular "space" is fixed in pulmonary hypertension; additional lung units cannot be recruited to handle the increased CO during exercise. V_D/V_T may also be elevated in individuals who use inappropriate breathing strategies. Small tidal volumes and high respiratory rates to recruit $\dot{V}_E$ in an otherwise healthy patient can yield falsely high ratios. Coaching a patient to increase tidal volume and use a more normal breathing pattern can alleviate a falsely elevated V_D/V_T ratio.

During exercise in healthy patients, $\dot{V}_A$ increases more than $\dot{V}_E$ as V_D/V_T decreases. In patients whose V_D/V_T ratio remains fixed or increases, adequacy of $\dot{V}_A$ must be assessed in terms of $Paco_2$ and not simply by the magnitude of $\dot{V}_E$.

CARDIAC OUTPUT DURING EXERCISE

There are several methods for calculating CO during exercise. Noninvasive methods include CO_2 rebreathing, soluble gas, and Doppler (ultrasound) techniques. Invasive methods measure CO by the direct Fick method or by thermal dilution. The invasive methods require placement of a pulmonary artery catheter (Criteria for Acceptability 7.5).

Noninvasive Cardiac Output Techniques

The CO_2 rebreathing technique (also termed the *indirect Fick method*) uses the Fick equation for CO_2:

$$\dot{Q}_T = \frac{\dot{V}co_2}{C\bar{V}CO_2 - CaCO_2}$$

where:

$\dot{Q}_T$ = CO, L/min
$\dot{V}co_2$ = CO_2 production calculated from exhaled gases
$Caco_2$ = arterial CO_2 content, calculated from $Paco_2$
$C\bar{V}CO_2$ = mixed venous CO_2 content, calculated from alveolar Pco_2 after rebreathing to allow equilibrium of alveolar gas with mixed venous blood

CRITERIA FOR ACCEPTABILITY 7.5
Cardiac Output During Exercise

1. If a noninvasive technique (e.g., soluble gas, CO_2 rebreathing) was used, were the laboratory's quality standards for the test satisfied?
2. For the Fick cardiac output method, the pulmonary artery catheter must be properly placed. For thermodilution, the catheter must also be properly placed; the proximal (injection) port must be in the right atrium with the thermistor in a pulmonary arteriole.
3. For Fick measurements, arterial and mixed venous blood should be drawn simultaneously over 15 to 30 seconds (or longer). Care should be taken to avoid dilution with flush solution; dilution can markedly alter content calculations and therefore cardiac output.
4. Oxygen consumption should be measured over the same interval as blood sampling for the Fick method.
5. Thermodilution measurements should be performed according to the manufacturer's recommendations, particularly in regard to the temperature of injectate and rate of injection.
6. Two or more acceptable measurements should be averaged, if possible; multiple measurements may not be practical during exercise.

The acetylene technique, also known as the *soluble gas technique,* can be performed with either closed-circuit (rebreathing) or open-circuit methods. This method depends on the rate of uptake of a soluble gas (e.g., acetylene) that has a low diffusion coefficient. The rate of uptake is directly proportional to the pulmonary blood flow. As long as there is no intracardiac or pulmonary shunt, pulmonary blood flow equals CO. Both of these breathing techniques correlate well with invasive techniques in healthy patients but have limited use in patients with maldistribution of ventilation. Another similar technology is termed the inert gas rebreathing technique that uses 0.5% nitrous oxide (N_2O) and 0.1% sulfur hexafluoride (SF_6) as the soluble and insoluble gases.

Instrumentation with Doppler technology to estimate CO works on the principle of measuring flow with an ultrasound signal directed at the arch of the aorta. A measurement of the diameter of the aorta is also made with echocardiography. These two measurements allow for the determination of CO (i.e., flow × cross-sectional area = total output). This method works well at rest and at low levels of exercise with a cycle ergometer, but motion artifact and increasing tidal volumes limit its usefulness at higher workloads.

Direct Fick Method

The direct Fick method is based on the measurement of O_2 consumption and arteriovenous content difference for O_2:

$$\dot{Q}_T = \frac{\dot{V}O_2}{C(a-\bar{v})O_2} \times 100$$

where:

$\dot{Q}_T$ = CO, L/min
$\dot{V}O_2$ = oxygen consumption, L/min (STPD)
$C(a-\bar{v})O_2$ = arterial-mixed venous O_2 content difference, mL/dL
100 = factor to correct $C(a-\bar{v})O_2$ to liters (content differences are normally reported in vol% or mL/dL)

$\dot{V}O_2$ is measured using one of the methods described previously. $C(a-\bar{v})O_2$ is obtained by measuring or calculating oxygen content in both arterial and mixed venous blood (see Chapter 6). Arterial and mixed venous blood specimens should be drawn simultaneously during the last 15 to 30 seconds of each exercise level. Oxygen consumption averaged over the same interval should be used for the calculation.

Thermodilution Method

Most pulmonary artery (Swan–Ganz) catheters include circuitry for the measurement of CO by thermodilution. A sensitive thermistor is placed near the tip of the catheter. A chilled saline solution (usually 10°–20°C) is injected through a catheter port located in the right atrium. The thermistor senses the change in temperature as the solution is pumped through the right ventricle and into the pulmonary artery. The computer then integrates the change in temperature and the time required for the change to occur, and CO is calculated.

The thermodilution method is typically used in critical care settings. However, it has also been used during exercise testing. Multiple measurements (two to four) should be made at each exercise level and the results averaged. Some automated systems allow other cardiopulmonary variables (e.g., ejection fraction) to be calculated as well.

Cardiac Output During Exercise

CO in healthy adults is approximately 4 to 6 L/min at rest. During exercise, it may increase to 25 to 35 L/min (Interpretive Strategies 7.5). CO is the product of HR and SV:

$$\dot{Q}_T = HR \times SV$$

where:

$\dot{Q}_T$ = CO, L/mL
HR = heart rate, beats/minute
SV = stroke volume, L/mL

In healthy, upright adults, SV is approximately 70 to 100 mL at rest. SV may be slightly higher if the patient is supine or semirecumbent because of increased venous return from the lower extremities. SV increases to 100 to 140 mL with low or moderate exercise. HR increases almost linearly with increasing work rate, as described earlier, so at low workloads, an increase in CO is caused by a combination of HR and SV. At moderate and high workloads, further increases in CO result mainly from increased HR. Derivation of SV (dividing $\dot{Q}_T$ by HR) is useful for quantifying poor cardiac performance in patients with coronary artery disease, cardiomyopathy, or other diseases that affect myocardial contractility.

Patients who are able to reach their predicted $\dot{V}O_2$ max and their predicted HRmax typically have normal CO and SV. A patient who has a reduced $\dot{V}_{O_2}$ max but achieves maximal predicted HR often has low CO because of low SV. Limited CO with increasing workload is often accompanied by early onset of anaerobic metabolism (anaerobic or ventilatory threshold). Reduced CO may be seen in both atrial and ventricular arrhythmias, valvular insufficiency, and cardiomyopathies.

INTERPRETIVE STRATEGIES 7.5

Cardiac Output During Exercise

1. Were cardiac output measurements acceptable by laboratory standards? If a pulmonary artery catheter was used, were the measurements reproducible within 10% (as applicable)? If not, interpret cautiously.
2. Did cardiac output increase appropriately with increasing workloads? If not, consider cardiomyopathy, myocardial hypokinesis, valvular insufficiency, and other outflow tract abnormalities.
3. Was stroke volume normal at rest? Did it increase at low and medium workloads?
4. Was there evidence of ischemic changes or arrhythmias (on ECG) that might explain reduced cardiac output?
5. Was cardiac output compromised by increased systemic or pulmonary vascular resistance?
6. If cardiac output was not available, did the O_2 pulse (surrogate for SV) increase appropriately with exercise?

In fit patients, SV is increased both at rest and during exercise. Endurance (aerobic) training normally results in increased SV. Other benefits of aerobic training include reductions in systolic BP and ventilation. Fit patients typically have a lower resting HR than their sedentary counterparts. Because HR (i.e., CO) is the factor that limits exercise in most individuals, fit patients reach a higher $\dot{V}_{O_2}$ max. Depending on the frequency, intensity, and duration of training, fit individuals are able to maintain a higher level or work for longer periods because of improved CO.

Symptom Scales

The measurement of RPE (or Borg scale) and other symptom scales can be essential for connecting

TABLE 7.8

Ratings of Perceived Exertion (Borg) Scales

Perceived Exertion Scale		Modified Perceived Exertion Scale	
6		0	Nothing at all
7	Very, very light	0.5	Very, very slight (just noticeable)
8		1	Very slight
9	Very light	2	Slight
10		3	Moderate
11	Fairly light	4	Somewhat moderate
12		5	Severe
13	Somewhat hard	6	
14		7	Very severe
15	Hard	8	
16		9	Very, very severe (almost maximal)
17	Very hard	10	Maximal
18			
19	Very, very hard		
20			

subjective symptoms and the physiologic responses to exercise. Rating scales, when they are discordant, can assist the physician in counseling the patient. There are two versions of the RPE scale, often referred to as the *Borg* and *modified-Borg scales* (Table 7.8). These scales are usually printed on a card or poster that the patient can see or point to during exercise testing. The scales should be reviewed with the patient before exercise begins. This is particularly important if exhaled gas is being collected because the patient may have a mouthpiece or facial mask in place. The patient should be able to indicate his or her level of exertion even without vocalizing. General symptom (visual analog) scales can be adapted to any chief complaint the patient may be expressing by simply using a scale of 0 to 4 and grading intensity from "nothing at all" to "severe." A patient complaining of lightheadedness or chest tightness can then alert the testing staff to his or her level of discomfort during the test using hand signals.

Quality of Test

General quality assurance and quality control of instrumentation are discussed in Chapter 11. However, the complexity of cardiopulmonary exercise testing warrants additional considerations including a quality system approach to testing. The CLSI's *A Quality Management Systems: A Model for Laboratories Services,* discussed in Chapters 1 and 12, incorporates the concept of the path of workflow process. This concept integrates pretest, test, and posttest assessments of processes that can affect any section across the path of workflow. Pretest processes include patient assessment, test request, patient preparation, and equipment preparation. Patient assessment, as it relates to cardiopulmonary exercise testing, might include a review of laboratory results, current medications affecting exercise performance (e.g., beta-blockers, digitalis), or orthopedic issues that may affect ergometer selection. Test processes include, but are not limited to, making sure the subject understands the purpose of the test and the expected effort, testing staff is competent in identifying normal and abnormal responses to exercise, and appropriate response to patient conditions to maintain patient safety. In the posttest period, posttest assessments (i.e., post-FVCs, BP), selecting data for analysis, and the reporting process all need to be considered.

Additional quality processes specific to exercise testing systems include monitoring phase-delay data, ergometer calibration, and biologic quality control (QC) data. The importance of phase delay was previously discussed in the chapter. Cycle ergometer calibration can be specific to the device; however, many of the new electronic ergometers cannot be calibrated without expensive adjunct hardware. Treadmill outputs can be easily validated. Speed can be assessed by knowing the belt length and timing belt revolutions with a stopwatch. Grade can be verified by dividing the length of the treadmill by the height (Fig. 7.16). The entire system can be monitored by performing biologic QC (BioQC). Several methods have been suggested; however, all include collecting steady-state data at rest and a predetermined submaximal workload(s). Determining an appropriate workload can

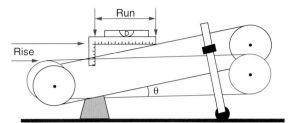

FIG. 7.16 Treadmill calibration. Calibration of treadmill grade using carpenter's square and level.

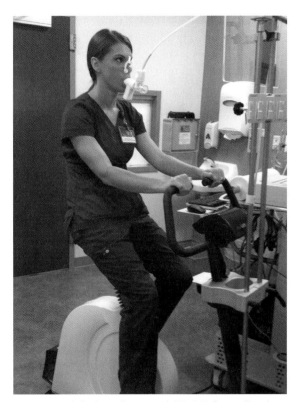

FIG. 7.17 Biologic quality control (BioQC) for cardiopulmonary exercise testing. BioQC subject performing test on cycle ergometer at rest, 25 watts, and 75 watts. Standard deviation, coefficient of variation, and absolute difference can all be monitored to ensure accurate and precise equipment function.

be achieved by having the BioQC subject perform a maximal test, identify the anaerobic threshold, and select a workload below the AT. Another suggested method has the subject perform steady-state exercise (5 minutes at each stage) at two workloads 50 watts apart (example 25 and 75 watts) (Fig. 7.17).

The expected oxygen consumption difference between the two workloads should be 500 mL because the normal $\dot{V}_{O_2}$-to-watt relationship is 10 mL/watt. Regardless of the method used, the data can be entered into a spreadsheet with the mean and 2 standard deviations calculated. The data can be monitored over time to identify "out-of-control" situations, which may not be recognized with a standard individual module (i.e., pneumotach and gas analyzer) calibration.

Interpretation Strategies

To interpret a study appropriately, the interpreter first needs to assess the degree of effort and determine whether the test is a maximal study (Table 7.9). Once the test has been qualified as maximal or submaximal, an algorithmic approach to data review and interpretation is essential (see Interpretive Strategies 7.2, 7.3, 7.4, and 7.5).

The following scheme can assist in a stepwise approach to data analysis:

- Determine maximal study (see Table 7.9)
  - $\dot{V}_{O_2}$max, $\dot{V}_{O_2}$/kg
- If reduced, why? Review the following responses:
  - Cardiovascular response (see Interpretive Strategies 7.2 and Criteria for Acceptability 7.5)
  - ECG, BP, CO, O_2 pulse, and symptoms
  - Ventilatory response (see Interpretive Strategies 7.2)

- Ventilatory reserve, breathing kinetics
- Gas exchange (see Interpretive Strategies 7.4)
  - A-a gradient, V_D/V_T, Pa_{CO_2}
- Metabolic response (see Interpretive Strategies 7.3)
- Anaerobic/ventilatory threshold, lactate
- Impression

SUMMARY

- The chapter examines the measurement of cardiopulmonary variables during exercise.
- Various protocols for assessing exercise responses are described, including treadmill and cycle ergometry methods and the 6MWT.
- Monitoring of the cardiovascular system, with a special concern for patient safety, is discussed.
- Techniques for measuring ventilation, oxygen consumption, carbon dioxide production, and the associated variables during exercise are delineated.
- The measurement of breathing kinetics and flow-volume analysis during exercise is described.
- Special emphasis is given to criteria for acceptability and interpretive strategies for the various measurements described.
- Assessment of blood gases and cardiac output is also discussed.

TABLE 7.9		
Determining Maximal Study		
***	Heart rate:	> 85%–90% of predicted
***	End exercise:	50%–80% $\dot{V}_E$/MVV or $\geq$ 90% $\dot{V}_E$/MVV or MVV – $\dot{V}_E$max $\leq$ 15 L/min suggesting ventilatory limitation
**	Sao$_2$:	< 80%
*	Metabolic work:	RER > 1.10 or lactate > 7 mmol/L
*	Clinical investigator:	Opinion of effort or early termination criteria met

* = Weighted variable.
Once single criterion or multiple criteria are met, test is graded as maximal study.

CASE STUDIES

CASE 7.1

HISTORY

The subject is a 54-year-old man complaining of dyspnea on exertion. Several months ago, he had an initial episode of SOB, which has worsened during the past 2 months. He has a 15 to 20 pack-year smoking history. He works as a foreman for a utility company and does not have any related environmental exposures. His laboratory results were all normal. His echocardiogram, chest radiograph, and computed tomography (CT) scan of the chest were also normal. His spirometry results are as follows.

PULMONARY FUNCTION TESTS
Personal Data

Sex:	Male, Caucasian
Age:	54 yr
Height:	69.3 in. (176 cm)
Weight:	195 lb. (88.4 kg; BMI 28.6)

BMI, Body mass index.

Spirometry

	Predicted		Control	
	Normal	LLN	Found	% Predicted
VC	4.73	> 3.89	5.12	108
FVC	4.73	> 3.89	5.03	106
FEV$_1$	3.74	> 3.06	4.19	112
FEV$_1$/FVC	79.1	> 69.9	83.3	
FEF$_{25\%-75\%}$	3.4	> 1.9	4.0	119
FEFmax	8.7	> 5.2	9.0	104
MVV	148	> 115	141	95

LLN, Lower limit of normal.

Technologist's Comments

Spirometry testing was performed, meeting criteria for acceptability and reproducibility.

QUESTIONS

1. What is the interpretation of the spirometry results?

Exercise Test

	Rest	AT	Max	Pred Max	% Pred Max
Exercise					
Workload (watts)		160	180		
Time (min:sec)	4:40	8:56	10:50		
$\dot{V}o_2$(L/min)	0.167	1.938	2.108	2.424	87
$\dot{V}o_2$ / kg (mL / kg)	1.9	21.9	23.9		
RER	0.80	1.07	1.13		
Cardiac Function					
Heart rate (beats/min)	78	139	156	175	89
Blood pressure (direct) (mm Hg)	145/90	235/110	235/110		
Oxygen pulse (mL/beat)	2.1	13.9	13.5		

	Rest	AT	Max	Pred Max	% Pred Max
Ventilation					
Minute ventilation (L/min)	6.7	56.0	69.3	141.0	49
Respiratory rate (per min)	14	20	23		
Tidal volume (mL, BTPS)	498	2803	2975		
Tidal volume/FVC (%)	10	56	59		
Vent equivalent for O_2 ($\dot{V}_E / \dot{V}_{O_2}$)	40.5	29.2	32.8		
Blood Gases					
Arterial pH	7.42	7.37			
Arterial P_{CO_2} (mm Hg)	38	39			
Arterial P_{O_2} (mm Hg)	82	98			
Arterial O_2 sat (%)	98	96			
Arterial bicarbonate (mEq/L)	24.0	22.0			
(A-a) gradient O_2 (mm Hg)	16.3	11.1			
$P_{(E_T-a)} CO_2$ (mm Hg)	−1.9	6.3			
V_D/V_T (%)	55	2.4			
Arterial lactate (mmoL/L)	0.7	4.9			

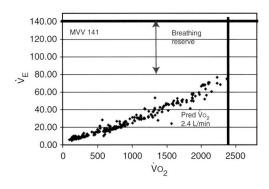

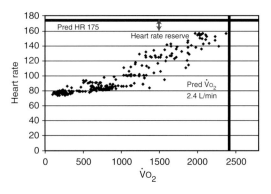

2. Was it a maximal study?
3. What is the interpretation of the following?
   a. Cardiovascular response
   b. Ventilation during exercise
   c. Gas exchange during exercise
   d. Oxygen consumption and ventilatory threshold during exercise
   e. Impression

DISCUSSION
Interpretation (Pulmonary Function)
Normal spirometry.

Interpretation (Exercise)
The subject exercised on a cycle ergometer to a maximum workload of 180 watts using a 20-watt incremental protocol. He terminated the test, complaining of SOB and leg fatigue. This appears to be a near-maximal study based on HR criterion.

Cardiovascular Response: HR increased from 78 to 156 beats/min. Electrocardiogram showed normal sinus rhythm at rest with rare PVCs with exercise. There is no evidence of ischemic changes. BP shows exercise-induced hypertension (i.e., elevated diastolic BP).

Ventilatory Response: There was a normal ventilatory reserve with normal breathing kinetics. Tidal volume increased to 59% of FVC.

Gas Exchange: Arterial blood gases were normal at rest and at exercise. The V_D/V_T ratio decreased appropriately with exercise. Maximal oxygen consumption and ventilatory threshold were within normal limits.

Impression: Normal study with the exception of exercise-induced hypertension.

Discussion of Subject's Exercise Response

The testing staff selected an incremental protocol of 20 watts/min based on what appeared to be a healthy subject with a predicted $\dot{V}o_2$ max of 2.424 L (increment based on $\dot{V}o_2$ = 2400 − 300/100 = 21). The test was determined to be a near-maximal study based on a heart rate response of 89% of predicted, a large ventilatory reserve, and a lactate level of 4.9 mmoL/L.

Cardiovascular Response: He had a normal HR response without significant ECG changes. His BP showed exercise-induced hypertension with an elevated diastolic pressure, which is the only abnormality during this test. His oxygen pulse increased from 2.1 to 13.5, which is consistent with an appropriate increase in stroke volume.

Ventilatory Response: His minute ventilation increased to 69.3 L, which was 49% of his MVV, resulting in a normal ventilatory reserve. He used appropriate breathing strategies, increasing his tidal volume to 59% of his forced vital capacity.

Gas Exchange: His resting blood gas values were within normal limits, with a resting V_D/V_T at 55 being somewhat elevated. However, this is most likely secondary to a low tidal volume–high breathing frequency anticipatory response rather than a physiologic abnormality. His blood gases remained normal through exercise, and his V_D/V_T decreased appropriately with exercise. Lactate increased from 0.7 to 4.9 mmoL/L.

Oxygen consumption and the ventilatory threshold were within normal limits.

Treatment

The primary physician was made aware of his exercise-induced hypertension. An exercise prescription was given.

CASE 7.2

HISTORY

A 69-year-old woman with a history of COPD seeks medical attention because of increased dyspnea on exertion. Her medical history includes a smoking history of 40 pack-years. She is currently using montelukast (Singulair), salmeterol (Serevent), and budesonide (Pulmicort). Her primary care physician orders a pulmonary function test and a chest radiograph. The chest radiograph is normal.

PULMONARY FUNCTION TESTS
Personal Data

Sex:	Female, Caucasian
Age:	69 yr
Height:	59 in. (149.9 cm)
Weight:	152 lb (68.9 kg; BMI 30.7)

Lung Volumes

	Predicted		Control		Post-Dilator[a]	
	Normal	LLN	Found	% Predicted	Found	% Change
TLC (Pleth)	4.24	>3.14	4.84	114		
VC	2.41	>1.67	1.95	81	2.08	+7
RV	1.84	<2.39	2.89[b]	158		
RV/TLC	43.3	<56.7	59.8[b]	138		
FRC		3.8				

Pleth, Plethysmograph, *RV*, reserve volume; *TLC*, total lung capacity.
[a] Bronchodilator was albuterol.
[b] Outside normal range.

Spirometry

	Predicted		Control		Post-Dilator[a]	
	Normal	LLN	Found	% Pred	Found	% Change
FVC	2.41	1.67	1.86	77	2.06	+11
FEV$_1$	1.97	>1.42	0.98[b]	50	1.23[b]	+25
FEV$_1$/FVC	81.8	>70.7	52.6[b]	59.5[b]		
FEF$_{25\%-75\%}$	2.1	>0.9	0.3[b]	15	0.4[b]	
FEFmax	4.9	>2.2	4.6	94	4.7	+3

[a] Bronchodilator was albuterol.
[b] Outside normal range.

Diffusing Capacity

	Predicted		Control	
	Normal	LLN	Found	% Pred
D$_{LCO}$sb	18.5	>12.0	11.8[a]	63
D$_{LCO}$ (adjusted for Hb = 14.4 g/dL)		19	11.8	62
$\dot{V}_A$	4.09	>3.14	3.88	95

[a] Outside normal range.

Technologist's Comments

Spirometry testing was performed, meeting criteria for acceptability and reproducibility.

QUESTIONS

1. What is the interpretation of the following?
   a. Prebronchodilator and postbronchodilator spirometry
   b. Lung volumes and diffusing capacity

Exercise Test

	Rest	Maximum	Pred Max	% Pred Max
Exercise				
Workload (watts)		70	110	
Time (min/sec)	3:20	7:01		
$\dot{V}o_2$ (L/min)	0.266	0.863	1.368	63
$\dot{V}o_2$/kg (mL/kg)	3.8	12.3		
RER	0.80	0.95		
Cardiac Function				
Heart rate (beats/min)	91	153	165	93
Blood pressure (direct) (mm Hg)	150/85	225/105		
Oxygen pulse (mL/beat)	2.9	5.6		
Ventilatory Response				
Minute ventilation (L/min)	11.3	30.8	44.0	70
Respiratory rate (per min)	17	30		
Tidal volume (mL, BTPS)	638	1026		
Tidal volume/FVC (%)	35	56		
Vent equiv for O$_2$ $\left(\dot{V}_E / \dot{V}o_2\right)$	47.1	35.8		

	Rest	Maximum	Pred Max	% Pred Max
Blood Gases				
Arterial pH	7.41	7.35		
Arterial P_{CO_2} (mm Hg)	40	47		
Arterial P_{O_2} (mm Hg)	66	63		
Arterial O_2 sat (%)	91	89		
Arterial bicarbonate	25.0	25.0		
(A-a) gradient O_2 (mm Hg)	29.0	31.1		
$P(_{ET}-a)$ CO_2 (mm Hg)	−6.2	−3.5		
V_D/V_T (%)	60	52		
Arterial lactate (mmoL/L)	0.6	3.9		

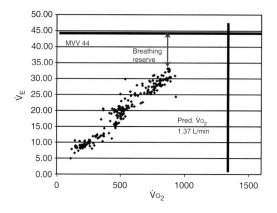
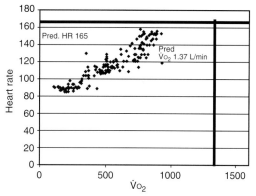

2. Was it a maximal study?
3. What is the interpretation of the following?
   a. Cardiovascular response
   b. Ventilation during exercise
   c. Gas exchange during exercise
   d. Oxygen consumption and ventilatory threshold during exercise
   e. Impression
4. Discuss the subject's exercise response.
5. What treatment might be recommended, based on these findings?

DISCUSSION
Interpretation (Pulmonary Function)
Spirometry is consistent with moderate to severe obstruction, with a significant response to bronchodilator. Her total lung capacity is within normal limits. However, there is an increase in her residual volume, consistent with air trapping. Her diffusing capacity is reduced, suggesting the presence of a pulmonary parenchymal or vascular abnormality.

Her primary physician ordered a cardiopulmonary exercise test to rule out an exercise-induced gas exchange abnormality and look for any evidence of concomitant cardiac disease.

Interpretation (Exercise)
The subject exercised on a cycle ergometer using a 10-watt incremental protocol to a maximum workload of 70 watts. She terminated the test complaining of SOB. This appears to be a maximal study based on both HR and ventilatory criteria.

Cardiovascular Response: The HR increased to a maximum of 153 beats/min, which was 93% of predicted. BP increased and showed borderline exercise-induced hypertension. The ECG displayed a normal sinus rhythm at baseline. There were no abnormalities suggestive of ischemic heart disease. Oxygen pulse increased with exercise but not to the level expected, suggesting a reduced stroke volume response to exercise.

Ventilatory Response: There is a slight reduction in the ventilatory reserve but normal breathing kinetics with an increase in tidal volume to 56% of the vital capacity.

Gas Exchange: ABGs at rest show an increase in the A-a gradient and an elevation in V_D/V_T. Exercise blood gases show an increase in $Paco_2$ consistent with ventilatory limitation and essentially no change in the A-a gradient. V_D/V_T remains high at 52%. Oxygen consumption is moderately reduced, and it appears that the subject did not reach anaerobiosis.

Impression: (1) Moderate reduction in exercise capacity, (2) ventilatory limitation with exercise-induced hypercapnia, (3) gas exchange abnormality at rest and with exercise, and (4) exercise-induced hypertension.

Discussion of the Exercise Response

A 10-watt incremental protocol was selected, based on a predicted $\dot{V}o_2$ max of 1.368 L ([1300−300]/100 = 10). The subject terminated the test, complaining of SOB. This appeared to be a maximal study based on HR and ventilatory criteria. Her cardiovascular response showed exercise-induced hypertension. Her oxygen pulse increased with exercise but appeared somewhat reduced. This suggests a reduced stroke volume. Another possible explanation for the reduced O_2 pulse is a defect in oxygen extraction. O_2 pulse is also directly related to arterio-venous content difference. Her ventilatory reserve was reduced, with an absolute difference of 13 L (44 L expected; 31 L actual). However,

her $\dot{V}_E/MVV$ ratio is still within normal limits. This is an excellent example of how a subject with a reduced MVV resulting from lung disease can have a normal ratio even though the overall ventilatory reserve is compromised. There should be an actual reserve of at least 10 to 15 L between the maximal expected and the achieved ventilation. The tidal volume increased appropriately with exercise to 56% of vital capacity, so her breathing kinetics is appropriate. She has a gas exchange abnormality at rest with an elevated V_D/V_T. Her gas exchange abnormality does not worsen with exercise. However, she does show progressive hypercapnia that is inappropriate during exercise and further supports that she is ventilation limited. Her V_D/V_T kinetics do not respond appropriately and stay essentially flat with exercise.

Treatment

The subject was enrolled in a pulmonary rehabilitation program. The following chart shows the improvement in her 6MWD after 6 weeks of enrollment.

Six-Minute Walk Test				
	Distance (ft)	Inspired Gas	Spo₂ (End Exercise)	RPE (6–20)
Initial test	1047	Room air	91%	17
6 weeks later	1425	Room air	91%	17

CASE 7.3

HISTORY

The subject is a 53-year-old office worker who was referred for evaluation of SOB. She has a 44 pack-year history of smoking and continued to smoke up to the time of her test. She has a morning cough that produces thick white sputum of 50 to 100 mL/day. Her chest radiograph shows increased vascular markings and mild hyperinflation. She was taking no medications at the time of this test. No familial history of lung disease or cancer was found, and she had no unusual environmental exposure.

PULMONARY FUNCTION TESTS
Personal Data

Sex:	Female, Caucasian
Age:	53 yr
Height:	65 in.
Weight:	131 lb

Spirometry					
	Predicted	Control	% Pred	Post-Dilator	% Change
FVC	3.35	3.24	97	3.34	3
FEV₁ (L)	2.53	1.49	59	1.56	7
FEV₁/FVC	0.76	0.46		0.47	
MVV (L/min)	97.9	52	53		
Raw (cm H₂O/L/sec)	0.6–2.4	2.22	–	2.1	–
sGaw (L/sec/cm/H₂O/L)	0.14–0.58	0.012	–	0.13	–

Lung Volumes (by Plethysmograph)

	Predicted	Control	% Pred
VC (L)	3.35	3.27	98
IC (L)	2.31	1.80	78
ERV (L)	1.04	0.99	95
FRC (L)	2.88	3.54	123
RV (L)	1.84	2.55	136
TLC (L)	5.20	5.82	112
RV/TLC (%)	35	44	—

Diffusing Capacity (Single Breath)

	Predicted	Control	% Pred
D_{LCO} (mL CO/min/mm Hg)	20	8.8	44
D_{LCO} (adj)	18.1	8.8	49
$\dot{V}_A$ (L)	—	5.67	—
KCO	3.85	1.55	—

Blood Gases (F_{IO_2} 0.21)

pH	7.38
$Paco_2$ (mm Hg)	43

Pao_2 (mm Hg)	59
Sao_2 (%)	85.1
Hb (g/dL)	11.7
COHb (%)	5.7

Technologist's Comments

All spirometric efforts were acceptable both before and after bronchodilator administration. Lung volume and D_{LCO} testing was performed acceptably. D_{LCO} was corrected for an Hb level of 11.7 and a COHb level of 5.7.

Three days later, a treadmill test was performed with an arterial catheter in place. The test was repeated with oxygen supplementation. Gas with an F_{IO_2} of 0.28 was prepared in a meteorologic balloon for the portion of the exercise test using O_2 (see the Exercise Test in Case Study 7.1).

QUESTIONS

1. What is the interpretation of the following?
   a. Prebronchodilator and postbronchodilator spirometry
   b. Lung volumes and diffusing capacity
   c. Room air blood gases at rest

Exercise Test

	Air		Oxygen (28%)			
Exercise Response	Rest	Exercise	Rest	Exercise	Predicted	% Pred
mph	0	1.5	0	1.5		
Grade (%)	0	0	0	0		
Time (min)	10	3	10	3		
$\dot{V}o_2$ (L)	0.310	0.835	0.279	0.986	1.858	53
$\dot{V}co_2$ (L)	0.303	0.743	0.251	0.916		
RER	0.98	0.89	0.90	0.93		
Spo_2 (%)	92	87	97	93	> 93	
Cardiac Response						
HR (beats/min)	90	110	92	105	167	66
Systolic BP (mm Hg)	130	145	134	145		
Diastolic BP (mm Hg)	85	88	90	90		
$\dot{V}o_2$/HR (mL/beat)	3.44	7.59	3.29	6.18		
Ventilatory Response						
Resp rate	16	28	13	20		
$\dot{V}_E$ (L)	10.2	23.4	6.2	16.6	52	44
$\dot{V}_A$ (L)	6.02	14.74	3.74	10.45		
V_T (L)	0.638	0.836	0.479	0.830		
$\dot{V}_E/\dot{V}o_2$ (L)	32.90	28.00	22.33	25.50		

Exercise Response	Air		Oxygen (28%)		Predicted	% Pred
	Rest	Exercise	Rest	Exercise		
Blood gases						
pH	7.45	7.39	7.39	7.38		
Pa_{CO_2} (mm Hg)	34	39	44	45		
Pa_{O_2} (mm Hg)	61	47	84	71		
Sa_{O_2} (%)	87.4	77.3	91.4	88.9		
COHb (%)	5.1	4.7	4.8	4.7		
$P(A-a)_{O_2}$ (mm Hg)	51	56	64	78		
V_D/V_T	0.41	0.37	0.40	0.37		

2. What is the interpretation of the following?
   a. Ventilation during exercise
   b. Gas exchange during exercise
   c. Blood gas levels during exercise
3. What is the cause of the subject's exercise limitation?
4. What treatment might be recommended, based on these findings?

DISCUSSION

Interpretation (Pulmonary Function Tests)

All spirometry, lung volume, diffusing capacity, and blood gas measurements were acceptable.

Spirometry results show an obstructive process with a well-preserved FVC. There is only a 5% improvement in the FEV_1 after bronchodilator administration. Lung volumes by plethysmography show increased FRC and RV, consistent with air trapping. TLC is close to normal, so there is little hyperinflation. D_{LCO} is decreased even after correction for Hb and COHb. ABGs on air show hypoxemia complicated by an elevated COHb.

Impression: Moderately severe obstructive disease with no significant response to bronchodilators. Air trapping is present, and D_{LCO} is severely decreased. Exercise evaluation for oxygen desaturation is recommended.

Interpretation (Cardiopulmonary Exercise Test)

The exercise test was performed in two parts; the first part of the test was stopped because the subject's Pa_{O_2} decreased to 46 mm Hg with an Sa_{O_2} of 77.3%. The second phase, using 28% oxygen, was terminated because of SOB. The subject tolerated very low workloads even with supplemental O_2.

Ventilation was slightly elevated at rest but increased normally. When given O_2, the subject's ventilation was slightly lower both at rest and at similar workloads. The V_D/V_T ratio was mildly elevated but decreased with exercise on both air and oxygen. The subject's minute ventilation was only 44% of her observed MVV after bronchodilator administration, indicating some ventilatory reserve.

The subject achieved a peak $\dot{V}_{O_2}$ of only 0.986 L/min on oxygen, which is 53% of her age-related predicted value of 1.858 L/min. This is consistent with moderately severe exercise impairment. The ventilatory equivalent for O_2 is within normal limits, and the O_2 pulse increased normally, although not to maximal values.

Blood gas analysis during exercise shows borderline hypoxemia at rest resulting from Pa_{O_2} of 61 mm Hg in combination with elevated COHb. Pa_{O_2} decreased to 47 mm Hg with only slight exertion. On 28% oxygen, the Pa_{O_2} improved to 84 mm Hg at rest but decreased as workload increased. Pa_{CO_2} increased slightly during oxygen breathing possibly because of respiratory depression. COHb was elevated, likely resulting from the subject's continued smoking. Pulse oximetry (Sp_{O_2}) during exercise shows readings higher than the actual saturation, presumably because of the elevated COHb.

The HR and BP responses were appropriate for the workloads achieved while breathing both air and oxygen. The low maximal HR suggests an exercise limitation other than cardiovascular pathology or deconditioning. The ECG was unremarkable.

Impression: Moderately severe exercise impairment is primarily caused by desaturation during exercise. Some ventilatory limitation is probably present. Desaturation is aggravated by an elevated COHb.

Cause of the Subject's Exercise Limitation

This subject characterizes an individual with obstructive lung disease in whom derangement of blood gases limits exercise more than impaired ventilation does. Her ventilation and gas exchange are close to normal at rest and at 1.5 mph, 0% grade. Pa_{O_2} is low, however, and decreases abruptly with just a small increase in workload. The decrease is severe enough that desaturation may occur with daily activities or during sleep. The elevated COHb further impairs O_2 delivery. Although a pulse oximeter was used during the exercise test, its readings were falsely high because of the elevated COHb. Even if pulse oximeter readings are corrected for COHb, a discrepancy often exists between Sp_{O_2} and Sa_{O_2} during exercise. This error in pulse oximeter readings may result from changes in blood flow at the sensor site or motion artifact during exercise. Desaturation might be expected because of her low DLCO. There is some evidence that DLCO values of less than 50% of predicted values are accompanied by exercise desaturation.

To evaluate the effect of oxygen therapy, a controlled trial of walking while breathing supplemental O_2 was performed. The subject breathed from a balloon containing gas blended to have an Fi_{O_2} of approximately 0.28. The most notable change was the increase in resting Pa_{O_2} from 61 to 84 mm Hg. However, the pattern of desaturation persisted. Her O_2 tension decreased dramatically, just as when she breathed room air. Because her Pa_{O_2} was elevated by the supplemental O_2, it remained above 55 mm Hg. This is the level at which serious symptoms of hypoxemia begin to occur. Supplemental O_2 also may be responsible for the decrease in ventilation exhibited by the subject at rest and during exercise. The mild increase in Pa_{CO_2} may be evidence of increased sensitivity to hypoxemia. When she breathes O_2, her respiratory drive decreases slightly, allowing CO_2 to increase. Abnormal $\dot{V}/\dot{Q}$ is the most likely explanation of desaturation observed in the subject. The bronchitic component of her obstructive disease results in shunting and venous admixture.

While breathing oxygen, she did not desaturate to a level at which hypoxemia might be considered as a cause of the exercise limitation. She also did not increase ventilation to her maximal level. This may suggest that deconditioning was responsible for the low maximal workload achieved. However, her HR and BP did not increase as is typical in significant deconditioning. Other possible causes for the low workload achieved while breathing oxygen may be inadequate subject effort, development of bronchospasm, or greatly increased work of breathing.

Treatment

The subject began a formal effort to stop smoking and eventually quit. She was also referred for pulmonary rehabilitation, which included bronchial hygiene, breathing retraining, and exercise with supplemental O_2. She began using nasal oxygen at 1 to 2 L/min for exertion. A follow-up evaluation was recommended 3 to 6 months after smoking cessation.

CASE 7.4

HISTORY

The subject is a 62-year-old woman complaining of dyspnea on exertion. Her medical history includes severe subglottic stenosis, which has been managed with several rigid dilatations over the past 2 years. She had a surgically corrected endarterectomy and a significant family history of coronary artery disease. Her current medications include metoprolol (Toprol), levothyroxine (Synthroid), and amlodipine (Norvasc). On physical examination, her lungs were clear to auscultation, and she was in no apparent distress.

Chest radiograph showed some narrowing of the subglottic trachea, with no significant change since 1 year ago.

PULMONARY FUNCTION TESTS
Personal Data

Sex:	Female, Caucasian
Age:	62 yr
Height:	62.5 in. (158.8 cm)
Weight:	179 lb (81.3 kg; BMI 32.3)

Lung Volumes

	Predicted		Control		Post-Dilator[a]	
	Normal	LLN	Found	% Pred	Found	% Change
TLC (Pleth)	4.82	>3.72	4.06	84		
VC	2.96	>2.22	2.28	77	2.42	+6
RV	1.86	<2.41	1.79	96		
RV/TLC	38.5	<50.5	44.0	114		
FRC			2.2			

[a] Bronchodilator was albuterol.

Spirometry

	Predicted		Control		Post-Dilator[a]	
	Normal	NNL	Found	% Pred	Found	% Change
FVC	2.96	>2.22	2.07[b]	70	2.20[b]	+6
FEV_1	2.4	>1.85	1.70[b]	71	1.78[b]	+5
FEV_1/FVC	81.2	>70.0	82.3		80.9	
$FEF_{25\%-75\%}$	2.3	>1.0	1.5	67	1.5	
FEFmax	5.5	>2.9	3.1	55	3.6	+17
FIFmax					1.5	
$FEF_{50\%}/FIF_{50\%}$					1.5	

[a] Bronchodilator was albuterol.
[b] Outside normal range.

Airway Function

	Predicted		Control	
	Normal	Range	Found	% Pred
sRaw	4.7	>7.9	5.5	117

Diffusing Capacity

	Predicted		Control	
	Normal	LLN	Found	% Pred
Dlco	20.9	>14.4	14.4	69
V_A	4.64	>3.72	3.58[a]	77

[a] Outside normal range.

Oximetry

	Predicted		Control	
	Normal	LLN	Rest	Exercise (Step 3 Min)
O_2sat	96	≥ 93	95	97
Pulse			66	104

Exercise Test

	Rest	Maximum	Pred Max	% Pred Max
Exercise				
Workload (watts)		60		
Time (min:sec)		7:00		
Oxygen saturation (%)	99	98		
$\dot{V}o_2$ (L/min)	0.191	0.801	1.674	48
$\dot{V}o_2$/kg (mL/kg)	2.3	9.9		
R	0.68	1.05		
Cardiac Function				
Heart rate (beats/min)	67	110	170	65
Blood pressure (cuff) (mm Hg)	122/60	148/72		
Oxygen pulse (mL/beat)	2.9	7.3		
Ventilatory Response				
Minute ventilation (L/min)	6.2	29.2	68.0	43
Respiratory rate (per min)	12	20		
Tidal volume (mL)	528	1564		
Tidal volume/FVC (%)	26	76		
Vent equiv for O_2 ($\dot{V}_E/O_2$)	34.7	36.7		

Technologist's Comments

Spirometry testing was performed, meeting criteria for acceptability and reproducibility.

QUESTIONS

1. What is the interpretation of the following?
   a. Prebronchodilator and postbronchodilator spirometry
   b. Lung volumes and diffusing capacity
2. Was it a maximal study?
3. What is the interpretation of the following?
   a. Cardiovascular response
   b. Ventilation during exercise
   c. Gas exchange during exercise
   d. Oxygen consumption and ventilatory threshold during exercise
   e. Impression
4. Discuss the subject's exercise response.
5. What treatment might be recommended, based on these findings?

DISCUSSION

Interpretation (Pulmonary Function)

Spirometry results show a nonspecific reduction in vital capacity and FEV_1 with a normal FEV_1/FVC ratio. Lung volumes were within normal limits. There was no response to the bronchodilator. The D_{LCO} was at the lower limit of normal. A cardiopulmonary exercise test was ordered with F-V loop analysis to determine whether there was flow limitation that would require repeat dilatation of the trachea, versus deconditioning or decreased exercise tolerance.

Interpretation (Exercise)

The subject exercised on a cycle ergometer to a maximal workload of 60 watts using a 10-watt protocol. The subject terminated the test complaining of SOB. This appears to be a submaximal study.

Cardiovascular Response: The HR increased to 110 beats/min, which was 65% of predicted. The ECG was a normal sinus rhythm at rest. During exercise, there were no arrhythmias and/or evidence of ischemic changes. The reduced HR response may also be secondary to the beta-blocker the subject was taking. BP and the O_2 pulse increased appropriately with exercise.

Ventilatory Response: There was an adequate ventilatory reserve; breathing kinetics were appropriate with increasing tidal volumes to 76% of the FVC. The tidal volume–to–FVC ratio is somewhat elevated at 76%, but this can be seen in individuals with reduced lung volumes.

Gas Exchange: Pulse oximetry was 99% at rest and 98% at end exercise, suggesting normal oxygen saturation.

Oxygen consumption in this submaximal study was 48% of predicted, and the ventilatory threshold could not be determined.

F-V loops were performed at rest, during warm-up, and at maximal workload. There was no evidence of either inspiratory or expiratory flow limitation compared with either the resting maximum F-V loop or the partial loops performed during exercise.

Impression: Submaximal study with reduced exercise tolerance and no evidence of flow limitation.

Discussion of Exercise Response

A 10-watt incremental protocol was selected based on a predicted $\dot{V}O_2$ max of 1.674 L ([1600 – 300]/100 = 13) and because of the subject's stated reduced exercise tolerance.

In evaluating whether a study represents maximal effort, five categories are examined. These are cardiovascular response, ventilatory response, oxygen saturation, metabolic parameters, and clinical observation (see Table 7.8). Her heart rate was 65% of predicted; $\dot{V}_E$ max reached 43% of her calculated MV. SpO_2 was 98%, and her metabolic work showed an RER of 1.05. Clinical observation revealed poor effort. These factors all suggest a submaximal study. On the basis of these findings, the study can still be interpreted accordingly.

Cardiovascular Response: HR response was reduced, either related to the poor effort or secondary to a beta-blockade effect.

Ventilatory Response: There was adequate ventilatory reserve based on both a normal ratio $\dot{V}_E$ max/MVV) and an absolute difference of 39 L. Tidal volume increased appropriately with exercise; however, it did comprise a significant portion of the FVC. This is often seen in individuals with restrictive patterns and/or reduced lung volumes.

Gas exchange analysis was limited to oxygen saturation, which was normal.

Oxygen consumption was 48% of predicted in this submaximal study, and the ventilatory threshold could not be determined. This is not surprising in a submaximal test.

Flow-Volume Loops: F-V loops showed no evidence of flow limitation. The resting graph is a plot of the maximal F-V loop versus her tidal breathing. The warm-up and 60-watt graphs demonstrate her tidal breathing plotted against both her resting maximal F-V loop (see F-V graphs) and partial loops performed during exercise.

Treatment

The purpose of this test was to discover whether the subject needed another surgical dilatation for subglottic stenosis. Visual inspection via bronchoscopy showed the area to be the same diameter as measured earlier. Despite this, she had an increase in dyspnea on exertion. The surgical procedure was deferred, based on the results of the F-V loop analysis during exercise. The subject was enrolled in a pulmonary rehabilitation program to improve her exercise tolerance.

SELF-ASSESSMENT QUESTIONS

Entry-Level

1. Which of the following are required to perform a 6MWT?
   1. Countdown timer
   2. Lap counter
   3. 30-ft unobstructed hallway
   4. Sphygmomanometer
   a. 1 and 2
   b. 1, 2, and 3
   c. 1, 2, and 4
   d. 2, 3, and 4

2. In an adult patient with a resting BP of 130/90, which of the following responses would be an indication to stop an exercise test?
   a. Systolic increase to 180, diastolic increase to 95
   b. Systolic increase to 255, diastolic increase to 130
   c. Systolic increase to 160, diastolic increase to 100
   d. Systolic remains at 130, diastolic decrease to 85

3. What cycle ergometer protocol should the technologist select, based on the information provided?

Pred HR	175	Pred $\dot{V}o_2$	2.40 L/min
Height	69 in.	Weight	190 lb
FVC	4.65 L	FEV_1	3.74 L

   a. 10 watts/min
   b. 15 watts/min
   c. 20 watts/min
   d. 25 watts/min

4. Which of the following is an indication for terminating a cardiopulmonary exercise test?
   a. Shortness of breath (Borg = 4)
   b. A 2-mm down-sloping ST-segment depression
   c. Five premature ventricular contractions per minute
   d. Failure of pulse oximeter sensor

5. This graph plots $\dot{V}_E$ and $\dot{V}co_2$ against $\dot{V}o_2$. At approximately what $\dot{V}o_2$ does the ventilatory threshold occur?

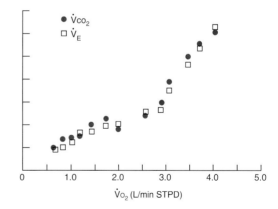

   a. 1.0 L/min
   b. 2.0 L/min
   c. 3.0 L/min
   d. 4.0 L/min

6. The "phase delay" between flow at the mouth and analysis of O_2 and CO_2 is necessary for calibration of a
   a. mixing chamber–type exercise system.
   b. rebreathing cardiac output system.
   c. standard Fick cardiac output determination.
   d. breath-by-breath exhaled gas analysis system.

Advanced

7. Which results from a maximal exercise test would be consistent for a patient who has severe COPD?
   1. $\dot{V}_E$/MVV 90%
   2. V_T/VC 48%
   3. V_D/V_T 12%
   4. A-a gradient 45
      a. 1 and 4
      b. 1 and 2
      c. 2, 3, and 4
      d. 1, 2, and 4

8. A 61-year-old woman with dyspnea on exertion has the following results from a cardiopulmonary exercise test:

	Rest	Maximal Exercise	Pred
HR	88	154	170
$\dot{V}_{O_2}$ (mL/kg)	4	17	23
$\dot{V}_E$ (L)	9.0	44.0	90.0
V_T (mL)	575	685	
RR (per min)	12	64	
V_D/V_T (%)	45	50	

These findings are most consistent with
   a. ventilatory limitation.
   b. pulmonary hypertension.
   c. inappropriate breathing strategy.
   d. pulmonary fibrosis.

9. Tidal breathing loops at different stages of exercise are plotted against the resting maximal F-V curve. Which of the following best describes the data?
   a. Inappropriate breathing strategy
   b. Dynamic hyperinflation
   c. No significant flow limitation
   d. Fixed obstruction

10. A patient has the following results of a cardiopulmonary exercise test (values in parentheses are percentages of predicted):

$\dot{V}_{O_2}$ max (L / min,STPD)	3.44	(97%)
HRmax (beats/min)	171	(95%)
$\dot{V}_E$ max (L / min,BTPS)	60	(47%)

Which of the following best describes these results?
   a. Mild aerobic impairment consistent with deconditioning
   b. Poor patient effort indicated by low maximal ventilation
   c. Moderate exercise impairment with ventilatory limitation
   d. Normal exercise response

11. A patient performs a symptom-limited maximal exercise test on a cycle ergometer using a ramp protocol of 20 watts/min. The ventilatory threshold is measured at 39% of the patient's peak $\dot{V}_{O_2}$. These findings are consistent with which of the following?
   a. Inappropriate ergometer protocol
   b. Poor patient effort
   c. Early onset of anaerobic metabolism
   d. Normal cardiovascular response

12. A patient has the following results of an exercise test:

	Maximal Exercise	Predicted
HR (beats/min)	119	159
ST change (mm)	0.5	<1
$\dot{V}_E$ (mL/min/kg)	10.2	22
$\dot{V}_E$ (L/min)	37	42
Pa_{O_2} (mm Hg)	53	>85

Which of the following clinical conditions is most consistent with these findings?
   a. COPD
   b. Poor patient effort
   c. Exercise-induced bronchospasm
   d. Coronary artery disease

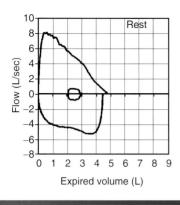
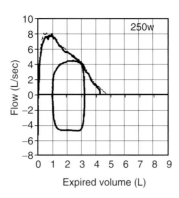
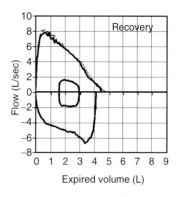

SELECTED BIBLIOGRAPHY

General References

American College of Sports Medicine. *Guidelines for exercise testing and exercise prescription* (10th ed.). Wolters Kluwer. Philadelphia PA.

American College of Sports Medicine. (2014). *Resource manual for guidelines for exercise testing and prescription* (7th ed.). Wolters Kluwer- Lippincott Williams & Wilkins Philadelphia PA.

Jones, N. L. (1997). *Clinical exercise testing* (4th ed.). Philadelphia, PA: WB Saunders.

Sietsema KE, Sue, DY, Stringer WW, Ward, SA. *Wasserman & Whipp's Principles of exercise testing and interpretation* (6th ed.). Wolters Kluwer. Philadelphia PA.

Weber, K. T., & Janicki, J. S. (1986). *Cardiopulmonary exercise testing: Physiologic principles and clinical applications*. Philadelphia, PA: WB Saunders.

Six-Minute Walk Test

An Official European Thoracic Society and American Thoracic Society Technical Standard. Field Walking Tests in Chronic Respiratory Disease. (2014). *European Respiratory Journal, 44,* 1428–1446.

Casanova, C., Celli, B. R., Barria, P., et al. (2011). on behalf of the Six-Minute Walk Distance Project (ALAT). The 6-minute walk distance in healthy subjects: Reference standards from seven countries. *European Respiratory Journal, 37,* 150–156.

Cote, C. G., Casanova, C., Marin, J. M., et al. (2008). Validation and comparison of reference equations for the 6-minute walk distance test. *European Respiratory Journal, 31,* 571–578.

Enfield, K., Gammon, S., Floyd, J., et al. (2010). Six-minute walk distance in patients with severe end-stage COPD. *Journal of Cardiopulmonary Rehabilitation and Prevention, 30,* 195–202.

Enright, P. L., & Sherrill, D. L. (1998). Reference equations for the six-minute walk in healthy adults. *American Journal of Respiratory and Critical Care Medicine, 158,* 1384–1387.

Reference Equations

Blackie, S. P., Fairbarn, M. S., McElvaney, G. N., et al. (1989). Prediction of maximal oxygen uptake and power during cycle ergometry in subjects older than 55 years of age. *American Review of Respiratory Disease, 139,* 1424–1429.

Cooper, D. M., & Weiler-Ravell, D. (1984). Gas Exchange Response to Exercise in Children. *American Review of Respiratory Disease, 129*(2), S47–S48.

Hansen, J.E., Sue, D.Y., and Wasserman, K., "Predicted values for clinical exercise.

Jones, N., Makrides, L., Hitchcock, C., et.al. "Normal standards for an incremental progressive cycle ergometer test, *American Review of Respiratory Disease,* vol. 131, no. 5, pp. 700–708, 1985.

Koch, B., Schaper, C., Ittermann, T., Spielhagen, T., et al. (2009). Reference values for cardiopulmonary exercise testing in healthy volunteers: The SHIP study. *Eur Respir J, 33,* 389–397.

Kokkinos, P., Kaminsky, L., Arena, R., Zhang, J., Myers, J. A new generalized cycle ergometry equation for predicting maximal oxygen uptake: The Fitness Registry and the Importance of Exercise National Database (FRIEND) European Journal of Preventive Cardiology April 2018.

Myers, J., Kaminsky, L. A., Lima, R., Christle, J. W., Ashley, E., & Arena, R. (2017). A Reference Equation for Normal Standards for VO2 Max: Analysis from the Fitness Registry and the Importance of Exercise National Database (FRIEND Registry) Progress in Cardiovascular Dz. *Elsevier.*, 21–29.

Neder, A., Nery, L., Peres, C., & Whipp, B. (2001). Reference Values for Dynamic Responses to Incremental Cycle Ergometry in Males and Females Aged 20 to 80. *Am J Respir Crit Care Med, 164,* 1481–1486.

Cardiovascular Monitoring During Exercise

Bruce, R. A. (1984). Value and limitations of the electrocardiogram in progressive exercise testing. *American Review of Respiratory Disease, 129*(Suppl.), S28.

Daida, H., Allison, T. G., Squires, R. W., et al. (1996). Peak exercise blood pressure stratified by age and gender in apparently healthy subjects. *Mayo Clinic Proceedings, 71,* 445.

Ventilation, Gas Exchange, and Blood Gases

Beaver, W. L., Wasserman, K., & Whipp, B. J. (1986). A new method for detection of anaerobic threshold by gas exchange. *Journal of Applied Physiology, 60,* 2020–2027.

Blackie, S. P., Fairbarn, M. S., McElvaney, N. G., et al. (1991). Normal values and ranges for ventilation and breathing pattern at maximal exercise. *Chest, 100,* 136–142.

Eschenbacher, W. L., & Mannina, A. (1990). An algorithm for the interpretation of cardiopulmonary exercise tests. *Chest, 97,* 263–267.

Johnson, B. D., Beck, K. C., Zeballos, R. J., et al. (1999). Advances in pulmonary laboratory testing. *Chest, 116,* 1377–1387.

Johnson, B. D., Weisman, I. M., Zeballos, R. J., et al. (1999). Emerging concepts in the evaluation of ventilatory limitation during exercise—the exercise tidal flow-volume loop. *Chest, 116,* 488–503.

Proctor, D. N., & Beck, K. C. (1996). Delay time adjustments to minimize errors in breath-by-breath measurement of VO_2 during exercise. *Journal of Applied Physiology, 81,* 2495–2499.

Yamaya, Y., Bogaard, H. J., Wagner, P. D., et al. (2002). Validity of pulse oximetry during maximal exercise in normoxia, hypoxia, and hyperoxia. *Journal of Applied Physiology, 92,* 162–168.

Standards and Guidelines

ACC/AHA Clinical competence statement on stress testing: A report of the American College of Cardiology/American Heart Association/American College of Physicians–American Society of Internal Medicine Task Force on Clinical Competence. (2000). *Journal of the American College of Cardiology, 36,* 1441–1453.

AHA. (2013). Exercise standards for testing and training: A Scientific Statement from the American Heart Association. (2013). *Circulation, 128,* 873–934.

American Association for Respiratory Care. Clinical practice guideline: Exercise testing for evaluation of hypoxemia and/or desaturation. (2001). *Respiratory Care, 46,* 514–522.

ATS/ACCP statement on cardiopulmonary exercise testing. (2003). *American Journal of Respiratory and Critical Care Medicine, 167,* 211–277.

Clinical and Laboratory Standards Institute (CLSI). Quality management system: A model for laboratory services, approved guideline. (2011). *QMS01-A4.* Wayne, PA: CLSI.

CLSI. Blood gas and pH analysis and related measurements, approved guideline. (2009). *C46-A2.* Wayne, PA: CLSI.

CLSI. Procedures for the collection of arterial blood specimens, approved standard. (2004). *H11-A4.* Wayne, PA: CLSI.

Recommendations for Clinical Exercise Laboratories: A Scientific Statement from the American Heart Association. (2009). *Circulation, 119,* 3144–3161.

Chapter 8

Pediatric Pulmonary Function Testing

KATRINA M. HYNES, MHA, RRT, RPFT

CHAPTER OUTLINE

LEARNING OBJECTIVES

After studying the chapter and reviewing the figures, tables, and case studies, you should be able to do the following:

Entry-level
1. State how the combined American Thoracic Society–European Respiratory Society (ATS-ERS) task force guidelines relate to pulmonary function testing and, specifically, spirometry in children.

2. Suggest techniques for approaching young children, gaining their confidence, and ensuring maximal effort.
3. Identify common technique and/or effort-related errors during forced vital capacity (FVC) maneuvers and the resultant effect on the reliability of testing.
4. Discuss the potential importance of examining both the expiratory and inspiratory loops during spirometry.
5. State the most common pharmaceutical agent used for bronchoprovocation testing and the steps involved in performing this challenge in children.
6. State limitations and considerations for equipment as they relate to testing in children for the measurement of lung volumes and diffusion capacity.
7. State the physiologic and testing effects that sedation may produce in infants.
8. Identify various passive techniques to evaluate pulmonary function in infants, toddlers, and preschool children.
9. State the components of lung volume measurements that can be obtained in well-sedated infants and the equipment necessary to make those measurements.

Advanced

1. According to ATS-ERS recommendations, the end-of-test criteria have been changed to end of expiratory flow, with a minimum of 1 second needed to calculate certain pediatric values (e.g., $FEV_{0.5}$ and $FEV_{0.75}$).
2. Discuss a scenario when the $FEV_{0.5}$ and $FEV_{0.75}$ may be a valuable parameter when performing spirometry in young children.
3. Explain the limitations of the $FEF_{25\%-75\%}$ in a young child performing spirometry.
4. Compare the appearance of the flow-volume loop in variable intrathoracic versus extrathoracic obstruction and fixed patterns of obstruction, and provide examples of pediatric disorders associated with each.
5. State the difference between direct and indirect methods of bronchoprovocation, and give examples of each.
6. Discuss problems associated with the delivery of pharmaceutical agents in pediatric patients, and state advantages and disadvantages of each.
7. Discuss the added benefit of performing lung volume measurements in pediatric patients to differentiate obstructive and restrictive components of disease.
8. Identify potential problems in obtaining diffusion capacity measurements in children, and relate the effect of potential errors to resultant data.
9. Discuss the role of passive mechanics in evaluating infants and toddlers.
10. Compare and contrast an adult plethysmograph and an infant plethysmograph.
11. State the purpose of performing the raised volume technique when measuring lung volumes in infants.
12. Define the components that comprise respiratory impedance (Z), and state how airway reactivity can be evaluated using these measurements.

KEY TERMS

airway resistance (Raw)
asynchrony
dynamic FRC
exhaled nitric oxide (eNO)
flow transient
forced oscillation technique (FOT)
Hering–Breuer reflex
impedance

impulse oscillometry (IOS)
interrupter technique (Rint)
lung clearance index (LCI)
malacia
multiple-breath washout (MBW)
passive occlusion technique
raised volume technique

rapid thoracoabdominal compression (RTC)
reactance (X_{rs})
resonant frequency
respiratory inductive plethysmography (RIP)
static compliance (C_{rs})
time constant
vocal cord dysfunction (VCD)

Pulmonary function testing in children is one of the most dynamic and challenging aspects of pulmonary physiology. Although technologic improvements have affected all areas of pulmonary function testing, the implications for testing children are especially evident. Improved accuracy and precision of flow sensors, combined with user-friendly computer software, make measurements of respiratory mechanics more easily obtainable. The range and sophistication of equipment are broad. Suitable systems are available for physician offices, hospital clinic settings, and clinical and research-oriented pulmonary function laboratories. Guidelines from the American Thoracic Society and the European Respiratory Society (ATS-ERS) have redefined the concepts of repeatability and reproducibility and have provided recommendations for the pediatric population. Recently, international workgroups have organized a global initiative to collect normative data and publish reference sets for a variety of pulmonary function tests (PFTs) that span broader age and ethnic groups. Infants and toddlers, of course, are unable to follow specific instructions. Respiratory measurements in this age group are limited to techniques independent of effort or that involve mechanical manipulation of the patient's chest. The specialized equipment and techniques needed for these measurements are discussed in the chapter. Preschool children present a different array of challenges for the clinician, and alternative techniques for measuring respiratory mechanics are available for young children. Standard measurements of pulmonary function are still the mainstay for children able to understand and cooperate with testing. The primary limiting factor for the pediatric patient, even into the teenage years, is the "effort and cooperation" component. The chapter focuses on practical tips, techniques, and guidelines for obtaining pulmonary function data in all age groups that are reliable and relevant in assessing respiratory ailments in children.

INFANT, TODDLER, AND PRESCHOOL PULMONARY FUNCTION TESTING

The challenge for diagnostic testing in infants, toddlers, and preschool children is their lack of comprehension of instruction. Even obtaining a value as simple as an oximetry reading may not be so simple in a crying young child or a wiggling baby. Toddlers may be capable of understanding simple instructions but can be fearful of the hospital environment, unfamiliar faces, or strange-looking equipment. Expecting full cooperation and maximal effort is unrealistic. Alternative methods of assessing pulmonary function have been developed. The ability to obtain forced flows and lung volume measurements remains the cornerstone of pulmonary function testing, even in the youngest patient. Modifications of technique and specialized equipment are necessary, however. Newer, less invasive methods of measuring tidal breathing mechanics, **airway resistance (Raw),** thoracoabdominal motion, impedance, and airway inflammation continue to be investigated and are promising techniques. Some of the techniques discussed in the following sections are available in clinical pediatric laboratories; however, other techniques are currently used primarily in the research arena. Clinical applications will be more apparent as experience and standardization of techniques are developed. Pediatric research trials grow in number yearly, and through these research trials, the relevance of the following procedures will be validated.

Purpose of Pulmonary Function Tests for Infants and Toddlers

Infant and toddler PFTs provide important data regarding growth of the lungs, identification of airflow obstruction, progression of a disease state, and response to therapeutic interventions. Infant PFTs require a significant time commitment and competent and patient clinicians. Commercially available equipment typically uses the most technically advanced flow sensors and analyzers that are able to accurately measure a range that extends to the gas volumes of the smallest newborn. Such technology may be expensive for a pulmonary laboratory to purchase. Before pursuing this type of testing, the laboratory should thoroughly evaluate its expectations and goals and the resources available to perform quality testing.

Performance of Pulmonary Function Testing in Infants and Toddlers

Newborn babies, older infants, and young toddlers are not capable of following the directions needed to perform conscious PFTs. Placing a mask on an infant is usually not tolerated and results in a screaming baby. Even a child who permits a mask over his or her nose and mouth invariably changes his or her breathing pattern (i.e., volume and frequency of breathing). Only premature babies and young newborns will tolerate a mask while sleeping. In these specific and rare instances, it may be possible to assess passive tidal breathing mechanics. More sophisticated PFTs that measure lung volumes and forced flows require the infant to be in a quiet sleep, fully relaxed, and spontaneously breathing. To accomplish this state of sleep and cooperation, the child must be sedated.

Sedation as an Important Consideration

Sedation of infants and toddlers is a common practice in pediatric hospitals because many procedures require a calm, motionless child. The hospital anesthesia department usually establishes procedures and protocols for sedation of children that follow The Joint Commission (TJC) guidelines. It is essential that established procedures be closely observed for the protection of the child, the pulmonary laboratory, and the hospital. The sedating agent chosen, the personnel needed, and the required recovery time all depend on the extent of testing needed and patient history. A straightforward test in an uncomplicated infant can be safely performed by minimal personnel with the use of an oral sedating agent, such as chloral hydrate (CH). At the other end of the spectrum may be an infant with an unstable airway, severe pulmonary compromise, or other organ complications. This scenario may warrant an anesthesiologist and sedation nurse in addition to the clinician(s) performing the test.

CH is a relatively safe and easy sedating medication to administer, although several other intravenous (IV) agents are available within the current armamentarium of drugs. The advantages of CH are that it is administered orally and may not require all the resources of a "sedation team." However, sedation of infants has become a highly regulated and supervised service of the anesthesia department. Many hospitals now require that any sedation, including CH, be given by sedation-certified physicians, nurses, or nurse anesthetists. CH, arguably once classified as a "conscious sedating agent," is now considered to produce unconscious sedation in the higher dosing ranges. Refer to institutional policies regarding dosing and drug administration. An important action of CH is that it generally maintains the infant's normal respiratory pattern. This is not the case for most IV sedation agents. Additionally, predicted reference sets for infant PFTs have almost exclusively been obtained using CH as the sedation agent. If a child sleeps well during this type of sedation and for ample time, he or she arouses easily by the end of the test. An unfortunate disadvantage of CH is that a large quantity of a very unpleasant medicine must be swallowed. The most common side effect of the oral dose sedation is vomiting. Recent studies recommend that infants younger than 6 months receive formula and solids for up to 6 hours before sedation, breast milk for up to 4 hours, and clear liquids for up to 2 hours. Children who are 6 months or older may receive solids and liquids for up to 6 hours and clear liquids for up to 2 hours before sedation. Crying and upset stomachs are also common side effects. Nevertheless, CH works very well in the majority of cases.

IV narcotics such as pentobarbital or secobarbital need to be administered and monitored by a sedation nurse or nurse anesthetist. The advantage of IV medications is that IV access is available if needed, and the medication can be titrated to the child's need. Additional options include ketamine and propofol. Both of these drugs require a physician and possibly an anesthesiologist or specially trained hospitalist to administer. The rapid onset of action and quick recovery make these attractive sedating agents but also require close monitoring for apnea. Although these alternatives exist, CH remains the preferred mode of sedation for infant PFTs.

Regardless of the agent chosen, safety is the primary concern. The child must be closely monitored throughout the entire procedure, including recovery. Because of the moderate level of sedation needed, hospital policies require that a pediatric physician trained in advanced cardiac life support (ACLS) be present. Written documentation of the sedation procedure is to be placed in the patient's medical record. A fully stocked crash cart should be nearby; a resuscitation bag and mask should be on the patient's bed. Loss of a patent airway is always possible with any sedating agent. It is also extremely important to remember that sleep induced with sedation is not natural sleep. Changes in respiratory pattern, depth of respiration, and breathing frequency should be noted. Interpretation of any test of respiratory mechanics should be made with the level of sedation in mind.

PF TIP 8.1

Sedated sleep in infants is never natural sleep, and respiratory measurements made during sedated sleep may be influenced by the altered sleep state.

When Children Are Too Old for Infant-Style Testing and Too Young for Standard Testing

Once toddlers reach ages 2½ to 3 years, changes are occurring that make it more difficult to perform the infant-style PFTs. The most obvious is that the child may "outgrow" the size of the plethysmograph. CH sedation may no longer be an option, with testing therefore requiring general anesthesia. IV sedatives (narcotics, ketamine, propofol) carry more risks, and the expense increases, with additional personnel required to deliver more complicated sedations. As a result, the risks and cost of sedation may outweigh the benefits of the test. Physiologic changes are also occurring as the infant grows through the toddler and preschool years. The child's chest wall becomes more rigid, and the Hering–Breuer reflex disappears. This makes several of the techniques discussed in the following sections available only to infants and small toddlers but unavailable to children in the 3-year-old to 5-year-old range. Young children also may be able to tolerate simple passive

mechanics without the need for sedation. Earlier in the chapter, spirometric measurements in young children were discussed. The following sections discuss several other available techniques to measure pulmonary mechanics. Some may be performed on any patient from infancy through adulthood, and some are developed specifically for infants, toddlers, and preschool children.

Lung Volume Measurement

As with measurement of lung volumes in adults, the lung volume compartments in the infant can be measured by several techniques, including gas dilution and whole-body plethysmography. Until recently, infant pulmonary research laboratories almost exclusively performed body plethysmography in infants. Only a few manufacturers produce commercially available body boxes for infants (Fig. 8.1). Whole-body plethysmography in an infant presents a unique set of challenges. The theory and technical aspects of measuring V_{TG}, previously discussed in Chapter 4, are essentially the same for adults and infants but with several additional caveats. The sedated infant is placed in a supine position with the nose and mouth surrounded by a tight-fitting mask with putty placed around the edges to create an airtight seal with a small dead-space volume.

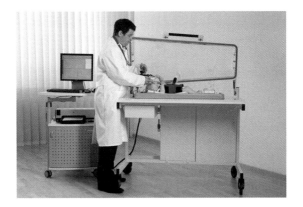

FIG. 8.1 Infant body plethysmograph. Whole-body infant plethysmograph directly measures V_{TG} (forced reserve capacity [FRC] at resting level). The infant body box also has the capability of obtaining passive mechanics and forced flows (partial and raised volume) and provides close estimation of fractional lung volumes. (The photograph of the infant body box is © 2021 Vyaire Medical, Inc.; Used with permission.)

Facemasks can cause trigeminal nerve stimulation and induce vagal reflexes that may alter the pattern of heart rate and rhythm or respiratory frequency and pattern. For this reason, exercise caution whenever using a facemask. Rapidly moving valves may make airway occlusions at end inspiration or end-expiration for determination of V_{TG} and Raw. The infant does not pant. However, tidal breaths may be shallow; therefore the pressure transducers and flow sensors must be critically precise and accurate. In addition, the infant body box is relatively small, and temperature changes can dramatically alter these measurements. Therefore the temperature in the box must be controlled and the air vented.

Signal-to-noise ratios are particularly critical in an infant plethysmograph. Although the child is motionless, safety features must permit rapid access to the box and the baby. The breathing apparatus should be easily removable in case the child is in distress or vomits. The advantage of plethysmography in infants is that it accurately measures V_{TG}, and thus forced reserve capacity (FRC) may be determined. Because the infant is not capable of performing a voluntary maximal inspiration or expiration, residual volume (RV) and total lung capacity (TLC) cannot be obtained in the traditional manner. However, if the infant pulmonary function system is capable of performing raised volumes and forced thoracic compressions, then a full set of fractional lung volumes can be estimated. A forced squeeze from TLC provides a volume close to a vital capacity (VC) measurement and can be used to calculate expiratory reserve volume (ERV), RV, TLC, FRC/TLC, and RV/TLC.

Multiple-Breath Washout Including Lung Clearance Index

Optional methods of determining lung volumes are available for infants, as well as for toddlers and young children. These include **multiple-breath washout (MBW)** techniques that use inert gases such as helium, sulfur hexafluoride (SF_6), and nitrogen. Additional information on these testing techniques is presented in Chapter 4.

The Cystic Fibrosis Foundation reported that MBW was "a valuable potential outcome measure for CF clinical trials in preschool-aged patients."

The American Thoracic Society (ATS) technical statement on MBW notes that these techniques are technically easy to perform. However, gas equilibration techniques have several disadvantages applicable to both infants and young children. Infants will still require sedation. Children ages 2 to 6 years may tolerate sitting in a chair with a mouthpiece/nose clips or facemask applied. Distractors to the awake child, such as a tablet computer or reading by a parent, are often necessary to obtain a quality test. Fussing and movement lead to leaks in the systems and may falsely elevate FRC values. In addition, steady breathing patterns without extreme changes in respiratory ranges are desired. When possible and practical, facemasks should be sealed with therapeutic putty. Dead space from the mask and valve switching apparatus should be taken into consideration. Adequate inspiratory flow with an appropriate inspired O_2 concentration should be available to the patient. Children with intrathoracic airflow obstruction may have poor ventilation distal to obstructed airways, causing an incomplete washout or equilibration and falsely low FRC values. The smaller the child, the smaller the radius of the airways, and superimposed obstruction from secretions or bronchospasm will further narrow the airway.

After completing an MBW test, different indices of ventilation inhomogeneity can be calculated, with the **lung clearance index (LCI)** being the most common. LCI is the cumulative expired volume (CEV) divided by the measured FRC (LCI = CEV/FRC).

The effect of sedation in infants may compound the problem and inhibit the natural sigh mechanism, resulting in atelectasis, hypoventilation, or hypoxemia. Monitoring end-tidal CO_2 is helpful in this regard. Infants do have an incredible ability to adjust their FRC, depending on their clinical status. Babies may respond to hypoxia by dynamically elevating their FRC to create an effect similar to positive end-expiratory pressure (PEEP), termed **dynamic FRC.** Grunting is a clinical sign that an infant may be hypoxic. In this situation, further sedation and supplemental O_2 tend to relax a child. It is possible to see consecutive FRC measurements decrease as the infant falls into a deeper sedation and static lung volume decreases to a resting FRC. Nevertheless, the measurement of FRC is an important parameter in pulmonary function testing. The preceding clinical scenarios should, however, be taken into account. The normal FRC range for an infant is between 15 and 25 mL/kg of weight and 2 and 3 mL/cm of length. Current recommendations state that three technically acceptable tests should be performed. The average of the three acceptable efforts is reported. Two technically acceptable tests are usable in the event a third maneuver is unattainable. The repeatability target is 10% of the mean. If the FRC differs from the median of all three tests by greater than 25%, the test should not be reported. The wait time between maneuvers should be a minimum of the total time it took the lungs to wash out. For example, if the washout time took 3.5 minutes, the operator would need to wait a minimum of 3.5 minutes before repeating the maneuver.

Passive Tidal Techniques to Measure Respiratory Mechanics
Passive Tidal Loops

Many studies have examined the passive tidal loops of infants and have attempted to differentiate normal tidal loops from loops associated with airflow obstruction. Fewer studies have concentrated on passive mechanics in preschool-aged children. Several parameters have been suggested to examine intrathoracic airflow obstruction during tidal breathing, such as t_{TPEF}/t_E (ratio of time to reach tidal peak flow to total expiratory time) and V_{PTEF}/V_E. Even recording simple measures such as tidal volume (V_T), respiratory rate, and minute ventilation may have some benefit. Passive loops are highly variable, however, and the degree of variability may differ for different age groups. They are especially subject to changes in upper airway tone, as may be seen with sedation or with laryngeal or diaphragmatic braking. As mentioned previously, infants can adduct their vocal cords (grunt) during exhalation to create a physiologic PEEP. Likewise, they have the ability to modulate their diaphragms and intercostal muscles in an attempt to dynamically elevate their FRC and improve oxygenation. Therefore the shape of tidal loops and the parameters used to describe the shape may change from

minute to minute. To ensure repeatability of measures, it is advisable to express these parameters as a mean of at least 10 consecutive breaths or at least 30 seconds of tidal breathing. The coefficient of variation (CV) should also be reported. Baseline passive measurements may then be compared with like parameters after any desired intervention (e.g., bronchodilator). As with standard pulmonary function testing, passive tidal loops are not maximal maneuvers. Therefore efforts have concentrated on techniques to identify flow limitation and quantify forced flow measurements.

Passive Compliance, Resistance, and Time Constants

The chest wall of the infant is extremely compliant, unlike that of an adult. It does not contribute significantly to the compliance of the total respiratory system. Measuring pulmonary mechanics in the infant takes advantage of this important difference. Noninvasive measures of respiratory system compliance, therefore, directly reflect the child's lung compliance. **Static compliance (C_{rs})** describes the elastic properties of the total respiratory system. The two components of C_{rs}, change in pressure and change in volume, are obtained. In simplest terms, *compliance* is defined as the change in volume divided by the change in pressure ($C = \Delta V/\Delta P$; see Chapter 4). In a quiet, relaxed baby (usually sedated), these parameters can be measured easily. The method is referred to as the **passive occlusion technique.** Rapid occlusion of the airway may occur once (single occlusion) at the end of a tidal breath or with multiple occlusions at different lung volumes. Young infants will hold their breath when their airway is occluded. This phenomenon is known as the **Hering–Breuer reflex** and is present in children until approximately 1 year of age. The occlusion creates an apneic pause and relaxes the respiratory muscles. During a single-breath occlusion and breath hold, alveolar pressure equalizes and can be measured by a pressure transducer at the airway opening (mouth). Once the occlusion valve opens, the child can passively exhale, and the exhaled volume can be measured by a flow sensor.

Airway resistance (Raw) can be easily calculated from the same maneuver. It reflects the nonelastic airway and tissue forces resisting gas flow. *Resistance* is defined as the change in driving pressure divided by flow (R = $\Delta P/\dot{V}$) and is described in centimeters of water per liter per second (cm H_2O/L/s). Raw is dependent on the radius length and the number of airways and varies with volume, flow, and respiratory frequency. With the maneuver described, the driving pressure is the plateau pressure (alveolar pressure) measured at the airway opening developed during the occlusion. Flow is the peak flow (discounting pneumotach artifact) measured from the passive exhalation. Refer to Fig. 8.2. The graphs on the left side of the page represent passive exhalation after occlusion. The graphs on the right depict

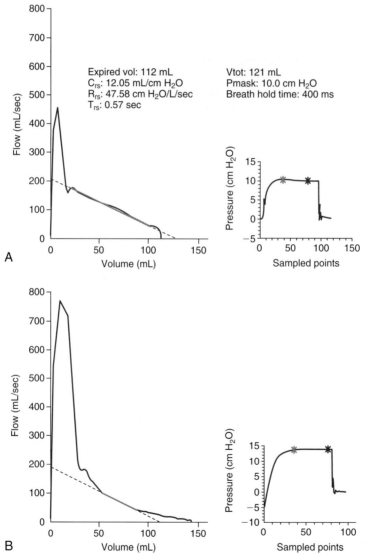

FIG. 8.2 Passive occlusion/exhalation mechanics in infants. (A) An infant's passive tidal exhalation after an airway occlusion. The slope of the curve is linear, and the infant exhales to a relaxed forced reserve capacity (FRC). (B) Passive tidal exhalation showing lungs with multiple time constants, meaning that the lung does not empty homogeneously.

the increase in airway opening pressure to plateau (alveolar) pressure during occlusion. A normal passive exhalation after occlusion in an infant without any lung disease is shown in Fig. 8.2A. Typically, the passive exhalation occlusion technique can be performed with little disturbance to the infant. However, infants with severe lung disease have an increased respiratory drive, and it may not be possible to induce a Hering–Breuer response.

The slope of the curve is linear as the baby exhales to a relaxed FRC. Children with airflow obstruction do not empty their lungs at a constant rate. The expiration may be forced with paradoxical movement of the diaphragm and belly. The accuracy of compliance and Raw measurements made under these conditions is poor. The exhaled curve may end abruptly with the child at an elevated FRC or may appear "scooped out" or curvilinear, as in Fig. 8.2B. The lungs do not empty homogeneously or uniformly and therefore have multiple time constants. One **time constant** represents the amount of time to expire approximately ⅔ of the V_T. Time constant (T_{rs} or τ) is easily calculated as compliance times resistance ($T_{rs} = C_{rs} \times R_{rs}$). Because respiratory system compliance is dependent on the lung volume at which it is measured, it may be important to "correct" the measured parameter by the infant's FRC. As mentioned earlier, dividing the Raw or actual compliance by the FRC yields specific compliance.

PF TIP 8.2

The diameter of the airway is an important determinant of flow. Inflammation or secretions in the airways of a young child can cause significant intrathoracic obstruction and profound clinical symptoms.

Single-breath passive measurement of compliance is not feasible in the toddler and older age groups. The chest wall develops more rigidity as the child ages and becomes an increasingly important factor in the overall measure of respiratory system compliance. Additionally, loss of the Hering–Breuer reflex makes equilibration of pressure from the alveolus to the mouth more difficult to achieve.

Compliance in infants can also be determined by other methods, including the insertion of an esophageal catheter or by weighted spirometry. Although inserting an esophageal catheter into an infant is usually not difficult, it is invasive, and the exact placement of the catheter may affect measurements. In addition, the distortion of pleural pressure in children with airflow obstruction causes associated artifactual changes, yielding inaccurate compliance values. Under ideal circumstances, when accurate pleural pressures are measured, total respiratory system compliance can be subdivided into the chest wall and lung compliance components.

Children undergoing intubation and ventilation represent an additional challenge when assessing pulmonary mechanics. Several of the parameters discussed can also be obtained in babies on ventilators; however, several technical and mechanical problems must be considered. The endotracheal tube represents a resistor and can limit flow and alter pressure readings at the airway opening. Endotracheal tubes in infants are generally uncuffed, and leaks around the tubes are common. Secretions in the endotracheal tube and water condensation in the tubing easily clog pneumotachometers. Ventilators offer a variety of operational modes, such as pressure or volume control, intermittent mandatory ventilation (IMV) or synchronized IMV (SIMV), and pressure support. Depending on the mode chosen, auxiliary flow through the ventilator circuit will result in inaccurate flow measurements at the child's airway. Children on ventilators are often sedated, and passive mechanics are dependent on the sleep state. For all the reasons stated, only experienced clinicians who are familiar with the child and the ventilator should do pulmonary mechanics on children undergoing ventilation. In addition, measurements made under artificial conditions (e.g., ventilator, PEEP) do not necessarily reflect the infant's own lung mechanics when not ventilated.

Thoracoabdominal Motion Analysis

One of the main disadvantages of all the measurements discussed in the preceding sections is that they involve the use of a mask or mouthpiece. Unfortunately, the presence of any foreign body in the airway is invasive and can alter breathing, especially passive tidal breathing. An advantage to this next technique is that it does not use any device at the mouth and can be considered truly noninvasive. Although the following techniques are not commonly performed in many clinical pediatric pulmonary function laboratories, they are central to the measurements made in a sleep laboratory. Observing the motion of the respiratory system can also provide valuable qualitative and quantitative assessment of pulmonary and chest wall mechanics. Recall the basic mechanics of breathing and the coordination of the diaphragm and respiratory muscles during the passive breathing cycle. During inspiration, the diaphragm contracts and flattens, which causes the abdomen to rise. Simultaneously, the intercostal muscles contract, pulling the ribs upward and forward. During passive expiration, the diaphragm and intercostal muscles relax, and the abdomen and chest fall. This synchronous movement of the abdomen and rib cage can be easily monitored by placing an expandable strain gauge or compliant elastic band around both the abdomen and the chest wall (rib cage). These devices differ as to how they are made and the method by which they make measurements. Although the devices differ, the principle is similar. This technique is not generally limited by size or age; therefore it can apply to infants, toddlers, older children, and even adults. The length of the strain gauges or bands is appropriate for the size of the patient. A popular example of this method is known as **respiratory inductive plethysmography (RIP)**. The band is elasticized and has coiled wire sewn through the band in a sinusoidal pattern. A very low-voltage alternating current is passed through the coils. As each band expands (as with inspiration), the coils are stretched, which alters the cross-sectional area of the bands and changes the inductance of the coiled wire. A positive voltage signal (upward deflection) can be visualized on the monitoring device for both the abdominal component and rib cage component (Fig. 8.3A). The change in the cross-sectional area is proportional to the expansion of the band and therefore the depth of the inspiratory maneuver. As passive exhalation occurs, the bands relax, and

the voltage signal drops (downward deflection), with the pattern producing a sinusoidal respiratory tracing. The movements of the rib cage and the abdomen are monitored simultaneously. Both components independently contribute to lung volume, and the sum of the two signals determines V_T.

The V_T is maximized when the rib cage and abdomen move in synchrony or are "in phase" with one another. The phase shift, Φ or phi, describes the **asynchrony** (or lack of synchrony) of the sinusoidal relationship between these two independent components. Both qualitative and quantitative information can be obtained from these tracings. A phase shift equal to 0 degrees denotes perfect synchrony. Fig. 8.3A is representative of normal, quiet breathing. The movements of the rib cage and abdomen are in complete unison or synchrony. The child's resultant V_T is the sum of the components of rib cage and abdominal movements. Fig. 8.3B represents a child with paradoxical breathing. Note that the rib cage tracing is moving in the opposite direction of the abdomen. The abdominal and rib cage components are out of phase with one another. If observing this child, one would see the abdomen appear to sink while the chest was rising. This is the extreme end of asynchrony; however, there are endless variations in the movements of the rib cage and abdomen between complete synchrony and asynchrony. The phase shift will increase from 0 degrees to a maximum of 180 degrees with complete paradoxical breathing. Refer to Fig. 8.3C. Notice the difference in the shape of the tracing of the abdominal component. There are asynchronous movements of the rib cage and abdomen in this child.

Phase shift, Φ, can also be represented on an X-Y recorder. The figures produced, known as *Lissajous figures* or *Konno–Mead loops*, graphically plot abdominal movement on the *x*-axis and rib cage movement on the *y*-axis. The arrows on the figures represent the direction of movement of the rib cage and abdomen during the respiratory cycle. Refer to the tracing in Fig. 8.3A. Perfect synchrony would produce a loop that appears to be a straight line oriented as depicted (Φ = 0 degrees). Fig. 8.3B is representative of a Konno–Mead loop that demonstrates paradoxical breathing. The phase shift for this loop is 153

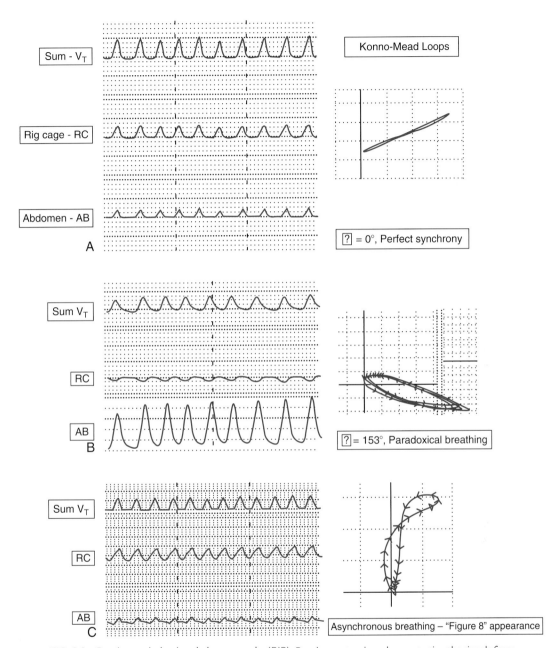

FIG. 8.3 Respiratory inductive plethysmography (RIP). Respiratory tracings demonstrating the signals from the rib cage (RC), abdomen (AB), and sum V_T (tidal volume). Accompanying each set of tracings is the corresponding Konno–Mead loop for (A) normal tidal breathing, (B) paradoxical breathing, and (C) asynchronous breathing and figure-eight Konno–Mead loop.

degrees, approaching the maximum of 180 degrees. The tracing in Fig. 8.3C represents an interesting Konno–Mead loop, as one can imagine from the asynchronous movements of the rib cage and abdomen. Notice that the figure is vertical and forms a figure eight. Unfortunately, Konno–Mead loops often form figure-eight patterns, which cannot be assigned a quantitative Φ value. There is also significant variation in the shape of Konno–Mead loops and Φ values in patients with normal and abnormal breathing patterns. The limitations of quantifying these loops make it impractical for clinical testing in a pulmonary function laboratory. Nevertheless, there is a wealth of physiologic information in these measurements, and they are a valuable tool in illustrating the relationship of rib cage movement to abdominal movement.

An important advantage of respiratory inductance plethysmography is that it is possible to calibrate the movement of the bands in quiet breathing to a flow signal from a pneumotachometer placed over the patient's mouth. This enables quantitative measurement of V_{TS} or minute ventilation over an extended period. The calibration period is very short, and the pneumotach is removed after the calibration period.

Additional Passive Techniques Available to Measure in the Preschool Child

Impulse Oscillometry

Impulse oscillometry (IOS) is also referred to as the **forced oscillation technique (FOT).** See Chapter 10 for a detailed description. A miniature loudspeaker is placed proximal to the device's flow sensor and produces forced oscillations of flow with a range of frequencies into the airway. They are sensed as popping pulsations as the child breathes tidally. The pressure oscillations generated by the sound waves are of two types: (1) those in phase with airflow, termed *resistance* (R_{rs}), and (2) those out of phase with airflow, termed **reactance (X_{rs})**. The reactance component is complex and relates to delays of pressure change caused by elastic components of the respiratory system, as well as inertia. The interaction of resistance and reactance constitutes respiratory **impedance** (Z_{rs}), or $Z_{rs} = R_{rs} + X_{rs}$.

The advantage of IOS is that it requires passive tidal breathing only. The patient is asked to breathe into a mouthpiece for approximately 30 to 60 seconds; however, only 15 to 20 seconds of stable data is required. Although it is often stated that IOS is a relatively easy test to perform, even for a small child, this is not necessarily the case. The child must sit still with a mouthpiece in his or her mouth and nose clips in place. The clinician's (or parent's) hands support the patient's cheeks and the floor of the mouth to prevent oscillations of the mouth. Gagging, swallowing, or coughing will interfere with accurate measurements. The tongue cannot move around or obstruct the mouthpiece. This can be a challenge in a 2-year-old or 3-year-old child, even for clinicians experienced in working with children. Often, several visits to the laboratory for practice are necessary to obtain repeatability in these young children. Three to five trials should be collected with a mean and CV reported. IOS should be performed before any spirometric maneuvers because the forced expirations may produce airway hyperreactivity. Several minutes should also be given between trials to allow the child to relax.

Refer to Fig. 8.4 for an example of the types of graphs that IOS measurements produce. Notice there is a graph for resistance (R_{rs}) measurements and reactance (X_{rs}) measurements. In both graphs, however, the x-axis is labeled as *Hz,* representing the multifrequency band of forced oscillations being emitted by the loudspeaker. Note in Fig. 8.3 that the resistance in this 12-year-old child's lung is higher at lower frequencies and falls as the frequency of oscillations increases. This phenomenon is known as *frequency dependence* and is a characteristic pattern for a child this age. In an adult, however, this would not be normal but more characteristic of peripheral airflow obstruction, as seen in a smoker. Caution is needed, however, in viewing resistance measurements at very low frequencies (e.g., 5 Hz) in children because of other confounding factors, such as the effect of the cardiac impulse on these measurements. Reactance measurements are even less understood. Researchers are interested in the curve that is formed by the reactance curve at 5 Hz and where it crosses "zero" reactance. The triangular region highlighted in the figure is known as *AX.*

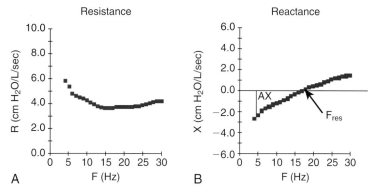

FIG. 8.4 Impulse oscillometry (IOS). Normal resistance and reactance tracings from a 12-year-old boy. (A) Note the frequency dependence of the resistance curve. (B) On the reactance curve, AX represents the area of the triangle depicted. F_{res} is the resonant frequency of the lung.

The larger the area of this region, the more abnormal the measurement, which may be related to airflow limitation. The point (Hz) that the reactance curve crosses the zero line is known as the **resonant frequency** of the lung (F_{res}). Because reactance at this point equals zero, only resistive forces are active and contributing to impedance. The resonant frequency (F_{res}) depicted in Fig. 8.4 is approximately 18 Hz.

Reference values for IOS have been collected in European children, and several ongoing studies in the United States are collecting data for additional predictive purposes. The clinical significance of IOS is yet unclear. Some researchers think that it will not provide any additional information, especially regarding peripheral airflow obstruction, for children who can be trained to do spirometry. However, there may be several scenarios in which IOS is beneficial. It may be helpful for any child who cannot perform spirometry or has a significant degree of central airway malacia. Forced flows, as with spirometry, cause compression and collapse in malacic airways, whereas IOS is a passive, tidal breathing maneuver. Patients may be able to serve as their own controls and perform this procedure serially at every clinic visit. Some laboratories have performed methacholine challenges with changes in IOS parameters as the endpoint. The sensitivity of this test may be greater than that of the FEV_1, especially with methacholine challenges, although its variability is somewhat greater.

Fig. 8.5 shows the results from a 5-year-old child performing IOS. She was unable to perform spirometry during a clinic visit to the pediatric pulmonologist. The child was very symptomatic with cough, but her pediatrician had never heard any wheezing in her lungs. Note on the data chart that the resistance and reactance measurements prebronchodilator all appear normal as a percentage of predicted. Postbronchodilator, note that the resistance measurements of R5, R10, and R20 all dropped in the range of 28% to 33%. Because of the variability of this test, it is necessary to see a percent change this high to interpret the results as a significant response to the bronchodilator. The 32% increase in reactance at 5 Hz (X5) along with the 64% decrease in AX and 42% decrease in resonant frequency (F_{res}) correlate with a decrease in resistance and a significant response to the bronchodilator. The first set of diagrams (see Fig. 8.5) again illustrates how resistance and reactance are graphed at the various frequencies or hertz. Observe the change in both graphs after the bronchodilator is administered. The postbronchodilator curve for reactance (red) drops vertically or downward, indicating a drop in Raw. The postbronchodilator curve for reactance moves to the left and upward. The two diagrams at the bottom of Fig. 8.5 are a second method of graphing IOS measurements. The axes are reversed, with frequency (Hz) on the vertical axis, and both resistance and reactance are graphed on the x-axis. The line on the left side of the zero point is represented

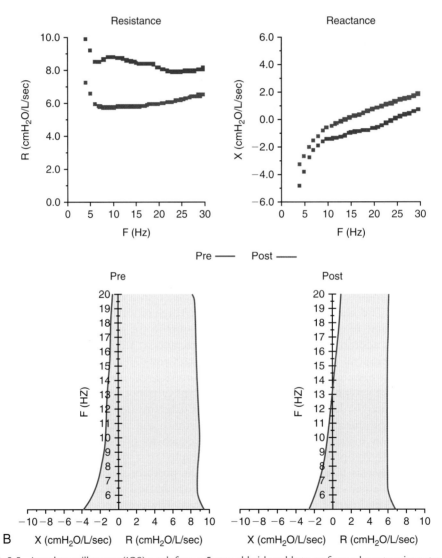

	REF	PRE	% REF	POST	% REF	% CHG
RS (cmH$_{20}$/L/sec)	9.68	9.42	97	6.68	69	−29
R10 (cmH$_{20}$/L/sec)	8.38	8.68	104	5.82	69	−33
R20 (cmH$_{20}$/L/sec)	7.00	8.24	118	5.94	85	−28
AX (cmH$_{20}$/L)	30.00	23.50		8.55		−64
X5 (cmH$_{20}$/L/sec)	−3.29	−3.24		−2.88		11
Frez (Hz)	24.14	25.30		14.76		−42
CO$_5$		0.64		0.66		
CO$_{10}$		0.93		0.90		

A

FIG. 8.5   Impulse oscillometry (IOS) result from a 5-year-old girl unable to perform adequate spirometry.

by reactance (X), and the line on the right side of zero is resistance (R). The graph is shaded between the two lines and has the appearance of a tree trunk. The higher the resistance and more negative the reactance, the wider the tree trunk. Notice postbronchodilator that the lines move closer to one another and to the zero point. The width of the tree trunk decreases as resistance falls and reactance increases (becomes less negative) postbronchodilator.

Interrupter Technique

The **interrupter technique (Rint)** is another method of measuring Raw in the very young child. It also involves passive tidal breathing, but as the name implies, the respiratory cycle is "interrupted" multiple times during the respiratory cycle. The child is seated in a position like IOS with the neck slightly extended ("sniffing" position). A clinician or parent supports the cheeks, and nose clips are in place. While the child is quietly breathing, flow is measured, and an interrupter valve closes rapidly at a preset flow or volume trigger. The valve remains closed for only 100 ms, so the child is barely able to feel these occlusions but can hear the valve closing. The principle of operation assumes a rapid equilibration of mouth pressure and alveolar pressure as the occlusions occur. Each measurement is calculated by dividing the driving pressure by the flow rate immediately before the occlusion. However, as with many physiologic measurements, other factors come into play. The resistance of the chest wall and the tissues of the lung are included in Rint measurements, so the results are not purely Raw. Rint measurements may be obtained during either inspiration or expiration, but it is still unclear whether a difference is significant. This technique has been used extensively in Europe for a considerable time but has remained primarily a research technique in the United States and abroad. Commercial devices are now available; however, predicted values are lacking in preschool children. The popularity of Rint will likely increase if the technique can show a clear clinical advantage in the pediatric population. Studies are ongoing as to the intersubject and intrasubject repeatability and reproducibility of Rint. As with IOS, this technique may serve as a clinical adjunct in assessing the bronchodilator response or with inhalation challenge protocols.

Forced Flow Techniques for Infants, Toddlers, and Preschool Children

Partial Expiratory Flow-Volume Curves

Flow is related to the volume of air in the chest during the forced exhalation. Stated simply, the larger the volume, the faster the flow. The advantage and reason for the repeatability of spirometry are that it is performed from TLC with every maneuver. As discussed earlier, with training sessions and reasonable patient effort, exhaled flows and volumes are repeatable in young children. However, if the child does not understand or cannot inhale to TLC, significant variability in flows and volumes will be observed. This is a common obstacle in the youngest of children. Traditional spirometric measurements (FVC, forced expiratory volume in the first second [FEV_1], peak expiratory flow [PEF]) may not be repeatable. These forced flows are not without merit, however. It is possible to relate these flows to a lung volume that the child can reproduce. This can be accomplished if the child is able to breathe quietly and relax for several breaths. More important, if he or she returns to a stable resting level with each exhalation, then this relaxed resting level represents the child's FRC. It is not necessary to measure FRC; rather, it represents a reference point (static lung volume) to which flow can then be related. After several tidal breaths, the child is asked to take a slightly deeper breath in and blow out as hard and long as possible. It does not matter how deep the breath is, but the forced exhalation must extend beyond the FRC point from the previous tidal breaths. Once the FRC point is identified, the flow corresponding to that point is then recorded. Because FRC is approximately 40% of TLC, flows at this relatively low lung volume correspond to flows such as $FEF_{25\%-75\%}$, $FEF_{50\%}$, and $FEF_{75\%}$ seen in standard spirometry. These flow rates are only as repeatable as the resting-level FRC. The technique may be of value in a cooperative child when assessing the response to bronchodilator therapy or performing a methacholine challenge, for example. If the child's tidal loops are highly variable, a stable FRC cannot be identified. The corresponding flow at FRC will not be reproducible in such instances. An additional confounding factor is the lack of predicted values for partial forced flows in the toddler age range. Because of the variability in testing, the trend has been to begin training in young children (age 3 years) to do full FVC maneuvers from TLC or traditional spirometry.

From a historical perspective, the technique of performing partial forced flow-volume (F-V) curves was the first attempt at obtaining forced flows in infants and dates to the late 1970s and the work of several notable respiratory physiologists. This technique is increasingly being replaced by measuring maximal forced flows from a raised lung volume close to TLC. The principle of the partial forced flows is like that described previously, but the infant must be sedated for complete relaxation. The child's chest is mechanically squeezed (or "hugged") by an inflatable jacket that surrounds the chest or by a bladder placed over the chest and upper abdominal region. The technique is referred to as **rapid thoracoabdominal compression (RTC)**. The flows that are generated are maximal

flows from within tidal range (partial forced expiratory flow). They are measured by a flow sensor (usually a pneumotachometer) attached to a mask placed on the infant's face. The lung volume that can be identified and referenced is the FRC. This is the resting level that the child passively exhales to with each tidal breath. Once the FRC point is identified on the y-axis (volume), a line can be drawn upward to intersect the F-V loop. The flow at this point is referred to as the *flow at FRC*, or *V̇ maxFRC*. Fig. 8.6 identifies these points.

It is important that several tidal loops are observed before the hugging maneuver to ensure that the infant returns with each breath to a stable resting level or FRC. The RTCs are done at progressively higher pressures until maximal flow at FRC from the child is attained. The pressures are generated from a large air reservoir connected to the hugging bag. The pressure within the hugging bag usually does not exceed 100 cm H_2O. A significantly lower pressure is transmitted across the chest wall to the lung tissue. With progressively higher hugging pressures, flow at FRC increases until flow limitation is reached. At this point, higher hugging pressures do not yield higher flows, and flow at FRC may in fact decrease. Reaching flow limitation

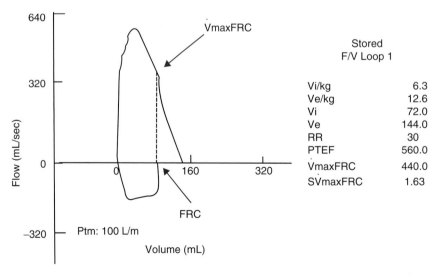

FIG. 8.6 Partial expiratory forced flow-volume (F-V) loop in an infant. Measurements include a V̇ maxFRC of 440 mL/sec and an S V̇ maxFRC of 1.63.

while doing these maneuvers is an important concept and is somewhat controversial. Because infants grow (length and weight) at such different rates and because males differ from females, the question often arises of whether flow limitation is achieved with partial forced flows. This question is especially difficult in infants with normal lung function. The problem is complicated when trying to identify normal flows for any particular child. Several infant research centers have published a collaborative study combining data from healthy infants, but technique-related differences still exist. It is recommended that PFT laboratories performing infant studies test a group of infants without respiratory difficulties to confirm that the normal values obtained concur with published reference norms. Although this type of comparison is desirable, some hospital internal review boards may not permit the sedation of infants for the collection of normative data. Another method of standardizing flow is to compare maximal flow at FRC with the actual FRC measured. This parameter is known as the *specific flow at FRC* (S$\dot{V}$maxFRC or $\dot{V}$maxFRC/ FRC) As discussed earlier, FRC serves as a static measured reference volume. Because flow increases with higher volumes, a fixed relationship or constant value, independent of age or height, can be determined for flow at that volume. This constant value is termed *specific flow,* and normal specific flow should equal or exceed 1.20 L/sec.

$$S\dot{V}maxFRC$$

$$\frac{\dot{V}maxFRC}{FRC}$$

PF TIP 8.3

Infant growth and development are highly variable. Because pulmonary function parameters such as flow rates, compliance, and resistance are directly related to lung volume, a method to standardize these parameters is recommended. The infant's measured FRC may be used to "volume correct" each parameter (e.g., specific flow at FRC).

Fig. 8.6 shows a partial forced expiratory flow-volume curve from an infant. An RTC was performed after a tidal inspiration. Parameters measured include a $\dot{V}$maxFRC of 440 mL/sec and an S$\dot{V}$maxFRC of 1.63. The specific flow at FRC was obtained by dividing the child's $\dot{V}$max FRC of 440 mL/sec by a previously measured FRC of 270 mL (from nitrogen washout).

Forced Flows From Raised Lung Volume

Success in standardization of spirometry has been dependent on the patient inspiring to TLC before performing a maximal expiration. This is the key to standardization in infants as well. Techniques have been developed to raise the volume of the infant's lungs before a rapid thoracoabdominal compression (RVRTC). This may be accomplished by stacking inspirations or by a method known as the **raised volume technique.** For this maneuver, a bias flow of air is provided to the child during inspiration. The exhalation port is simultaneously occluded, raising the intrathoracic pressure and volume in the child's lungs. A pressure of $+30$ cm H_2O is required to inflate the infant's lung to near TLC. Once inflated, the child is then permitted to passively exhale. After several cycles of inflation and deflation, the child's P_{CO_2} decreases, relaxing the child further. The final inflation is then followed by a forced compression from the inflatable jacket. The maneuver is repeated at an increasingly higher jacket pressure until expired volume and flows maximize at midlung volumes. The advantage of this method compared with partial forced flows is that the expired volume is nearly an FVC measurement. The traditional FEV_1 is not measured because the infant reaches residual volume before 1 second of exhalation occurs. However, the volume expired in 0.5 second or 0.75 second can be calculated and is analogous to the FEV_1 in standard spirometry. Fig. 8.7 shows several F-V curves obtained after RTCs (from raised lung volume) are superimposed. Progressively higher squeeze pressures do not yield higher flows or volumes, indicating that flow limitation has been met. In addition, a partial F-V curve (from a lower lung volume)

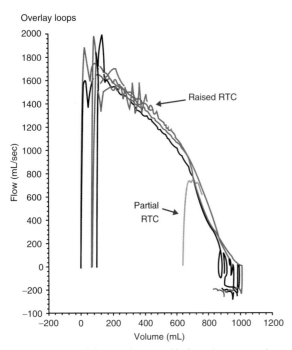

Overlay loops

FIG. 8.7 Raised lung volume rapid thoracic compressions (RTCs). Flow-volume (F-V) curves obtained after RTCs from raised lung volume (RVRTC) are superimposed. In addition, a partial F-V curve (from a tidal breath) is superimposed in the diagram.

is superimposed on the diagram. The F-V curve in this example is from a child with normal lung function. Compare this to the F-V loop pictured in Fig. 8.8. This infant PFT report is representative of a 1-year-old child with cystic fibrosis and mild intrathoracic airflow obstruction.

Note that the report resembles that of a standard PFT for an older child except that the FEV_1 is replaced with the $FEV_{0.5\%}$. Although the FVC, $FEV_{0.5}$, and $FEV_{0.5\%}$/FVC are within the normal percent-predicted range, the flows from lower lung volumes (i.e., $FEF_{75\%}$ and $FEF_{85\%}$) are reduced. TLC and FRC are within percent-predicted values. The RV and RV/TLC are mildly elevated, consistent with mild air trapping. Also note that the values for forced flows may be represented as a Z score. This is a statistical method comparing test results to normative data that is growing in popularity in the pediatric pulmonary function world and is now recommended by the ATS-ERS focus group

for infants and preschool children. It is thought that Z scores more accurately reflect normative data in pediatrics because of varying growth rates for age and sex differences. Refer to the Evolve site (http://evolve.elsevier.com/Mottram/Ruppel/) for a discussion of means, standard deviation, and confidence ranges. One standard deviation equals 1 Z score. Two ($\pm$) standard deviations from the mean, in a positive or negative direction, is generally considered to be within the limits of normal, or the 95% confidence range. This would be represented by a Z score of ± 2.0. Refer again to Fig. 8.8, and notice that the parameters that have normal percent-predicted values also have Z scores close to zero. The $FEF_{75\%}$ and $FEF_{85\%}$, however, have reduced percent-predicted values, and their Z scores are greater than –2.0, both indicative of values outside of the normal range.

Forced Deflation Technique

As with the RTC technique, the forced deflation techniques also produce maximal expiratory F-V (MEFV) curves. The method, however, is exactly the opposite of the positive pressure generated during the RTC method. Instead, a negative pressure is applied to the airway opening, and the lungs are deflated quickly. This technique is usually reserved for intubated infants in a critical care setting and performed by clinicians and physicians familiar with its possible complications. The size of the endotracheal tube may limit flow. The child must be maximally sedated and paralyzed, and therefore the child's lungs must be ventilated between maneuvers. Before the deflation, the lungs of the infant are manually inflated to TLC with approximately $+30$ to $+40$ cm H_2O. This inflation is performed four times with a breath hold of 2 to 3 seconds at TLC. The airway is then switched into a source of negative pressure (approximately –30 to –40 cm H_2O). Air is evacuated for a maximum of 3 seconds or until expiratory flow ceases (i.e., residual volume is reached). As the lungs empty, an F-V curve is produced, and flows at lower lung volumes are analyzed. The lungs are then reinflated with 100% O_2, and the procedure is repeated until flow limitation is obtained.

	PRE	% PRED	Z score
FVC (mL)	360	94	−0.37
$FEV_{0.5\%}$ (mL)	271	91	−0.65
$FEV_{0.5\%}/FVC$	0.75	96	−0.54
$FEF_{25\%}$ (mL/sec)	1142	116	
$FEF_{50\%}$ (mL/sec)	561	84	−0.86
$FEF_{75\%}$ (mL/sec)	175	52	−2.22
$FEF_{85\%}$ (mL/sec)	83	42	−2.61
$FEF_{25\%-75\%}$ (mL/sec)	458	75	−1.34

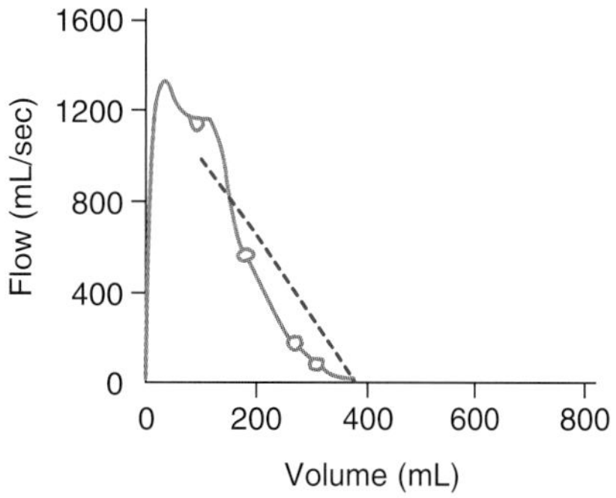

	PRE	% PRED
TLC (mL)	550	97
FVC (mL)	360	86
ERV (mL)	39	68
FRC_{pleth} (mL)	231	108
RV (mL)	192	127
RV/TLC	0.35	126
FRC/TLC	0.42	

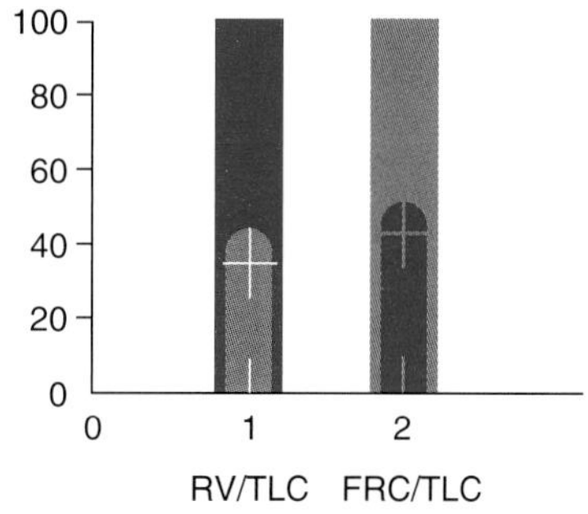

FIG. 8.8 Infant pulmonary function test (PFT) report. PFT test results from a 1-year-old child with cystic fibrosis. The report details forced flows from raised lung volumes and lung volume determination via plethysmography.

PF TIP 8.4

Normative data may be viewed with a variety of statistical methods. Z scores are an alternative method of viewing standard deviation from the mean. A Z score of ±2.0 approximates 2 standard deviations from the mean, otherwise referred to as the 95% confidence range. (See Chapter 13.)

SPIROMETRY

Spirometry, by far, is the most common type of PFT performed in the pediatric population. Understanding how to teach children to perform this test well will help ensure that the physician will use and interpret this tool to treat his or her patient. The basics of spirometry apply to both pediatrics and adults (see Chapter 2). The same principles for testing and equipment are used. The indications for testing are similar, although disease processes in pediatrics often differ. The anatomy and physiology of the respiratory system change significantly from the infant to the young child and to the older adolescent. As for adults, the primary goals of spirometry are the following:

1. To identify the presence of an obstructive defect or a restrictive pattern of flow
2. To quantify the degree of the abnormality
3. To test for a response to a bronchodilator

Spirometry in pediatrics, however, has several pitfalls and special challenges. These can be addressed by approaching the challenges with specific examples.

Age Considerations for Children Performing Spirometry

Age considerations are a common concern that cannot be addressed until spirometry is attempted. Children as young as 2.5 years have the potential to perform the maneuver but with limitations. As a result, according to the ATS-ERS Standardization

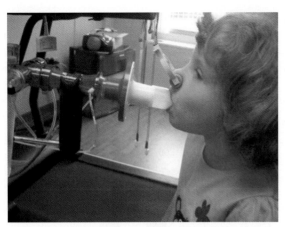

FIG. 8.9 A 5-year-old child performing spirometry for the first time.

of Spirometry 2019 Update, individuals performing pediatric PFTs should receive specific training and competencies, initially and ongoing, to work with this population. Published data from several sources suggest that preschool children can perform technically repeatable FVC maneuvers within 10%. Introducing spirometry to children at a young age often yields remarkable results within only a few training sessions. Fig. 8.9 shows a 5-year-old child performing spirometry for the first time.

The ATS-ERS Technical Statement on Pulmonary Function Testing in Preschool Children more clearly define acceptable and repeatable spirometry in this young age group. The most difficult part of spirometry for a young child is to continue to exhale once the initial blast of air occurs. Small children do not understand how to sustain applied pressure to their chest and abdomen once they feel their lungs are empty. These guidelines include identify premature termination of the maneuver by comparing the flow at termination to that of peak flow. For children aged 6 years or younger, a usable $FEV_{0.75}$ may be obtained from a maneuver with early termination after 0.75 second. Likewise, a usable FEV_1 can be obtained when early termination occurs after 1 second.

As with current recommendations, the highest FVC and FEV_1 (or $FEV_{0.5}$ and $FEV_{0.75}$) should be reported, and the selection of "best" curve should be based on the sum of FVC and FEV_1.

Additionally, a close look at the extrapolated volume is recommended. Because children have smaller lung volumes, the extrapolated volume during spirometry may exceed the criterion of <5% of the FVC (or 0.100 L) currently stated in ATS-ERS guidelines. In young children, an expiratory curve with an extrapolated volume as high as 80 mL or 12.5% (whichever is greater) should be reexamined but need not necessarily be excluded.

Although it is desirable to have at least two repeatable maneuvers, even a single satisfactory trial provides important information. However, learning variability and lack of repeatability should be noted. Other testing modalities available in assessing young children are discussed later in the chapter.

Published guidelines from the ATS-ERS task force offer more realistic expectations for young children. There is not an age at which all children, without exception, can perform technically acceptable spirometry. The ATS-ERS guidelines suggest that certain F-V curves may be usable, if not technically acceptable. Consider Fig. 8.10A. This is the first experience for this 5-year-old child in the pulmonary lab. On multiple attempts, her FEV_1 was repeatable with the best curve, as shown. Note, however, that exhalation is incomplete and expiratory time is short (slightly over 1 second). Therefore the FVC values are underestimated and the FEV_1/FVC is inaccurate. The curves, however, meet criteria for satisfactory start of test and are free of artifact for at least the first second. These classify as usable F-V loops, although they are not technically perfect.

PF TIP 8.5

An ATS-ERS technical statement defines the criteria required for the usability of a maneuver. This is important in young children or patients of any age who cannot complete the full FVC maneuver in order to report parameters such as $FEV_{0.5}$ and $FEV_{0.75}$.

As long as the patient blows for at least 1 second and that first second is free of artifact, the F-V loops and values may be used for interpretation.

Spirometry	PRED	LLN	PRE	% PRED	POST	% PRED	% CHG
			A		B		
FVC (L)	1.57	1.29	1.25	80	1.41	90	13
FEV_1 (L)	1.41	1.16	1.21	86	1.38	98	13
FEV_1/FVC (%)	90	81	97	**	97	**	**
$FEF_{25\%-75\%}$ (L/sec)	**	**	1.45	**	1.76	**	21
PEFR (L/sec)	3.53	2.54	2.77	79	3.46	98	25
FET 100% (sec)	**	**	1.21	**	1.54	**	**

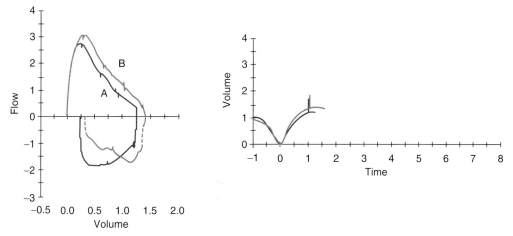

FIG. 8.10 Results of first-time spirometry in a 5-year-old patient. (A) Prebronchodilator. (B) Postbronchodilator.

Values such as $FEV_{0.5}$ or $FEV_{0.75}$ would be considered usable. Caution is suggested in interpreting the FEV_1/FVC, based on an incomplete expiratory maneuver where FVC may be underestimated. It is certainly understood that this may not represent the child's maximal effort; however, identifying that this young child's FEV_1 and other parameters are repeatable and within the normal range for her age is valuable information for the pulmonologist. The shape of the postbronchodilator F-V loop in maneuver B in Fig. 8.10 is similar to that of maneuver A, but larger. There is a proportional increase in both FVC and FEV_1, which suggests the child took a deeper breath before performing the FVC maneuver. A learning effect can be seen even during the first session of working with a young child and should definitely be considered when interpreting this study. Although a bronchodilator response should not be ruled out, it is likely that a learning effect was responsible for most of the improvement. It should be emphasized that spirometry is

an effort-dependent test that requires cooperation and attention from the child. Equally important are the experience and patience of a well-trained pulmonary function clinician. Children who are mentally delayed or not capable of following directions may not perform adequate spirometry at any age, regardless of the coach or clinician. Patients who are not feeling well or having chest pain, for example, may follow instructions but not perform maximally.

Ensuring Maximal Effort on the Part of the Child

First, gain the child's confidence, and do not rush into testing. Children are fearful that the testing will hurt. When possible, reassure the child by carrying on a conversation that is directed toward the child. Provide a child-friendly environment that includes but is not limited to colored walls, interesting wall art (Fig. 8.11A), and the use of window clings on a body plethysmograph (see Fig. 8.11B)

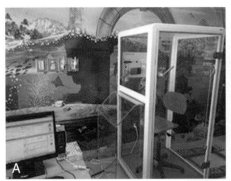
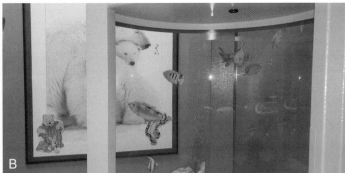
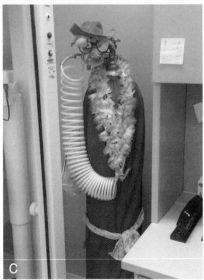

FIG. 8.11 (A) Kid-friendly environment with wall art. (B) Kid-friendly environment with window clings on body plethysmograph. (C) "Clyde," a medical gas cylinder dressed up to create a fun and welcoming testing environment.

to reduce the child's level of anxiety and fear. Some clinicians even dress up a medical gas cylinder, such as "Clyde," who resides in the pulmonary function laboratory at the Dartmouth-Hitchcock Medical Center (see Fig. 8.11C), as a fun distraction that creates a comfortable atmosphere. As illustrated in Fig. 8.12 try some "blowing" games with the very young child before approaching the PFT equipment. The use of a pinwheel is often successful. It teaches the child the need to take a big breath and blow fast. Additionally, have the child try to continue to blow until the pinwheel stops turning. This important step reinforces a complete exhalation. Demonstrate the test and reassure the child that it

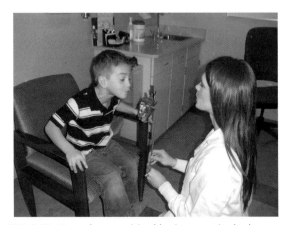

FIG. 8.12 Young boy practicing blowing on a pinwheel.

is easy and fun. Pinwheels also make an excellent and inexpensive prize for the patient when testing is over. If a pinwheel is unavailable, a tissue will substitute, although it is a bit harder. Demonstrate blowing the tissue as high as possible and keeping the tissue suspended for as long as possible.

Once the child has practiced several times, move the child to the PFT machine and prepare for testing. The child should be seated, and the clinician should be at eye level with the child. A smaller chair or a raised footstool should be provided for the child in the event the child is unable to put his or her feet flat on the floor. See Box 8.1 for a list of suggestions that will break the ice and get things going in a positive direction. The use of nose clips is recommended, depending on the age and cooperation of the child. The anatomy of the nasopharyngeal structures in younger children is such that the use of nose clips may not be necessary. If the child is willing to wear nose clips, encourage him or her to do so.

Many pulmonary function systems offer two mouthpiece techniques for performing spirometry: "closed" and "open" techniques. Each offers advantages and disadvantages. Attempt the technique with which laboratory clinicians are most comfortable and consistent. For the closed technique, have the child sit with nose clips in place and the mouthpiece situated securely. Ask the patient to breathe tidally for several breaths. This offers the opportunity to observe the child and ensure that the seal around the mouthpiece is tight. It also gives the child a feeling of security that he or she will get plenty of air through the mouthpiece. The child should be reassured during tidal breathing that he or she is doing very well. If the spirometer permits real-time visualization of flow, the clinician may show the child that he or she is "drawing pictures" with his or her breathing. It is essential to gain the child's confidence and offer praise whenever possible. It is important to talk the child through the maneuver. Use simple words and phrases, for example, "Breathe in, breathe out"; "Take easy, little baby breaths"; or "One more little breath. Now take a giant breath in." The clinician should be vocal and use his or her hands and arms to demonstrate. The intonation of the voice should mimic the action, for example, "easy, gentle breaths" in a soft voice versus "big, fast, and long breath" in a louder tone. Sometimes having the child race with another

---

BOX 8.1   TIPS FOR SUCCESS WITH SPIROMETRY IN PEDIATRIC PATIENTS

1. Greet the child, introduce yourself, and engage in conversation.
   - Compliment the child on a pretty dress or cool T-shirt.
   - Ask about vacations, school, sports activities, and so forth.
   - Ask whether the child would like to play a "blowing game" on the computer.
2. Demonstrate the test.
   - Blow on a tissue, pinwheel, or similar toy.
   - Reassure the child how easy the test is.
3. Encourage the child to sit up straight and hold the flow sensor upright.
   - Use nose clips if possible, but compromise if necessary.
   - Achieve the same eye level of the child.
4. Be expressive with body language.
   - Change the intonation of your voice and be enthusiastic.
   - Use your hands to emphasize action.
5. Use words the child can understand, and keep directions simple.
   - "Breathe in, breathe out."
   - "Take little baby breaths."
   - "Take a giant breath in until you feel ready to burst!"
   - "Blast the air out! Keep blowing until it comes out of your toes!"
6. Think like a kid!
   - "Race" with the child to see who can blow longer.
   - Pretend it is the child's birthday and he or she must blow out the same number of candles as his or her age.
7. Be prepared to try different techniques (open versus closed) and offer rest periods.
8. Offer praise and prizes.
   - High-fives
   - "Best Blower of the Day" awards
   - Small toys and stickers
   - Smiley faces or A+ on pulmonary function testing records
9. Be patient! Know when to quit—repeated efforts can be frustrating and counterproductive for the next visit.

clinician is helpful. Again, the use of the pinwheel or tissue can reinforce what is expected of a young patient while the test is actually going on.

PF TIP 8.6

For spirometry, different catchphrases can help the child more clearly understand instructions. Examples include the following:
- "Take a big breath in until you feel like a balloon ready to burst!"
- "Punch that air out like an elephant fell on your belly!"
- "Keep blowing until the air comes out of your toes!"
- Be creative and think like a kid!

If the child is having particular difficulty, changing the technique may lead to success. At times, tidal breathing may confuse the child. Have the patient get onto the mouthpiece, immediately take a maximal breath in, and blast the air out. Alternatively, use a different mouthpiece or try the open technique. The child may have a sensitive gag reflex or, for unclear reasons, become anxious with tidal breathing. With the open technique, the child should first be instructed to hold the mouthpiece close to his or her face, perhaps supported on the cheek. Next, open the mouth wide, take in the deepest breath possible, place the mouthpiece in the mouth, and immediately blow out. The disadvantage of this technique is that air may be lost as the child tries to get the mouthpiece into his or her mouth and form a seal. To aid in a complete exhalation, the clinician can place his or her hands on the child's belly. As the patient exhales, *gently* press on the stomach. This reinforces a smooth and continuous expiratory maneuver. Once the child is more comfortable performing spirometry, transition to a closed-mouthpiece technique without any assistance from the clinician.

Although eight FVC maneuvers is the upper limit for most adults, more than eight attempts may be required when testing children. The testing operator should be in tune to the child's enthusiasm and effort to avoid exhausting or discouraging the child from future testing.

Importance of Effort

One of the biggest challenges with children is ensuring a maximal breath in before the forced expiration. The concept is simple: The more air in, the more air out. The operator should strive to get the child to breathe in as deeply as possible and observe the child's chest excursion. Movement of the shoulders upward without chest excursion is common and can fool the clinician into believing it is a maximal inspiratory capacity. This may also be a pitfall when comparing prebronchodilator and postbronchodilator spirometry. Fig. 8.13 is from a 5-year-old patient performing spirometry for the first time. The prebronchodilator spirometry (see maneuver A in Fig. 8.13) appears to be normal and was repeatable. Post bronchodilators, both FVC and FEV_1, improve significantly (see Fig. 8.13). The increase in FVC and FEV_1 is very symmetric, similar to the last example presented (see maneuver A in Fig. 8.10). A learning effect cannot be ruled out. However, the shape of the F-V curve is very different with postbronchodilator spirometry. This is an example of a situation where the change in $FEV_{0.5}$ might be more helpful in assessing intrathoracic airflow obstruction than the change in FEV_1.

The child is at a low lung volume when 1 second is reached (close to FVC), and the FEV_1 is not reflective of airflow changes that are occurring at midlung volumes. It is critically important to realize that all the action has already taken place by the time 1 second has elapsed. Parameters such as $FEV_{0.5}$ or $FEV_{0.75}$ should be assessed in these young children, although standards and guidelines for interpretation are not available. Contrast the results shown in Fig. 8.13 with those in Fig. 8.14. In this example of a 7-year-old child, both FVC and FEV_1 increase with postbronchodilator spirometry; however, the increase in FEV_1 is proportionately higher, which also increases the FEV_1/FVC ratio. Although a learning effect may have influenced this example, it is evident that mild airflow obstruction is completely reversed. Once a child has learned the technique and is capable of performing spirometry, the results are remarkably repeatable. The ATS-ERS technical statement now bases the repeatability of FVC and

Spirometry	PRED	LLN	PRE	% PRED	POST	% PRED	% CHG
			A		B		
FVC (L)	1.29	1.07	1.21	94	1.36	106	13
FEV$_1$ (L)	1.26	0.96	1.14	91	1.31	104	15
FEV$_1$/FVC (%)	89	79	94	**	96	**	**
FEF$_{25\%-75\%}$ (L/sec)	**	**	1.38	**	2.29	**	65
PEFR (L/sec)	2.68	1.93	2.73	102	3.48	130	27
FET 100% (sec)	**	**	1.8	**	2.93	**	**

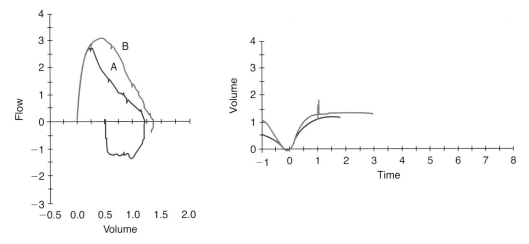

FIG. 8.13   First-time spirometry in a 5-year-old patient. (A) Prebronchodilator. (B) Postbronchodilator.

Spirometry	PRED	LLN	PRE	% PRED	POST	% PRED	% CHG
			A		B		
FVC (L)	1.41	1.15	1.26	89	1.36	97	9
FEV$_1$ (L)	1.26	1.02	0.96	76	1.24	98	28
FEV$_1$/FVC (%)	90	81	77	**	91	**	**
FEF$_{25\%-75\%}$ (L/sec)	**	**	0.79	**	1.65	**	109
PEFR (L/sec)	3.46	2.49	2.33	67	2.93	85	26
FET 100% (sec)	**	**	6.74	**	7.03	**	**

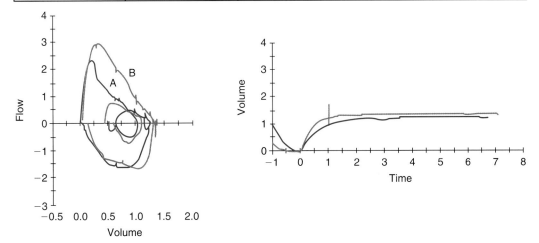

FIG. 8.14   Spirometry in a 7-year-old patient. (A) Prebronchodilator spirometry in a child showing mild intrathoracic airflow obstruction. (B) Postbronchodilator response.

FEV$_1$ on age. In children aged > 6 years, FVC and FEV$_1$ repeatability should be within 0.150 L. For children ≤ 6 years, repeatability of the largest and next-largest FVC and FEV$_1$ should be within 0.100 L, or 10% of the highest value, whichever is greater. A full description of the updated grading system for FEV$_1$ and FVC can be found in Chapter 2.

PF TIP 8.7

In children aged > 6 years, FVC and FEV$_1$ repeatability should be within 0.150 L. For children ≤ 6 years, repeatability of the largest and next-largest FVC and FEV$_1$ should be within 0.100 L, or 10% of the highest value, whichever is greater.

Once a maximal inspiration is accomplished, most young children do not have difficulty blowing out forcefully. As for adult spirometry, the clinician should minimize hesitation before the forced maneuver that may create a time-zero or back-extrapolated volume error. The back-extrapolated volume must be < 5% of the FVC or 0.100 L, whichever is greater. Do not encourage a breath hold. Delayed exhalation can result in a poor peak flow measurement and falsely raise the FEV$_1$. Fig. 8.15 demonstrates this volume-extrapolation or time-zero error.

Maneuver A in Fig. 8.15 is an acceptable effort. Note how maneuver B in Fig. 8.15 has an exhalation delay. This results in the curve appearing tilted to the right, which can falsely elevate timed parameters.

Obtaining a maximal peak flow can actually be more difficult in an adolescent. Teenage children can often be reluctant to perform maximally unless strongly encouraged to do so. This may be caused by chest pain, embarrassment, or fear that something is wrong with them. Occasionally, this poor effort may be related to typical teenage angst or attention-seeking motivation. A sensitive and perceptive clinician can often combine the right amount of compassion with the necessary verbal encouragement to obtain optimal results. Variability caused by effort alone may be especially important if the patient is performing serial measurements, as in a methacholine challenge. A change in treatment regimen or admission to the

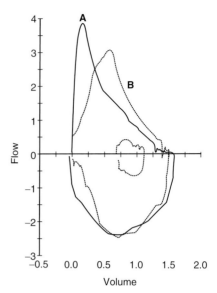

FIG. 8.15 Spirometry in a child showing effects of effort. (A) An acceptable forced vital capacity (FVC) effort. (B) Poor technique, resulting in delayed exhalation.

hospital is often based on spirometric changes; therefore repeatability is critical.

Length of Exhalation for a Child During an FVC Maneuver

The ATS-ERS Standardization of Spirometry 2019 Technical Statement no longer recognizes exhalation time (e.g., minimum 6 second exhalation) as an acceptability criterion for an FVC maneuver. It simply focuses on the end of forced expiration (EOFE) based on reaching a plateau of zero flow for 0.025 L in 1 second.

PF TIP 8.8

EOFE criteria state that the subject exhales (1) until there is a change of less than 0.025 L in volume for at least 1 second (a "plateau"), or (2) the subject has achieved an FET of 15 seconds, or (3) the subject cannot expire long enough to achieve a plateau and the same FVC is achieved with each maneuver.

Because children have lung volumes that are significantly smaller than adult lung volumes, it is common for their lungs to become completely empty in only 2 or 3 seconds. A coached forced inspiratory maneuver should be initiated once the expiratory curve reaches a plateau, regardless of exhalation time (see later discussion of inspiratory vital capacity [IVC]). With instruction, practice, and maturation, the child can learn to continue the expiration; however, this may not be possible on the first several visits to the lab. This does not invalidate the FVC maneuvers but requires that the testing be evaluated carefully. Maneuvers A in Fig. 8.16 represent three prebronchodilator F-V loops superimposed over each other. Although this young child does not meet the EOFE criteria, the FEV_1 and shape of the F-V loop are remarkably repeatable. Postbronchodilator, in maneuvers B in Fig. 8.16, the F-V loops are significantly improved and repeatable.

Children who are severely obstructed, like their adult counterparts, may have the ability to exhale for an extended time. Fig. 8.17 shows the F-V loop and volume–time tracing of a 10-year-old girl with cystic fibrosis. This child is able to sustain expiration for 15 seconds. However, the additional volume

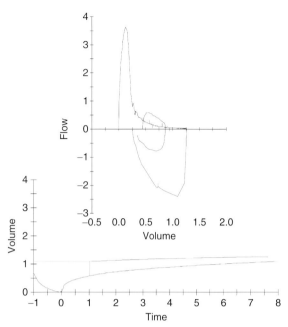

FIG. 8.17 Flow-volume (F-V) loop and volume–time tracing of a 10-year-old girl with cystic fibrosis. Note prolonged exhalation and severe airflow obstruction.

measured in this prolonged expiration is small and may exhaust the child when performing the test. She approaches a flow plateau at approximately 7 to 8 seconds, and the maneuver can be terminated at this point. The spirometry is certainly still valid for interpretation if terminated before zero flow occurs. Many decisions regarding the acceptability of PFT results require good judgment from the clinician and careful interpretation from the physician.

Reliability of $FEF_{25\%-75\%}$ in Children

Historically, $FEF_{25\%-75\%}$ has been used to evaluate flow from the small airways. More precisely, the $FEF_{25\%-75\%}$ should be considered a measurement of flow at lower lung volumes, not merely flow from medium-sized and smaller airways. As in adults, the variability of the $FEF_{25\%-75\%}$ is greater than that of the FVC and FEV_1. Because children may be even less repeatable at baseline, the reliability of this measurement in pediatric testing may be questionable. In addition, if the child does not fully exhale to RV, $FEF_{25\%-75\%}$ may be artificially elevated because of reduced vital capacity. If it is reported,

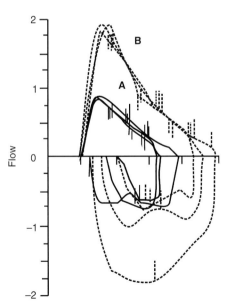

FIG. 8.16 Repeatability of efforts in a young child. (A) Prebronchodilator spirometry that is repeatable, although the end-of-test criteria are not met (see text). (B) Postbronchodilator spirometry in the same patient, again demonstrating repeatability of improvement.

the FEF$_{25\%-75\%}$ in a pediatric subject should be interpreted with caution, especially in a young child. A substantially greater change postbronchodilator is needed using FEF$_{25\%-75\%}$ before a change can be considered significant, as shown in Fig. 8.13. The change in the shape of the F-V loop, as well as the change in FEF$_{25\%-75\%}$ of 65%, is certainly suggestive of a reversal of airflow obstruction. An FEF$_{25\%-75\%}$ that improves by more than 35% to 45% after a bronchodilator may be indicative of airway reactivity, but again, caution is advised when considering this parameter. Repeatability of the FEF$_{25\%-75\%}$ is more reliable in older children and teenagers. As previously noted, FEF$_{25\%-75\%}$ can be reduced for several reasons that are not always related to peripheral airway disease. Refer to Fig. 8.18. This F-V loop is from a 17-year-old patient who had tracheal stenosis after a prolonged intubation as a young child. The FEF$_{25\%-75\%}$ of this curve is severely reduced, as is the FEV$_1$. The reduction is not caused by peripheral airway obstruction but by a large, fixed airway obstruction.

Maximal Voluntary Ventilation

In a cooperative child, the maximal voluntary ventilation (MVV) can be a useful measure of muscle strength, as well as maximal ventilation (see Chapter 2). If the child has significant muscle weakness, he or she may not be able to perform this maneuver. The MVV may also be used before a maximal exercise test to identify the maximal level of ventilation of which the child is capable. Comparing the minute ventilation at maximal O$_2$ consumption with the MVV obtained before exercise can identify ventilatory limitation during exercise.

Parameters of the Inspiratory Flow-Volume Loop

Spirometry yields both a measured volume and a variety of expiratory and inspiratory flows, including FEF$_{25\%}$, FEF$_{50\%}$, FEF$_{75\%}$, FEF$_{85\%}$, FIF$_{50\%}$, and the FEF$_{50\%}$/FIF$_{50\%}$ ratio. Each flow parameter relates to a particular lung volume and may have some interpretation benefits. These flows, like the FEF$_{25\%-75\%}$, are less repeatable than the FEV$_1$ and FVC and do not have any reference values. The FEF$_{50\%}$/FIF$_{50\%}$ ratio may be helpful in classifying airflow obstruction: intrathoracic, extrathoracic, or fixed (see Chapter 2). Unlike the expiratory limb of the F-V loop, the inspiratory limb has not been well characterized in pediatric subjects. There are several reasons for this; however, the most important are energy expenditure and effort dependence. Expiration from TLC is far more repeatable because of the elastic recoil of the lung. The FEF$_{50\%}$ occurs in the portion of the expiratory limb that is considered effort independent. The inspiratory limb, conversely, is effort dependent and energy dependent for the entire maneuver. Therefore optimal patient effort is vital for analyzing the inspiratory loop. A great deal of important

Spirometry	PRED	LLN	PRE	% PRED
FVC (L)	3.72	3.06	2.89	78
FEV$_1$ (L)	3.31	2.72	1.13	34
FEV$_1$/FVC (%)	89	80	39	**
FEF$_{25\%-75\%}$ (L/sec)	3.86	2.62	0.54	14
PEFR (L/sec)	6.82	4.9	1.55	23
FET 100% (sec)	**	**	8.55	**

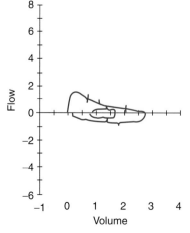

FIG. 8.18   Spirometry in a 17-year-old girl with severe airflow obstruction resulting from tracheal stenosis.

information can be obtained from an appropriately performed maneuver. Too often, the inspiratory limb is ignored. When teaching children how to perform spirometry, certainly the emphasis is on expiration. Once it is mastered, attention should be paid to the inspiratory maneuver as well.

The 2019 ATS-ERS Spirometry Technical Statement defines inspiratory volume as a quality indicator for the acceptability of efforts. When the inspiratory volume at the end of the maneuver exceeds the FEV, the subject does not reach TLC before blowing out. The maneuver is not acceptable if the inspiratory volume exceeds the FVC by more than 0.100 L or 5% of FVC, whichever is greater.

PF TIP 8.9

Assuming maximal effort is given by the child for the entire maneuver, the inspiratory limb of the F-V loop can give valuable information regarding extrathoracic obstruction in pediatric patients.

The aperture, or opening, through the vocal cords is approximately the same at both 50% of expiratory vital capacity (EVC) and 50% of IVC. Therefore the $FEF_{50\%}/FIF_{50\%}$ ratio should not be greater than 1.0. A ratio greater than 1.0 suggests an extrathoracic obstruction; however, this relationship has not been closely studied or reported in pediatric patients. Conversely, an $FEF_{50\%}/FIF_{50\%}$ ratio of less than 1.0 may be normal or may represent significant intrathoracic obstruction. In addition, a ratio close to normal is possible if significant obstruction is seen on both inspiration and expiration (fixed obstruction), yielding a ratio of 1.0. Fig. 8.18 demonstrates the effect of tracheal stenosis in a 17-year-old patient on the shape of the F-V loop and the resulting $FEF_{50\%}/FIF_{50\%}$ ratio. This highlights the importance of correlating the F-V loop with the child's clinical picture and symptoms.

Fig. 8.19 shows examples of F-V loops with differing $FEF_{50\%}/FIF_{50\%}$ ratios and the shape of the loops represented by those ratios. Although $FEF_{50\%}/FIF_{50\%}$ may not always discriminate between intrathoracic and extrathoracic airflow obstruction, the importance of extrathoracic obstruction should

not be underestimated. Laryngeal webs, subglottic stenosis, tracheal malacia, and other lesions of the laryngeal-tracheal airway are important causes of upper airway obstruction in the pediatric population. In addition, the vocal cords represent a major "choke point" to airflow. The cords may have a structural abnormality, such as nodules or granulomas, or may become edematous, as in croup. The recurrent laryngeal nerve may be damaged, resulting in inappropriate movement or paralyzed cords. These conditions are generally easy to diagnose with direct visualization of the vocal cords. **Vocal cord dysfunction (VCD)** may also be responsible for poor abduction (opening) of the vocal cords during inspiration.

Role of Vocal Cord Dysfunction

VCD has become increasingly recognized as a reason for shortness of breath (SOB), in addition to throat and sternal chest pain, often mimicking asthma. Adolescents who are competitive athletes or are exceptionally goal oriented and children who have stress-related disorders are at highest risk. Unfortunately, VCD is highly variable and may be detectable only when the patient is stressed in a manner that provokes the condition. The term *VCD* has sparked controversy among pediatric pulmonologists. Perhaps the term is not the most important consideration but rather the understanding that the vocal cords and larynx are very complex structures. There are likely many scenarios, some consciously controlled and others unconsciously controlled, that lead to the malfunction or inappropriate movement of the vocal cords. In very severe forms, "clipping" or truncation of the inspiratory loop with a completely normal expiratory loop is the classic presentation (see Fig. 8.19E). The child may or may not sound very stridorous during inspiration. The patient may try to speak while inspiring in short, gasping sentences. More common is a completely normal-appearing child with normal expiratory loops but highly variable inspiratory loops. Some inspiratory loops may be normal ($FEF_{50\%}/FIF_{50\%} < 1.0$); however, many are often abnormal, with an $FEF_{50\%}/FIF_{50\%}$ greater than 1.0.

VCD is an example of a disorder in which the variability in the patient's inspiratory loop

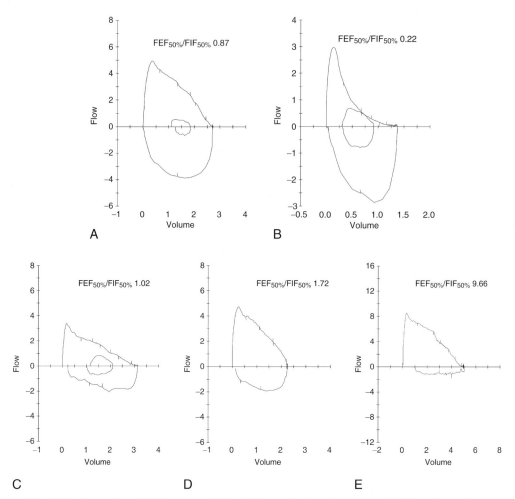

FIG. 8.19   Flow-volume (F-V) loops and $FEF_{50\%}/FIF_{50\%}$ ratios in various types of airflow obstructions. (A) Normal. (B) Expiratory airflow obstruction. (C) Fixed airflow obstruction. (D) Extrathoracic airflow obstruction. (E) Extrathoracic airflow obstruction with severe clipping of the inspiratory flow pattern.

is the hallmark of the dysfunction (Fig. 8.20A). Figure 8.20A shows the baseline loops from one patient, a 15-year-old teenager. Note how different all the inspiratory loops look. Some have a triangular-shape appearance; some have the more classic flat, truncated appearance; and others have multiple inflection points. The inspiratory volume may be limited, giving a short, gasping type of inspiratory loop. A more normal inspiratory loop may appear among many abnormal loops (see Fig. 8.20A, Trial 4). This is important to capture when possible. It indicates that the child can perform normal inspiratory loops, and the problem is likely more dynamic in nature—that is, a vocal cord malfunction. If there is a structural upper airway abnormality, the inspiratory loops should all look abnormal and similar in shape. Structural obstructions are usually more fixed in nature, with expiratory clipping also present. Refer again to the example of fixed airflow obstruction shown in Fig. 8.19.

Bronchoprovocation testing can sometimes provoke VCD; however, conclusive evidence of inappropriate movement of the vocal cords should be visualized through a laryngoscope, ideally during an episode. Because laryngoscopy may not be practical or available, a series of well-performed F-V

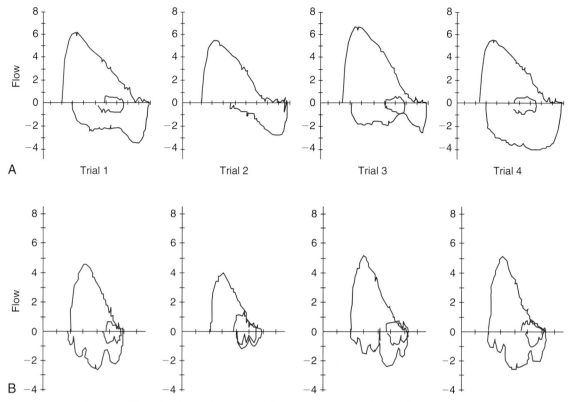

FIG. 8.20 Variability in inspiratory loops. (A) Trials 1 to 3, 15-year-old girl with different forms of inspiratory clipping; trial 4, closer to normal. (B) Multiple involuntary inflection points.

loops may be helpful in making this presumptive diagnosis. It should be noted that VCD, on the milder side of the spectrum, is primarily a diagnosis of exclusion, and the absence of inspiratory clipping on F-V loops does not rule out the diagnosis. It is important to emphasize that effort, technique, and learning play a major role in the shape of inspiratory loops. In young children, it may require several sessions, on different days, with abnormal inspiratory loops consistently obtained, before the diagnosis of VCD can be suggested.

Under certain circumstances, very unusual inspiratory loops can be seen in multiple trials that are not related to effort or technique. Consider Fig. 8.20B. These loops were obtained from a patient with excessive secretions and laryngospasm. F-V loops are rarely diagnostic as a single test but certainly can suggest and support other diagnoses that are being considered.

VCD Combined With Airflow Obstruction

To further complicate matters, VCD is often seen in children with asthma. The relationship between these two disorders is not fully understood. There is certainly some similarity in symptoms, primarily SOB, chest pain, and/or throat pain. However, some children who experience both asthma and VCD can distinguish between the two disorders. Refer to Fig. 8.21A. These loops are from a child with known asthma who was experiencing symptoms of SOB and chest pain. The expiratory loops show very mild (if any) airflow obstruction. However, the inspiratory flow loops are variable and abnormal, as described in the earlier section. Vice versa, in Fig. 8.21B, note the characteristic "scooping" appearance of severe expiratory airflow obstruction. This is accompanied by a normal-appearing inspiratory loop. Note that the relationship of FEF_{50}/FIF_{50} is skewed when the

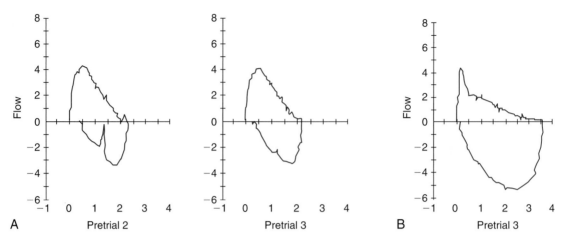

FIG. 8.21   Same trial as in Fig. 8.20 (15-year-old girl with inspiratory clipping). (A) Mild intrathoracic air-flow obstruction with abnormal inspiratory loops. (B) Severe expiratory airflow obstruction with normal inspiratory loop.

expiratory loop is not normal. The FEF_{50}/FIF_{50} ratio discussed earlier is no longer valid in the face of expiratory obstruction. This ratio also does not hold true when the inspiratory loops are not complete, full loops or are very irregular in shape.

FVC-Induced Bronchospasm

The ATS-ERS recommendations emphasize the importance of repeatability of the FVC and FEV_1. In some instances, patients cannot reproduce these parameters, and effort is not the reason. Fig. 8.22 shows an example of such an instance. If only a single (best) F-V loop (trial 1) were reported to the physician, the interpretation would state that this patient has airflow obstruction. However, the next successive maneuvers performed by this 15-year-old with asthma show a progressive decline in both flow and volume (see Fig. 8.22). These successive trials reveal progressively significant drops in FEV_1 and FEV_1/FVC, which are not repeatable with trial 1. This pattern is an extremely important clue to the hyperreactivity of the patient's airway and demonstrates FVC-induced bronchospasm, some-times also termed *FVC-induced worsening* (Fig. 8.22, Table 8.1). Simply performing repeated forced maneuvers may cause a subject with hyperreactive airways to become suddenly more obstructed. In such an instance, the operator should stop testing the patient and administer a bronchodilator. If the patient's report included only his or her best

prebronchodilator and postbronchodilator spirometry, it would completely omit this important information and might prevent necessary changes in his or her medication regimen.

An interesting but opposite phenomenon may be seen in the spirometry of a patient with mild asthma. Deep inspirations may cause progressive bronchodilation with improving FEV_1 and FEV_1/FVC. This is a beneficial compensatory mechanism and is likely similar to the athlete with asthma who is able to "run through" his or her asthma with bronchodilation during exercise. After exercise, V_{TS} decreases, airway temperature changes, and bronchoconstriction may be provoked.

PF TIP 8.10

Variability (or lack of repeatability) in both inspiratory and expiratory spirometric efforts may be important for identifying diseases such as asthma and VCD. Reporting or displaying all F-V loops can assist in the data interpretation. The operator performing the test should look for characteristic patterns of variability and include appropriate data in the final report.

Airway Malacia

Unusual F-V curves may be extremely helpful in providing clues to the location of fixed or variable obstruction. One scenario common in pediatrics

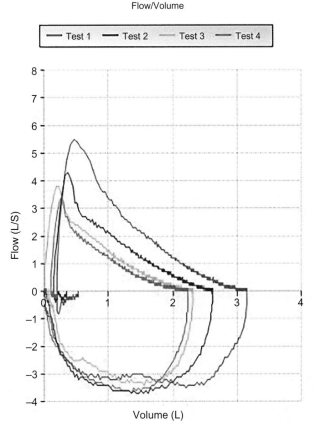

Flow/Volume

— Test 1   — Test 2   — Test 3   — Test 4

FIG. 8.22   Repeated spirometry maneuvers in a 15-year-old patient with asthma demonstrating broncho-spasm induced by forced vital capacity (FVC).

TABLE 8.1

FVC-Induced Worsening

Result	1	2	3	4	5	6
FVC (L)	3.48	3.30	3.07	2.79	2.97	2.76
FEV$_1$ (L)	2.53	2.12	2.01	1.62	1.77	1.56
FEV$_1$/FVC	0.73	0.64	0.65	0.58	0.60	0.57
PEF (L/sec)	6.80	5.75	5.58	4.42	4.98	4.02

FVC, Forced vital capacity; *FEV$_1$,* forced expiratory volume in the first second; *PEF,* peak expiratory flow.

is tracheal and/or bronchial malacia. **Malacia** refers to an airway (or more than one airway) that is soft and pliable because of a lack of supportive connective or cartilaginous tissue. Depending on the location (intrathoracic, extrathoracic, or both), these airways may collapse during inspiration or be compressed during exhalation. Tracheal or

bronchomalacia in infants may produce significant stridor and "noisy breathing," especially when the baby is excited or crying. With time and growth, the airways stiffen and are less prone to collapse.

For older children, airway malacia may produce some bizarre-shaped F-V curves. Refer to Fig. 8.23. These F-V loops are from a 12-year-old child with a

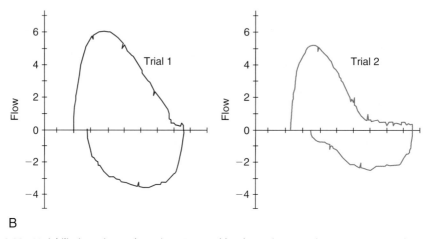

	REF	Trial 1	Trial 2	% CHG
FVC (L)	2.95	3.31	3.38	2
FEV$_1$ (L)	2.58	2.93	2.13	-27
FEV$_1$/FVC (%)	86	89	63	
FEF$_{25\%-75\%}$ (L/sec)	2.91	2.91	0.98	-66
PEF (L/sec)	5.43	6.01	5.13	-15

A

B

FIG. 8.23   Variability in expiratory loops in a 12-year-old male. Trial 1, normal expiratory curve with minimal airway closure at end-exhalation. Trial 2, Central airway closure with significant effect on FEV$_1$ and FEF$_{25\%-75\%}$.

malacic left mainstem bronchus. Trial 1 represents a forced exhalation that is normal in shape. Trial 2 is from the same patient during the same testing session. Notice the rapid drop in flow rate, followed by a flattening, or shelf-like, appearance in the curve. Blowing harder caused critical compression at the malacic segment and resulted in a sudden decrease in flow rate, or **flow transient.** Note the reduction in FEV$_1$, as well as FEF$_{25\%-75\%}$, from trial 1 to trial 2. This represents another example of the inadequacy of looking solely at one or two parameters instead of considering the entire picture. The shape of the curve in trial 2 is characteristic of two lungs emptying at different time constants. One lung empties normally during forced exhalation, whereas the other lung takes considerably longer to empty because of the central intrathoracic obstruction present. Obtaining repeatable and acceptable F-V loops in the face of airway malacia can be challenging. Although not always successful, taking extra time with the child to try different breathing techniques or different mouthpieces may result in a more normal expiratory loop.

DIFFUSION CAPACITY

The diffusion capacity (D$_{LCO}$) in the pediatric population can be an important indicator of gas transport difficulties at the alveolar level. This may be caused by problems with perfusion of the pulmonary capillary bed, bleeding within the lung, or thickening of the alveolar-capillary membrane. Several serious pediatric disorders fall into these categories, and the D$_{LCO}$ may provide an answer to a very specific question. Examples of pediatric pulmonary diseases that may produce a reduced D$_{LCO}$ include pulmonary fibrosis (primary disease or secondary to radiation treatment or chemotherapy), immunologic disorders (scleroderma, systemic lupus erythematosus), bronchiolitis obliterans, pulmonary edema, and hematologic disorders. An abnormally high D$_{LCO}$ may be seen in acute hemorrhagic bleeds, as in pulmonary vasculitis. The single-breath D$_{LCO}$ is the most common method used for assessing diffusion capacity. The problems already discussed in performing pulmonary function studies in the pediatric patient are compounded for this test. However, the guidelines and recommendations offered by the ATS-ERS for DLCO testing in adults are also applicable to pediatrics (see Chapter 3). The single-breath maneuver is difficult for small children to perform and often requires several sessions of practice. Even older children may have difficulty accomplishing the important components of the DLCO maneuver. These components include emptying to residual volume before a deep inspiration; obtaining an IVC of at least 85% of FVC; a relaxed breath hold of 8 to 12 seconds; and a smooth, complete exhalation. In addition, other technical considerations may alter results, such as inappropriate mechanical or anatomic dead-space corrections. The demand valve used for the inspiration of test gas should be sensitive enough to open easily with use by a child. Unfortunately, children who cannot perform a breath hold are generally not able to perform this test well.

Other confounders that alter the measurement of DLCO are abnormal levels or types of hemoglobin. Children who require repeated DLCO measurements may have conditions that cause anemia (e.g., chemotherapy, sickle cell disease, transplantations). Reduced circulating hemoglobin reduces the raw measurement of DLCO. Conversely, chronic hypoxemia may produce a secondary polycythemia that increases circulating hemoglobin and may increase the raw measurement of diffusion capacity. The presence of carboxyhemoglobin (COHb), methemoglobin (MetHb), or fetal hemoglobin will decrease the ability of hemoglobin to bind with carbon monoxide and reduce the diffusion capacity. It should not be assumed that pediatric patients do not smoke. Certainly, teenagers should be asked whether they smoke and told honestly that smoking may affect the results of the test. If the patient has been smoking before testing, a COHb level can be obtained to correct for carbon monoxide already present in the circulating blood. Correction of DLCO for hemoglobin is an essential component in analyzing the diffusion capacity of the lung (see Chapter 3).

As with adults, diffusion capacity is dependent on the size of the lungs. An estimation of lung size known as the *alveolar volume* (VA) is also made during the single-breath maneuver. In addition to carbon monoxide, the test gas also contains an inert gas such as helium, methane, or neon that is used

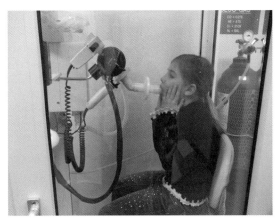

FIG. 8.24 Girl holding cheeks with hands while performing lung volume test.

to estimate VA by a dilution method. The VA can be compared with the TLC obtained by other methods, such as plethysmography, but should be a lesser value. Calculated VA does not account for dead-space ventilation as plethysmographic TLC measurements do. As with all gas dilution techniques, VA will be increasingly underestimated as airflow obstruction worsens. Refer again to Fig. 8.24. Recall that the patient discussed in Fig. 8.24A is a young man with advanced cystic fibrosis. The raw DLCO is reduced, but DLCO/VA (KCO) is in the normal range. This patient's VA is only 2.31 L compared with the TLC of 4.83 L—more than 50% less. It is important to understand that the VA will measure only lung volume with communicating airways (i.e., adequate ventilation). The ratio DLCO/VA (KCO) also reflects diffusion capacity only in well-ventilated areas of the lung. Compare this to the patient with systemic scleroderma in Fig. 8.24B. The raw DLCO is severely reduced, consistent with the diffusion block and fibrosis associated with scleroderma of the lung. Lung tissue that is less affected has a diffusion capacity within normal limits; thus the DLCO/VA (KCO) is 76% predicted. The VA of 0.91 L is closer to the TLC value of 1.55 L, reflecting the primary restrictive component of her disease. In a purely restrictive disease, the VA may come close to the TLC. Recall, however, that this patient also has ventilation defects.

Predictive or normative sets for the diffusion capacity in pediatrics are limited and based on small groups of children. This, unfortunately, makes interpretation of the diffusion capacity even more difficult in the pediatric population. Caution should be taken in interpreting all parameters of the diffusion capacity. Consideration should be given to the child's technique and repeatability of the maneuvers, technical equipment limitations, and normative sets used for comparison.

RESPIRATORY MUSCLE STRENGTH

Measurement of muscle strength can be an important parameter in the pediatric population. Children have a variety of congenital and acquired neuromuscular disorders and thoracic deformities that reduce the strength of the diaphragm and intercostal muscles. Examples of neuromuscular diseases include, but are not limited to, muscular dystrophies, spinal muscle atrophy, meningomyeloceles, Guillain-Barré syndrome, myasthenia gravis, trauma-related paralysis, and steroid-induced myopathies. Thoracic deformities include scoliosis, kyphoscoliosis, pectus excavatum or carinatum, and undefined congenital syndrome abnormalities.

Maximal Respiratory Pressures

The measurement of maximal inspiratory pressure (MIP) and maximal expiratory pressure (MEP) may help (1) identify the degree of weakness and (2) follow the progression of the specific disorder. See Chapter 10 for a discussion of the technique for performing MIP and MEP. In children, it may be necessary to attach a mask and one-way valve to the pressure manometer and apply the mask snugly to the child's face. It may also be necessary to hold the mask in place until the child becomes air hungry and feels a need to gasp for air. It is understandable why this test is so unpopular with children. A similar measurement of spontaneous inspiratory strength may be made while a child is undergoing mechanical ventilation, and this parameter is often referred to as the *negative inspiratory force* (NIF). Although the measurement of inspiratory strength may ultimately be involuntary, the expiratory strength measurement (MEP) is completely effort dependent. The child cannot be forced to push as hard as possible; he or she must choose to do so. For this reason,

MEP results should be viewed cautiously. Predicted values have been defined in children and adolescents aged 8 to 19 years old. Trending serial measurements often provide information that is more useful once the child is accustomed to the test.

Maximal respiratory pressure is a useful marker of respiratory muscle weakness. In patients with Duchenne muscular dystrophy (DMD), VC begins to decline by approximately 8% to 8.5% each year after 10 to 12 years of age. Patients develop chronic alveolar hypoventilation. Weakened respiratory muscles create a spiral-down effect that leads to a reduction in chest wall compliance caused by micro-atelectasis, diminishing the lung capacity and impairing the patient's ability to cough. As a result, airway secretions cannot be sufficiently eliminated, thus putting the patient at increased risk for mucus plugging, which can cause atelectasis and pneumonia. Nearly 90% of respiratory failures in this patient population are developed suddenly because of impaired airway clearance and during recurrent chest colds as a result of ineffective cough. Therefore improving the effectiveness of cough is the most important pulmonary hygiene therapy for these patients. For this reason, and because the expiratory muscles play the most basic and important role in producing a functional cough flow, much research and a great deal of interest focus on the relationship between expiratory muscle strength and cough.

Cough Peak Flows

Cough peak flow (CPF) has been identified as an effective test to assess muscle weakness in pediatric patients with neuromuscular disease. The CPF is the maximum airflow generated during a coached-cough maneuver after a maximal inspiration. The technique can be performed using a facemask or mouthpiece with nose clips and is reported in liters/minute. Reference values have been reported in children ages 4 to 18 years of age. Studies have demonstrated that CPF should be > 160 L/min for cough to effectively clear secretions. In patients with DMD, PCF < 270 L/min is used in conjunction with reduced FVC and MEP results to institute assisted-coughing interventions.

Sniff Nasal Inspiratory Pressures

Sniff nasal inspiratory pressures (SNIPs) have been deemed effective in the assessment of respiratory muscle weakness. The technique involves measuring nasal pressure in an occluded nostril during a maximal sniff performed through the contralateral nostril. Reference values have been defined for children 6 to 17 years of age. Studies have described SNIP as a possible earlier marker of decline in respiratory muscle strength than vital capacity in young patients with DMD.

LUNG VOLUMES

Lung volume measurements in the pediatric population are extremely valuable and often reveal information not obtained from spirometry only. Not all children need lung volume determination. It is preferable that the child be comfortable performing spirometry before attempting lung volumes, but many children adapt easily to a new test situation. The choice of techniques for measuring lung volume is like that with adults. Lung volume determination through gas dilution techniques often underestimates lung volumes in patients with obstructive airway disease. This problem becomes even more relevant in the pediatric population because the size of the airway is smaller and easier to obstruct. Helium dilution or nitrogen washout may not be as well tolerated as body plethysmography. Problems with keeping a mouth seal and breathing a dry gas for several minutes make these techniques less desirable. Conversely, a child who performs even less-than-optimal spirometry may "jump" into the body box and attempt the maneuvers. Many commercial body plethysmographs require minimal effort in determining thoracic gas volume (V_{TG}). Vigorous panting is no longer required to obtain V_{TG}. With most systems, limited panting or only tidal breathing is necessary. Some commercial systems permit the clinician to adjust the timing and duration of the panting to minimize patient discomfort. Technical advances in body plethysmography, the ease and versatility of making measurements, and the accuracy of the measurement make this technique the preferred choice for lung volumes in pediatric patients. A detailed description of the functioning of a body plethysmograph is included in Chapter 4.

> **PF TIP 8.11**
>
> The versatility and accuracy of commercially available body plethysmographs make this method of lung volume determination the preferred technique even in the pediatric population. Children are generally not fearful of a plethysmograph and typically do not experience claustrophobia.

First Step

The first step in performing plethysmography in the pediatric population is getting the child into the body box. This is usually not a major obstacle. In many cases, the child has been to the pulmonary function laboratory on previous occasions and is familiar with the environment and personnel. The child often asks, "What's that?" This becomes an opportunity to appeal to the child's imagination. A body box, in a child's eye, can be a spaceship or Cinderella's coach. Sometimes the child sits in the body box only on the first or second visit, but ultimately, this is a valuable experience. It may be possible to have the parent also sit in the body box and perform some testing until the child feels comfortable alone. The instructions should be kept simple and be demonstrated to the child. In many instances, the child will perform adequately without the need to modify instructions. Too many instructions can lead to confusion. A mouthpiece and nose clips are required for testing in the body box. The instructions can be modified if the child pouches his or her cheeks, producing open loops rather than closed loops during panting, by supporting the cheeks during the test, as shown in Fig. 8.25. The door should be opened periodically to let the child rest and converse with the clinicians or parent. If you open the door to the body box throughout the test, be sure to allow it to stabilize each time you close the door for a minimum of 1 minute to ensure thermal equilibration and eliminate the potential for drift. Children requiring O_2 should also be

Spirometry	PRED	LLN	PRE	% PRED
FVC (L)	3.42	2.84	1.11	32
FEV$_1$ (L)	3.01	2.48	0.62	21
FEV$_1$/FVC (%)	88	78	56	**
FEF$_{25\%-75\%}$ (L/sec)	3.42	2.32	0.21	6
PEFR (L/sec)	5.99	4.31	2.07	35
FET100% (sec)	**	**	9.2	**

Lung volumes	PRED	LLN	PRE	% PRED
VC (L)	3.42	2.84	1.11	33
TLC (L)	4.45	3.92	4.83	109
FRC$_{PL}$ (L)	2.19	1.84	3.88	177
RV (L)	1.01	0.68	3.72	368
RV/TLC (%)	24	**	77	**
IC (L)	**	**	0.95	**
ERV (L)	**	**	0.14	**

Diffusion capacity	PRED	LLN	PRE	% PRED
D$_{LCO}$ (mL/mm Hg/min)	22.9	**	14.1	61
D$_L$ Adj (mL/mm Hg/min)	22.9	**	15.2	66
D$_{LCO}$/V$_A$	6.45	**	6.06	94
V$_A$ (L)	**	**	2.31	**

A

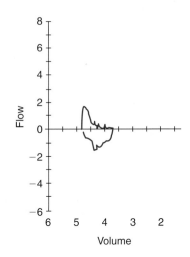

Spirometry	PRED	LLN	PRE	% PRED
FVC (L)	3.98	3.27	2.47	62
FEV$_1$ (L)	3.55	2.92	2.16	61
FEV$_1$/FVC (%)	89	80	87	**
FEF$_{25\%-75\%}$ (L/sec)	4.05	2.75	2.74	68
PEFR (L/sec)	7.61	5.47	5.45	71
FET100% (sec)	**	**	6.36	**

Lung volumes	PRED	LLN	PRE	% PRED
VC (L)	3.98	3.27	2.62	66
TLC (L)	5.49	4.65	3.31	60
FRC$_{PL}$ (L)	2.72	2.12	1.66	61
RV (L)	1.33	0.91	0.69	52
RV/TLC (%)	23	**	21	**
IC (L)	**	**	1.65	**
ERV (L)	**	**	0.97	**

B

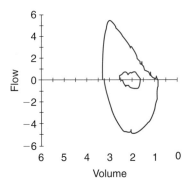

NOTE: **denotes predicted value and/or LLN not available.

FIG. 8.25 Pulmonary function studies in pediatric patients demonstrating obstruction and restriction. (A) Data from a 15-year-old boy with advanced cystic fibrosis. (B) Data from a 10-year-old girl with systemic scleroderma.

(Continued)

Spirometry	PRED	LLN	PRE	% PRED
FVC (L)	1.72	1.41	0.78	45
FEV$_1$ (L)	1.51	1.22	0.71	47
FEV$_1$/FVC (%)	88	79	92	**
FEF$_{25\%-75\%}$ (L/sec)	1.93	1.29	1.33	69
PEFR (L/sec)	4.14	2.97	3.15	76
FET100% (sec)	**	**	6.98	**

Lung volumes	PRED	LLN	PRE	% PRED
VC (L)	1.72	1.41	0.78	45
TLC (L)	2.47	**	1.55	63
FRC$_{PL}$ (L)	1.21	**	0.88	73
RV (L)	0.64	**	0.77	120
RV/TLC (%)	26	**	50	**
IC (L)	**	**	0.67	**
ERV (L)	**	**	0.11	**

Diffusion capacity	PRED	LLN	PRE	% PRED
DL$_{CO}$ (mL/mm Hg/min)	16.5	**	4.4	27
DL Adj (mL/mm Hg/min)	16.5	**	4.5	27
DL$_{CO}$/V$_A$	6.41	**	4.85	76
V$_A$ (L)	**	**	0.91	**

C

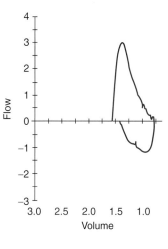

FIG. 8.25, CONT'D

given a break between trials to replace their cannula or mask until their oxygenation is back to baseline.

Important Plethysmographic Parameters

The tests performed and parameters examined depend on the reason for performing the study and on the ability of the child. In young children, obtaining a stable resting level and reproducible FRC may be all that can be accomplished. Once spirometry is mastered, the child can quickly learn to perform a full IC and VC in the body box. In a clinical setting, a skilled clinician and user-friendly software allow data to be edited as necessary to provide TLC, FRC, RV, and RV/TLC. It is important that the operators understand when and how to average data versus deleting data and when to accept the best test data. This is especially true with pediatric patients, who may not reproduce the entire maneuver with each trial.

Although spirometry is the first test performed in many patients, spirometry alone may not accurately predict lung volumes in children. Fig. 8.25 demonstrates case presentations of obstructive and restrictive lung disease. Note that predicted values, as well as the lower limit of normal (LLN), are presented. In some reference sets, the LLN is not available and is indicated with asterisks (**).

The case in Fig. 8.25A is a 15-year-old white male with advanced cystic fibrosis. Severe obstruction is evident in the spirometry data. Both FEV$_1$ and FEV$_1$/FVC are reduced, consistent with an obstructive disorder. Lung volume measurements confirm the severity of obstruction and air trapping. Although the TLC is within normal limits, FRC, RV, and RV/TLC are significantly elevated.

A 10-year-old African American girl has systemic scleroderma (see Fig. 8.25B). The FVC and FEV$_1$ are severely reduced with a normal FEV$_1$/FVC ratio, suggesting a restrictive pattern. Her F-V loop has a very restrictive appearance (witch's hat). Scleroderma is a generalized disease that can cause shrinkage of any of the connective tissues in the body. When the lungs are affected, the disease presents as a restrictive disorder with a gas exchange abnormality, as noted by the reduction in the subject's D_{LCO}.

Are lung volumes necessary? The cases in Fig. 8.25A and B demonstrate the use of lung volumes in further characterizing the abnormalities seen in spirometry. In the case of the 15-year-old boy with cystic fibrosis, the lung volumes depict the presence of hyperinflation. In the 10-year-old girl with systemic scleroderma, the presence of a restrictive disorder is confirmed.

Role of Measurement of Airway Resistance

The measurement of Raw during plethysmography may be an option to characterize airway function. Raw is measured while having the patient pant before closing a shutter or valve to obtain the V_{TG} so that specific airway conductance (sGaw) or specific Raw (sRaw) can be calculated. Patients, including children, tend to pant at an elevated lung volume. In other words, they do not return to the resting expiratory level with every pant and progressively increase their chest volume. If V_{TG} is measured at the very end of the maneuver, it will be artificially elevated. Although this is not the patient's true FRC, the application software makes a correction and reports separate values for V_{TG} and FRC. Raw should always be reported and interpreted at the lung volume at which it was measured (i.e., using V_{TG} to calculate sRaw and sGaw). Except in trained patients, Raw tends to be less reproducible than other pulmonary function parameters. Measurement of Raw may complicate and prolong the test and may not be necessary for routine testing. However, Raw can be significantly increased in patients with extrathoracic obstruction, central airway intrathoracic obstruction, and diffuse peripheral obstruction. Many laboratories find the measurement of Raw, sRaw, and sGaw helpful during methacholine challenges. Because the variability of these measurements is greater, a greater change is required to meet clinical significance. Whereas a decrease of 20% in FEV_1 is considered a positive response to methacholine, a corresponding increase of 35% to 40% in sRaw/sGaw is required. The measurement of airways resistance may be a more sensitive test and may identify changes in airflow earlier in the challenge.

BRONCHOPROVOCATION CHALLENGES

As with adults, children can be exposed to a variety of inhaled, ingested, or topically applied substances to challenge the airways. The purpose of any challenge study is to identify and/or stage the level of airway hyperreactivity. Examples of conditions that cause bronchoconstriction in children are asthma, gastroesophageal reflux, and anaphylactic reactions. Airway hyperreactivity may range from a very mild condition that produces only intermittent cough to sudden death from status asthmaticus or life-threatening anaphylaxis. Therefore it can be very important to identify whether a child's airway has the potential to react to a substance that provokes bronchoconstriction and/or stage the level of reactivity. Negative bronchoprovocation challenges are also very helpful in ruling out organic causes of airway reactivity, such as asthma. Children can be very susceptible to psychological causes of airflow obstruction. Many pediatric patients with VCD, hyperventilation syndromes, psychogenic cough, and tic disorders have been incorrectly diagnosed as having asthma. With the ability to challenge the patient's airways in a variety of ways, it is possible to rule out airway hyperreactivity and consider these other causes of cough, SOB, chest pain, and so forth. Many children misdiagnosed with asthma are treated needlessly and unsuccessfully with bronchodilators, histamine antagonists, and inhaled steroids. Labeling a child with an incorrect diagnosis has far-reaching effects, including possible morbidity from medications, as well as the cost of medications and medical insurance issues. Therefore establishing a valid diagnosis is vital, and bronchoprovocation challenges have become a common and invaluable tool in pediatric pulmonary laboratories.

The question arises: Which type of bronchoprovocation challenge is best? The answer, unfortunately, is unclear. Examples of provocative agents include methacholine, histamine, adenosine, cold air, hyperventilation, exercise, and allergen challenges. The mechanism of the bronchoconstriction differs with the agent administered, and each type of bronchoprovocation study has its own level of sensitivity and specificity. The definitions of these terms get quite confusing, but the commonsense approach is easier to understand. If a test is specific, the predictive value of that test is high. For example, a patient who has a positive exercise challenge test has a high probability that he or she truly has exercise-induced bronchospasm (EIB). Exercise, in this case, very specifically elicits the bronchospasm, consistent with asthma. Unfortunately, tests that are specific often have a lower sensitivity. Exercise, although quite specific, is a poorly sensitive test. Many patients with mild hypersensitivity—for instance, mild asthma—test negative with exercise. The exercise challenge does not elicit the symptoms of hyperreactivity, even though the patient has the disease. This is also referred to as a *false-negative test.* Methacholine, on the other hand, is a substance that has a high sensitivity. This bronchoprovocation agent correctly identifies patients with hyperreactive airways, even if only mild hyperreactivity exists. If a patient tests negative with a methacholine challenge, there is an extremely high probability that the patient does not have asthma. Therefore there are few false-positive tests. The "perfect" bronchoprovocation agent would have as high of a level of sensitivity and specificity as possible, balanced with a few false negatives or false positives. Of course, perfect does not exist, so finding the agent that best balances these concepts is our task. It may require that the patient completes more than one type of challenge to find the right answer.

Bronchoprovocation agents can be broadly divided into direct and indirect stimuli. Direct bronchochallenge testing is most commonly used, and the agent acts specifically and directly on targeted smooth muscle receptor sites. Airway hyperresponsiveness leads to bronchoconstriction of the smooth muscle and resultant narrowing of the airways. Examples of direct bronchoprovocation agents include methacholine and histamine. Indirect bronchoprovocation agents most often cause a release of mediators from inflammatory cells, such as mast cells and eosinophils. In turn, these mediators also cause smooth muscle contraction. Indirect stimuli producing inflammation include exercise, eucapnic voluntary hyperventilation (EVH), adenosine, mannitol, and hypertonic saline.

Traditionally, methacholine chloride has been considered to be the "gold standard" for bronchoprovocation testing. If a conclusive answer is not obtained, the physician may then choose to test the patient with a stimulus that has a different mode of action. For example, a common complaint in adolescents is SOB and chest tightness with exercise. The specific question posed by the physician might be: Does this child have EIB? If symptoms present only while the child is exercising, the logical provocation study to perform first would be an exercise stress test. Most pediatric laboratories will admit, however, that only a small percentage of children performing exercise actually exhibit EIB. This type of provocation study is very specific but not very sensitive. Recall that exercise is an indirect method of provoking bronchospasm and may be influenced by the type of exercise performed (running vs. swimming vs. gymnastics, for example). The environment may contribute to the provocation. Is the child running outdoors during allergy season? Is the child swimming in a chlorinated indoor pool? Do the temperature of the air and humidity affect the response, such as cold ice rinks versus hot, humid football fields? It is not unusual for a child with intermittent or mild persistent asthma to test negative during an exercise challenge in a controlled laboratory environment.

The next step might then be a methacholine challenge, a direct stimulus, which is less specific than exercise but more sensitive for eliciting bronchospasm. The child with a negative exercise challenge may well have a positive methacholine challenge, although likely positive in the mild or borderline range. Should the physician skip the exercise challenge and move directly to a methacholine challenge? This decision is up to the physician and is dependent on the question he or she is asking. There is neither a right or wrong answer nor a right or wrong challenge to perform. The use of an alternative provocation agent, such as EVH and mannitol, should also be considered, depending on the laboratory's resources. Specific protocols for each type of challenge should be established by the pulmonary laboratory and approved by the medical director. These methods are described in Chapter 9. Whichever provocation agent is used, it is important that the child be capable of performing serial spirometry at specific time intervals in a repeatable manner. Challenges can be time intensive. The child should be continually monitored for signs of fatigue or waning effort. Because children can become fatigued or easily distracted with prolonged testing, abbreviated protocols have been published. In some pediatric laboratories, challenges on very young children who cannot perform spirometry are obtained. Techniques for monitoring Raw and reactance, such as IOS, have been successfully used in children who are 3 years of age or older who cannot perform spirometry adequately. See Fig. 8.26 and the IOS discussion to follow later in the chapter. Challenge tests are considered a supervisory level II. As a result, a physician must be present or immediately available. Challenges in pediatric patients are not recommended in any facility where clinicians are unfamiliar or inexperienced with children. A fully stocked emergency cart is also essential. Patient safety and well-being are always the number-one priority.

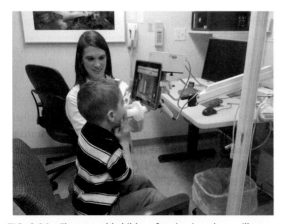

FIG. 8.26 Five-year-old child performing impulse oscillometry (IOS). The patient is wearing a nose clip, supporting the cheeks, and making a tight seal with his lips at the mouthpiece. The clinician is distracting the child with the use of a movie to aid in calming the patient's breathing during the data-acquisition period.

PULMONARY EXERCISE STRESS TESTING

Pulmonary function laboratories are asked to perform exercise stress tests for the following reasons: (1) to assess exercise intolerance, (2) to rule out exercise limitation in patients with known pulmonary or cardiac disease, and (3) to assess EIB. Protocols for exercise are as varied as protocols for inhalation challenges. The protocol used is often geared toward answering a specific question. Refer to Chapters 7 and 9 for examples of specific exercise protocols.

VCD is often elicited when a child is exercising and should be considered as a possible component of a subject's complaint of SOB and chest tightness. Performing a pulmonary or submaximal exercise test will produce enough stress for the child to evoke his or her symptoms. Inspiratory stridor may be audible with more severe VCD. Children who exhibit VCD tend to recover very quickly after the stress of exercise. F-V loops may be performed throughout exercise to aid in defining the abnormality. However, F-V loos do not specifically characterize the location of the abnormality. The use of flexible bronchoscope/rhinoscope to visualize the upper airway architecture during exercise has been shown to help identify whether or not a structural abnormality exists. Neither VCD nor exercise-induced bronchospasm is mutually exclusive. Although each diagnosis may occur without the other, it is common to have a child with both EIB and VCD. It is important to understand that pulmonary function testing does not always distinguish the role that VCD plays in the child's symptomatology. Clinical correlation by an experienced clinician and physician is key to correctly diagnosing true EIB versus VCD, exercise-induced hyperventilation, technique-related problems, or comorbid conditions.

PF TIP 8.12

Protocols for exercise stress tests may vary according to the patient being studied and the indication for testing. Different protocols may yield differing results, and the interpretation of exercise stress tests may differ depending on the test performed. Careful examination of FVLs during exercise can be helpful in identifying an abnormality.

The indication for a maximal cardiopulmonary exercise test (CPET) is to evaluate how well the respiratory and cardiovascular systems work together. The clinical question asked is often whether the child has normal exercise tolerance. If not, is the child limited by the lungs (ventilatory limitation), the heart (cardiovascular limitation), or both? The American Heart Association (AHA) has published guidelines on CPET in the pediatric age group. Box 8.2 lists the common reasons for pediatric CPET and specific clinical applications according to the AHA.

Maximal tests are performed with a full 12-lead electrocardiogram (ECG), pulse oximetry, and a mouthpiece or mask in place to measure ventilation, oxygen consumption, and carbon dioxide production (see Chapter 7 for a detailed discussion of indications, protocols, analysis, etc.). The use of an ergometer versus a treadmill may be a laboratory preference. Maximal oxygen consumption is usually slightly higher on a treadmill. The advantage of an ergometer, however, is that the child's upper body is relatively still while the legs cycle. This decreases movement of the head and leaks around the mouthpiece. Pulse oximetry is often problematic during exercise because of movement of the arms and fingers. With cycle ergometry, however, less whole-body motion produces fewer artifacts. The cycle ergometers typically used in pediatric testing can be modified to fit varying body sizes using saddle height, crankshaft length, and handlebar adjustments (Fig. 8.27).

Unless a plateau in oxygen consumption ($\dot{V}O_2$) can be identified, the highest level reached is termed *peak oxygen consumption*.

BOX 8.2 COMMON REASONS FOR PEDIATRIC CARDIOPULMONARY EXERCISE TESTS AND SPECIFIC CLINICAL APPLICATIONS

Common Reasons for Testing

- To evaluate specific signs and symptoms induced by exercise
- To assess or identify abnormal responses to exercise
- To assess efficacy of specific medical or surgical treatments
- To assess functional capacity for athletic and vocational activities
- To evaluate prognosis
- To establish baseline data for rehabilitation

Specific Clinical Applications

- Cardiac disorders
- Aortic stenosis
- Cardiomyopathy
- Tetralogy of Fallot, Ebstein's anomaly
- Coarctation of the aorta
- Prolonged QT syndrome
- Pulmonary
- Asthma
- Cystic fibrosis
- Chest wall (e.g., pectus excavatum)
- Vocal cord dysfunction
- Others
- Obesity
- Neuromuscular disease
- Exercise-induced syncope (e.g., postural orthostatic tachycardia syndrome [POTS])

Adapted from Paridon, S. M., Alpert, B. S., Boas, S. R., et al. (2006). Clinical stress testing in the pediatric age group: a statement from the American Heart Association Council on Cardiovascular Disease in the Young, Committee on Atherosclerosis, Hypertension, and Obesity in Youth. *Circulation, 113,* 1905–1920.

EXHALED NITRIC OXIDE AND NASAL NITRIC OXIDE

The measurement of **exhaled nitric oxide (eNO)** through the mouth and nasal nitric oxide (NO) is a technique now used in children. This procedure is an attractive alternative in the pediatric population because it does not involve any forced mechanics and is relatively simple to accomplish. The child is asked to take a single maximal breath in, followed by a prolonged exhalation through a restricted orifice in the mouth (Fig. 8.28). Alternately, nasal NO is measured from exhaled air through the nasal passage. Abnormally low values of nasal NO are found in children with primary ciliary dyskinesia (PCD). NO is a normally occurring substance found in reproducible levels in exhaled air. Levels of NO have been shown to significantly increase in tissues that are inflamed. The measurement of eNO has therefore been proposed as an index of airway inflammation, such as occurs in asthma. The clinical use of eNO, as well as nasal NO, in the pediatric population is still under investigation. As with IOS and Rint, eNO may be an important adjunct to serially follow asthma exacerbations in children and the effects of various drug regimens to control these exacerbations. Several limitations to this technique need to be addressed, including the collection of

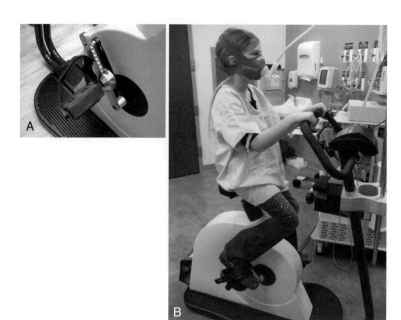

FIG. 8.27 (A) An adjustable pedal crankshaft used to test smaller patients when performing cardiopulmonary exercise tests (CPETs). (B) An 8-year-old female positioned on a cycle ergometer with a facemask interfaced with a pneumotachometer to measure exhaled air.

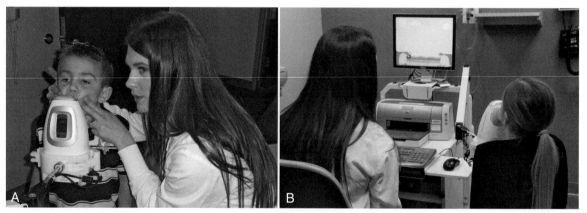

FIG. 8.28 (A) Clinician coaching and actively assisting a 5-year-old male in successfully performing an exhaled nitric oxide test. (B) Clinician passively coaching an 8-year-old female using an interactive software incentive program.

normative data and standardization of the technique. There is a range of normal changes with age, and it is important not to "overinterpret" results. It is generally believed that an eNO greater than 25 ppb is above the upper limit of normal in children. A comprehensive discussion of eNO measurements can be found in Chapter 10.

REFERENCE SETS AND PREDICTED VALUES FOR PEDIATRICS

Reference sets in the pediatric population have been well defined for spirometry and other lung function parameters. The Global Lung Function

Initiative has predicted values for spirometry, diffusion of the lung, and lung volumes that incorporate the pediatric age groups from 3 to 5 ages and older. A comprehensive review of these values is presented in Chapter 13.

ARTERIAL BLOOD GASES

An arterial blood gas is a valuable measurement of pulmonary function. Regardless of what spirometry, lung volumes, or D_{LCO} reveals, Pa_{O_2} and Pa_{CO_2} ultimately signify how well the lungs are performing. Pediatricians tend not to order a blood gas analysis as frequently as physicians who treat adults because of the challenges of drawing arterial blood in the pediatric population. Pulse oximetry can often be substituted for a blood gas for O_2 saturation and a capillary blood gas obtained for P_{CO_2}. There are definite indications, however, for obtaining arterial blood gases. Examples are (1) impending ventilatory failure, (2) prior problem with anesthesia or sedation, and (3) impending thoracic surgery in a child unable to perform routine PFTs. Children tolerate arterial punctures much better with reassurance and local anesthesia at the puncture site. The use of topical lidocaine (4%)/prilocaine cream or subcutaneous lidocaine (1%) is extremely helpful. See Chapter 6 for the details of the procedure.

SUMMARY

- The chapter describes techniques for performing PFTs in pediatric patients.
- Common lung function tests (e.g., spirometry, lung volumes, D_{LCO}) and other, more specialized tests are discussed, with attention to how these measurements differ in the pediatric population.
- For each category of tests, relevant questions are posed to relate pediatric testing to adult testing.
- Special emphasis is given to how the clinician should approach testing in young children and adolescents.
- Measurement of lung volumes, forced flows, and passive breathing mechanics in infants and preschool children is described, along with the highly specialized techniques required to obtain data from these patients.
- Special problems related to standards for testing, including guidelines from the ATS-ERS, are addressed.

CASE STUDIES

CASE 8.1

HISTORY

A 13-year-old African American female is well known to the pediatric pulmonary clinic and has a diagnosis of persistent, severe asthma complicated by a component of VCD. She presented today in the physician's office for a regular visit, stating she was having a "bad asthma" day. Her school held a fire drill earlier in the morning, and the students had to stand outside in cold air for 10 to 15 minutes. Pulse oximetry in the office revealed an O_2 sat of 96%. Prespirometry and postspirometry data were requested by her physician. The results of her spirometry are as follows:

Prebronchodilator

PRE BD	REF	LLN	BEST	% REF	Trial 1	Trial 2	Trial 3
FVC	3.18	2.44	2.15	68	2.15	1.99	1.85
FEV$_1$	2.84	2.21	1.10	39	1.10	0.97	0.71
FEV$_1$/FVC	89	78	51	**	51	49	38
FEF$_{25\%-75\%}$	3.57	2.14	0.65	18	0.65	0.54	0.36
PEF	6.49	4.40	1.94	30	1.94	1.80	1.29

A

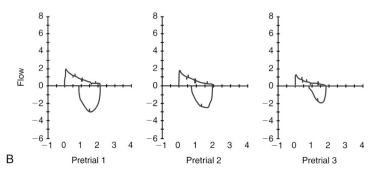

B   Pretrial 1   Pretrial 2   Pretrial 3

Postbronchodilator

POST BD	REF	LLN	BEST	% REF	Trial 1	Trial 2	Trial 3	Trial 4	% CHG
FVC	3.18	2.44	2.66	84%	1.81	1.90	2.54	2.66	24
FEV$_1$	2.84	2.21	1.98	70%	1.21	1.36	1.88	1.98	80
FEV$_1$/FVC	89	78	74	**	67	72	74	74	**
FEF$_{25\%-75\%}$	3.57	2.14	1.53	43%	0.75	0.98	1.45	1.53	137
PEF	6.49	4.40	4.45	69%	2.95	3.49	4.08	4.45	130

C

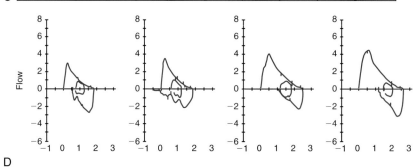

D

QUESTIONS

1. What do the results of the best prebronchodilator spirometry reveal?
2. What additional information do the prebronchodilator spirometry trials indicate?
3. Evaluate the entire F-V loop prebronchodilator.
4. What do the results of the best postbronchodilator spirometry reveal?
5. What additional information do the postbronchodilator spirometry trials indicate?
6. Evaluate the entire F-V loop post bronchodilator.

DISCUSSION

The results of prebronchodilator spirometry indicate that the subject has severe airflow obstruction. The ratio of the FEV_1/FVC tells us that airflow obstruction exists, and the FEV_1 of 39% tells us the severity of the obstruction is severe. Notice that the best results are essentially those of trial 1. For trial 2, the FEV_1 declined further, as did the FEV_1/FVC ratio. By trial 3, the FEV_1 had dropped approximately 400 mL and the ratio had worsened to 38%. The subject had an audible expiratory wheeze. This is a great example of a subject who has maneuver-induced bronchospasm from performing serial forced maneuvers. It is not necessary, and could be harmful, to have the subject continue to perform spirometry to meet criteria for repeatability. Indeed, the subject stated she felt worse after each maneuver. The inspiratory loops for this subject are also all abnormal. Note that the subject is not able to inspire fully after a forced maneuver. This could be an effort problem but is more likely physiologic. With so much bronchospasm occurring during forced exhalations, the more peripheral airways are likely collapsing during expiration and are unable to recruit and expand completely during inspiration. The bottom line, however, is that this subject is having severe airflow obstruction and needs a fast-acting bronchodilator.

Postbronchodilator, there is certainly a significant response to the bronchodilator. The FEV_1 improved by 80%, and even the FVC improved by 24%. The spirometry has not normalized, however. The FEV_1/FVC ratio is still below the LLN; therefore airflow obstruction still exists. The FEV_1 is now mildly reduced at 70% predicted, so the level of obstruction can be denoted as mild. Recall that the improvement in FEV_1 postbronchodilator is the change that occurred from her best prebronchodilator trials. If the calculations are made from her lowest FEV_1 prebronchodilator, what would the change in FEV_1 be? The answer is 179%! The change in FEV_1 is calculated by subtracting her lowest FEV_1 (0.71 L) from her best postbronchodilator FEV_1 (1.98 L) and dividing by the lowest FEV_1 (1.98 − 0.71 ÷ 0.71 × 100). Note again all the postbronchodilator trials. Her first several trials are quite variable, with FEV_1 ranging from 1.21 to 1.88 L, and only the last two trials are repeatable. The airways may be continuing to respond to the albuterol and dilating further. VCD also needs to be considered at this point. The subject's inspiratory maneuvers are not full and maximal. Recall that incomplete and triangular-shaped inspiratory loops are consistent with VCD. Trial 2 is particularly suspicious for VCD. Note that the inspiratory volume is greater than the expiratory volume. The flow rate at end inspiration is almost imperceptible. This is clearly abnormal.

HISTORY

The subject discussed previously returns to the emergency room 3 weeks later. She is admitted with a diagnosis of an asthma exacerbation. PFTs were obtained later that day. The operator observed the subject while performing the first several trials and noted that her chest excursion did not appear maximal. The operator first encouraged the subject to take maximal inspirations, with some improvement. The operator then suggested trying an open-mouth technique on the last two trials. The results of the spirometry trials are as follows, with superimposed volume–time tracings and F-V loops.

Prebronchodilator

PRE BD	REF	BEST	% REF	Trial 1	Trial 2	Trial 3	Trial 4	Trial 5	Trial 6	Trial 7
FVC	3.18	3.16	99	1.54	1.80	1.68	2.23	2.50	3.05	3.16
FEV_1	2.84	2.12	75	1.20	1.13	0.97	1.38	1.56	2.00	2.12
FEV_1/FVC	89	67	**	78	63	58	62	63	67	67
$FEF_{25\%-75\%}$	3.57	1.40	39	1.06	0.71	0.56	0.83	0.93	1.38	1.40
PEF	6.49	4.66	72	2.29	2.06	2.13	2.76	4.08	4.47	4.66

A

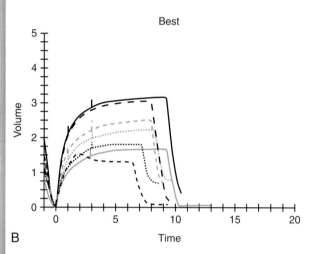

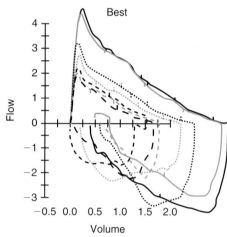

B

QUESTIONS

1. What do the multiple trials done on this subject indicate, and how does this fit into her clinical picture?
2. What accounts for improvement in spirometry in trials 6 and 7?
3. How could these results change a physician's treatment plan?

DISCUSSION

Once again, the variability in trials is noted. It is very important to observe the subject when abnormal spirometry is obtained. In this case, reminding the subject to take maximal inspirations had a marginal effect on improving the spirometry values (trials 4 and 5). Completely changing the technique made a significant difference for this subject (trials 6 and 7). Recall that this subject has a history of VCD with abnormal inspiratory loops on previous tests. Some of the inspiratory loops on this test are complete full loops, but some are not. Some have that truncated, triangular inspiratory loop discussed in the chapter. It is likely that the subject was not taking maximal breaths in the initial trials. Observing the subject helps identify if this is simply an effort problem or if the subject is using his or her throat and accessory muscles instead of the diaphragm and intercostal muscles. Changing to an open-mouth technique (subject takes a maximal breath first and then places mouthpiece in mouth and exhales maximally) altered her mechanics of breathing and minimized her VCD. There is a dramatic improvement in her spirometry in trials 6 and 7. It is possible there is the presence of bronchial dilatation from the multiple trials performed. The subject still has mild airflow obstruction, and this must be addressed by her physician. However, if one of the first several trials were reported as best, the child would likely have been treated differently and perhaps hospitalized for a longer period. It was extremely important for the operator to recognize how the subject's technique was affecting the results and to attempt methods to obtain better results.

CASE 8.2

HISTORY

The two subjects presented in this case have sternal deformities. Subject A is a 13-year-old male with pectus carinatum and no other medical diagnosis. Subject B is a 9-year-old female with pectus excavatum. However, this young lady also has multiple other musculoskeletal deformities, including spondylosis, thoracic and costovertebral dystrophy, and kyphoscoliosis. Her thoracic deformities warranted the insertion of titanium rib implants several years ago. Both subjects are presenting to their pulmonologist's office with complaints of increasing SOB during exercise.

PFTs for subjects A and B are presented on the following pages.

QUESTIONS

1. Compare and contrast the results of both sets of PFTs.
2. From the results presented, is there basis to explain SOB with exercise for either subject?
3. Is further testing warranted for either subject?

DISCUSSION

Subject A has pectus carinatum (also known as *pigeon breast*), a straightforward and uncomplicated sternal deformity. Spirometry is within normal limits and without significant response to a bronchodilator. For lung volumes, the TLC and FRC are slightly above the upper limit of normal but in proportion to the spirometry values. There is no evidence of air trapping. This PFT is representative of what is generally seen in a subject with either pectus carinatum or pectus excavatum alone. A bronchodilator response may be seen in subjects with an asthmatic component but is not seen in this young man.

Subject B is a far more complicated case. Her pectus excavatum is in combination with several other thoracic and skeletal deformities, which exacerbates her dysfunctional pulmonary mechanics several-fold. Her spirometry has a restrictive pattern. The FVC and FEV_1 are both severely and proportionately reduced but with an increased FEV_1/FVC ratio. Her expiratory loop is very tall and narrow with a peak flow and $FEF_{25\%-75\%}$ within normal limits. This is the expected shape of the F-V loop with severe restrictive disease. Restrictive disease cannot be identified by spirometry alone. Lung volumes are needed to confirm the restrictive component. Indeed, her TLC is reduced, indicating a moderately restrictive component.

However, note that the FRC is within normal limits and the RV and RV/TLC are mildly increased. This is likely caused by the extensive deformity of her chest cage and the mechanical inability for her to completely empty her lungs. Her PFTs indicate a restrictive process.

Spirometry	REF	LLN	PRE BD	% REF	POST BD	% REF	% CHG
FVC (L)	4.38	3.50	5.13	117	5.11	117	0
FEV$_1$ (L)	3.70	2.95	4.09	111	4.29	116	5
FEV$_1$/FVC (%)	85	10	80	**	84	**	**
FEF$_{25\%-75\%}$ (L/sec)	3.82	2.31	3.68	96	4.31	113	17
PEF (L/sec)	7.49	5.30	8.81	118	8.73	117	−1

Lung Volumes	REF	LLN	PRE BD	% REF
VC (L)	4.41	3.85	5.13	116
TLC (L)	5.62	4.95	6.64	118
FRC (L)	2.78	2.36	3.42	123
RV (L)	1.19	0.81	1.51	127
RV/TLC (%)	23	19	23	**

A

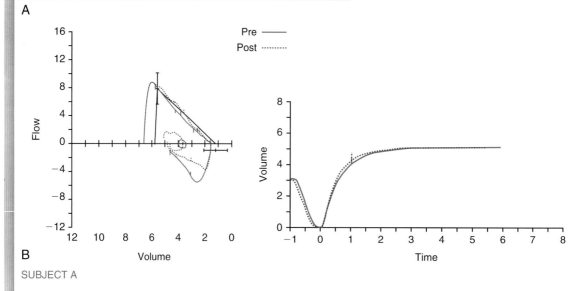

B

SUBJECT A

For subject A, SOB with exercise cannot be explained by the PFT results alone. However, a cardiopulmonary exercise stress test might be indicated to evaluate oxygen consumption, O$_2$ pulse, or possibly a ventilatory limitation. Further cardiac evaluation may be indicated.

Subject B has severely abnormal PFTs. As she grows, her chest cage may not be growing with her because of the rigid titanium implants.

Spirometry	REF	LLN	PRE BD	% REF	POST BD	% REF	% CHG
FVC (L)	1.57	1.17	0.59	38	0.62	40	5
FEV$_1$ (L)	1.46	1.13	0.56	38	0.55	37	-2
FEV$_1$/FVC (%)	89	10	94	**	88	**	**
FEF$_{25\%-75\%}$ (L/sec)	2.01	1.30	1.67	83	2.09	104	25
PEF (L/sec)	3.29	2.31	2.63	80	2.61	79	-1

Lung Volumes	REF	LLN	PRE BD	% REF
VC (L)	1.63	1.35	0.60	37
TLC (L)	2.21	1.87	1.33	60
FRC (L)	1.08	0.84	0.96	89
RV (L)	0.59	0.40	0.73	124
RV/TLC (%)	26	22	55	**

A

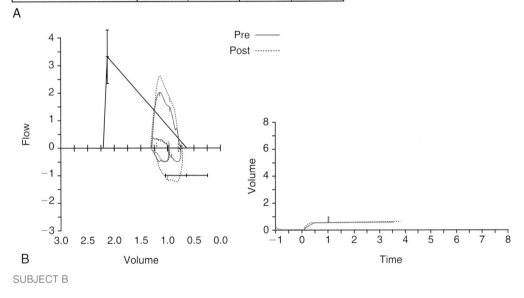

B

SUBJECT B

Her respiratory system is likely performing less efficiently with time. It is also impossible to guess what effect the abnormal chest, sternal, and rib structures are producing on the larger bronchial airways, as well as the thoracic vessels and the heart itself. This subject requires extensive imaging of her chest and a full cardiac workup.

She would also benefit from a cardiopulmonary exercise stress test, although she may have difficulty performing a maximal study. A baseline arterial blood gas would also help define her respiratory and ventilatory deficiencies.

SELF-ASSESSMENT QUESTIONS

Entry-Level

1. A 7-year-old child has an FVC of 0.95 L. ATS-ERS recommends or suggests which of the following?
   1. The repeatability of his FVC maneuvers be within 150 mL.
   2. The repeatability of his FEV_1 be within 100 mL.
   3. Exhalation time reaches a flow plateau of 0.025 L.
   4. Volume extrapolation errors are insignificant in children younger than 10 years.
      a. 1, 2, 3
      b. 2, 3
      c. 1 only
      d. 2, 3, 4

2. An 11-year-old boy performs technically acceptable and repeatable spirometry. His FVC reveals a value of 3.5 L (119% of predicted). and FEV_1 is 2.30 (92% of predicted). These spirometric values indicate
   a. normal spirometry.
   b. mild obstructive component.
   c. mild restrictive component.
   d. severe obstructive component.

3. Which of the following statements regarding ATS-ERS recommendations for spirometry most applies to children > 6 years old?
   a. The best F-V curve is based on the curve with highest addition of FVC and FEV_1, but the best values for each parameter should be independently reported.
   b. The curve with the best peak flow should be reported.
   c. The F-V loop with the best FEV_1 should be reported.
   d. The best F-V curve is based on the curve with the highest addition of FVC and $FEF_{25\%-75\%}$, but the best values for each parameter should be independently reported.

4. A 4-year-old child is performing spirometry for the first time. The child is capable of performing similar F-V loops several times; however, his best expiratory time is 2 seconds, and there is a change of less than 0.025 L in volume for 1 second. Which of the following statements is true regarding the spirometry?
   a. The test meets all current ATS-ERS recommendations.
   b. The F-V loops produced may be used for calculating the $FEF_{25-75\%}$.
   c. The loops are not usable because a true FVC cannot be obtained.
   d. Only the one best PEF rate is reportable.

5. Inspiratory loops in children
   a. should be essentially ignored because of effort limitation.
   b. are not valuable in assessing expiratory volume.
   c. can be a valuable component of the F-V loop when performed maximally.
   d. can be examined for evidence of intrathoracic airflow obstruction.

6. Asynchrony of the respiratory system occurs
   a. when the chest wall (rib cage) and abdomen are moving in unison.
   b. during normal passive tidal breathing.
   c. during any forced maneuver.
   d. with paradoxical movement of the chest wall and diaphragm.

7. Indirect methods of bronchoprovocation include which of the following?
   1. Methacholine challenges
   2. Exercise challenges
   3. Eucapnic voluntary ventilation
   4. Mannitol challenges
      a. 1, 2
      b. 2, 3, 4
      c. 4 only
      d. 3, 4

8. Which of the following strategies may lead to successful teaching of spirometry in a young child?
   1. Patience
   2. Persistence until the child gets the test performed correctly
   3. Praise for efforts the child makes
   4. Prizes or small trinkets as reward for child's efforts
      a. 1, 2, 3
      b. 1, 3, 4
      c. 1, 3
      d. 1, 2, 3, 4

9. Which of the following is a *false* statement regarding reference or predicted values?
   a. The greater the number of "normal" patients of each sex in a reference set, the more likely the regression equations will be accurate.
   b. Entering a child's height as 50 in. gives a predicted value similar to entering the child's height as 50 cm.
   c. PFT data may be expressed as percent predicted, the 95th confidence interval, or Z score.
   d. Age, height, ethnicity, and weight are all used in the calculation of predicted values.

10. What is the most common effect on the F-V curve when children have known VCD?
   a. Flattening of the inspiratory curve
   b. Fixed obstruction
   c. No effect on flow volume curve
   d. Flattening of the expiratory curve

Advanced

11. A 12-year-old child with advanced cystic fibrosis has lung volume determination by two methods, plethysmography and nitrogen washout. Which of the following outcomes would be expected?
   a. The FRC from the nitrogen washout and the V_{TG} from plethysmography would be comparable.
   b. The FRC from the nitrogen washout would likely be underestimated because of poor equilibration of gas in the thorax of an obstructed patient.
   c. The V_{TG} from plethysmography would greatly overestimate FRC because of hyperinflation and air trapping.
   d. The FRC from nitrogen washout would likely be overestimated because of inherent leaks in the system.

12. Primary pulmonary hypertension in children is characterized by decreased perfusion to the lung, but FVC and TLC are within normal limits. Assuming a normal hemoglobin of 14.0, the expected results from performing diffusing capacity would reveal which of the following?
   a. Increased Raw, D_{LCO}, increased D_L/V_A
   b. Normal Raw and D_{LCO} but reduced D_L/V_A
   c. Reduced Raw and D_{LCO} but normal D_L/V_A
   d. Normal Raw but reduced D_{LCO} and D_L/V_A

13. The ease of obtaining repeatable forced flow measurements in infants may be affected by which of the following?
   1. Sleep state
   2. Type of sedation used
   3. Age/size of child
   4. Technical and equipment considerations
      a. 1, 3, 4
      b. 2, 3
      c. 3, 4
      d. 1, 2, 3, 4

14. During tidal breathing, a sedated infant has a passive single-breath occlusion performed. The peak flow immediately after occlusion is 360 mL/sec, the occlusion plateau is 9.0 cm H_2O, and the passive exhaled volume is 144 mL. This child's respiratory system compliance can be calculated as which of the following?
   a. 4 mL/cm H_2O
   b. 13 mL/cm H_2O
   c. 16 mL/cm H_2O
   d. Not enough information available to calculate

15. Which of the following does *not* affect IOS results?
   a. Child's head position
   b. Use of nose clips
   c. Child's breathing pattern
   d. All of the above will affect IOS results.

16. During EVH, which of the following parameters should be kept constant and in normal physiologic range?
   a. Respiratory rate
   b. ET_{CO_2}
   c. Heart rate
   d. Tidal volume

17. A young child who is unable to perform spirometry might have both IOS and eNO measurements made. Which combination of values would suggest that the child is having an acute flare-up of his or her asthma and allergies?
   a. eNO = 10 ppb, R5Hz = 160% predicted
   b. eNO = 0 ppb, R5Hz = 50% predicted
   c. eNO = 20 ppb, R5Hz = 100% predicted
   d. eNO = 150 ppb, R5Hz = 200% predicted

18. Which of the following testing maneuvers triggers the Hering–Breuer reflex?
    a. Panting maneuvers during plethysmographic measurements
    b. Impedance measurements during IOS testing
    c. Passive occlusion measurements in infants
    d. FVC maneuvers
19. A bronchodilator response using IOS would cause which of the following changes?
    1. An increase in the resonant frequency
    2. A decrease in AX
    3. A decrease in R5, R10, and R20
    4. A less negative reactance (X5)

a. 1, 3
b. 2, 3
c. 2, 4
d. 2, 3, 4

20. A 10-year-old boy with a history of DMD is undergoing multiple discharge assessments. He performs a CPF maneuver. Which of the following results would give confidence that the child should be able to affectively clear secretions at home?
    a. 50 L/min
    b. 100 L/min
    c. 75 L/min
    d. 175 L/min

SELECTED BIBLIOGRAPHY

Spirometry

Crenesse, D., Berlioz, M., Bourrier, T., et al. (2001). Spirometry in children aged 3 to 5 years: Reliability of forced expiratory maneuvers. *Pediatric Pulmonology, 32,* 56–61.

Krowka, M. J., Enright, P. L., Rodarte, J. R., et al. (1987). Effect of effort on measurement of forced expiratory volume in one second. *American Review of Respiratory Diseases, 136,* 829–833.

Redding, G. J., Praud, J. P., & Maye, O. H. (2011). Pulmonary function testing in children with restrictive chest wall disorders. *Pediatric allergy and immunology pulmonology, 24*(2), 89–94.

Predicted Values and Reference Equations

Hankinson, J. L., Odencrantz, J. R., & Fedan, K. B. (1999). Spirometric reference values from a sample of the general U.S. population. *American Journal of Respiratory and Critical Care Medicine, 159,* 179–187.

Ip, M. S., Ko, F. W., Lau, A. C., et al. (2006). Hong Kong Thoracic Society. Updated spirometric reference values for adult Chinese in Hong Kong and implications on clinical utilization. *Chest, 129,* 384–392.

Quanjer, P. H., Stanojevic, S., Cole, T. J., et al. (2012). Multi-ethnic reference values for spirometry for the 3-95-yr age range: The global lung function 2012 equations. *European Respiratory Journal, 40,* 1324–1343.

Quanjer, P. H., Stocks, J., & Cole, T. J. (2011). Influence of secular trends and sample size on reference equations for lung function tests. *European Respiratory Journal, 37,* 658–664.

Stanojevic, S., Graham, B., Cooper, B., et al. (2017). Official ERS technical standards: Global Lung Function Initiative reference values for the carbon monoxide transfer factor for Caucasians. *European Respiratory Journal, 50.*

Stanojevic, S., Wade, A., Stocks, J., & Cole, T. J. (2009). Spirometry centile charts for young Caucasian children. The Asthma UK Collaborative Initiative. *American Journal of Respiratory and Critical Care Medicine, 180,* 547–552.

Hulzebos, E., Takken, T., Reijneveld, E. A., Mulder, M., & Bongers, B. C. (2017). *Reference Values for Respiratory Muscle Strength in Children and Adolescents.* Respiration: Karger.

Stefanutti, D., & Fitting, J-W. (1999). Sniff Nasal Inspiratory Pressure: Reference Values in Caucasian Children. *American Journal of Respiratory and Critical Care Medicine, 159,* 107–111.

Vocal Cord Dysfunction and Obstructing Upper Airway Lesions

Davis, R. S., Brugman, S. M., & Larsen, G. L. (2007). Use of videography in the diagnosis of exercise-induced vocal cord dysfunction: A case report with video clips. *Journal of Allergy and Clinical Immunology, 119,* 1329–1331.

McFadden, E. R., Jr., & Zawadski, D. K. (1996). Vocal cord dysfunction masquerading as exercise-induced asthma: A physiologic cause for "choking" during athletic activities. *American Journal of Respiratory and Critical Care Medicine, 153,* 942–947.

Perkins, P. J., & Morris, M. J. (2002). Vocal cord dysfunction induced by methacholine challenge testing. *Chest, 122,* 1988–1993.

Watson, M. A., King, C. S., Holley, A. B., et al. (2009). Clinical and lung-function variables associated with vocal cord dysfunction. *Respiratory Care, 54*(4), 467–473.

Weinberger, M., & Abu-Hasan, M. (2007). Pseudo-asthma: When cough, wheezing, and dyspnea are not asthma. *Pediatrics, 120,* 855–864.

Respiratory Muscle Strength

Bianchi, C., & Baiardi, P. (2008). Cough Peak Flows: Standard Values for Children and Adolescents. *American Journal of Physical Medicine & Rehabilitation, 87,* 461–467.

Birnkrant DJ, Bushby K, Bann CM, Alman BA et. al. Diagnosis and management of Duchenne muscular dystrophy, part 2: respiratory, cardiac, bone health, and orthopaedic management. Lancet Neurology Vol April 17, 2018. P347-361.

Gauld, L., & Boynton, A. (2005). *Pediatric Pulmonology, 39,* 457–460.

Neve, V. C. J., & Edme, J. (2013). Sniff nasal inspiratory pressure in the longitudinal assessment of young Duchenne muscular dystrophy children. *European Respiratory Journal, 42,* 671–680.

Exercise Stress Testing

Abu-Hasan, M., Tannous, B., & Weinberger, M. (2005). Exercise-induced dyspnea in children and adolescents: If not asthma then what? *Annals of Allergy, Asthma, and Immunology, 94,* 366–371.

Heinle, R., Linton, A., & Chidekel, A. S. (2003). Exercise-induced vocal cord dysfunction presenting as asthma in pediatric patients: Toxicity of inappropriate inhaled corticosteroids and the role of exercise laryngoscopy. *Pediatric Asthma Allergy Immunology, 16*(4), 215–224.

Paridon, S. M., Alpert, B. S., Boas, S. R., et al. (2006). Clinical stress testing in the pediatric age group: A statement from the American Heart Association Council on Cardiovascular Disease in the Young, Committee on Atherosclerosis Hypertension, and Obesity in Youth. *Circulation, 113,* 1905–1920.

Pulmonary Function Testing in Infants and Very Young Children

Aurora, P., Stocks, J., Oliver, C., et al. (2004). Quality control for spirometry in preschool children with and without lung disease. *American Journal of Respiratory and Critical Care Medicine, 169,* 1152–1159.

Castile, R., Filbrun, D., Flucke, R., et al. (2000). Adult-type pulmonary function tests in infants without respiratory disease. *Pediatric Pulmonology, 30,* 215–227.

Davis, S. D. (2003). Neonatal and pediatric respiratory diagnostics. *Respiratory Care, 48*(4), 367–385.

Debley, J., Filbrun, A. G., & Subbarao, P. (2011). Clinical applications of pediatric pulmonary testing: Lung function in recurrent wheezing and asthma. *Pediatric Allergy and Immunology Pulmonology, 24*(2), 69–76.

Hoo, A. F., Dezateux, C., Hanrahan, J. P., et al. (2002). Sex-specific prediction equations for max FRC in infancy. *American Journal of Respiratory and Critical Care Medicine, 165,* 1084–1092.

Jones, M., Castile, R., Davis, S., et al. (2000). Forced expiratory flows and volumes in infants—normative data and lung growth. *American Journal of Respiratory and Critical Care Medicine, 161,* 353–359.

Lesnick, B. L., & Davis, S. (2011). Infant pulmonary function testing: Overview of technology and practical considerations—new current procedural terminology codes effective 2010. *Chest, 139*(5), 1197–1202.

Lum, S., Bush, A., & Stocks, J. (2011). Clinical pulmonary function testing for children with bronchopulmonary dysplasia. *Pediatric Allergy and Immunology Pulmonology, 24*(2), 77–88.

Nuttall, A., Velasquez, W., Beardsmore, C. S., & Gaillard, E. A. (2019). Lung clearance index: assessment and utility in children with asthma. *Eur Respir Rev 2019, 28.* 190046.

Ren, C. L., Robinson, P., & Ranganathan, S. (2014). Chloral hydrate sedation for infant pulmonary function testing. *Pediatric Pulmonology, 49*(12), 1251–1252. https://doi.org/10.1002/ppul.23012.

Subbarao, P, Milla, C, Aurora, P, Davies, JC, Davis, SD, Hall, GL, et al. (2015). Multiple-breath washout as a lung function test in cystic fibrosis: A Cystic Fibrosis Foundation Workshop report. *Ann Am Thorac Soc, 12,* 932–939.

Oscillometry and Nitric Oxide

Buchvald, F., & Bisgaard, H. (2001). FeNO measured at fixed exhalation flow rate during controlled tidal breathing in children from the age of 2 years. *American Journal of Respiratory and Critical Care Medicine, 163,* 699–704.

Smith, H. J., Reinhold, P., & Goldman, M. D. (2005). Forced oscillation technique and impulse oscillometry. *European Respiratory Society*, *31*, 72–105.

Standards and Guidelines

American Thoracic Society. (2018). An Official American Thoracic Society Technical Statement: Preschool Multiple-Breath Washout Testing. *American Journal of Respiratory and Critical Care Medicine*, *197*(5), e1–e19.

American Thoracic Society. (2011). An Official ATS Clinical Practice Guideline: Interpretation of Exhaled Nitric Oxide Levels (FE_{NO}) for Clinical Applications. *American Journal of Respiratory and Critical Care Medicine*, *184*, 602–615.

American Thoracic Society/European Respiratory Society. (2019). An official American Thoracic Society and European Respiratory Society Technical Statement: Standardization of Spirometry 2019 Update. *American Journal of Respiratory and Critical Care Medicine*, *200*(8).

American Thoracic Society/European Respiratory Society. (2007). An official American Thoracic/ European Respiratory Society statement: Pulmonary function testing in preschool children. *American Journal of Respiratory and Critical Care Medicine*, *175*(12), 1304–1345.

American Thoracic Society/European Respiratory Society. (2005). ATS/ERS Statement: Raised volume forced expirations in infants: Guidelines for current practice. *American Journal of Respiratory and Critical Care Medicine*, *172*, 1463–1471.

An Official American Thoracic Society Workshop Report. (2013). Optimal lung function tests for monitoring cystic fibrosis, bronchopulmonary dysplasia, and recurrent wheezing in children less than 6 years of age. *American Thoracic Society*, *10*(2), S1–S11.

Stanojevic, S., Kaminsky, D. A., Miller, M., et al. (2021). ERS/ATS technical standard on interpretive strategies for routine lung function tests. *European Respiratory Journal* (in press).

ATS/ERS Taskforce, Wanger, J., Clausen, J. L., Coates, A., et al. (2005). Standardisation of the measurement of lung volumes. *European Respiratory Journal*, *26*, 511–522.

ERS Taskforce, Palange, P., Ward, S. A., Casaburi, R, et al. (2007). Recommendations on the use of exercise testing in clinical practice. *European Respiratory Journal*, *29*, 185–209.

European Respiratory Society/American Thoracic Society. (2013). ERS/ATS Consensus Statement: Consensus statement for inert gas washout measurement using multiple- and single-breath tests. (2013). *European Respiratory Journal*, *41*, 507–522.

European Respiratory Society/American Thoracic Society. 2017. (2017). ERS/ATS standards for single-breath carbon monoxide uptake in the lung. *European Respiratory Journal*, *49*.

General References

Hall, G., et al. (2018). Special Considerations for Pediatric Patients. *Pulmonary Function Testing: Principles and Practice*, 249–269. Springer.

Pfaff, J. K., & Morgan, W. J. (1994). Pulmonary function in infants and children. *Pediatric Clinics of North America*, *41*(2), 401–423.

Stocks, J., Sly, P. D., Tepper, R. S., et al. (1996). *Infant respiratory function testing*. New York, NY: Wiley-Liss.

Chapter 9

Bronchoprovocation Challenge Testing

CHAPTER OUTLINE

LEARNING OBJECTIVES

After studying the chapter and reviewing the figures, tables, and case studies, you should be able to do the following:

Entry-level

1. Describe two methods of performing bronchial challenge tests.
2. Identify a positive response to a methacholine challenge test.
3. List two indications for bronchoprovocation testing.
4. Select an appropriate protocol to test for exercise-induced bronchospasm.

Advanced

1. Describe direct versus indirect challenge mechanisms.
2. Interpret the various cut points for determining a positive challenge test.
3. Describe the dilution process for the preparation of methacholine doses.
4. Understand the physiologic determinants of exercise-induced bronchospasm.

KEY TERMS

1-minute tidal breathing method
eucapnic voluntary hyperventilation (EVH)
exercise-induced bronchospasm (EIB)

five-breath dosimeter method
histamine
mannitol
methacholine

provocative concentration (PC_{20})
provocative dose (PD_{20})

Diagnosis or evaluation of specific pulmonary disorders requires that appropriate tests be performed. Specialized tests often consist of standard tests performed under special conditions to evaluate a response to a condition or medication, such as performing forced vital capacity (FVC) maneuvers or pulmonary mechanics measurements (e.g., resistance or conductance) after inhalation challenge, hyperventilation, or exercise to quantify airway reactivity. In this chapter, we will review the various agents and conditions that elicit a hyperreactive airway response in subjects sensitive to the specific challenge.

BRONCHOPROVOCATION CHALLENGE TESTING

Bronchial challenge testing is used to identify and characterize airway hyperresponsiveness (AHR). AHR is an increased sensitivity and exaggerated response to nonallergenic stimuli, resulting airway narrowing. Although AHR is most often associated with asthma, it may be present in other diseases that cause airway inflammation or obstruction. Challenge tests may be performed in patients with symptoms of bronchospasm who have normal pulmonary function studies or uncertain results of bronchodilator studies. Bronchial challenge can also be used to assess changes in the hyperreactivity of the airways or to quantify the severity of hyperreactivity. Bronchial challenge tests are sometimes

used to screen individuals who may be at risk from environmental or occupational exposure to toxins.

Several commonly used provocative agents can be used to assess airway hyperreactivity. These include the following:
- Methacholine challenge
- Histamine challenge
- Mannitol challenge
- Eucapnic voluntary hyperventilation
- Exercise challenge (with either cold or room-temperature gas)

Each of these agents may trigger a bronchospasm but in slightly different ways.

Bronchoprovocation tests are classified as *direct* or *indirect* based on their mechanism of action (see Fig. 9.1 and Table 9.1).

Histamine and methacholine act directly on the smooth muscle cells of the airways to cause bronchoconstriction and AHR. Indirect bronchoprovocation tests, such as mannitol, act by inducing the release of bronchoconstricting mediators.

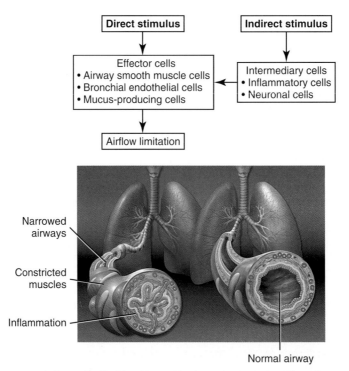

FIG. 9.1 Direct versus indirect stimuli of the airways. There are two categories of bronchoprovocation tests, those that act directly on smooth muscle and those that cause the airways to narrow indirectly by a release of endogenous mediators.

TABLE 9.1	
Agents Commonly Used in Bronchial Provocation Testing	
Direct Stimuli	**Indirect Stimuli**
Methacholine	Mannitol
Histamine	Adenosine (AMP)
Prostaglandins	Exercise
Leukotrienes	Eucapnic voluntary hyperventilation (EVH)
	Hypertonic saline

Hyperventilation, either at rest or during exercise, results in heat and water loss from the airway. This provokes a bronchospasm in susceptible patients. With each of these agents, pulmonary function variables are assessed before and after exposure to the challenge. Forced expiratory volume in the first second (FEV_1) is the variable most commonly used. Other flow measurements, in addition to airway resistance (Raw) and specific conductance (sGaw), may also be evaluated before and after the challenge. Additional parameters that have been used to assess the response to a bronchial challenge include breath sounds and forced oscillation measurements of resistance and reactance (see Chapter 10).

Methacholine Challenge

Bronchial challenge by inhalation of methacholine is performed by having the patient inhale increasing doses of the drug. All subjects will show a change in airway caliber with increasing concentrations of methacholine. Patients who have hyperresponsive airways demonstrate these changes at low doses of inhaled methacholine. This dose–response relationship permits the sensitivity of the airways to be quantified.

9.1   How To …

Perform a Bronchoprovocation Inhalation Challenge Test

1. Tasks common to all procedures:
   a. Calibrate and prepare equipment.
   b. Review order.
   c. Introduce yourself and identify patient according to institutional policies.
   d. Describe and demonstrate procedure.
2. Verify compliance with pretest instructions (Table 9.2), and note discrepancies. Test may need to be rescheduled.
3. Perform acceptable and repeatable baseline spirometry.
   a. Determine eligibility to test (e.g., $FEV_1 > 60\%-70\%$ predicted [exercise challenges] or 1.5 L).
   b. Determine FEV_1 target for PD_{15} or PD_{20}, depending on the challenge agent ($FEV_1 \times 0.8$ of 0.85, depending on the challenge agent).
   c. Determine recovery FEV_1 (baseline $FEV_1 \times 0.90$).
4. Formulate the dose concentrations based on the challenge agent and manufacturer's instructions. Some agents may be formulated and not require additional mixing.
5. Deliver initial dose based on the protocol/agent selected (may include diluent or 0-mg drug).
   a. Administer via dosimeter, tidal breathing, and/or dry-powder inhaler.
   b. Recalculate new target FEV_1 based on the "new baseline" FEV_1 obtained after the diluent or 0-mg administration (new baseline $FEV_1 \times 0.8$ of 0.85, depending on the challenge agent).
6. Measure FEV_1 at 30 and 90 seconds (airway resistance optional); a complete FVC manuever is not required.
   a. If either is greater than target FEV_1, move to next dose level.
   b. If the larger of the two manuevers is less than target FEV_1, stop test and administer a bronchodilator.
7. Measure postbronchodilator FEV_1.
   a. If greater than target recovery FEV_1 and the subject is symptom-free, he or she can be dismissed.
   b. If less than target recovery FEV_1, follow lab protocol, which may include administering another dose of bronchodilator.
8. Calculate PD_{15} or PD_{20} concentration.
9. Report data and note comments related to test quality.

TABLE 9.2

Withholding Medications Before Bronchial Challenge

Common to Direct and Indirect Challenges

Short-acting beta-agonist agents (e.g., albuterol)	6–8 hours
Long-acting beta-agonist agents (e.g., salmeterol)	36 hours
Ultra long-acting (e.g., indacaterol)	48 hours
Anticholinergic agents (ipratropium)	24 hours
Long-acting muscurinics	>168 hours
Standard theophylline preparations	12–24 hours
Indirect challenges only	
Inhaled corticoid steroids (e.g., budesonide)	6 hours
Cromones	4 hours
Leukotriene synthesis inhibitors	12–16 hours
Antihistamines	72 hours
Caffeine-containing drinks (cola, coffee)	6 hours
Vigorous exercise	4 hours

Adapted from 2017/2018 European Respiratory Society (ERS) Technical Standards for Bronchial Challenge Testing.

BOX 9.1   METHACHOLINE DOSING SCHEDULES

Dose Quadrupling Schedule (4× Increase)	Dose Doubling Schedule (2× Increase)
0.0625 mg/mL	0.031 mg/mL
0.250 mg/mL	0.0625 mg/mL
1.0 mg/mL	0.125 mg/mL
4.0 mg/mL	0.25 mg/mL
16.0 mg/mL	1.0 mg/mL
	2.0 mg/mL
	4.0 mg/mL
	8.0 mg/mL
	16.0 mg/mL

Spirometry and sometimes sGaw are measured after each dose. Most clinicians consider the test result positive when inhalation of methacholine precipitates a 20% decrease in FEV_1. The methacholine concentration at which this 20% decrease occurs is called the **provocative concentration (PC_{20}).** If the accumulative dose is measured, it would be termed the **provocative dose (PD_{20}).** The newest technical standard prefers using a dosing-versus-concentration scheme and reporting the PD_{20} versus the PC_{20}. In the doses used (Boxes 9.1 and 9.2; see also Box 9.4), healthy subjects do not display decreases greater than 20% in FEV_1. Therefore the methacholine challenge test is highly specific for airway hyperreactivity. Many patients who have asthma experience a 20% reduction in FEV_1 with doses of <400 μg. Bronchial hyperresponsiveness may also be seen in other pulmonary disorders such as chronic obstructive pulmonary disease (COPD), cystic fibrosis, and bronchitis.

Patients to be tested should be asymptomatic, with no coughing or obvious wheezing. Recent upper or lower respiratory tract infections may alter airway responsiveness, so bronchial challenge testing may need to be deferred. Their baseline FEV_1 should be normal or at least greater than 60% to 70% of their expected value. For patients with known obstruction or restriction, FEV_1 should be close to their highest previously observed value. Obvious airway obstruction (e.g., $FEV_{1\%} < 60\%$) is a contraindication to testing. A subject with an absolute $FEV_1 \le 1.5 L$ is at risk that a large drop in FEV_1 after a methacholine challenge might leave the individual with a compromised lung function. Bronchial challenge may be indicated in obstructed patients if the clinical question is related to the degree of responsiveness. Box 9.3 lists the contraindications to a bronchial challenge testing.

If the patient has been taking medication to mediate a lung condition, the medications should be withheld according to the schedule listed in Table 9.2. Other medications or substances can

BOX 9.2   SUGGESTED DOSING SCHEME USING A COMMON NEBULIZER AND 1-MINUTE TIDAL BREATHING

Concentration	0.0625 mg/mL	0.250 mg/mL	1.0 mg/mL	4.0 mg/mL	16.0 mg/mL
Hudson RCI MicroMist	1.81 μg	7.26 μg	29.03 μg	116.10 μg	464.4 μg

Courtesy Methapharm Inc., Brantford, ON, Canada.

affect the validity of the challenge as well. All medications being taken at the time of testing should be recorded to assist in the evaluation of the test results.

Baseline spirometry is performed to establish that the patient's FEV_1 is greater than 60% to 70% of predicted or the previously observed best value. Patients who demonstrate obstruction based on reduced $FEV_{1\%}$ or other flows typically do not require challenge testing. However, obstructed patients may be tested to establish the degree of hyperreactivity. Patients who have a restrictive process (i.e., reduced FEV_1, FVC, and total lung capacity [TLC]) may also be tested for coexisting AHR. If a patient is unable to perform acceptable and repeatable baseline spirometry (i.e., FEV_1), changes after an inhalation challenge may be impossible to interpret. In these situations, other parameters (e.g., sGaw or oscillatory resistance) that are less dependent on patient effort may be preferable as an end point.

Two methods of delivering methacholine to the airway are the **five-breath dosimeter method** and the **1-minute tidal breathing method**. A dosimeter can provide a true "quantitative" challenge test by delivering a consistent dose of the drug. The dosimeter (or nebulizer) is activated during inspiration, either automatically (by a flow sensor) or manually (by the technologist). A standardized driving pressure (typically 20 psi) and activation time (0.5–0.9 seconds) allow a fixed volume of aerosol to be generated for

each breath. By limiting the period of aerosol production, the last part of the inhalation carries the aerosol into the lung. The 2017 technical standard notes that if using this method, the subject should be instructed not to take a deep breath but rather a "usual" tidal breath.

The 1-minute tidal breathing method is the preferred method of methacholine delivery. A small-volume nebulizer is used to generate the methacholine aerosol (Fig. 9.2). The nebulizer's dose output must be characterized to calculate the delivered dose. This includes knowing the concentration (inhaled mass), the percentage of particles < 5 μm (respirable fraction), and the time in minutes (inhalation time):

$$\text{Dosage delivered} = \text{inhaled mass} \times \text{respirable fraction} \times \text{inhalation time}$$

Because the output of each nebulizer varies by manufacturer and model, the delivered dosage must be characterized using this formula.

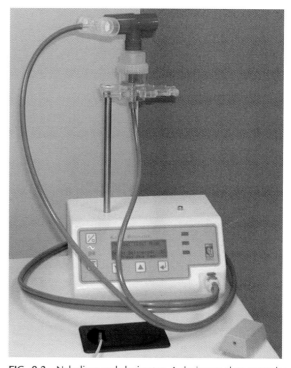

FIG. 9.2 Nebulizer and dosimeter. A dosimeter that controls the flow of gas to the nebulizer is also shown. The dosimeter provides a timer so that nebulization occurs for a specific time (e.g., 0.6 seconds), depending on the nebulizer used and its specific output. This dosimeter senses the patient's inspiratory effort and triggers flow automatically; some require manual actuation.

Two dosing routines are commonly used for a methacholine challenge (see Box 9.1 and 9.2). One routine uses a quadrupling (4×) increase in methacholine concentration, and the other method uses a doubling dose (2×). For each of these regimens, the highest dose is 16 mg/mL, and the dilutions can be easily prepared from a stock solution starting with 100 mg of dry methacholine (Table 9.3). The stock solution is prepared by dissolving the powdered drug in a saline diluent. A preservative (0.4% phenol) may be added to the solution but is not required. Methacholine concentrations from 0.025 to 25.0 mg/mL are stable after mixing and may be kept for 5 months if refrigerated at 2°C to 8°C (36°F–46°F). An alternate dosing scheme is provided with the form of methacholine that has been approved by the U.S. Food and Drug Administration (FDA; Provocholine, Methapharm, Ontario, Canada). This dosing schedule uses methacholine concentrations of 0.025, 0.25, 2.5, 10, and 25 mg/mL and is designed for use with the five-breath dosimeter method. Methacholine should be prepared by a pharmacist or individual trained in preparing drugs using a sterile technique. Appropriate precautions should be taken when handling dry-powder methacholine. Vials of methacholine should be carefully marked with labels that clearly identify the concentration.

Five-Breath Dosimeter Method

Methacholine is prepared according to the desired dosing scheme. Methacholine may be stored under refrigeration but should be brought to room temperature before administration. Baseline spirometry is performed.

The patient begins by inhaling five breaths of nebulized diluent, usually normal saline. The diluent step is optional but provides a means of checking that the patient understands the procedure and that

TABLE 9.3

Preparation of Methacholine for Two Common Dosing Schedules[a]

Methacholine	Diluent (0.9% NaCl)	Dilution
Doubling Dosage		
100 mg (dry powder)	6.25 mL	16.0 mg/mL
3 mL of 16.0 mg/mL	3 mL	8.0 mg/mL
3 mL of 8.0 mg/mL	3 mL	4.0 mg/mL
3 mL of 4.0 mg/mL	3 mL	2.0 mg/mL
3 mL of 2.0 mg/mL	3 mL	1.0 mg/mL
3 mL of 1.0 mg/mL	3 mL	0.5 mg/mL
3 mL of 0.5 mg/mL	3 mL	0.25 mg/mL
3 mL of 0.25 mg/mL	3 mL	0.125 mg/mL
3 mL of 0.125 mg/mL	3 mL	0.0625 mg/mL
3 mL of 0.625 mg/mL	3 mL	0.031 mg/mL
Quadrupling Dosage		
100 mg (dry powder)	6.25 mL	16.0 mg/mL
3 mL of 16.0 mg/mL	9 mL	4.0 mg/mL
3 mL of 4.0 mg/mL	9 mL	1.0 mg/mL
3 mL of 1.0 mg/mL	9 mL	0.25 mg/mL
3 mL of 0.25 mg/mL	9 mL	0.0625 mg/mL

[a]For each schedule, 6.25 mL of saline is added to dry-powder methacholine. Subsequent dilutions then use 3 or 9 mL of saline added to 3 mL of the previous dilution.

the system is working properly. If the diluent step is performed, the FEV_1 after the diluent becomes the "control," and the target FEV_1 for a positive test is 80% of this value. If the diluent step is omitted, the target FEV_1 is 80% of the baseline spirometry value. The breath should be like a tidal breath, focusing on not inspiring to TLC. The patient should be wearing a nose clip to ensure the breath is completed. The dosimeter should be triggered as inspiration begins; this may be done manually or automatically. The nebulizer should be activated for 0.5 to 0.8 seconds, depending on the output of the nebulizer, to deliver the desired dose. Again, the inspiration should emulate a normal breath, ensuring the subject does not take a deep or maximal breath. Inhalations are repeated for five breaths, lasting 2 minutes or less.

Spirometry is then repeated at approximately 30 and 90 seconds after the last inhalation. A timer or stopwatch is useful for staging the maneuvers. The FEV_1 maneuver should be acceptable and may be repeated, if necessary. The manuevers do not need to be a complete manuever (a.k.a. exhaling until completely empty). Full flow-volume (F-V) loop maneuvers may be useful for detecting changes in inspiratory flow that may occur (e.g., vocal cord dysfunction [VCD]). If Raw and sGaw are also measured, the patient should be seated in the plethysmograph and the door closed as soon as spirometry has been completed. With practice and careful timing, spirometry and resistance measurements can be completed within about 5 minutes after each dose of methacholine.

The largest FEV_1 after each dose should be reported. If airway resistance/conductance measurements are made, the average of two acceptable panting maneuvers should be reported. If FEV_1 decreases less than 20% or specific conductance (sGaw) decreases less than 35% to 40%, the next highest dose is administered. If FEV_1 decreases more than 20%, the challenge is complete. Signs and symptoms (e.g., coughing, wheezing, chest tightness) related to asthma should be recorded. A beta-agonist bronchodilator should be administered and spirometry repeated after a 10-minute delay.

1-Minute Tidal Breathing Method

As noted earlier, the 1-minute tidal breath technique is the preferred method of testing because it does not require the subject to take deep breaths, thus eliminating the broncho-protective effect associated with these maneuvers. In this method, normal relaxed breathing is used as the patient inhales the aerosol. Methacholine is usually prepared in 10 doses of doubling concentrations (see Box 9.1, Box 9.2, and Table 9.3). If the methacholine has been refrigerated, it should be allowed to come to room temperature for 30 minutes. A nebulizer that has been characterized should be used.

The patient should hold the nebulizer upright and breathe quietly through the mouthpiece with a nose clip in place. A facemask may be used in place of a mouthpiece, but the nose clip should not be omitted (nose clip may be placed over the mask). A filter may be placed on the expiratory limb of the nebulizer circuit to limit the amount of methacholine released in aerosol form in the testing area. A timer or stopwatch should be used to ensure that the breathing interval is exactly 1 minute long.

As in the dosimeter method, spirometry is repeated at 30 and 90 seconds after the end of the 1-minute tidal breathing interval. If a diluent step is included, the target FEV_1 (for a positive response) is 80% of the largest value obtained after the diluent. If the diluent step is omitted, the target FEV_1 is 80% of the baseline value. Patients with highly reactive airways may have a positive response (e.g., a 20% decrease in FEV_1) to the diluent. The FEV_1 maneuvers should be completed at 30 and 90 seconds. A complete FVC maneuver is not required, although once the target FEV_1 has been obtained, some laboratories do perform a full FVC manuever to note any effects on VC. If Raw or sGaw is to be measured, those measurements should be performed as quickly as possible after spirometry. If FEV_1 decreases less than 20%, the next highest dose should be administered. If FEV_1 decreases by 20% or more, the challenge is complete. A beta-agonist bronchodilator should be administered to reverse the bronchospasm and spirometry repeated after 10 minutes.

Spirometry or plethysmographic measurements are the most commonly used end points for bronchial challenge tests. For each parameter, the percentage of decrease is calculated as follows:

$$\%\text{Decrease} = \frac{x - y}{x} \times 100$$

where:

x = control FEV_1 (baseline or after diluent)
y = current FEV_1 after methacholine inhalation

This change is sometimes reported as a negative value (e.g., –20%) to indicate a fall in the FEV_1.

A 20% or greater decrease in the FEV_1 is considered a positive response based on the last dose used (see Interpretative Strategies 9.1). The same equation may be used to calculate changes in airway resistance or specific conductance. A decrease of 35% to 45% in sGaw is consistent with increased bronchial responsiveness. In patients suspected of having VCD, complete F-V loops may be helpful. VCD is sometimes mistaken for asthma in patients referred for bronchial challenge testing. Limitation of inspiratory flow (with little or no change in FEV_1) is usually observed in VCD.

Several methods of quantifying the results of the challenge are commonly used. The concentration of methacholine that results in a 20% decrease (PD_{20}) can be calculated from the last and second-to-last doses administered:

$$PD_{20} = antilog\left[\log D_1 + \frac{(\log D_2 - \log D_1)(20 - R_1)}{R_2 - R_1} \right]$$

where:

D_1 = second-to-last methacholine dose

D_2 = final methacholine dose (causing 20% or greater decrease)

R_1 = percent decrease in FEV_1 after D_1

R_2 = percent decrease in FEV_1 after D_2

PD_{20} calculated in this way provides a single index of bronchial responsiveness. PD_{20} may also be identified directly from a graph in which the change in FEV_1 is plotted against the log concentration of methacholine (Fig. 9.3).

Provocative concentrations for other variables, such as sGaw, can be calculated similarly by substituting the appropriate percentage for 20 in the preceding equation and substituting the percent

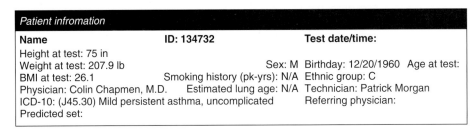

Patient infromation		
Name	**ID: 134732**	**Test date/time:**
Height at test: 75 in		
Weight at test: 207.9 lb		Sex: M Birthday: 12/20/1960 Age at test:
BMI at test: 26.1	Smoking history (pk-yrs): N/A	Ethnic group: C
Physician: Colin Chapmen, M.D.	Estimated lung age: N/A	Technician: Patrick Morgan
ICD-10: (J45.30) Mild persistent asthma, uncomplicated		Referring physician:
Predicted set:		

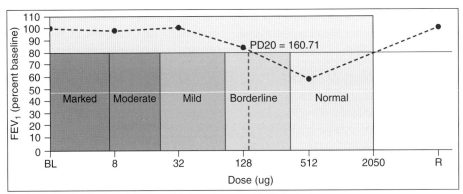

Challenge grade: *PD20 of 160.71 indicates borderline airway hyper-responsiveness*

Stage	Dosage	FVC	% BL	FEV1	% BL	Level notes
Baseline		6.99		5.10		
Diluent		—	—	—	—	0
Level 1	8	6.96	—	4.99	−2	1 No response
Level 2	32	6.94	−1	5.12	—	2 No response
Level 3	128	5.92	−15	4.30	−16	3 Subject feeling tight
Level 4	512	5.11	−27	2.96	−42	4 Significant response
Level 5	2050	—	—	—	—	5
Recovery	Albuterol	7.06	1	5.13	1	

FIG. 9.3 Methacholine challenge test. Results of data gathered during a bronchial challenge test are shown. The dosage of the challenge agent (methacholine, in this case) is plotted on the *x*-axis. Forced expiratory volume in the first second (FEV_1; or other variable) is plotted on the *y*-axis. The first point represents the baseline FEV_1 (5.10 L in this example). FEV_1 after each dose of methacholine is plotted until a decrease of 20% or greater occurs. In this example, FEV_1 decreased by more than 20% with a dose of 510 µg. A vertical line drawn from the point at which the dose–response curve crosses the 20% line defines the PD_{20} (160.7 µg). The patient is then given an inhaled bronchodilator to reverse the effect of the provocative agent, and the response is plotted.

decrease for that variable for R_1 and R_2. Note that this calculation requires that at least two doses of methacholine have been given. If FEV_1 decreases 20% after the diluent or the first dose of methacholine, PC_{20} should be reported as less than the lowest concentration administered. If FEV_1 does not decrease by at least 20% after the highest dose, PD_{20} should be reported as greater than the final dose based on the delivery dose of the nebulizer. See Interpretive Strategies 9.1. Airway responsiveness to methacholine can be described using the PD_{20}. Most patients referred for bronchial challenge testing have a history or symptoms suggestive of asthma but not a definite diagnosis. For these patients, if FEV_1 decreases less than 20% at the highest dose (PC_{20} or PD_{20}), bronchial responsiveness is probably normal, and asthma is unlikely. For patients whose FEV_1 decreases 20% or more at low doses of methacholine ($PC_{20} < 1.0\,mg/mL$ or $PD_{20} < 6\text{–}25\,\mu g$), the diagnosis of asthma is highly likely. For patients with PC_{20} values from 1 to $16\,mg/mL$ or PD_{20} from 100 to $400\,\mu g$, the diagnosis of asthma must be considered based on the pretest probability of asthma, the history of symptoms, and other possible causes for bronchial hyperreactivity. In practice, patients who have a PC_{20} or PD_{20} of greater than 8 to $16\,mg/mL$ and 200 to $400\,\mu g$, respectively, often do not have asthma. Patients who have a negative methacholine challenge ($PC_{20} > 16\,mg/mL$; $PD_{20} > 400\,\mu g$) may have asthma that has been suppressed by antiinflammatory medications or occupational asthma that is triggered by a specific agent. Patients with allergic rhinitis and smokers with COPD often have bronchial hyperreactivity but not asthma.

PF TIP 9.2

Some patients whose FEV_1 drops 20% or more at low doses of methacholine may not have asthma. Hyperreactive airways are also found in some patients with COPD who smoke or in patients who have allergic rhinitis. A negative methacholine challenge (i.e., a decrease in FEV_1 of <20% at the highest dose) may occur in patients who have asthma that has been suppressed by antiinflammatory medications. Some patients with asthma may have their asthma triggered by exposure to a specific agent, such as cold, dry air.

INTERPRETIVE STRATEGIES 9.1

Bronchial Challenge Tests

1. Were the pretest instructions adhered to (medication withholding schedule, etc.)?
2. Was the challenge agent administered appropriately?
3. For histamine and methacholine, was the delivered dose defined?
4. For mannitol, was the proper inhalation technique using the DPI performed?
5. For exercise, did the patient maintain an appropriate workload for > 4 minutes (preferably 6 minutes)?
6. For hyperventilation, did the patient maintain the target level of ventilation for 6 minutes?
7. Were the FEV_1 maneuvers performed at the correct intervals (30–90 sec)?
8. Were spirometric efforts acceptable and repeatable before and during the challenge? If not, interpret very cautiously or not at all.
9. For histamine and methacholine challenge, was there a 20% decrease in FEV_1 after inhaling diluent? If so, test result is positive. Was there a 20% decrease in FEV_1 after inhalation of the agonist? If so, test result is likely positive, and PC_{20} or PD_{20} should be used to categorize the degree of hyperresponsiveness. Was there at least a 35% decrease in sGaw (preferably 50%)? If so, test result is likely positive.
10. For mannitol, was there a 15% or greater decrease in the FEV_1 after inhalation or a 10% incremental fall in FEV_1 between two consecutive mannitol doses? If so, the test is positive. A PC_{15} can be calculated if the former occurs.
11. For exercise or hyperventilation challenge, was there a 10% decrease (prefer 15%) in FEV_1 after challenge? If so, test is positive.
12. Were there signs or symptoms of airway hyperreactivity (coughing, wheezing, and shortness of breath)? If so, test suggests bronchial hyperresponsiveness.
13. Were the results borderline? If so, consider repeat testing in the future.
14. Were symptoms present despite little or no change in FEV_1? Consider additional measurements such as sGaw or related conditions such as VCD.

A number of physiologic factors can affect the sensitivity and specificity of methacholine challenge testing. **Methacholine** causes a constriction of bronchial smooth muscle. In healthy individuals, taking a deep breath before performing the

FVC maneuver may cause bronchodilation for several minutes. In patients who have mild asthma, a similar response is sometimes observed. In patients who have severe asthma, the bronchodilating effect of a deep inspiration is reduced; a deep breath may actually cause bronchoconstriction. Because of this differing response, FEV_1 discriminates between those who have and those who do not have asthma.

Spirometry (i.e., FEV_1) may not detect a response in all patients. Raw or sGaw may be more sensitive in detecting hyperreactive airways in some individuals or used in subjects unable to perform acceptable spirometry maneuvers. Because Raw and sGaw are more variable than FEV_1 in healthy subjects, a larger change after the methacholine challenge is required to demonstrate hyperreactive airways. A decrease in sGaw of 35% to 45% may be considered a positive methacholine response. Some individuals with asthma symptoms may have primarily large airway changes in response to methacholine. These changes may manifest themselves as a decrease in sGaw or blunting of the inspiratory limb of the F-V loop. Although PEF is useful for monitoring asthma, it is less reproducible and more effort-dependent than FEV_1 for detecting changes after a bronchial challenge.

Technical factors can also make methacholine challenge tests difficult or impossible to interpret (see Criteria for Acceptability 9.1). Changes in FEV_1 after a bronchial challenge are usually not diagnostic in patients who cannot perform acceptable and reproducible baseline spirometry. Variable efforts by the patient may produce a false-positive test result (apparent reduction in FEV_1 but not AHR). The FEV_1 values obtained at 30 and 90 seconds after each dose of methacholine should be similar. Although the staging maneuvers do not need to be complete FVC maneuvers, they should still meet the criteria for an acceptable effort, with the exception of the end of forced expiration (EOFE; see Chapter 2). The usual repeatability criteria (FEV_1 efforts within 150 mL) may not be met because of the effects of methacholine. The FEV_1 reported for each dose of methacholine should be the largest value obtained at that level.

CRITERIA FOR ACCEPTABILITY 9.1

Bronchial Challenge Tests

1. The subject adhered to the medication withholding schedule and pretest instructions.
2. The subject should also be free of upper or lower respiratory infection.
3. Spirometric or plethysmographic efforts must meet standard criteria for acceptability and repeatability. For adults, the two largest FEV_1 measurements should be within 150 mL before the challenge (within 100 mL if the VC is 1.0 L or less). sGaw measurements should be within 10% before the challenge. During the challenge, acceptable efforts should be obtained; repeatability is desirable but may not be attained.
4. For methacholine challenges, the nebulizer's delivered dose has been characterized.,
5. For mannitol, the medication and administration technique should be performed according to the manufacturer's instructions. For exercise challenges, the patient should attain at least 80% to 90% of the predicted maximal heart rate (or $\dot{V}o_2$ max, if measured). This level should be maintained for 6 minutes. Ventilation should increase to 40% to 60% of the maximal voluntary ventilation (MVV; $FEV_1 \times 35$). Measurement of $\dot{V}_E$ is recommended.
6. For hyperventilation challenges (cold or ambient air), the target ventilation level should be maintained for the specified interval (dependent on protocol used). For the **eucapnic voluntary hyperventilation (EVH)** test, a target ventilation of $30 \times FEV_1$ for 6 minutes is recommended. For all challenge protocols, clinical signs and symptoms (e.g., presence or absence of coughing, wheezing) should be documented.

Adapted from 2017/2018 European Respiratory Society (ERS) Technical Standards for Bronchial Challenge Testing.

The spirometer used should meet the minimal standards set by the American Thoracic Society–European Respiratory Society (ATS-ERS; see Chapter 11). It should provide spirometric tracings or F-V loops for later evaluation.

Methacholine challenge testing is a safe procedure. The main risk to the patient is that severe bronchospasm may occur, so a physician experienced in treating acute bronchospasm should be immediately available. The technologist administering the bronchial challenge test should be thoroughly familiar with the procedure and with the signs and symptoms of a bronchospasm. It has been suggested that a minimum of 4 days of training and 20 supervised tests are needed to achieve proficiency in bronchoprovocation testing. The technologist must know when to stop the test and how to administer bronchodilators to reverse an acute bronchospasm. The technologist should also be proficient in the delivery of the medications used for reversal of the bronchospasm (e.g., albuterol and epinephrine) and for resuscitation, and these should be immediately available in the event of an adverse reaction. Because of the risks involved, some laboratories require written consent from the patient. The test should be administered in a well-ventilated room to protect other patients and the technologist from exposure. The addition of a filter to the exhalation port of the nebulizer may help reduce the volume of aerosolized methacholine in the room. Technologists with a known sensitivity to methacholine should not perform this procedure unless appropriate methods are used to avoid exposure to the drug.

Histamine Challenge

Aerosolized histamine extract (histamine phosphate) may be used for a bronchial challenge in a manner similar to a methacholine challenge. **Histamine** produces bronchoconstriction by an uncertain pathway. Antihistamines or H_1-receptor antagonists can block the response to histamine. Histamine-induced bronchospasm is also partially blocked by most classes of bronchodilators. Histamine differs from methacholine in its side effects, half-life, and cumulative effects. Flushing and headache are two common side effects of histamine inhalation. The peak action of histamine occurs within 30 seconds to 2 minutes, which is similar to that observed in methacholine. Recovery of baseline function is significantly shorter for histamine than for methacholine. The action of histamine, unlike that of methacholine, is thought to be less cumulative.

Patient preparation for a histamine challenge is similar to that used for methacholine (see Table 9.2). Antihistamines and H_1-receptor antagonists should be withheld for 48 hours before testing.

Various dosing regimens for a histamine challenge have been proposed. Box 9.4 lists one dosing protocol for a histamine challenge. These increments approximately double the concentration of drug at each level. The same criteria as those used for baseline spirometry in a methacholine challenge are observed. Diluent may be administered first to determine a control value for FEV_1.

If FEV_1 does not decrease by more than 10%, then five breaths of the first dilution are administered. Spirometric measurements are performed immediately and repeated at 3 minutes. A response is considered positive if FEV_1 decreases by 20% or more below the control at 3 minutes. If there is a negative response (FEV_1 decreases < 20%), the next dose is given, and measurements are repeated.

The results of a histamine challenge are reported in a manner similar to that described for methacholine, with the exception of using PC_{20} rather than PD_{20}.

Histamine, like methacholine, is relatively safe if testing follows the procedures described. Baseline and control values should always be established (see Criteria for Acceptability 9.1). Bronchial challenge should always begin with a low concentration of drug. The range of concentrations used should be appropriate for the patient tested. For adult patients in whom AHR is the suspected diagnosis, the dosing schedules previously described are recommended. Patients who have a positive response to a histamine challenge recover more quickly than those tested with methacholine. Histamine challenge can be repeated within 2 hours after the patient has returned to the baseline level of function.

BOX 9.4   HISTAMINE DOSING SCHEDULE
• 0.03 mg/mL
• 0.06 mg/mL
• 0.12 mg/mL
• 0.25 mg/mL
• 1.00 mg/mL
• 2.50 mg/mL
• 5.00 mg/mL
• 10.00 mg/mL

Mannitol Challenge

Mannitol is a hypertonic stimulus, and inhalation increases the osmolarity of the airways, which subsequently leads to the release of inflammatory mediators from mast cells and basophils. This leads to airway narrowing similar to that observed with hypertonic saline and exercise challenge tests. Mannitol is a sugar alcohol and is delivered by a special DPI. The DPI is trademarked as the Osmohale inhaler device and is a component of the testing kit (Aridol-Methapharm, ON Canada; Fig. 9.4).

The testing kit includes the drug packaged in capsules, which contain the mannitol in the desired doses. These capsules load into the DPI device, so there is not a need for additional specialized equipment or drug mixing. The dose scheme is listed in Table 9.4. Patient preparation for the mannitol

TABLE 9.4
Mannitol Dose Steps for Bronchial Challenge Testing with Aridol

Dose (#)	Dose (mg)	Cumulative Dose (mg)	Capsules per Dose
1	0	0	1
2	5	5	1
3	10	15	1
4	20	35	1
5	40	75	1
6	80	155	2 × 40 mg
7	160	315	4 × 40 mg
8	160	475	4 × 40 mg
9	160	635	4 × 40 mg

Adapted from the Aridol package insert.

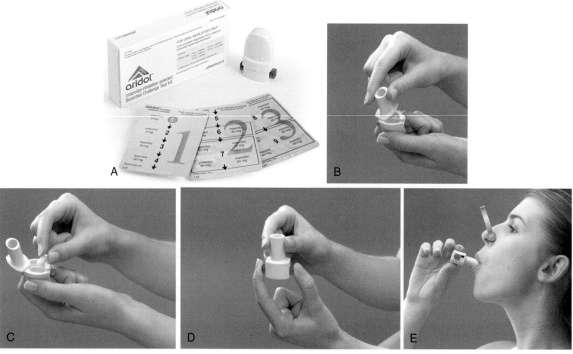

FIG. 9.4 Mannitol challenge testing. (A) Aridol kit with dry-powder inhaler (DPI) and capsules containing dosing scheme. (B) Twist the DPI to open the capsule chamber. (C) Insert the appropriate capsule into the holding chamber (do not use rubber gloves). (D) Puncture the capsules only once by depressing both puncture tabs. (E) Have the subject exhale, place the mouth on the DPI with the head slightly tilted, take a controlled deep breath, and then hold for 5 seconds. Set a timer for 60 seconds. After the 60 seconds, perform a forced vital capacity (FVC) maneuver. (Courtesy of Methapharm. Brantford, ON, Canada.)

challenge is similar to that used for methacholine (see Table 9.2). Mannitol is contraindicated in patients with known hypersensitivity to mannitol or to the gelatin used to make the capsules. According to the manufacturer's package insert, it is for patients ages 6 years or older who do not have apparent clinical asthma. The most common adverse reactions (rate $\geq 1\%$) were headache, pharyngolaryngeal pain, throat irritation, nausea, cough, rhinorrhea, dyspnea, chest discomfort, wheezing, retching, and dizziness. Special testing requirements are listed in Box 9.5; otherwise, the technique is similar to other inhaled challenge testing. Performance of acceptable spirometry with the largest FEV_1 at least 60% of predicted is required for test performance. After the administration of 0 mg mannitol, FEV_1 is measured, and if it is not within 10% of the baseline, the test is terminated. The 0-mg dose FEV_1 then becomes the baseline value, and the target FEV_1 is calculated:

$$\text{Target } FEV_1 = \text{highest baseline value} \left(0\, mg\right) \times 0.85$$

A *positive* response may be achieved in two ways; greater than 15% fall in FEV_1 from the baseline

(using the post–0-mg FEV_1 as the baseline) or an incremental fall in FEV_1 of greater than or equal to 10% (between two consecutive mannitol doses). A *negative* test is when a cumulative dose of 635 mg of mannitol has been administered and the patient's FEV_1 has not fallen by greater than or equal to 15% from the baseline.

Mannitol has been shown to have the same sensitivity and specificity as methacholine testing.

Exercise Challenge

Exercise-induced bronchospasm (EIB) is typified by a hyperreactive airway response (e.g., bronchospasm) during or immediately after vigorous exercise. Exercise-induced asthma (EIA) was at one time used to describe this hyperreactive response to exercise; however, asthma is a disease and not a sign or symptom. Therefore *EIB* has been accepted as the more appropriate term. EIB is related to heat and water loss from the upper airway that accompanies increased ventilation during exercise. The exercise challenge is considered an *indirect* test because it depends on the response of airway smooth muscle to bronchoconstricting mediators released from airway inflammatory cells. Evaluation of EIB may be helpful in the following instances:

1. In patients who have shortness of breath on exertion but exhibit normal resting pulmonary function
2. In symptomatic patients in whom other bronchial provocation tests (e.g., methacholine challenge) produce negative or ambiguous results
3. In patients with known EIB in whom therapy is being evaluated
4. In screening patients where some risk to those with asthma might be involved (e.g., athletics, military service)

Patients referred for exercise challenge should be evaluated by means of an appropriate history and physical examination. The evaluation should include a resting electrocardiogram (ECG) to ascertain potential contraindications to exercise testing (see Chapter 7). Patient preparation and the medication withholding schedule are listed in Table 9.2. Before exercise, the patient's FEV_1 should not be less than 70% of the predicted value. Patients with overt obstruction usually do not require an exercise

---

BOX 9.5	SPECIAL MANNITOL TESTING INSTRUCTIONS

- The dry-powder inhaler (DPI) is for single patient use only.
- Pierce the capsule once by holding the inhaler in an upright position and fully depressing both piercing buttons on the sides of the inhaler simultaneously. A second puncture may cause the capsule to split/fragment.
- During challenge, subjects should exhale away from the Osmohaler to minimize humidity effects on the dry powder.
- Do not wear rubber/latex gloves when administering the test and handling mannitol because they may increase static and inhibit the capsule movement within the inhaler (removing the capsule with a twizer may be required).
- The subject should use a special inhalation technique, with the head tilted slightly (see Fig. 9.4E).
- Inhalation of mannitol can cause coughing.
- Challenge test time is critical, and prolonged intervals between doses may affect results—perform forced vital capacity (FVC) maneuvers 1 minute after drug administration.

challenge to demonstrate airway hyperreactivity. Patients should refrain from vigorous exercise for 4 hours before the test because there is a refractory period after exercise. Patients referred for EIB testing should be free from respiratory infections for 3 to 6 weeks before testing.

PF TIP 9.3

The normal response to exercise is for the FEV_1 (and specific conductance) to increase slightly. Patients who have EIB usually have a decrease in flows (FEV_1). When an increase is expected, a decrease of 10% to 15% is consistent with airway hyperreactivity. Some patients have a much greater decrease in response to even moderate exercise, so the pulmonary function technologist should be prepared to reverse severe bronchospasm.

Either a treadmill or a cycle ergometer may be used. The rapid increase in ventilation or heart rate (HR) during treadmill running makes it the preferable test; however, a cycle ergometer can be used effectively, provided that the work rate is increased rapidly. Exercise should be vigorous enough to elicit work rates of 80% to 90% of the patient's predicted HR or 40% to 60% of the target ventilation for a minimum of 4 minutes but ideally 6 minutes. The patient's response to an increasing workload should be monitored through continuous ECG and blood pressure (BP) monitoring. A pulse oximeter should be used to determine whether oxygen (O_2) desaturation occurs with exercise. Because pulse oximetry is not always accurate during exercise, an arterial line may be indicated if there is a high probability that exercise desaturation will occur. The pulse oximeter should be left in place in the postexercise phase to detect desaturation that may occur with a bronchospasm.

Measurement of variables such as minute ventilation $\left(\dot{V}_E\right)$ and tidal volume (V_T) may be helpful in assessing the ventilatory load imposed by the exercise. Measurement of F-V curves during exercise may be a useful adjunct in assessing the ventilatory response to increasing workloads

(see Chapter 7). A spirometer that meets ATS-ERS requirements (see Chapter 11) is necessary. Resuscitation equipment, as described in Chapter 7, should be available.

Because EIB is related to heat and water loss from the upper airway, environmental conditions should be controlled. The room temperature should be less than 25°C (75°F), with relative humidity of 50% or less. The patient should wear nose clips, even if exhaled gas is not collected, to reduce gas conditioning by nasal airflow. Ambient temperature, relative humidity, and barometric pressure (P_B) should be recorded. The patient should breathe dry gas from a compressed air source using a reservoir bag (see section on EVH testing later in the chapter).

Low-intensity exercise for 1 to 2 minutes allows the evaluation of ventilatory and cardiovascular responses to work. As soon as a normal cardiovascular response is observed, the workload should be increased rapidly over a 2- to 3-minute period until the patient attains 85% of predicted maximal HR or predicted maximal O_2 consumption ($\dot{V}O_2$). Alternately, the minute ventilation ($\dot{V}_E$) may be used as a target for exercise intensity if exhaled gas is collected. Ventilation should reach 40% to 60% of the patient's predicted MVV. The treadmill or cycle ergometer can be adjusted to increase or decrease the workload to maintain the correct intensity for the desired length of time.

In most instances, a short period of moderately heavy work is all that is required to trigger EIB. The goal is to have the patient exercise at high intensity for 4 to 6 minutes, with a total exercise duration of 6 to 8 minutes. Bronchospasm usually occurs immediately after the exercise, not during it, unless the test is extended over a longer interval (see Criteria for Acceptability 9.1). Repeated testing should be delayed for 4 hours because of a "refractory period" during which the severity of the bronchoconstriction lessens. This response is presumably caused by the release of catecholamines during exercise. An extended warm-up period before the actual exercise may also protect the airways and lessen subsequent bronchoconstriction (see section on EVH testing later in the chapter).

9.2   How To ...

Perform an Exercise Challenge Test

1. Tasks common to all procedures:
   a. Calibrate and prepare equipment.
   b. Review order.
   c. Introduce yourself and identify patient according to institutional policies.
   d. Describe and demonstrate procedure.
2. Regardless of the methodology selected, the subject should wear a nose clip to alleviate the moisture pathway provided by the nose.
   a. Select ergometer type.
   b. Calculate target heart (predicted HR × 0.85). The technologist may need to adopt a more symptomatic approach if the subject is on a beta-blocker or calcium channel blocker or has a bundle branch block or a pacemaker.
   c. The calculated target minute ventilation is 40% to 60% of the predicted MVV (estimated as FEV_1 × 40).
3. After a brief warm-up period, rapidly increase the workload to elicit the desired HR or $\dot{V}_E$ response. This should occur over a 2- to 3-minute period.
   a. It is common to "overshoot" a workload the subject can sustain for 4 to 6 minutes. Depending on the subject's HR, $\dot{V}_E$, and/or subjective response to the workload, it may have to be adjusted downward to allow the subject to complete the target exercise time.
   b. Monitor the subject's ECG, BP, and chest discomfort scales for indices of early termination (see Chapter 7).
4. After completion of the steady-state exercise, reduce the workload for a brief cool-down. Continue to monitor the ECG, BP, and symptoms.
5. Perform postexercise FVC maneuvers at 5-minute intervals (i.e., at 5, 10, 15, and 30 minutes).
   a. If results are equal to or less than the target FEV_1, administer the bronchodilator. If greater than the target recovery FEV_1 and the subject is symptom-free, the subject can be dismissed.

Baseline spirometry values are established before testing. The patient should be able to perform acceptable and repeatable FEV_1 measurements. Inability to perform acceptable spirometry will make the interpretation of postexercise changes difficult. The baseline FEV_1 value is also the control. After exercise, spirometry is performed at 1 to 2 minutes and then every 5 minutes as the selected variable (usually FEV_1) decreases to a minimum. For spirometry, the highest value of acceptable measurements is recorded; FEV_1 should be repeatable. The preferred method of reporting the response to exercise is the following:

$$\%\text{Decrease} = \frac{x - y}{x} \times 100$$

where:

x = baseline value (FEV_1)
y = lowest observed postexercise value

As in methacholine challenge testing, the fall in FEV_1 is sometimes presented as a negative number (e.g., –10%) to indicate a decrease. Similarly, an increase in FEV_1 (as observed in healthy subjects after exercise) may be represented as a positive value even though the preceding calculation produces a negative number if y is greater than x. Testing should be continued until the FEV_1 returns to the baseline. Maximal decreases are typically seen in the first 5 to 10 minutes after cessation of exercise. A decrease in FEV_1 of 10% to 15% is consistent with increased airway sensitivity. Allowing the FEV_1 to fall to its lowest point provides an estimate of how severe the response to exercise has been. Spontaneous recovery usually occurs within 20 to 40 minutes. Some laboratories administer a beta-agonist to reverse the bronchospasm as soon as a threshold (e.g., 10%–15% decrease) has been reached. The FEV_1 should return to near baseline values whether or not a bronchodilator is administered.

PF TIP 9.4

EVH testing may be a good substitute for EIB testing. High levels of eucapnic ventilation produce heat and water loss from the upper airway that is similar to the losses that occur with exercise. By setting a target ventilation that represents a significant fraction of the patient's maximal value (i.e., $FEV_1 \times 30$), airway hyperreactivity can be demonstrated. High levels of ventilation are not always achieved during exercise, especially if patients are limited by their maximal HR or by deconditioning.

Severe bronchospasm may occur after exercise, and the technologist performing the test should be prepared to manage it. If the bronchospasm is severe, it should be reversed using an inhaled bronchodilator. FEV_1 should return to within 10% of the pretest baseline value. Administration of a bronchodilator may also be useful in assessing borderline decreases in FEV_1 (< 10%) after the exercise challenge. Patients who show a minimal decrease after exercise may improve dramatically with an inhaled bronchodilator, suggesting increased airway responsiveness.

Patients who have VCD or other upper airway abnormalities are often referred for EIA tests. F-V curves (including maximal inspiratory flows) should be performed if the history or physical examination suggests these disorders. Measurement of tidal breathing loops during exercise (see Chapter 7) may also help define the pattern of ventilatory limitation.

One potential problem with using exercise to elicit EIB is that the level of exercise chosen may not mimic real-world triggers. Sedentary patients may not attain a level of ventilation high enough to trigger EIB when exercising at 85% of their maximal HR. Patients who are very fit (e.g., elite athletes) may require high workloads to reach 85% of their predicted HR or to increase their ventilation significantly. Measurement of $\dot{V}_E$ during exercise may be needed to determine the level of ventilation attained. Patients whose asthma is triggered by cold, dry air may not show a maximal response if tested under standard laboratory conditions. EIB may be evaluated using hyperventilation with either cold or ambient-temperature gas. These techniques eliminate the need for more complicated exercise testing. Hyperventilation (with a target ventilation level) may be more sensitive in detecting airway hyperreactivity than exercise testing.

Exercise testing with cold air can also be performed using the same exercise protocols as described earlier but requires specialized equipment to refrigerate and dry inspired gas (TurboAire Challenger, VacuMed, Ventura, CA). This equipment delivers cold, dry air to the airways (relative humidity of 0% and temperature of $-20°C$). In patients with symptoms specifically associated with exercise in the cold, exercise challenge while breathing cold, dry air may be useful to enhance the sensitivity and specificity of the response versus testing at room temperature (Fig. 9.5).

Eucapnic Voluntary Hyperventilation

AHR may also be assessed by having the patient breathe at a high level of ventilation. At one time, the International Olympic Committee Medical Commission expressed a viewpoint that EVH was the optimal laboratory challenge to confirm that an athlete has EIB. However, the commission's 2008 recommendations only state that bronchoprovocation testing is required in the absence of baseline airflow limitation.

EVH testing requires the use of carbon dioxide mixed with room air to prevent respiratory alkalosis (i.e., true hyperventilation) during the test. This gas mixture allows high levels of ventilation with little change in pH.

Patients to be tested with EVH should withhold medications as suggested in Table 9.2, including those for indirect challenge testing. Baseline spirometry is performed to ascertain that airway obstruction is not present. For ventilation challenges, the baseline FEV_1 is the control value with which subsequent measurements will be compared.

If cold air is to be used, the mixture is passed through a heat exchanger or over a cooling coil. These devices lower the temperature and remove water vapor from the gas. Gas temperatures are reduced to a subfreezing level in the range of $-10°C$ to $-20°C$. The relative humidity is usually near 0%.

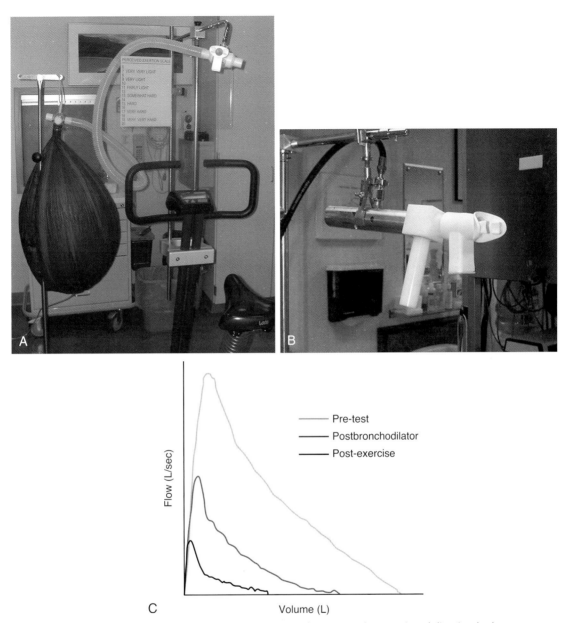

FIG. 9.5 Exercise challenge testing. (A) Using a compressed air source via reservoir and directional valve. (B) Using a TurboAire Challenger, a device that delivers cold, dry air. (C) Forced vital capacity (FVC) values before and after exercise challenge, with a significant reduction in flow and volume after exercise and suboptimal return to baseline after the first dose of bronchodilator.

The study uses medical dry air from a reservoir with an admixture of 5% CO_2, balance room air, that enables the subject to breathe at high ventilation without the adverse consequences of hypocapnia. The subject is instructed to perform voluntary hyperventilation for 4 to 6 minutes, aiming at a target ventilation of 85% of MVV and a minimum ventilation of 60% of MVV. Spirometry or sGaw is then measured at fixed intervals after the hyperventilation (e.g., 5, 10, and 30 minutes; Fig. 9.6).

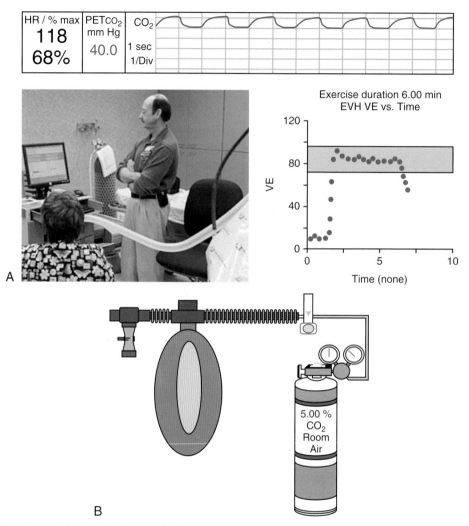

FIG. 9.6   Breathing circuit for eucapnic voluntary hyperventilation (EVH). (A) A gas containing 5% CO_2, 21% O_2, and balance N_2 is directed through a precision high-flow flowmeter to a reservoir bag. Flow is adjusted to a target ventilation level, such as 30 times the patient's forced expiratory volume in the first second (FEV_1). (B) The patient is coached according to the required predetermined ventilation. The test is continued for a predetermined interval, usually 6 minutes.

A commercial system is available that uses a large reservoir bag for the hypercarbic gas mixture, gas analyzer, and pneumotach, which then gives feedback to the technologist and patient, via the data-acquisition screen, on maintaining the predetermined ventilation (see Fig. 9.6).

For both the cold-air and room-temperature protocols, if no decrease in FEV_1 occurs within 30 minutes after hyperventilation, the test may be considered negative. The percentage decrease is calculated just as for methacholine challenge testing, as described previously. A decrease of 10% is consistent with some degree of airway hyperreactivity (see Criteria for Acceptability 9.1). EVH in healthy subjects usually results in bronchodilatation. Therefore a 10% decrease is abnormal and highly specific for increased bronchial responsiveness. Some patients with asthma may experience significant decreases in FEV_1 (20%–60%). Bronchospasm should be reversed with inhaled bronchodilators and the reversal documented with spirometry. The technologist performing the procedure should be prepared to manage severe bronchospasm if it occurs.

Raw and sGaw can be measured easily when hyperventilation tests are used. Because the airway challenge is applied once, the patient can remain in the body plethysmograph for measurements at defined intervals.

Both exercise testing and EVH techniques correlate well with the results of methacholine challenge tests, although they are slightly less specific. If multiple levels of ventilation are evaluated, a dose–response curve can be constructed. However, the single challenge is less complicated and can be used to evaluate patients with suspected asthma, particularly EIA.

SUMMARY

· Bronchial challenge tests can be done with several different agents, all of which test the airway responsiveness in slightly different ways.
· Methacholine challenge is the most commonly used standardized test of airway hyperreactivity.
· Mannitol is an indirect agent used to assess bronchial hyperreactivity. It is standardized and easy to use.
· Exercise testing can be specifically used to evaluate exercise-induced bronchospasm.
· Hyperventilation tests with cold or room-temperature air mimic the ventilatory load that occurs with exercise.

CASE STUDIES

CASE 9.1

HISTORY

The subject is a 39-year-old white woman who has recently experienced episodes of "choking and coughing." She was referred by her primary care physician, who suspected reactive airway involvement. The subject relates that cigarette smoke and strong odors seem to bring on the episodes. She has never smoked and has no history of lung disease. She had some childhood allergies that disappeared at puberty. There is no history of lung disease in her immediate family. The subject was not taking any medications at the time that she was tested.

PULMONARY FUNCTION TESTS
Personal Data

Sex:	Female
Age:	39 yr Caucasian
Height:	66 in. (168 cm)
Weight:	130 lb (59 kg)

Exhaled NO[a]

	Actual	Predicted
FE_{NO} (ppb)	97	< 35

[a] Measured at 50 mL/sec.

Spirometry

	Pre-Drug	LLN	Predicted	%
FVC (L)	3.71	3.24	3.97	93
FEV_1 (L)	2.96	2.62	3.24	91
$FEV_{1\%}$ (%)	80	73	83	
MVV (L/min)	106		110	96
Raw (cm H_2O/L/sec)	2.37		0.6–2.4	
sGaw (L/sec/cm H_2O/L)	0.14	0.12		

LLN, Lower limit of normal.

Methacholine Challenge[a]

Methacholine (mg/mL)	FEV_1	% Control	sGaw	% Control
Baseline	2.96	—	0.14	—
Control	2.92	100	0.14	—
0.0625	2.93	100	0.13	93
0.25	2.90	99	0.11	79
1.0	2.75	94	0.11	79
4.0	2.41	83	0.09	64
16.0	1.99	68	0.08	57

[a] Five-breath dosimeter method.

Technologist's Comments

Exhaled NO measurements were acceptable and repeatable. All spirometry and body box efforts were acceptable and reproducible. The subject complained of "chest tightness" near the end of the test; some scattered wheezes were heard on auscultation.

QUESTIONS

1. What is the interpretation of the following?
   a. Exhaled nitric oxide (see Chapter 10)
   b. Spirometry
   c. Airway resistance and specific conductance
2. What is the interpretation of the methacholine challenge?
3. Are these findings related to the subject's symptoms?
4. What treatment might be recommended, based on these findings?

DISCUSSION
Interpretation (Pulmonary Function)

Spirometry before and during the inhalation challenge was performed acceptably, as were maneuvers in the body plethysmograph. Spirometry results are within normal limits. Raw and sGaw are close to the limits of normal, suggestive of airflow obstruction.

Interpretation (Methacholine Challenge)

The methacholine challenge test is positive, with a PC_{20} of approximately 5.2 mg/mL. The test was terminated because the subject's FEV_1 decreased below 80% of the control value with the final dose of methacholine. sGaw decreased in a similar fashion, with a 36% decrease (64% of control) at the 4-mg/mL dose and a 43% decrease (57% of control) at the maximal inhaled dose. Wheezing was present on auscultation for the last two methacholine doses, and the subject experienced symptoms similar to her chief complaint when the test became positive.

Impression: Normal lung function with a positive methacholine challenge consistent with hyperreactive airway disease.

Cause of Symptoms

This subject is an ideal candidate for a bronchial challenge test. Her baseline pulmonary function studies are within normal limits, but her exhaled nitric oxide level strongly suggests inflammation of the airways. Her complaint of episodic coughing and choking suggests some form of hyperreactive airway abnormality. Many subjects who have an asthmatic response to inhaled irritants complain of cough as the primary symptom; wheezing may or may not be present.

If obvious airway obstruction were present on the baseline spirometry, the challenge test would have been contraindicated. A simple before-bronchodilator and after-bronchodilator trial may have been sufficient to demonstrate reversible obstruction. Methacholine challenge testing may be used in subjects with known obstruction to quantify the degree of ARH. In this case the objective of the test was to determine whether the subject had hyperreactivity.

FEV_1 is commonly used as the index of obstruction for inhalation challenge tests because it is simple to perform and highly reproducible. Raw and sGaw are sometimes used to define the extent of airway reactivity. sGaw is sensitive and reproducible and may be used to quantify changes occurring during challenge testing. A decrease of at least 35% to 45% in sGaw may be considered indicative of a positive response. As was observed in this subject, sGaw may actually decrease more rapidly than FEV_1. In some instances, peak expiratory flow (PEF) may decrease as the challenge is performed, particularly if the large airways are involved.

The results of a methacholine challenge test should be interpreted cautiously. The subject should be free of symptoms at the time of the test. Beta-agonist, anticholinergic, or methylxanthine bronchodilators that may influence the results must be withheld before testing. Some long-acting beta-agonists may need to be withheld for several days before testing. These conditions were met in this subject because she was not taking any medications. Because both FEV_1 and sGaw fell markedly with a PC_{20} of less than 8 mg/mL, the test can be interpreted as positive with some certainty. The subject appears to have airway inflammation. The cause of the subject's symptoms appears to be asthma triggered by inhaled irritants as described in her history.

Treatment

The subject was started on an inhaled corticosteroid (fluticasone). She was also given a portable peak flow meter. The subject was instructed in its use, and her PEF correlated well with that measured during spirometry. She was told to use the device every morning and evening or when symptoms appeared. Any significant change in PEF was treated with a beta-agonist bronchodilator through a metered-dose inhaler. Subsequent reports indicated that her peak flow fell in excess of the level demonstrated on the challenge, but symptoms were promptly relieved with the use of the inhaler. Her $F_{E_{NO}}$ while taking inhaled corticosteroids was measured during a follow-up visit at 25 ppb. This finding suggests that her underlying airway inflammation was being adequately managed at her current dose.

CASE 9.2

HISTORY

A 38-year-old woman's complaint is shortness of breath while jogging or playing tennis. She has been physically active for several years but recently had a "chest cold" that took 4 weeks to resolve. She smoked for approximately 2 years while in high school. She works as a teacher and has no unusual environmental exposures. Family history includes an older sister who has chronic bronchitis. She is not currently taking any medications. Her health maintenance organization referred her for evaluation of possible exercise-induced bronchospasm.

PULMONARY FUNCTION TESTS

Personal Data

Sex:	Female
Age:	38 yr, Caucasian
Height:	62 in. (158 cm)
Weight:	119 lb (54 kg)

Eucapnic Voluntary Hyperventilation			
	Baseline	5 Min	Postbronchodilator
FEV$_1$ (Pred: 2.64 L)	1.97	1.25	1.92
% Predicted	75	47	73
% Change	0	−37	−3
FVC (Pred: 3.37 L)	2.71	2.07	2.8
% Predicted	81	61	83
% Change	0	−24	3
PEF (Pred: 6.0 L/sec)	5.5	2.8	3.65
% Predicted	91	46	61
% Change	0	−49	−33

Technologist's Comments

All spirometry maneuvers were performed acceptably before and after hyperventilation. She hyperventilated at 60 L/min for 6 minutes. There were audible wheezes immediately after hyperventilation.

QUESTIONS

1. What is the interpretation of the following?
   a. Baseline spirometry
   b. Response to EVH
   c. Response to the bronchodilator
2. Are the findings related to the cause of the subject's symptoms?
3. What other tests might be indicated?
4. What treatment might be recommended, based on these findings?

DISCUSSION

Interpretation

All spirometric maneuvers were performed acceptably. Baseline spirometry results are close to the LLN, with a mildly decreased FEV$_1$. After EVH, there were significant decreases in FEV$_1$, FVC, and peak flow at 5 minutes. After an inhaled bronchodilator, FEV$_1$ returned to prechallenge levels, and FVC increased. Peak-flow recovery was somewhat slower.

Impression: Borderline normal spirometry results with a positive EVH test consistent with hyperreactive airways.

Cause of Symptoms

This subject is typical of an adult who begins experiencing breathlessness with increased physical activity and seeks medical attention. Her complaints suggest EIB. The development of this problem may or may not be related to her recent chest infection.

EVH is an appropriate way to challenge the airways in cases such as this. The subject breathed a mixture of 5% CO_2, 21% O_2, and balance N_2 for 6 minutes. The target level of ventilation was set at 30 times her FEV$_1$, or approximately 60 L/min. Spirometry was repeated 5 minutes after hyperventilation. In this case, the subject experienced a significant decrease in FEV$_1$, FVC, and PEF (see following figure). Because of the marked decrease in FEV$_1$, additional postchallenge measurements (at 10 and 15 minutes) were omitted. Four inhalations of albuterol through a metered-dose inhaler with a spacer reversed the obstruction, although PEF recovered only partially.

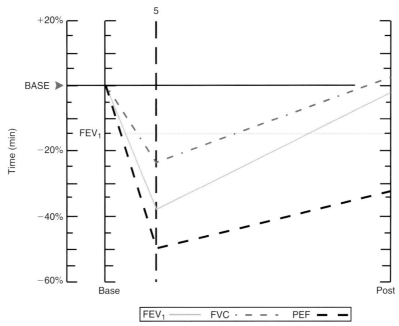

Eucapnic voluntary hyperventilation (EVH) graph. Forced vital capacity (FVC), forced expiratory volume in the first second (FEV₁), and peak expiratory flow (PEF) are plotted after a bronchial challenge maneuver. In this subject, there was a marked decrease in all three variables at 5 minutes (a positive test result). The graph also plots the reversal of the induced bronchospasm by inhaled bronchodilator.

Other Tests

EVH challenges the airways by inducing heat and water loss with increased ventilation. This is the same physical stimulus that may be responsible for EIB. The subject, in this case, could have been tested using exercise as the challenge agent. However, EVH is simpler and takes less time. In addition, EVH may be more sensitive in detecting EIB than exercise testing itself. Exercise tests are often performed with subjects working at 80% to 90% of their maximal HR for 6 to 8 minutes. In many subjects, particularly if they are sedentary, the workload that produces this elevation in HR may not induce a high enough level of ventilation to provoke bronchospasm. EVH, using a target of 30 times the FEV_1, produces a level of ventilation approximately 75% of MVV.

Treatment

The subject was given a beta-agonist bronchodilator to be used as pretreatment before exercise. She reported significant improvement in her symptoms. A trial regimen of cromolyn sodium also reduced the occurrence of symptoms associated with athletic activities.

SELF-ASSESSMENT QUESTIONS

Entry-Level

1. A patient with symptoms of chest tightness and cough while playing basketball is referred for bronchial challenge. In addition to spirometry before/after the challenge, which of the following protocols would be most appropriate?
   1. Treadmill exercise for 4 to 6 minutes at 85% of predicted maximal HR
   2. Cycle ergometer ramp test at 50 W/min
   3. EVH at 30 × FEV_1 for 6 minutes
   4. EVH at MVV × 5 minutes
      a. 1 and 3 only
      b. 2 and 4 only
      c. 2 and 3 only
      d. 1 and 4 only

2. A 35-year-old woman performs a methacholine challenge using the five-breath dosimeter protocol. The following data are recorded:

	FEV_1
Baseline	2.95 L
Diluent	3.01 L
Concentration/dose	
0.0625 mg/mL (1.81 µg)	2.89 L
0.250 mg/mL (7.26 µg)	2.75 L
1.0 mg/mL (29.03 µg)	2.70 L
4.0 mg/mL (116.10 µg)	2.51 L
16.0 mg/mL (464.4 µg)	2.35 L

Based on these results, the PC_{20} is
a. less than 0.0625 mg/mL.
b. between 1.0 and 4.0 mg/mL.
c. between 4.0 and 16.0 mg/mL.
d. greater than 16.0 mg/mL.

3. A patient who complains of shortness of breath is referred for a bronchial challenge test. Baseline spirometry shows the following results:

	Predicted	LLN	Actual
FVC (L)	3.56	2.75	3.01
FEV_1 (L)	2.89	2.18	2.12
FEV_1/FVC (%)	81	71	70
PEF (L/sec)	7.8	5.5	5.7
Raw (cm H_2O/L/sec)	1.5		2.4
sGaw (L/sec/ cm H_2O/L)		0.12	0.10

Based on these results, the pulmonary function technologist should take which action?
a. Perform a methacholine challenge using the five-breath dosimeter method.
b. Perform a methacholine challenge using the 1-minute tidal breathing method.
c. Do an exercise test for 6 to 8 minutes with postexercise spirometry.
d. Administer a bronchodilator and repeat spirometry after 15 minutes.

4. After inhalation of methacholine, a patient has spirometry and specific conductance measured. Which of the following changes are consistent with a positive methacholine challenge test?
a. FEV_1 decreased 10%, sGaw increased 10%
b. FEV_1 decreased 15%, sGaw increased 35%
c. FEV_1 decreased 25%, sGaw decreased 50%
d. FEV_1 increased 5%, sGaw decreased 25%

5. A patient is performing a mannitol challenge test. The subject performs acceptably, and repeatable spirometry with the measured FEV_1 is 3.50 L. After administration of the 0-mg mannitol dose, spirometry is performed, with a measured FEV_1 of 3.38 L. What should the technologist do next?
a. Discontinue the test secondary to the subject's decline in FEV_1 from the baseline.
b. Conclude that the calculated target FEV_1 is 2.98 L.
c. Conclude that t calculated target FEV_1 is 2.87 L.
d. Repeat baseline spirometry before proceeding.

Advanced

6. What is the mechanism of airway hyperreactivity when performing an exercise challenge test?
a. Increases the osmolarity of the airway
b. Stimulates H_1-receptor antagonists
c. Secondary to increased ventilatory demand
d. Loss of heat and water from the airways

7. A patient is performing a mannitol challenge test with the following results:

Mannitol Dose	FEV_1	Mannitol Dose	FEV_1
Baseline spirometry	3.95 L	40 mg	3.79 L
0 mg	3.86 L	80 mg	3.67 L
5 mg	3.88 L	160 mg	3.73 L
10 mg	3.85 L	160 mg	3.65 L
20 mg	3.86 L	160 mg	3.33 L

What is the interpretation of the test?
a. A negative test with a cumulative dose of 635 mg
b. A negative test with a maximal dose of 160 mg
c. A positive test with a 15% decline from the baseline FEV_1
d. A positive test with a 10% decline in FEV_1 after the third 160-mg dose

8. Why are mannitol and EVH considered to be in the same general category of bronchoprovocation testing?
1. They both cause heat and water loss of the airway through osmolarity.
2. They both act on the airways via indirect stimulation.
3. They both cause the release of inflammatory mediators.

4. They both cause direct stimulation of the smooth muscle of the airways.
   a. 1 only
   b. 2 and 3
   c. 3 and 4
   d. 1 and 4

9. A subject performs an exercise challenge test. He is a 57-year-old male. The exercise consisted of breathing dry air via a directional valve connected to a reservoir bag filled from a compressed air tank. After a 1-minute warm-up period, the subject performs 6 minutes of steady-state exercise at 75 watts on a cycle ergometer. The subject's HR was 140 bpm during the exercise period. Spirometry was performed at the baseline and 5 minutes postexercise, with the following results:
   Baseline FEV_1 is 2.89 L.
   Postexercise FEV_1 is 2.58 L.
   How would you interpret the test results?
   a. Positive exercise challenge with an 11% decline
   b. Negative challenge because there is not a 15% decline
   c. Test not conducted correctly because minute ventilation was not assessed
   d. Inconclusive test

10. Which of the following results suggest that a patient may have asthma?
   1. 12% or 200-mL increase in postbronchodilator FEV_1 (whichever is greater)
   2. 20% decrease in FEV_1 after inhaling 4 mg/mL of methacholine
   3. 9% fall in FEV_1 after 8 minutes of exercise at 90% of the predicted HR
   4. 17% fall in FEV_1 after administration of 315 mg of mannitol
   a. 1 and 4 only
   b. 2 and 3 only
   c. 1, 2, 4
   d. 2, 3, 4

SELECTED BIBLIOGRAPHY

Bronchial Challenge

Allen, N. D., Davis, B. E., Hurst, T. S., & Cockcroft, D. W. (2005). Difference between dosimeter and tidal breathing methacholine challenge: Contributions of dose and deep inspiration bronchoprotection. *Chest, 128,* 4018–4023.

Anderson, S. D., & Branman, J. D. (2003). Methods for "indirect" challenge tests including exercise, eucapnic voluntary hyperpnea, and hypertonic aerosols. *Clinical Reviews in Allergy and Immunology, 24,* 27–54.

Argyros, G. J., Roach, J. M., Hurwitz, K. M., et al. (1996). Eucapnic voluntary hyperventilation as a bronchoprovocation technique. *Chest, 109,* 1520–1524.

CHEST series: Airway hyperresponsiveness in asthma: Its measurement and clinical significance. Eight distinctive articles addressing AHR. (2010). *Chest, 138*(Suppl. 2).

Cockcroft, D. W., Davis, B. E., Todd, D. C., & Smycniuk, A. J. (2005). Methacholine challenge: Comparison of two methods. *Chest, 127,* 839–844.

Joos, G. F., O'Conner, B., Anderson, S. D., et al. (2003). Indirect airway challenges. *European Respiratory Journal, 21,* 1050–1068.

Storms, W. W. (2003). Review of exercise-induced asthma. *Medicine and Science in Sports and Exercise, 35,* 1464–1470.

Guidelines and Standards

Coates, AL, Wanger, J, & Cockcroft, DW. (2017). Culver4 BH, et al. ERS technical standard on bronchial challenge testing: general considerations and performance of methacholine challenge tests. *Eur Respir J, 49.*

Hallstrand, TS, Leuppi, JD, Joos, G, Hall, GL, Carlsen, KH, Kaminsky, DA, et al. (2018). ERS technical standard on bronchial challenge testing: pathophysiology and methodology of indirect airway challenge testing. *Eur Respir J, 52.*

Chapter 10

Specialized Tests and Evaluations

KATRINA M. HYNES, MHA, RRT, RPFT

CHAPTER OUTLINE

LEARNING OBJECTIVES

After studying the chapter and reviewing the figures, tables, and case studies, you should be able to do the following:

Entry-level

1. Describe the indications for respiratory muscle strength testing.
2. Understand the various methods available to assess respiratory muscle strength.
3. Define the pathophysiology of an elevated exhaled nitric oxide (eNO) result.
4. Identify the normal range for eNO values.
5. Understand the difference between open- and closed-circuit calorimetry.
6. List two indications for preoperative pulmonary function testing.

Advanced

1. Evaluate the clinical implications of an elevated level of eNO.
2. Understand the equation of motion and its relevance to forced oscillatory technique.
3. Judge the reliability of metabolic measurements.
4. Select appropriate tests to evaluate disability in either chronic obstructive pulmonary disease (COPD) or pulmonary fibrosis.

KEY TERMS

basal metabolic rate (BMR)
continuous-flow canopy
elastance (E)
eosinophilic inflammation
exhaled nitric oxide (eNO)
fast Fourier transform (FFT)
forced oscillation technique (FOT)

fraction of expired nitric oxide
($F_{E_{NO}}$)
Harris–Benedict equations
head hood
impulse oscillometry (IOS)
indirect calorimetry
inertia (I)

maximal expiratory pressure (MEP
or $P_{E}max$)
maximal inspiratory pressure (MIP
or $P_{I}max$)
respiratory exchange ratio (RER)
respiratory muscle strength testing
resting energy expenditure (REE)

Diagnosis or evaluation of specific pulmonary disorders requires that appropriate tests be performed. Specialized tests, such as those described in this chapter, are often used to further define a specific condition. They may also involve a simple modification of the standard tests performed under special conditions. The clinical question asked regarding a patient might be whether he or she qualifies for disability or whether it is safe to undergo surgery. Spirometry, lung volumes, diffusing capacity (D_{LCO}), or blood gas analysis may be required to answer these questions.

Specialized tests covered in this chapter include respiratory muscle strength, **exhaled nitric oxide (eNO)**, **forced oscillatory technique (FOT)**, and metabolic measurements. Respiratory muscle strength measurements, such as **maximal inspiratory pressure (MIP or $P_{I}max$)** and **maximal expiratory pressure (MEP or $P_{E}max$),** might assist in characterizing neuromuscular diseases. Measurement of eNO provides a sensitive and highly repeatable method for evaluating airway inflammation. It can be used to detect **eosinophilic inflammation,** which is common in asthma, and to evaluate response to treatments such as inhaled corticosteroids. Forced oscillatory technique (also known as **impulse oscillometry [IOS]**) provides a unique way to evaluate airway function. It provides a measurement of airway resistance in spontaneously breathing subjects and can be used in conjunction with bronchodilator evaluation or bronchial challenge. Metabolic measurements are widely used to assess caloric needs and nutritional support in a variety of patients. The methods used are similar to those used in gas exchange measurements during exercise. Specialized calculations allow for a precise description of the nutritional status of the patient.

RESPIRATORY MUSCLE STRENGTH TESTING

Maximal Respiratory Pressures

Description

Forced maneuvers during spirometry require the patient to give a maximal effort, as well as to have normal muscle function. Respiratory muscle strength is also critical in supporting adequate ventilation and airway protection (e.g., cough), hence the need for **respiratory muscle strength testing.** Muscle function is best assessed by the measurement of maximal inspiratory and expiratory pressures. MIP, also reported as $P_{I}max$, is the lowest pressure developed during a forceful sustained inspiration against an occluded airway. It is usually measured after a maximal expiration (near residual volume [RV]). It is recorded as a negative number in cm H_2O. MEP, also reported as $P_{E}max$, is the highest pressure that can be developed during a forceful sustained expiratory effort against an occluded airway. It is usually measured after a maximal inspiration (near total lung capacity [TLC]) and reported as a positive number in cm H_2O.

Technique

The patient is connected to a valve, shutter apparatus, or the pulmonary function testing system with a mouthpiece (a flanged mouthpiece may facilitate testing in subjects with excessive muscle weakness) and nose clip in place. The mouthpiece can be placed in the mouth or the lips pressed against the mouthpiece opening, as would be done with a bugle, thus the early term for the procedure, "bugles" (Fig. 10.1). Regardless of the mouth–device interface used, there should be a tight fit so that the

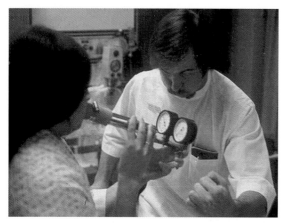

FIG. 10.1   Classic bugle. A simple and historical method of measuring maximal inspiratory and expiratory pressures involves the use of a small metal tube with a fixed leak and pressure gauges. During the expiratory maneuver, the subject would blow into the device with his or her lips within the mouthpiece, earning it the name "bugle testing."

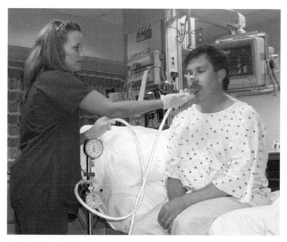

FIG. 10.2   Volumes and pressures. Measurement of vital capacity and respiratory muscle strength at the bedside.

patient can exert maximal pressure. The airway is occluded by blocking a port in the valve or by closing a shutter. In either system, a small, fixed leak is introduced between the occlusion and the patient's mouth. The leak may be a small opening, such as a large-bore needle, or created by the pulmonary function testing system in the hardware. The leak eliminates pressures generated by the cheek muscles during the MEP maneuver by allowing a small amount of gas to escape the oral cavity. Likewise, the leak prevents glottis closure during the MIP maneuver. The incorporation of this small leak does not significantly change lung volume or the pressure measurement.

Pressure may be measured using a manometer, an aneroid-type gauge, or a pressure transducer. The pressure-monitoring device should be linear over its range. It should be able to record pressures from -200 cm H_2O to approximately $+200$ cm H_2O. Pressure transducers are typically used in pulmonary function testing systems, with the output incorporated into a data-acquisition screen and algorithms used to calculate the sustained pressure. If a manometer or aneroid gauge is used, the operator directly observes the pressure and records it.

This type of monitoring is common in the hospital, where measurements of vital capacity and respiratory pressures are used to assess ventilatory adequacy (Fig. 10.2). The operator should record the plateau pressure that the patient can maintain for 1.5 seconds.

For the MIP test, the patient is instructed to expire maximally. Monitoring expiratory flow or having the patient signal helps determine when maximal expiration has been achieved. Then the airway is occluded as described. The patient inspires maximally and maintains the inspiration for 1.5 seconds. The first portion of each maneuver is disregarded because it may include transient pressure changes that occur initially (Fig. 10.3). The most negative value from at least three efforts that vary less than 20% is recorded, although a clinical trial may require a tighter repeatability (e.g., $< 15\%$).

MEP is recorded similarly. The patient inhales as much as possible and then exhales maximally against the occluded airway for 1.5 seconds. Longer efforts should be avoided because cardiac output can be reduced by the high thoracic pressures (e.g., Valsalva maneuvers) that are sometimes developed. MEP is usually larger than MIP in healthy patients.

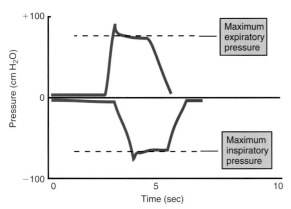

FIG. 10.3 Maximal inspiratory pressure (MIP) and maximal expiratory pressure (MEP). These tracings plot the respective pressures recorded in cm H_2O against time on a single graph. MIP shows a downward or negative deflection. MEP shows a positive or upward deflection. Each maneuver is conducted with the airway occluded (see text). The occlusion is maintained for a short interval (1.5 seconds), and any initial transient tracings are discarded.

BOX 10.1   SUGGESTED INDICATIONS FOR RESPIRATORY MUSCLE STRENGTH TESTING

- Amyotrophic lateral sclerosis
- Paralyzed diaphragm
- Fibromyalgia
- Dermatomyositis (myositis)
- Muscular dystrophy
- Chronic fatigue syndrome
- Guillain-Barré
- Phrenic nerve damage
- Peripheral neuropathy
- Multiple sclerosis (if muscle weakness)
- Spinal injury (paraplegia, quadriplegia)
- Myasthenia gravis
- Postpolio syndrome
- Polymyalgia rheumatica
- Polymyositis
- Stroke
- Cerebral palsy

The pressure-monitoring device should be able to withstand the higher pressure without damage. The most positive value from at least three efforts that vary less than 20% is recorded, although clinical trials may require a tighter repeatability (e.g., <15%; Criteria for Acceptability Box 10.1). Initial pressure transients during the MEP are disregarded. Both MIP and MEP require patient cooperation and effort. Low values may reflect a lack of understanding or insufficient effort.

Significance and Pathophysiology

Maximal respiratory pressure results are used to assist the clinician in identifying respiratory muscle weakness. Refer to Box 10.1 for a list of indications. MIP primarily measures inspiratory muscle strength. Healthy adults can generate inspiratory pressures of greater than -50 cm H_2O in women and -75 cm H_2O in men. Decreased MIP is seen in patients with neuromuscular disease or diseases involving the diaphragm, intercostals, or accessory muscles. MIP may also be decreased in patients with hyperinflation, such as in emphysema, where the diaphragm is flattened by the increased volume of trapped gas in the lungs. The intercostals and accessory muscles may also be compromised by injury to or diseases of the chest wall. Patients with chest wall or spinal deformities (e.g., kyphoscoliosis) may also have reduced inspiratory pressures. MIP is sometimes used to assess patient response to strength training of respiratory muscles. MIP is often used in the assessment of respiratory muscle function in patients who need ventilatory support.

CRITERIA FOR ACCEPTABILITY 10.1

MIP/MEP

1. Pressure plateau of 1.5 seconds should be obtained.
2. At least three MIP and three MEP maneuvers should be performed.
3. The largest value from three acceptable efforts that vary less than 20% is recorded.

MEP measures the pressure generated during maximal expiration. It depends on the function of the abdominal muscles and accessory muscles of respiration and the elastic recoil of the lungs and thorax. Healthy adults can generate

MEP values greater than $+80$ cm H_2O in women and greater than $+100$ cm H_2O in men. MEP may be decreased in neuromuscular disorders, particularly those resulting in generalized muscle weakness. Another common disorder that results in the reduction of MEP is high cervical spine fracture. Damage to nerves controlling abdominal and accessory muscles of expiration can dramatically reduce MEP. However, MIP may be preserved in these patients.

Reduced MEP often accompanies increased RV, as seen in emphysema. A low MEP is associated with the inability to cough effectively. Inability to generate an adequate cough may complicate chronic bronchitis, cystic fibrosis (CF), or other diseases that result in excessive mucus secretion.

Accurate measurement of MIP and MEP depends largely on patient effort. The operator should carefully instruct the patient on how to perform the maneuver. Low values may result if the patient fails to inhale or exhale completely before the airway is occluded. Some patients may show increased MIP or MEP with repeated efforts (training effect). Others may demonstrate decreasing pressures with repeated efforts (muscle fatigue). The best efforts should be repeatable within 20% or 10 cm H_2O, whichever is greater. Widely varying pressures for either MIP or MEP should be assessed carefully before interpretation.

Cough Peak Flow
Description
Cough peak flow (CPF) has been used in the assessment of pediatric patients with neuromuscular disease. Mucociliary clearance is dependent on an effective cough. CPF can be used in patients with neuromuscular disease to assess their ability to generate an effective cough.

Technique
The methodology is simple. It can be performed using a spirometer or peak flow meter. To perform the maneuver, the patient should be placed in a seated position. The operator instructs the patient to take in a full inspiration and then cough as forcibly as he or she can into the device by way of a mouthpiece or facemask. Similar to

spirometry, a nose clip is not required but may be used. The patient should be coached to perform three to five efforts. The highest CPF value should be reported.

Significance and Pathophysiology
The normal range can vary significantly and correlates with the age, height, and gender of a subject. Normal values range from 130 to 950 L/min in males and from 110 to 660 L/min in females. Clinical algorithms for Duchenne muscular dystrophy (DMD) have noted that assisted coughing should be implemented when the forced vital capacity (FVC) < 50% predicted and the CPF < 270 L/min, or MEP < 60 cm H_2O.

Sniff Nasal Inspiratory Pressures
Description
Sniff nasal inspiratory pressure (SNIP) can be used as an alternative or complementary test to MIP. Instrumentation can be sophisticated, from computer incentive screens to simple handheld devices (Fig. 10.4). Measurement limitations include nasal obstruction or collapse during the maneuver. Several articles have compared the test method to

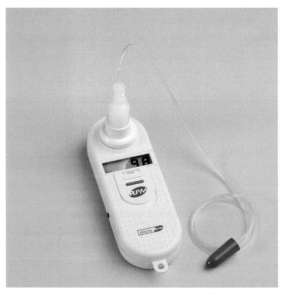

FIG. 10.4   Handheld device for measuring sniff nasal inspiratory pressure (SNIP). (Courtesy Vyaire Medical, Mettawa, IL.)

sniff pressures measured using an esophageal catheter, with good correlation in subjects with neuromuscular disease.

Technique

The measurement is performed by occluding a nostril during a maximal sniff maneuver performed through the contralateral nostril from functional residual capacity (FRC) or RV. In the contralateral nostril, a nasal olive with a central catheter is connected to a pressure transducer.

Significance and Pathophysiology

A sniff nasal inspiratory force of less than 40 cm H_2O has been shown to predict mortality in patients with amyotrophic lateral sclerosis (sensitivity 97%, specificity 79%).

EXHALED NITRIC OXIDE

Description

Measurement of eNO provides a simple and noninvasive method for assessing airway inflammation. Common reasons for measuring the **fraction of expired eNO ($F_{E}NO$)** include:

- Establish the correct diagnosis of asthma in corticosteroid-naïve patients
- Differentiate COPD from asthma
- Predict a favorable response to corticosteroids
- May be useful in the titration of anti-inflammatory medication in patients with asthma, and in maintenance of asthma control
- Monitor asthma medication adherence

Although it is not a single diagnostic test for asthma, it provides supportive evidence in diagnosing and monitoring lung diseases characterized by eosinophilic inflammation. In 2021 the ATS published a clinical practice guideline (CPG) which suggests that $F_{E}NO$ should be used in addition to usual care in patients with asthma in whom treatment is being considered. $F_{E}NO$ can be measured with a sensitive chemiluminescent or electrochemical analyzer (see Chapter 11). $F_{E}NO$ is reported in parts per billion (ppb). Because the measurement is dependent on flow during exhalation, the flow (in liters per second) may be subscripted to the term (e.g., $F_{E}NO_{0.05}$ represents the $F_{E}NO$ measured at a flow of 0.05 L/sec). Nitric oxide (NO) is also sometimes measured from the nasal cavities, including the sinuses, as a marker of nasal inflammation.

> ### PF TIP 10.1
>
> Exhaled nitric oxide levels are typically elevated by airway inflammation in patients who have asthma. However, $F_{E}NO$ may be reduced in patients who smoke. Smokers who also have asthma may show an elevated $F_{E}NO$ that is not as high as it would be if they were not currently smoking. Smoking status may be an important factor in detecting airway inflammation when the $F_{E}NO$ is near the upper limit of normal.

Techniques

$F_{E}NO$ can be measured either online or offline. The methods for each type of collection differ slightly in adults and children. Online measurements sample exhaled gas continuously at the mouth; offline measurements collect exhaled air in a sampling device for later analysis.

Online $F_{E}NO$

Before measuring $F_{E}NO$, patients should refrain from smoking, eating, or drinking (except water) for at least 1 hour before testing. Measurement of eNO should be performed before other tests such as spirometry, methacholine challenge, or exercise testing. Any recent infections, as well as the current medication regimen, should be recorded at the time of testing.

Because NO is produced in the airways (and in the alveoli), it is important that the patient inhale NO-free gas. This is accomplished by having the subject inspire through an NO scrubber. The ambient NO level should be recorded as well. The patient should be instructed to exhale to RV and then insert the mouthpiece and inspire over a 2- to 3-second interval to TLC. A nose clip is not used; this lessens the possibility that the much higher nasal NO will accumulate and contaminate the lower airway sample.

Without breath holding, the patient then exhales slowly and evenly while exhaled gas is sampled continuously. To prevent contamination of the exhalate with nasal NO, the patient exhales against an expiratory resistance while receiving feedback to maintain positive pressure at the mouth (Fig. 10.5). This positive pressure (usually about +5 cm H_2O) causes the velum in the posterior pharynx to close, preventing nasal NO from entering the air stream. The fractional concentration of NO in the exhaled gas varies inversely with the flow. To standardize online measurements, an exhaled flow of 0.05 L/sec (i.e., 50 mL/sec) ± 10% is recommended (Criteria for Acceptability Box 10.2). This flow allows dead-space gas to be exhaled and a plateau in NO to be observed in about 10 seconds in adults. The correct flow can be maintained by using a pressure-sensitive flow controller and providing visual feedback to the subject. Current commercially available instrumentation (see Chapter 11) uses visual incentives to ensure standardized flow/pressure and will mark a maneuver as not meeting acceptability criteria if flow/pressure is not maintained.

$F_{E_{NO}}$ is measured from the plateau of the single-breath exhalation profile (see Fig. 10.5). The plateau phase may slope up or down slightly. The exhalation should last long enough to establish this plateau (> 6 seconds for adults and children older than 12 years, > 4 seconds for children ages 12 years and younger). Two points should be chosen on the plateau that represent a 3-second interval (about 0.15 L) in which the $F_{E_{NO}}$ varies less than 10%. The $F_{E_{NO}}$ is the mean concentration over this 3-second interval. For $F_{E_{NO}}$ values of 10 ppb or less, variability of 1 ppb NO may be used in place of the 10% criteria. A minimum of 30 seconds should elapse between repeated measurements with the subject breathing air (off the NO sampling circuit).

At least two acceptable measurements of $F_{E_{NO}}$ that agree within 10% of each other should be averaged for the final report value. Three acceptable measurements should be averaged if $F_{E_{NO}}$ is measured at multiple flow rates.

Offline $F_{E_{NO}}$

Offline measurements of NO allow the gas to be collected away from the analyzer, making more efficient use of the analyzer. Potential problems with offline measurements include contamination with gas from the upper airway, errors caused by storing the sample, and lack of feedback to the patient regarding technique during gas collection.

The patient inhales through an NO scrubber or from a reservoir with NO-free gas. After inhaling to TLC, the patient exhales his or her vital capacity (VC) into an appropriate sampling device without breath holding. Expiratory resistance (+5 cm H_2O) is added, just as is done for online measurements, to minimize contamination by nasal NO. Flow is usually controlled by monitoring the back-pressure in the system; flows of 0.35 L/sec ± 10% are recommended to allow the VC to be collected in a reasonable interval. The sample is collected in a balloon made of polyester (Mylar) or a similar material impermeable to NO and large enough

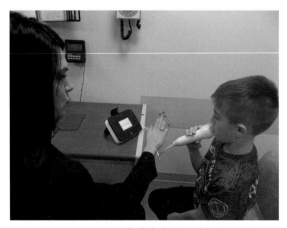

FIG. 10.5 Measurement of exhaled nitric oxide ($F_{E_{NO}}$). The upper graph shows three efforts in which flows are measured at the mouth. The subject exhales against a slight resistance to close the velum in the oropharynx. Visual feedback in the form of a computer display helps the patient maintain a constant pressure and thereby a constant flow at the recommended 0.05 L/sec. The lower graph displays the $F_{E_{NO}}$ values for the three maneuvers over 10 seconds of exhalation. Exhaled NO rises to a plateau, and the $F_{E_{NO}}$ concentration is measured over a 3-second (i.e., 0.15 L) window from the plateau.

to accommodate the adult's VC. Offline samples should be analyzed within 12 hours. Exhaled nitric oxide can be performed in children able to perform the single-breath maneuver and is described in Chapter 8.

Nasal Nitric Oxide

Although various methods of sampling nasal NO have been described, the recommended method uses transnasal airflow in series. In this technique, air is aspirated into one naris and out the opposite side, where NO is sampled. The subject exhales against a resistance of approximately 10 cm H_2O while air is aspirated at a constant flow rate. As for the measurement of $F_{E_{NO}}$ from the lower airways, exhalation against resistance closes the velum in the posterior pharynx to prevent contamination of the sample. Airflow of 0.25 to 3.0 L/min is used for nasal NO measurements. Flows in this range allow a plateau in the NO signal within 20 to 30 seconds in most adults. The flow used for NO analysis, along with the transnasal flow, should be recorded (Fig. 10.6).

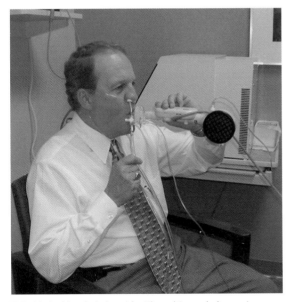

FIG. 10.6 Nasal nitric oxide. The subject exhales against a resistance of approximately 10 cm H_2O while air is aspirated at a constant flow rate using a nasal olive.

CRITERIA FOR ACCEPTABILITY 10.2

Exhaled Nitric Oxide

1. Patient should be free of respiratory tract infections; no eating, drinking, or smoking for 1 hour before testing. Exhaled NO should be measured before spirometry or bronchial challenges.

Online Measurement

2. Patient should inhale NO free air to TLC within 2 to 3 seconds.
3. Patient should exhale against + 5 cm H_2O resistance at a constant flow of 0.05 L/sec (50 mL/sec) ± 10%.
4. Duration of exhalation should be more than 6 seconds for adults and children older than 12 years (> 4 seconds for children ages 12 years and younger).
5. There should be a plateau in the NO signal, and $F_{E_{NO}}$ should be measured from a 3-second window in which NO does not vary by more than 10% (1 ppb for $F_{E_{NO}}$ < 10 ppb).
6. Thirty seconds should elapse between repeated measurements.
7. $F_{E_{NO}}$ value reported should be the average of at least two acceptable measurements that agree within 10% of each other.

Offline Measurement

8. Patient should inspire at least two tidal breaths of NO-free air, then a VC breath, and exhale against resistance (+ 5 cm H_2O) into a suitable reservoir without breath holding.
9. Flow of 0.35 L/sec ± 10% should be maintained throughout exhalation of the VC.
10. Reservoir should be sealed immediately and NO analyzed within 12 hours.

Adapted from American Thoracic Society and European Respiratory Society. (2005). ATS-ERS recommendations for standardized procedures for the online and offline measurement of exhaled lower respiratory nitric oxide and nasal nitric oxide—2005. *American Journal of Respiratory and Critical Care Medicine 171,* 912–930.

Significance and Pathophysiology

Normal values for $F_{E_{NO}}$ depend largely on the flow at which gas is sampled during analysis. At a standardized flow of 0.05 L/sec (50 mL/sec), healthy adults show $F_{E_{NO}}$ values of 10 to 30 ppb, whereas in children, the values are slightly lower (5–15 ppb). $F_{E_{NO}}$ actually increases with increasing age in children. The upper limit of normal in adults is approximately 35 ppb (25 ppb in children) when $F_{E_{NO}}$ is measured using standardized methods and flows (50 mL/sec). An eNO in the 35-50 ppb should be interpreted cautiously, whereas values >50 ppb (35 ppb in children) can be considered diagnostic of eosinophilic inflammation. $F_{E_{NO}}$ appears to be related to airway size; thus it tends to be slightly higher in males than in females.

Exhaled NO appears to correlate most closely with eosinophilic inflammation in the airways. Because this type of inflammation is characteristic of bronchial asthma, measurement of $F_{E_{NO}}$ can be viewed as a surrogate for measuring eosinophils in induced sputum samples, bronchoalveolar lavage, or bronchial biopsy in patients who have asthma. These correlations persist when inflammation is treated, making $F_{E_{NO}}$ an excellent tool for monitoring therapy.

Some studies have indicated a correlation between $F_{E_{NO}}$ and bronchial hyperresponsiveness, as measured by the PC_{20} from methacholine or histamine challenge. However, many studies show little or no correlation between eNO and hyperresponsiveness. These conflicting findings may result because eosinophilic inflammation is characteristic mainly in atopic individuals. Responsiveness to methacholine appears to correlate with forced expiratory volume in the first second (FEV_1), whereas increased $F_{E_{NO}}$ correlates with other markers of inflammation.

Although pulmonary function tests (PFTs), including bronchial challenge, are considered a standard method for diagnosing and assessing asthma, there appears to be little correlation between these measures and airway inflammation. In general, most tests of lung function do not correlate with levels of eNO. Changes in NO during periods of exacerbation tend to occur more rapidly than changes in pulmonary function indices (e.g., FEV_1). Spirometry and bronchial challenge tests can reduce the level of eNO, so if both procedures are to be performed on a patient, $F_{E_{NO}}$ should be measured first.

$F_{E_{NO}}$ is reduced by corticosteroids' effects on airway inflammation. Numerous well-designed studies have demonstrated that steroid therapy, including inhaled corticosteroids, can be monitored and evaluated using $F_{E_{NO}}$ as a marker of inflammation. $F_{E_{NO}}$ does not appear to be reduced by either short-acting or long-acting β-agonists, either alone or in combination with inhaled corticosteroids. $F_{E_{NO}}$ may also be reduced in some patients treated with leukotriene modifiers.

Because of the correlation between $F_{E_{NO}}$ and airway inflammation and the known antiinflammatory effects of inhaled corticosteroids, eNO has several potential uses in asthma diagnosis and management. $F_{E_{NO}}$ can be used as a simple diagnostic screening tool to differentiate asthma from other conditions (e.g., chronic cough). Exhaled NO compares favorably with bronchial challenge tests (methacholine, exercise) in terms of sensitivity and specificity in detecting asthma. Patients who have an elevated NO level typically respond to corticosteroid therapy. $F_{E_{NO}}$ is therefore a good tool to evaluate response to antiinflammatory therapy. Failure of $F_{E_{NO}}$ to decrease with steroid treatment suggests that the patient may be unresponsive to standard therapy or that the patient may be noncompliant with the recommended treatment. Some studies have suggested that the dosage of inhaled corticosteroids can be optimized with $F_{E_{NO}}$ to guide therapy.

Patients who have chronic obstructive pulmonary disease (COPD) often show normal levels of $F_{E_{NO}}$. However, some studies have shown increased NO in patients with COPD. These differences may be related to the presence or absence of eosinophilic inflammation in patients with COPD. Many patients with COPD respond poorly to inhaled corticosteroids; measurement of $F_{E_{NO}}$ may provide an indicator as to whether eosinophilic inflammation is present and whether the patient may respond to steroid therapy. $F_{E_{NO}}$ may also be increased in pulmonary diseases that are characterized by inflammatory changes, such as chronic bronchitis, chronic cough, sarcoidosis, pneumonia, alveolitis, bronchiolitis obliterans syndrome (BOS), and bronchiectasis.

$F_{E_{NO}}$ is typically decreased in smokers, even though smoking causes airway inflammation. The physiologic explanation for the reduction in NO levels in smokers is unclear. Cigarette smoking may decrease the production of NO by epithelial cells lining the airways. Exhaled NO levels are also usually lower than normal in patients who have CF.

There is abundant evidence confirming that the levels of NO in CF are not only affected by nitric oxide synthase 2 (NOS_2) but also include arginase activity, superoxide levels, S-nitrosothiol metabolism, and denitrification pathways/prokaryotic nitrogen oxide metabolism. It is important to consider these various determinants when interpreting $F_{E_{NO}}$ in CF. Nasal NO levels are typically much higher than eNO. Values from 100 ppb up to more than 1000 ppb have been reported. Most of the nasal NO appears to be produced by the epithelial cells in the paranasal sinuses. Patients with allergic rhinitis show elevated levels of NO that appear to be responsive to nasal corticosteroids. One disease in which nasal NO measurements may be particularly useful is primary ciliary dyskinesia (PCD). Patients who have PCD have much lower levels of nasal NO (Interpretive Strategies Box 10.1).

INTERPRETIVE STRATEGIES 10.1

Exhaled Nitric Oxide

1. Was the measurement of $F_{E_{NO}}$ (online or offline) performed acceptably? Were at least two measurements repeatable within 10%? If not, interpret cautiously or not at all.
2. Are there any pretest factors that might influence the results? Eating, drinking, or smoking within 1 hour of testing? Signs and/or symptoms of respiratory tract infection? If so, interpret cautiously or not at all.
3. If the $F_{E_{NO}}$ is above the upper limit of normal (> 35 ppb for adults, > 25 ppb for children at 0.05 L/sec), suspect eosinophilic inflammation of the airways and/or alveolitis. In a symptomatic patient, steroid-responsive airway inflammation is also likely. Consider clinical correlation, particularly if the patient is taking corticosteroids or other antiinflammatory medications. Consider steroid unresponsiveness, inappropriate dosing, or noncompliance with prescribed therapy.
4. If $F_{E_{NO}}$ is much lower than the normal range (15–25 ppb in adults, 5–20 ppb in children at 0.05 L/sec), eosinophilic airway inflammation is unlikely; consider clinical correlation (pulmonary or systemic hypertension, heart failure, ciliary dyskinesia, cystic fibrosis). Also consider other factors associated with reduced NO levels (active or passive smoking, bronchoconstriction, alcohol consumption).
5. For intermediate $F_{E_{NO}}$ (25–50 ppb in adults, 20–30 ppb in children), interpret with caution. Interpretation will depend on whether it is being used diagnostically for a symptomatic steroid-naïve subject or whether the decrease or increase of $F_{E_{NO}}$ is being measured over time to evaluate the efficacy and dosing strategy for the medication prescribed.
6. For persistently high $F_{E_{NO}}$ (> 50 ppb in adults, 35 ppb in children), consider poor adherence to inhaled corticosteroids (ICSs), poor inhaled drug delivery, or continued exposure to allergens.

FORCED OSCILLATION TECHNIQUE

One way to measure the mechanical properties of the respiratory system is to apply an oscillating flow of gas to the system and measure the resulting pressure response. This method is commonly called the *FOT*. When the forced oscillations are applied at the mouth and the resulting pressure oscillations are measured at the mouth, the output is known as *input impedance*. When the oscillations are applied around the body in a closed body plethysmograph and the resulting pressures are measured at the mouth, the output is known as *transfer impedance*.

PF TIP 10.2

The FOT is particularly useful for measuring changes in the airways of patients who may be unable to perform spirometry or body plethysmography. This includes subjects such as young children (see Chapter 8) or those with physical limitations that prevent them from performing tests that require effort and coordination (i.e., FVC).

The impedance of the respiratory system (Zrs) represents the net force that must be overcome to move gas in and out of the respiratory system (upper airway, lungs, and chest wall). Applying oscillatory flow is appropriate because that is how we breathe, in a regular in-and-out fashion. Imagine the lungs modeled as a stiff pipe (the airways) with a balloon on the end (the alveoli). The pressure required to push gas down the pipe and into the balloon must overcome three basic forces: the

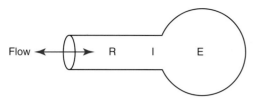

FIG. 10.7 Equation of motion. Measuring the pressure, flow, and volume generated at the mouth during breathing, one can solve for the parameters resistance (R), elastance (E), and inertia (I) that define the mechanical characteristics of the model.

resistance (R) of the pipe; the **elastance (E)**, or stiffness, of the balloon; and the **inertia (I)** of the gas itself (Fig. 10.7). Stated mathematically, the pressure necessary to move gas down the pipe and into the balloon is as follows:

$$Pressure = R\left(V^Y\right) + E\left(V\right) + I\left(V^{YY}\right)$$

where:

V = volume
V^Y = flow
V^{YY} = acceleration

This is known as the *equation of motion* for the system. Impedance depends not only on these three variables, R, E, and I, but also on the frequency of the oscillation. At low frequencies, I is negligible, R is less important, and E is dominant. At higher frequencies, R and I become more important.

Frequency is also important because the lung tissues have viscoelastic mechanical properties that change with the frequency of motion.

To measure Z, one could apply flow at various single frequencies and measure the resulting pressures generated at each frequency. Alternatively, one could apply a flow signal consisting of many different frequencies at once and then use a mathematical function known as the **fast Fourier transform (FFT)** to break down the output into unique sine waves, each of its own frequency. Despite involving complex mathematics with real and imaginary numbers, computers have made this method quick and accurate, and it has become the technique most commonly used (Fig. 10.8A).

Traditional devices use loudspeakers pulsating at different predetermined frequencies to generate the broadband flow signals (Fig. 10.9A). One commercially available device (see Fig. 10.9B) generates the broadband flow signal by an electronically controlled deflection of an internal speaker to create an impulse of flow containing many frequencies, although the frequencies analyzed range from 5 to 35 Hz. The more common of these frequencies are 5 and 20 (e.g., R_{rs5}, R_{rs20}, X_{rs5}, X_{rs20}). For all devices, the flow signal can be applied during quiet spontaneous breathing and thus requires little subject effort or cooperation. Once performed, the output is recorded in two parts: the part of Z that

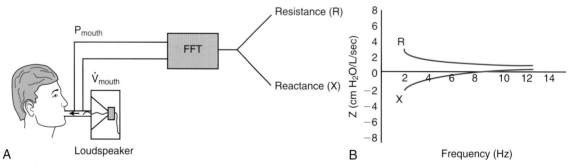

FIG. 10.8 Measurement and display of respiratory system impedance (Zrs). (A) A typical apparatus for measuring input Zrs involves a loudspeaker generating a flow signal consisting of many simultaneous frequencies. These pulsations are delivered to the mouth while mouth pressure (P_{mouth}) and flow ($\dot{V}_{mouth}$) are measured. These measurements are then processed using the fast Fourier transform (FFT). (B) The real (R) and imaginary (X) parts of Zrs are shown in relation to frequency. R is frequency dependent, falling to lower values with higher frequency.

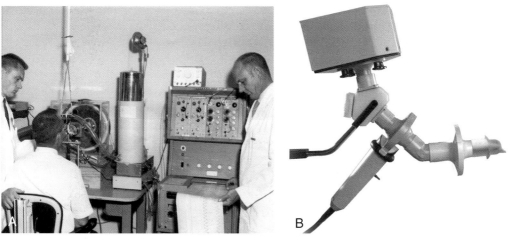

FIG. 10.9 (A) Mayo Clinic pulmonary physiology lab in the 1960s testing forced oscillation technique (FOT) using a loudspeaker and recorder. (B) A built-in loudspeaker generates an impulse of flow containing a wide range of frequencies (5–35 Hz). Courtesy Vyaire Medical, Mettawa, IL.)

is in phase with the flow signal, which represents the real part of the Z and is caused by flow-resistive properties of the respiratory system, R_{rs}; and the part that is out of phase with the flow signal, called the *reactance (X)*, which represents the imaginary part of Z and encompasses E and I. These real and imaginary parts are plotted against frequency, as shown in Fig. 10.8B.

In most clinical applications, the FOT is used to measure R_{rs} and X_{rs}. Because the technique is non-invasive, fast, and easy, it can be applied in many situations where other methods of measuring the resistance of the respiratory system (R_{rs}) are difficult or cumbersome. These situations include use in pediatric patients or others who cannot perform the panting maneuvers to measure Raw by the body box technique. However, as with Raw measured in the body box, the maneuver does require some degree of subject cooperation, including cheek holding to reduce the effect of facial noise in the signal (Fig. 10.10). The R_{rs} derived from the FOT has been shown to be sensitive to bronchoconstriction and bronchodilatation and thus can be used to assess airway hyperresponsiveness. An important disadvantage of the technique is that unless an esophageal balloon is placed to measure transpulmonary pressure, the R_{rs} measured is not of the lungs alone

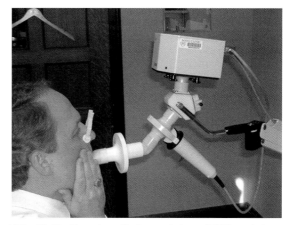

FIG. 10.10 Forced oscillation technique (FOT) technique. Cheek holding during forced oscillation technique (FOT) testing reduces the effect of the upper airway.

but of the entire respiratory system, thus including the upper airway and chest wall. The upper airway, in particular, can markedly influence the measurement because of its high compliance and the propensity for glottis interference. The European Respiratory Society (ERS) FOT technical statement cites a positive response to bronchodilator in both adults and children as –40% in R_{rs5}, or +50% in X_{rs5}.

10.1 How To ...

Perform an FOT Procedure

1. Tasks common to all procedures:
   a. Calibrate and prepare equipment.
   b. Review order.
   c. Introduce yourself and identify patient according to institutional policies.
   d. Describe and demonstrate procedure.
   e. When describing procedure, include a description of the "gentle puffing" the device will create while the patient breathes normally.
2. Verify compliance with pretest instructions (same as spirometry; see Chapter 2); test may need to be rescheduled if patient is noncompliant.
3. Have the subject place the mouthpiece, ensuring the tongue is under the mouthpiece, and breathe quietly for 30 to 60 seconds.
   a. Neck should be slightly extended.
   b. Support his or her cheeks with the hands to prevent pressure changes induced by the mouth.
4. Evaluate the quality of the tracings (i.e., artifact, stable baseline).
5. Perform three maneuvers that are repeatable; coefficient of variation (CV) within 10% for adults and 15% for children. Report the mean.
6. Report results and note comments related to test quality.

PREOPERATIVE PULMONARY FUNCTION TESTING

Preoperative pulmonary function testing is one of several means available to clinicians to evaluate surgical candidates at risk for developing respiratory complications. Preoperative testing, in conjunction with history and physical examination, electrocardiogram (ECG), and chest x-ray examination, may be indicated for any of the following reasons:

1. To estimate postoperative lung function in candidates for pneumonectomy or lobectomy
2. To plan perioperative care (preoperative preparation, type and duration of anesthetic during surgery, postoperative care) to minimize complications
3. To enhance the estimate of risk involved in the surgical procedure (i.e., morbidity and mortality) derived from history and physical examination

The need for preoperative pulmonary function testing is controversial. Some studies show increased odds of postoperative complications related to low FEV_1, hypoxemia, low D_{LCO}, hypercarbia, or low $\dot{V}O_2$. Other studies show little relationship between pulmonary function and postoperative risk, especially for general surgical and cardiovascular operations. Many investigations, both prospective and retrospective, have identified that the risk of postoperative pulmonary complications is highest in thoracic procedures, followed by upper and lower abdominal procedures. Postoperative pulmonary complications may occur in as many as 25% to 50% of major surgical procedures. Patients who have pulmonary disease are at higher risk in proportion to the degree of their pulmonary impairment. Specific tests, such as spirometry or D_{LCO}, seem to be most useful in candidates for lung resection or esophagectomy. Preoperative testing is also indicated for patients undergoing surgical procedures designed to alter lung function, such as lung volume reduction surgery (LVRS) or correction of scoliosis.

Preoperative pulmonary function testing may be indicated in patients who have the following:

1. A smoking history
2. Symptoms of pulmonary disease (e.g., cough, sputum production, shortness of breath)
3. Abnormal physical examination findings, particularly of the chest (e.g., abnormal breath sounds, ventilatory pattern, respiratory rate)
4. Abnormal chest radiographs or computed tomography (CT) scans

PF TIP 10.3

The value of pulmonary function studies to predict perioperative complications is controversial. Some studies have shown that FEV_1, D_{LCO}, Pao_2, and $Paco_2$ are useful in assessing preoperative risk. Other studies have shown no clear indicators of postoperative complications. PFTs seem to be most useful in patients undergoing lung resection or esophagectomy. FEV_1 and D_{LCO} have been used to predict postoperative lung function in lung resection.

Preoperative testing may also be indicated in patients who are obese ($>30\%$ above ideal body weight), advanced in age (usually >70 years of age), have a history of respiratory infections, or are markedly debilitated or malnourished.

In surgical candidates, the primary purpose of pulmonary function testing is to reveal preexisting pulmonary impairment. VC may decrease more than 50% from the preoperative value in thoracic or upper abdominal procedures. This places individuals with compromised function at risk of having atelectasis and pneumonia. Table 10.1 lists preoperative risk criteria for select lung function parameters. Postoperative decreases in FRC and increases in closing volume (CV) may lead to ventilation-perfusion $(\dot{V}/\dot{Q})$ abnormalities and hypoxemia. Abnormal ventilatory function related to the central control of respiration or to the ventilatory muscles may also play a role in postoperative complications.

Certain tests of pulmonary function appear to be better predictors of postoperative complications. These tests should be used both for risk evaluation and to assist in planning the perioperative care of the individual.

Spirometry

Obstructive disease can be easily identified with simple spirometry. A significant percentage of patients who may develop postoperative problems can be detected with minimal screening. Patients who have reduced FVC, with or without airway obstruction, typically have an impaired ability to cough effectively when VC decreases further during the immediate postoperative period. The FEV_1 is also used to predict postoperative pulmonary function in lung resection or pneumonectomy.

Bronchodilator Studies

Operative candidates with airway obstruction should also be tested with bronchodilators. Postbronchodilator values for FVC and FEV_1 may be used in estimating surgical risk. There may be significantly less risk if the patient's airway obstruction is reversible. Bronchodilator studies are similarly helpful in planning perioperative care. Bronchodilator therapy or inhaled corticosteroids may improve the patient's bronchial hygiene both before and after surgery.

Blood Gas Analysis

Arterial blood gas (ABG) analysis is helpful in assessing patients with documented lung disease to determine the response to pulmonary changes that occur postoperatively. Pa_{O_2} is generally not a good predictor of postoperative problems. Individuals with hypoxemia at rest usually also have abnormal spirometry results and therefore are at risk. Pa_{O_2} may improve postoperatively in patients undergoing thoracotomy for lung

---

TABLE 10.1			
Preoperative Pulmonary Function			
Test	Increased Postoperative Risk	High Postoperative Risk	Candidate for Pneumonectomy[a]
FVC	$<50\%$ of predicted	<1.5 L	
FEV_1	<2.0 L or 50% of predicted	<1.0 L	>2.0 L
MVV		<50 L/min or 50% of predicted	>50 L/min or 50% of predicted
Pa_{CO_2}		>45 mm Hg	
$\dot{V}O_2$ max	15–20 mL/min/kg	<15 L/min/kg	
Predicted postoperative FEV_1			>0.8 L/min

FEV_1, Forced expiratory volume in the first second; FVC, forced vital capacity; MVV, maximal voluntary ventilation.
[a]Values in this column determine whether the patient is to be considered a candidate for lung resection (see text).

resection if the resected portion contributed to $\dot{V}/\dot{Q}$ abnormalities. $Paco_2$ appears to be the most useful blood gas indicator of surgical risk. Some studies have shown that a $Paco_2$ above 45 mm Hg, in combination with airway obstruction and pulmonary symptoms (e.g., wheezing, cough), presents an increased risk of postoperative morbidity and mortality.

Exercise Testing

Exercise studies can accurately predict patients at risk. Individuals who cannot tolerate moderate workloads often have airway obstruction or similar ventilatory limitations. Patients who have an O_2 uptake $(\dot{V}O_2)$ of greater than 20 mL/min/kg typically have a low incidence of cardiopulmonary complications. Those unable to attain a $\dot{V}O_2$ of 15 mL/min/kg have an increased risk of postoperative complications.

Diffusing Capacity (DLCO)

A few studies have indicated that a low percent predicted postoperative diffusing capacity is an independent indicator of increased morbidity and mortality in patients undergoing lung resection. An accurate assessment of diffusing capacity is important in selecting patients who may be candidates for LVRS.

In addition to routine pulmonary function studies, several other tests are used in predicting postoperative lung function in candidates for pneumonectomy or lobectomy. These procedures are normally used in combination with spirometry and blood gas analysis.

Perfusion and V̇ / Q̇ Scans

Lung scans are particularly useful in estimating the remaining lung function in patients likely to require removal of all or part of a lung. Split-function scans are performed. These allow partitioning of the lungs into right and left halves or into multiple lung regions. Although ventilation-perfusion scans give the best estimate of overall function, simple perfusion scans yield similar information. Lung scan data, in the form of regional function

percentages, are used in combination with simple spirometric indices to calculate the patient's postoperative capacity. An example follows:

$$\text{Postoperative } FEV_1 = \text{Preoperative } FEV_1 \times \\ \%\text{Perfusion to unaffected regions}$$

This calculation is termed the *predicted postoperative FEV₁*, or ppo-FEV_1.

Patients whose postoperative FEV_1 is less than 800 mL are typically not considered surgical candidates. Resection of any lung parenchyma resulting in an FEV_1 of less than 800 mL would leave the patient more severely impaired. One exception to this general guideline occurs in patients referred for LVRS. These candidates are usually patients with end-stage COPD, often with FEV_1 values less than 800 mL and significant air trapping. Removal of poorly ventilated lung tissue often results in an improvement in spirometry, with significant increases in both FVC and FEV_1.

PULMONARY FUNCTION TESTING FOR SOCIAL SECURITY DISABILITY

PFTs are one of several means of determining a patient's inability to perform certain tasks. Respiratory impairment and disability, however, are not synonymous. Respiratory impairment relates to the failure of one or more of the functions of the lungs as measured by pulmonary function studies. Disability is the inability to perform tasks required for employment and includes medically determinable physical or mental impairment. The impairment must be expected to either result in death or last for at least 12 months. Impairment in children must be comparable to that which would disable an adult.

PFTs used to determine impairment leading to disability should characterize the type, extent, and cause of impairment. Pulmonary function testing may not completely describe all factors involved in the disabling impairment. Other factors involved may be age, educational background, and patient motivation. The energy requirements of the task in question also affect the level of disability.

Determination of the level of impairment caused by pulmonary disease usually includes history and physical examination, chest x-ray examination, other appropriate imaging techniques, and PFTs.

> **PF TIP 10.4**
>
> PFTs are often used in assessing disability from lung disease. Because tests such as FVC and FEV_1 are effort dependent, it is important that all tests meet established criteria for acceptability and repeatability. The calibration and testing criteria, including repeatability, for Social Security disability tests may differ from current clinical recommendations, and the laboratory staff should verify these criteria before testing.

Physical examination does not allow measurement of disabling symptoms but is useful in grading shortness of breath. Shortness of breath is the most prominent feature of respiratory impairment. Shortness of breath, like pain, is subjective. Tachypnea, cyanosis, and abnormal respiratory patterns are not indicative of the extent of impairment but may be helpful in interpreting pulmonary function studies.

Chest x-ray studies do not correlate well with shortness of breath or pulmonary function studies except in advanced cases of pneumoconiosis (i.e., "dust" diseases). The absence of usual findings in the pneumoconiosis may be helpful in excluding occupational exposure to toxins as part of the impairment.

Pulmonary function studies should be objective, reproducible, and, most important, specific to the disorder being investigated. Impairments caused by chronic respiratory disorders usually produce irreversible loss of function because of ventilatory impairment, gas exchange abnormalities, or a combination of both.

Forced Vital Capacity and Forced Expiratory Volume

Spirometry is the most useful index for the assessment of impairment caused by airway obstruction.

The test should not be performed unless the patient is stable. The reported FVC and FEV_1 should be the largest values obtained from at least three acceptable maneuvers. The two largest FVC values and FEV_1 values should be repeatable within 5% or 0.1 L, whichever is greater. Peak flow should be achieved early in the expiration, and the spirogram should show gradually decreasing flow throughout the breath. Spirometry should be repeated after inhaled bronchodilator if the patient's FEV_1 is less than 70% of the predicted value. Spirometric efforts, before and after bronchodilators, should meet these repeatability criteria. Standing height without shoes should be used for comparison of measured values with limits for disability (Table 10.2). In case of marked spinal deformity, arm span measurement should be used (see Chapter 1).

Computation of the FEV_1 should be done with back-extrapolated volumes (see Chapter 2). The spirogram is acceptable if the back-extrapolated volume is less than 5% of the FVC, or 0.1 L, whichever is greater. Each maneuver should be continued for at least 6 seconds or until there is no detectable

TABLE 10.2

Forced Expiratory Volume (FEV) and Forced Vital Capacity (FVC) Values for Disability Determinations

Height Without Shoes (cm)	$FEV_1 \leq$ (L); Age $\leq$ 20		FVC $\leq$ (L); Age $\leq$ 20	
	Male	Female	Male	Female
< 153.0	1.20	1.05	1.50	1.30
153.0 to < 159.0	1.35	1.15	1.65	1.40
159.0 to < 164.0	1.40	1.25	1.75	1.50
164.0 to < 169.0	1.50	1.35	1.90	1.60
169.0 to < 174.0	1.60	1.45	2.00	1.70
174.0 to < 180.0	1.75	1.55	2.20	1.85
180.0 to < 185.0	1.85	1.65	2.30	1.95
185.0 or more	1.90	1.70	2.40	2.00

Adapted from U.S. Social Security Administration. (n.d.). Disability evaluation under Social Security. ssa.gov/disability/professionals/bluebook/3.00-Respiratory-Adult.htm#3_00D4.

change in volume for the last 2 seconds of the maneuver. It is unacceptable to report FEV_1 when only a flow-volume (F-V) curve is recorded. A volume–time tracing from which FEV_1 can be measured is *required*. All lung volumes and flows must be reported in liters (L) at body temperature, pressure, and saturation (BTPS).

Volume calibration of the spirometer should agree to within 1% of a 3-L syringe. If spirometer accuracy is less than 99% but within 3% of the calibration syringe, a calibration correction factor should be used (see Chapter 12). If a flow-sensing spirometer is used, linearity should be documented by performing calibration at three different flows (3 L/6 sec, 3 L/3 sec, and 3 L/1 sec). The volume–time tracing should have the time sensitivity marked on the horizontal axis and the volume sensitivity marked on the vertical axis. The paper speed should be at least 20 mm/sec and the volume excursion at least 10 mm/L to allow manual calculation of the FEV_1 and FVC. The manufacturer and model of the spirometer should be stated in the report (Criteria for Acceptability Box 10.3).

Diffusing Capacity

The D_{LCO} is useful in determining impairment because of chronic impairment of gas exchange in both obstructive and restrictive disorders. The single-breath method should be used. The standard criteria for acceptability and repeatability for the D_{LCO} maneuver may be applied (see Chapter 3). However, the inspiratory vital capacity (IVC) should be at least 85% of the patient's best VC and the breath-hold time between 8 and 12 seconds. Your total exhalation time must be less than or equal to 4 seconds, with a sample collection time of less than 3 seconds. If your FVC is at least 2.0 L, the washout volume must be between 0.75 L and 1.0 L. If your FVC is less than 2.0 L, the washout volume must be at least 0.5 L. At least two acceptable D_{LCO} measurements within 3 mL CO (STPD)/min/mm Hg of each other or within 10% of the highest value should be performed; the mean of the two values should be reported. The reported value should be uncorrected for hemoglobin (Hb), but abnormal Hb or carboxyhemoglobin (COHb)

values should be reported. The report should also include legible graphics of each acceptable maneuver.

CRITERIA FOR ACCEPTABILITY 10.3

Disability Testing

1. Spirometer must show a 3-L calibration within 1% or corrected within 3%. Flow-based spirometers should be calibrated at three different flows to demonstrate linearity. The manufacturer and model of spirometer should be stated.
2. All FVC maneuvers should be recorded before and after the bronchodilator challenge. Time scale must be at least 20 mm/sec and volume scale at least 10 mm/L. FEV_1 may not be calculated from an F-V tracing.
3. There must be at least three acceptable FVC maneuvers before the bronchodilator; the two largest values (FVC, FEV_1) should be within 5% or 0.1 L, whichever is greater.
4. The spirogram must show peak flow early in expiration with a smooth, gradually decreasing flow. The maneuver is acceptable if the effort continues for at least 6 seconds or if there is a plateau with no change in volume for 2 seconds. The FEV_1 should be measured using back-extrapolation; the back-extrapolated volume should be less than 5% of FVC or 0.1 L, whichever is greater.
5. Postbronchodilator studies should be performed if FEV_1 is less than 70% of predicted. Postbronchodilator testing should be done 10 minutes after administration of the drug. The name and dose of the drug should be included in the report.
6. D_{LCO} testing (if performed) should meet all required testing elements as described. D_{LCO} uncorrected for Hb is reported.
7. Exercise testing (if performed) should be for 4 to 6 minutes at a workload of approximately 5 metabolic equivalents (METs). Blood gas samples should be obtained at rest and during exercise.
8. Statements regarding the patient's ability to understand directions, as well as effort and cooperation, should be included with all tests.

Adapted from U.S. Social Security Administration. (n.d.). Disability evaluation under Social Security. ssa.gov/disability/professionals/bluebook/3.00-Respiratory-Adult.htm#3_00D4.

Arterial Blood Gases

Although blood gas results are objective, they are largely nonspecific in determining impairment. Blood gases should be obtained while the subject is breathing room air (Table 10.3) without supplemental oxygen. The resting ABG report includes the name of the patient, the date of the test, and either altitude or city and state of the test site. Only the Pao_2 and the $Paco_2$ values are required to be reported. Blood gases may be assessed during exercise. If performing ABGs with exercise, see the Exercise Testing section later in this chapter. Blood gas analysis should be performed by a laboratory certified by a state or federal agency.

Pulse Oximetry

Pulse oximetry measures SpO_2, the percentage of oxygen saturation of blood hemoglobin. Pulse oximetry is used (either at rest, during a 6-Minute Walked Test [6MWT], or after a 6MWT) to evaluate respiratory disorders.

The following are requirements for pulse oximetry:
- Patient is medically stable at the time of the test.
- Pulse oximetry measurement must be recorded while breathing room air, that is, without oxygen supplementation.
- Pulse oximetry measurement must be stable, meaning the range of SpO_2 values (i.e., lowest to highest) during any 15-second interval cannot exceed 2 percentage points.
- When multiple measurements are performed (e.g., at rest and after a 6MWT), the lowest SpO_2 value is reported.

The pulse oximetry report must include the following information:
- Name, the date of the test, and either the altitude or both the city and state of the test site.
- A graphical printout showing the SpO_2 value and a concurrent, acceptable pulse wave.

Exercise Testing

Patients considered for exercise evaluation should first have resting blood gas evaluation, either sitting or standing. A steady-state exercise test (see Chapter 7) is then performed, preferably with a treadmill. The patient should

TABLE 10.3
Arterial Oxygen Tension and Pulse Oximetry for Disability Determinations

	Less Than 3000 Feet Above Sea Level	3000–6000 Feet Above Sea Level	More Than 6000 Feet Above Sea Level
PCO_2 (mm Hg)	PO_2 (mm Hg)	PO_2 (mm Hg)	PO_2 (mm Hg)
30 or below	65	60	55
31	64	59	54
32	63	58	53
33	62	57	52
34	61	56	51
35	60	55	50
36	59	54	49
37	58	53	48
38	57	52	47
39	56	51	46
40 or above	55	50	45
Pulse oximetry	$SpO_2 \leq 87\%$	$SpO_2 \leq 85\%$	$SpO_2 \leq 83\%$

Adapted from U.S. Social Security Administration. (n.d.). Disability evaluation under Social Security. ssa.gov/disability/professionals/bluebook/3.00-Respiratory-Adult.htm#3_00D4.

exercise for 4 to 6 minutes at an O_2 consumption rate $(\dot{V}O_2)$ of approximately 17.5 mL/min/kg (approximately 5 METs) breathing room air. An equivalent workload should be used for cycle ergometry (e.g., 75 W for a 175-lb patient). Blood gas samples should be drawn at this workload to determine whether significant hypoxemia is present (see Table 10.3). If the patient does not desaturate at this level, a higher workload can be used to determine exercise capacity. If the patient cannot achieve a workload of 5 METs, a lower workload can be selected to determine exercise capacity.

ECG should be monitored continuously throughout the exercise evaluation and in the immediate postexercise period. Blood pressure and an ECG should be recorded during each minute of exercise. An ABG should be drawn during the final 2 minutes of the steady-state workload. It may be helpful to measure $\dot{V}O_2$, $\dot{V}CO_2$, and $\dot{V}_E$. Either the altitude or both the city and the state of the test site should be included in the report to assist with interpretation of blood gas values.

In reporting impairment for the purpose of determining disability, the remaining functional capacity is as important in determining the patient's ability to perform a certain task as the percentage of lost function. Some statement of the patient's ability to understand and cooperate during pulmonary function measurements should accompany the tabular and graphic data.

Limits for determining disability based on respiratory impairment have been set for the United States by the U.S. Social Security Administration. Criteria are set according to the disease category (see Interpretive Strategies 10.1). COPD is evaluated by comparing FEV_1 with the values in Table 10.2. Restrictive ventilatory disorders are evaluated by comparing FVC with the values in Table 10.2. Impaired gas exchange is evaluated by comparing PaO_2 with the values in Table 10.3. Disability caused by asthma is also evaluated with FEV_1. Episodes of asthma (requiring emergency treatment or hospitalization) occurring at least every 2 months or at least six times per year may also be evidence of disability (Criteria for Acceptability 10.3 and Interpretive Strategies 10.2).

INTERPRETIVE STRATEGIES 10.2

Disability Testing

1. Were spirometry, diffusing capacity, blood gases, and exercise tests performed acceptably? If not, interpret very cautiously or not at all.
2. Was FEV_1 less than the predicted limit for the patient's height? If so, disabling obstruction is likely.
3. Was FVC less than the predicted limit for the patient's height? If so, disabling restrictive disease is likely.
4. Was the D_{LCO} (if measured) less than or equal to the cut point listed in Table 10.4 for the patient's specific height and gender?
5. Was the patient's PaO_2, measured while clinically stable on two occasions at least 3 weeks apart but within 6 months, equal to or less than published limits (adjusted for $PaCO_2$ and altitude)? If so, disabling hypoxemia is present.
6. Was PaO_2 equal to or less than published limits during steady-state exercise (less than or equivalent to 5 METs) breathing room air? If so, disabling hypoxemia is present.
7. Are lung function measurements consistent with history, physical examination, chest x-ray study, and other imaging techniques?

TABLE 10.4

Diffusing Capacity Values for Disability Determinations

Height Without Shoes (cm)	Males $D_{LCO} \leq$ (mL CO (STDP)/ min/mm Hg)	Females $D_{LCO} \leq$ (mL CO (STDP)/ min/mm Hg)
< 153.0	9.0	8.0
153.0 to < 159.0	9.5	8.5
159.0 to < 164.0	10.0	9.0
164.0 to < 169.0	10.5	9.5
169.0 to < 174.0	11.0	10.0
174.0 to < 180.0	11.5	10.5
180.0 to < 185.0	12.0	11.0
185.0 to more	12.5	11.5

STDP, Standard temperature, pressure, dry.

METABOLIC MEASUREMENTS: INDIRECT CALORIMETRY

Description

Measurements of $\dot{V}O_2$, $\dot{V}CO_2$, and the **respiratory exchange ratio (RER)** may be used to determine **resting energy expenditure (REE).** REE is usually expressed in kcal/day (kcal/day). These measurements allow nutritional assessment and management. In combination with measurements of urine urea nitrogen (UUN), **indirect calorimetry** allows calories to be partitioned among various substrates (e.g., fat, carbohydrate, protein).

Techniques

Indirect calorimetry may be performed with either an open-circuit or a closed-circuit system to measure O_2 consumption ($\dot{V}O_2$), CO_2 production ($\dot{V}CO_2$), and RER. The open-circuit method is more commonly used in clinical practice.

Open-Circuit Calorimetry

The exchange of O_2 and CO_2 may be measured by recording the fractional differences of O_2 and CO_2 between inspired and expired gas. These measurements are accomplished with a mixing chamber, a dilution system, or a breath-by-breath system similar to those used for expired gas analysis during exercise (see this chapter). $\dot{V}O_2$ and $\dot{V}CO_2$ are measured as described for exercise testing with a mixing chamber and breath-by-breath systems. $\dot{V}_E$, V_T, and f_b (respiratory rate) may be measured simultaneously. In systems that use the dilution principle, a constant flow of gas is mixed with expired air. The dilution of CO_2 is then used to calculate ventilation. Connection to the patient may be made by a standard directional breathing valve with a mouthpiece and nose clips. A ventilated hood or canopy (Fig. 10.11A) may also be used. Almost all metabolic measurement systems provide for connection to a mechanical ventilator circuit (Fig. 10.11B).

A hood or canopy allows long-term measurements without direct connection to the patient's airway. The hood is ventilated by drawing a flow of gas through it that exceeds the patient's peak inspiratory demand (40 L/min is usually adequate). Ventilation can be calculated by measuring the change in flow into and out of the hood during breathing ("bias" flow).

Connection to a ventilator requires a means of measuring exhaled volume along with fractional concentrations of both inspired and expired gas. Breath-by-breath metabolic measurement systems usually sample gas at the patient–ventilator connection.

Closed-Circuit Calorimetry

The simplest type of closed-circuit calorimeter is one that measures $\dot{V}O_2$ volumetrically. The patient rebreathes from a closed system that contains a spirometer filled with O_2. CO_2 is scrubbed from the circuit using a chemical absorber. A recorder

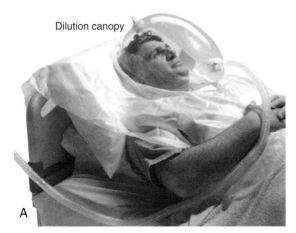

Dilution canopy

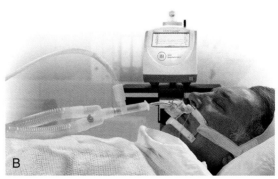

FIG. 10.11 (A) Resting energy expenditure (REE) performed using a continuous-flow canopy. (Courtesy Vyaire Medical, Mettawa, IL.) (B) REE performed with the subject on the ventilator. The gas collection system and pneumotach are integrated into the patient's ventilator circuit. (Courtesy MGC Diagnostics, Saint Paul, MN.)

is used to measure the decrease in spirometer volume, equal to the rate of O_2 uptake $(\dot{V}O_2)$. A similar approach uses a closed spirometer system to measure the volume of O_2 added as the patient rebreathes and consumes O_2. $\dot{V}O_2$ is equal to the volume of O_2 that must be added per minute to maintain a constant volume. CO_2 production cannot be measured with a closed-circuit system unless a CO_2 analyzer is added to the device. $\dot{V}_E$, V_T, and f_b may all be determined from volume excursions of the spirometer. Closed-circuit systems may be used with spontaneously breathing patients by means of a simple breathing valve and mouthpiece. The use of a closed-circuit calorimeter with a mechanical ventilator requires that the spirometer system be connected between the patient and ventilator. The ventilator then "ventilates" the spirometer, which, in turn, ventilates the patient. This technique usually requires a bellows-type spirometer in a fixed container so that the positive pressure generated by the ventilator can compress the bellows. The volume delivered by the ventilator (V_I) must be increased to compensate for the volume of gas compressed in the closed-circuit spirometer during positive pressure breaths.

Performing Metabolic Measurements

The primary purpose of indirect calorimetry is to estimate REE over an extended period, usually 24 hours. To extrapolate the values obtained during the sampling period, the patient's condition during the measurement is critical (Criteria for Acceptability 10.4). The calorimeter or metabolic cart should be calibrated at least daily, preferably before each test. Gas analyzers should be calibrated using gas concentrations appropriate for the clinical situation. Sample lines and gas-conditioning devices (absorbers) should be checked before each test. If calibration or testing produces questionable values, the device should be checked against a known standard. Burning ethanol or other material with a fixed respiratory quotient (RQ) can be used. A large-volume syringe can be used to simulate a patient with $\dot{V}O_2$ and $\dot{V}CO_2$ values near zero. Alternately, biologic controls can be used to check the precision of the calorimeter.

10.2   How To ...

Perform REE Study (Open Circuit)

1. Tasks common to all procedures:
   a. Calibrate and prepare equipment.
   b. Review order.
   c. Introduce yourself and identify patient according to institutional policies.
   d. Describe and demonstrate procedure.
2. Verify compliance with pretest instructions.
   a. Postabsorptive state, for example, 12 hours after the last meal
   b. Effect of eating a meal increases the metabolic rate by 46%, which does not disappear for 12 hours
3. Preliminary rest period of 20 minutes
4. Place the device on the subject or inline (ventilator) with the subject.
5. Remind the subject to breathe quietly/normally during the test (if spontaneously breathing)
   a. Hyperventilation during the test will increase the RER (RQ).
6. Subject should be recumbent.
7. Observations:
   a. Record the time the rest period begins.
   b. Record heart rate and respiratory rate at least twice.
   c. Note respiratory rate characteristics.
   d. Note shallow, deep, forced, regular, or irregular.
   e. Temperature and blood pressure (BP) measured 10 minutes into rest period.
   f. Muscular activity should be recorded.
8. Posttest data assessment
   a. RER (RQ) less than 0.7 indicates an error in the measurement; greater than 1.0 indicates a nervous patient.
   b. Ideally, average 10 minutes of steady-state data.
9. Report results and note comments related to test quality.

PF TIP 10.5

Estimation of caloric needs for a 24-hour period from a metabolic study requires that the measurements be made with the patient in a steady state. The short interval during which measurements are made (usually 5–20 minutes) should be free of interruptions that may alter the patient's metabolic rate. These include ventilator changes or suctioning. Nutritional support (if given) should be continuous, and the patient should be resting.

CRITERIA FOR ACCEPTABILITY 10.4

Indirect Calorimetry

1. Appropriate calibration of gas analyzers and volume transducers should be documented before each test.
2. RER (RQ) should be within the normal physiologic range of 0.7 to 1.0.
3. Measured $\dot{V}O_2$ and $\dot{V}CO_2$ values should vary by no more than 5% or less for a 5-minute data collection; longer data-collection intervals may be necessary if the variability is greater than 5%.
4. Data should be collected for a minimum of 5 minutes with minimal variability.
5. RER (RQ) values should be consistent with the patient's current nutritional intake.
6. Documentation should include the patient's medications, nutritional support, body temperature at time of test, and ventilatory support setting (if applicable).
7. The patient should be resting, with no bolus feedings or pharmacologic stimulants or depressants. There should be no physical therapy, airway care, or major ventilator changes immediately before the assessment.
8. If a stable FIO_2 cannot be achieved, REE may be estimated from the $\dot{V}CO_2$ with an assumed RER (RQ) of 0.85.
9. If a 24-hour urine urea nitrogen (UUN) is collected for substrate use, it should be concurrent with the metabolic study.

Adapted from American Association for Respiratory Care. (2004). Clinical practice guideline: Metabolic measurements using indirect calorimetry during mechanical ventilation—2004 revision & update. *Respiratory Care, 49*, 1073–1079.

Pretest instruction should include fasting after midnight in the outpatient subject or for 2 to 4 hours before the test starts in a hospitalized patient. If the inpatient is receiving either enteral or parenteral feedings, the feedings should be in continuous rather than bolus form. Information about the type and amount of nutritional support in the previous 24 hours may be helpful in interpreting test results. Drugs or substances that alter metabolism should be avoided. Substances such as caffeine and nicotine are particularly common stimulants. Theophylline-based drugs may also increase metabolic rate. The subject should refrain from exercise. Typically, these tests are performed in the morning hours to try to reduce the amount of activity performed before testing. The patient should be recumbent or supine for 20 to 30 minutes before beginning measurements and should stay quiet during the test. Ideally, the patient should be awake and alert during testing. The testing apparatus should not cause discomfort or exertion for the patient, which is the reason canopy testing is ideal for this procedure because breathing valves, mouthpieces, and nose clips may alter the patient's breathing pattern. The patient should be in a neutral thermal environment. Special corrections may be required for patients who are febrile or hypothermic. The patient's temperature at the time of the test should be recorded, along with a temperature history of the previous 24 hours. Temperature changes of 1°C can result in a 13% change in REE. Data collection should continue long enough to establish a stable baseline and verify steady-state conditions (Fig. 10.12). Ten to 15 minutes of stable readings for $\dot{V}O_2$ and $\dot{V}CO_2$ may be required, but an adequate measurement can be obtained in as short an interval as 5 minutes. Common indicators of steady-state conditions are the parameters assessed as part of the metabolic study. $\dot{V}O_2$ and $\dot{V}CO_2$ should not vary more than 5% from the mean value measured during the test (at least 5 minutes). RER values should be within the normal physiologic range (0.7–1.0). If the patient does not achieve steady-state conditions, a longer test interval may be required to average representative periods of metabolic activity. Patients on ventilators should be in a stable condition. Leaks in the ventilator circuit, around cuffed endotracheal tubes, or from chest tubes or bronchopleural fistulas may invalidate measurements of RER (RQ) and REE. No ventilator adjustments should be made 1 to 2 hours before the test period. Modifications in minute ventilation or FIO_2 settings can cause gross changes in the patterns of gas exchange, particularly in patients with pulmonary disease. The ventilator must have a stable delivered O_2 concentration; FIO_2 settings greater than 0.60 may result in erroneous $\dot{V}O_2$ measurements. Appropriate valves may need to be used for ventilator modes that involve continuous gas flow.

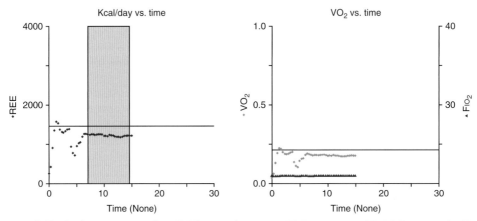

FIG. 10.12   Resting energy expenditure (REE). Pretest heart rate = 55. Temperature = 35.4°C. Pump speed = 25. Steady state achieved.

Metabolic Calculations

The **Harris–Benedict equations** are commonly used to estimate REE:

Men:
$$REE(kcal/24\,hr) = 66.47 + 13.75W + 5H - 6.76A$$

Women:
$$REE(kcal/24\,hr) = 655.1 + 9.56W + 1.85H - 4.68A$$

where:

W = weight, kilograms
H = height, centimeters
A = age, years

The REE by these formulas was originally described as the **basal metabolic rate (BMR).** These equations may be used to estimate the caloric expenditure in normal individuals under conditions of minimal activity. BMR in these circumstances is related to lean body mass. To determine the optimum level of caloric intake, BMR must be adjusted upward because trauma, surgery, infections, and burns all cause the REE to increase.

The Weir equation is used to calculate REE from respiratory gas exchange and urinary nitrogen:

$$REE(kcal/24\,hr) = 5.68\dot{V}O_2 + 1.59\dot{V}CO_2 - 2.17\,UUN$$

where:

$\dot{V}O_2$ is expressed in mL/min (STPD)
$\dot{V}CO_2$ is expressed in mL/min (STPD)

UUN = urine urea nitrogen (g/24 hr)
If UUN is unknown, REE may be calculated

Indirect calorimetry by the open-circuit method provides measures of both O_2 consumption and CO_2 production. As previously mentioned, RER is the ratio $\dot{V}CO_2/\dot{V}O_2$. Under steady-state conditions, RER approximates the mean RQ at the cellular level. RQ normally varies from 0.70 to 1.00, depending on the substrates being metabolized. Carbohydrate oxidation produces an RQ near 1.0, fat oxidation produces an RQ near 0.70, and protein oxidation produces an RQ of 0.82. RQ attributable to carbohydrates and fats may be determined by subtracting $\dot{V}O_2$ and $\dot{V}CO_2$ derived from protein. This form of the RQ is termed the *nonprotein RQ*, or *RQnp*, and is calculated as follows:

$$RQnp = \frac{1.44\dot{V}CO_2 - 4.754UUN}{1.44\dot{V}O_2 - 5.923UUN}$$

where:

$\dot{V}CO_2$ is expressed in mL/min
$\dot{V}O_2$ is expressed in mL/min
UUN = urine urea nitrogen (g/24 hr)
1.44 = factor to convert mL/min to L/24 hr

Because CO_2 production varies with O_2 uptake, deviations of the RQ from the average value of 0.85 result in differences of less than 5% in the calculation of REE if only $\dot{V}O_2$ and RQ are used. Indirect calorimetry by the closed-circuit (volumetric) method takes advantage of this small difference by assuming a fixed RQ (usually 0.85) and measuring only $\dot{V}O_2$. Open-circuit calorimetry is usually limited to measurements on patients whose F_{IO_2} is 0.6 or less. However, $\dot{V}CO_2$ can be measured on these patients and $\dot{V}O_2$ estimated, again by assuming an RQ of 0.85. This method provides a means of estimating caloric needs even though $\dot{V}O_2$ cannot be measured accurately.

UUN is obtained from a 24-hour urine collection. Because protein metabolism accounts for only a small portion of total calories per day (approximately 12%), omission of the UUN in the Weir equation changes the calculated REE by only 2%.

The Consolazio equations can be used to determine energy expenditure from gas exchange $\left(\dot{V}O_2,\dot{V}CO_2\right)$, UUN, and the caloric equivalents of carbohydrates, fats, and proteins:

$$CHO = 5.926\,\dot{V}CO_2 - 4.189\,\dot{V}O_2 - 1.539\,UUN$$

$$FAT = 2.432\,\dot{V}O_2 - 2.432\,\dot{V}O_2 - 1.943\,UUN$$

$$PRO = 6.250\,UUN$$

where:

CHO = carbohydrates oxidized in grams/24 hours
FAT = fat oxidized in grams/24 hours
PRO = protein oxidized in grams/24 hours

From the grams of each substrate used, the kcal derived from that source can be computed:

$$Carbohydrates\,(in\,kcal) = 4.18\,carbohydrates\,(in\,grams)$$

$$Fat\,(in\,kcal) = 9.46\,fat\,(in\,grams)$$

$$Protein\,(in\,kcal) = 4.32\,protein\,(in\,grams)$$

$$Total\,(in\,kcal) = carbohydrate + fat + protein$$

The percentage of calories from each substrate may also be calculated by dividing the kcal derived from that substrate by the total kcal. Because the Consolazio equations are intended for analysis of normal substrate partitioning, RQ values outside of the range of 0.70 to 1.00 will result in negative values for either carbohydrates or lipids (fat). These negative values are erroneous if RER does not equal RQ (i.e., the patient is not in a metabolic steady state).

Significance and Pathophysiology

See Interpretive Strategies 10.3. Indirect calorimetry assesses nutritional status in patients whose daily energy needs are altered by disease, injury, or therapeutic interventions. REE accounts for approximately two-thirds of the daily energy requirements in healthy patients. The Harris–Benedict equations, or similar predictive equations, are commonly used to estimate REE. Various factors can be used to adjust estimated REE to account for additional caloric needs imposed by the patient's clinical status. This approach works well in many patients. However, the metabolic requirements of critically ill patients vary widely. Indirect calorimetry is indicated for patients who do not respond favorably to traditional methods of nutritional assessment and support. Indirect calorimetry can be used to detect undernourishment, overnourishment, or the use of inappropriate substrates (Box 10.2).

BOX 10.2   INDICATIONS FOR INDIRECT CALORIMETRY[a]

1. Head trauma or paralysis
2. Chronic obstructive pulmonary disease (COPD)
3. Cachexia
4. Eating disorders (e.g., anorexia nervosa, bulimia nervosa)
5. Multiple trauma
6. Acute pancreatitis
7. Patients in whom height or weight is indeterminate
8. Poor response to enteral or parenteral support
9. Patients receiving total parenteral nutrition at home
10. Transplant patients
11. Morbidly obese patients
12. Patients with demonstrated hypermetabolism or hypometabolism
13. Patients on prolonged mechanical ventilation who are unable to eat

[a]Risk or stress factors known to interfere with the calculation of energy expenditure.

Undernourishment or starvation can occur during acute or chronic illness. It may be detected by caloric expenditure in excess of caloric intake (negative energy balance). Both fat stores and protein from muscle breakdown may contribute to metabolism during periods of undernourishment. Indirect calorimetry is often used, along with measurement of body weight, triceps skinfold measurements, and other approximations of energy reserves. These measurements allow for the planning of nutritional therapy to replenish diminished reserves.

Overnourishment occurs when any substrate is supplied in excess of the energy requirements. Overfeeding is most deleterious when the patient's nutritional status is already adequate. Excess lipid or carbohydrate calories are stored as fat, which may place stress on one or more organ systems (e.g., liver).

Patients who have pulmonary disease present a special dilemma. Excessive carbohydrate intake results in increased CO_2 production because the RER (RQ) of carbohydrates is 1. For patients in respiratory failure, excess CO_2 production increases the ventilatory load on the respiratory system. Adjustments in substrate use can be made after the nonprotein RER (RQ) is determined by indirect calorimetry. Lipids (i.e., fats) are typically substituted for glucose so that the RER (RQ) can be reduced while the caloric intake is maintained. Patients in respiratory failure may also experience atrophy of ventilatory muscles. Substrate analysis can be used to assess N_2 balance related to the breakdown of muscle protein. Substrate analysis permits measurement of the nutritional requirements necessary to maintain N_2 balance.

Technical considerations involved in indirect calorimetry include the accuracy of gas analysis and measurement of expired volume during the test (open-circuit methods). The most common problem during metabolic measurements is the attainment of a true steady state. Only if the measurements are made under steady-state conditions is the metabolic rate representative of caloric expenditure over 24 hours. Hyperventilation resulting from connection to a mask or mouthpiece, or from ventilator manipulation, occurs frequently. **Head hoods** or **continuous-flow canopies** can eliminate much of the stimulation associated with connection to the metabolic measurement system (see Fig. 10.11A) but cannot be used for patients on mechanical ventilators. Hoods or canopies may also cause hyperventilation in awake, alert patients. An RER greater than 1.0 should always be evaluated in relation to $\dot{V}_E$ and end-tidal CO_2. Abnormally high $\dot{V}_E$ and low end-tidal CO_2 values may indicate hyperventilation. RER values in excess of 1.0 that cannot be explained as hyperventilation may be caused by the storage of excess calories as fat (lipogenesis). RER values between 0.67 and 0.70 may occur in ketosis caused by extreme fasting or diabetic ketoacidosis. However, more commonly, low RER values (<0.67) signal improper calibration of the CO_2 or O_2 analyzers. Inaccurate calibration or improper performance of gas analyzers can result in RER values outside of the usual metabolic range of 0.70 to 1.0.

Special problems may be encountered in performing metabolic measurements on patients requiring mechanical ventilatory support. A common difficulty relates to measurements of O_2 consumption in patients receiving supplemental O_2. Measurement of $\dot{V}O_2$ by respiratory gas exchange requires analysis of the difference between inspired and expired O_2 along with $\dot{V}_E$. In patients breathing room air, inspired FIO_2 is constant. Many O_2-blending systems, such as those used on ventilators, may not provide a constant fraction of inspired O_2. Large differences in calculated $\dot{V}O_2$ may result from small fluctuations in FIO_2, even if FEO_2 remains relatively constant. Small differences in inspired and expired volumes (resulting from the RER) are corrected by adjusting the inspired fraction of O_2, according to the following equation:

$$\frac{\left(1 - FEO_2 - FECO_2\right)}{1 - FIO_2} \times FIO_2$$

This correction of inspired FIO_2 for gas balance in the lung (i.e., the Haldane transformation) limits the accuracy of the open-circuit method of determining $\dot{V}O_2$. As FIO_2 increases, the value in the denominator of the equation becomes smaller. Even with very accurate gas analyzers, the measurement of the differences between FIO_2 and FEO_2 (when FIO_2 is above 0.60) is variable. Breath-by-breath analysis of exhaled gas can reduce the problem of variable FIO_2 by measuring the fractional gas concentrations at the patient's airway and computing $\dot{V}O_2$ and $\dot{V}CO_2$ for individual breaths. Indirect calorimetry by the volumetric method (i.e., a closed system) avoids this problem by measuring the actual volume of O_2 removed during rebreathing. Allowing the patient to breathe from a reservoir bag containing an elevated FIO_2 (typically < 0.60) can usually accommodate measurement of $\dot{V}O_2$ and $\dot{V}CO_2$ in spontaneously breathing patients who require supplemental O_2.

If a stable FIO_2 cannot be achieved (as is often the case when it is > 0.60), REE can be estimated from the $\dot{V}CO_2$. If an RER (RQ) of 0.85 is assumed, $\dot{V}O_2$ can be estimated by dividing the $\dot{V}CO_2$ by the RER (RQ) and then solving the Weir equation (see this chapter). This method will underestimate the REE when the RER (RQ) is greater than 0.85, with a maximal error of about 25% if the RER (RQ) is really 1.20. Similarly, the REE will be overestimated

for RER (RQ) values less than 0.85, with a maximal error of approximately 19% if the RER (RQ) is 0.67.

Other considerations involved in metabolic measurements of ventilated patients include the effects of positive pressure on gas analysis and on volume determination. Analysis of O_2 and CO_2 in the ventilator circuit must take into account the effect of positive-pressure breaths on the gas analyzers. Depending on the sampling method used, positive-pressure swings during each breath may generate falsely high partial-pressure readings. Closed-circuit calorimetry places a volumetric device in the breathing circuit between the ventilator and the patient (Fig. 10.11B). The volume delivered by the ventilator must be increased to accommodate the higher compressible gas volume in the circuit, approximately 1 mL/cm H_2O for each liter of added volume.

SUMMARY

- Respiratory muscle strength testing can be a helpful tool in characterizing neuromuscular disease and other abnormalities that affect the diaphragm and abdominal muscles.
- Exhaled nitric oxide (FE_{NO}) provides a noninvasive means of measuring eosinophilic inflammation of the airways. FE_{NO} may be useful in the diagnosis and management of diseases characterized by inflammation, such as asthma.
- Forced oscillatory technique uses high-frequency oscillations to measure the mechanical properties of the respiratory system, in particular, resistance and impedance. It is especially useful in children or subjects who cannot perform conventional PFTs such as spirometry.
- Preoperative testing and disability testing use spirometry, lung volumes, diffusing capacity, blood gases, and exercise testing. Each test examines a specific aspect of either preoperative risk or respiratory impairment that prevents work.
- Metabolic measurements, specifically indirect calorimetry, provide a means of assessing nutritional status and support. They may be particularly useful in the evaluation of patients who do not respond adequately to estimated nutritional needs.

CASE STUDIES

CASE 10.1

HISTORY

A 27-year-old auto mechanic is referred to the pulmonary function laboratory by his physician. His chief complaint is "breathing problems." He describes breathlessness that occurs suddenly and then subsides. He has no other symptoms and no history of lung disease. He does not have a family history of lung disease. He is a current smoker and has smoked, on average, one pack of cigarettes per day for the past 10 years (10 pack-years). He has no unusual environmental exposure. He claims that gasoline fumes sometimes bring on the episodes of shortness of breath.

PULMONARY FUNCTION TESTING
Personal Data

Sex:	Male
Age:	27 yr
Height:	68 in. (173 cm)
Weight:	150 lb (68.2 kg)

Spirometry				
	Before Drug	Predicted	LLN	% Predicted
FVC (L)	3.80	5.21	4.32	73
FEV_1 (L)	3.70	4.30	3.55	86
FEV_1/FVC	0.97	0.83	0.73	—
$FEF_{25\%-75\%}$ (L/sec)	4.62	4.49	2.94	103
$FEF_{50\%}$ (L/sec)	4.81	6.01	—	80
$FEF_{75\%}$ (L/sec)	3.12	3.33	—	94
MVV (L/min)	77	146	—	53

FEF, Forced expiratory flow, *LLN*, lower limit of normal, based on National Health and Nutrition Examination Survey (NHANES) III; *MVV*, maximal voluntary ventilation.

Respiratory Pressures			
	Before Drug	Predicted	% Predicted
MIP (cm H_2O)	–118	–128	92
MEP (cm H_2O)	57	240	24

Technologist's Comments

None of the FVC maneuvers was acceptable; they did not last 6 seconds or show an obvious plateau. Best FVC values were not within 150 mL. Inspiratory efforts were variable. In total, eight maneuvers were attempted. Respiratory pressure measurements were variable. The subject had difficulty completing all maneuvers.

QUESTIONS

1. What is the interpretation of the following?
   a. Spirometry
   b. Low value for MEP
   c. Variability of the subject's efforts
2. What is the cause of the subject's symptoms?

3. What other tests might be indicated?
4. What treatment might be recommended, based on these findings?

DISCUSSION

Interpretation

All spirometry maneuvers and respiratory pressures are unacceptable because of poor subject effort or technical errors. The subject's best effort shows a reduced FVC. The FEV_1 is normal, and the FEV_1/FVC is above the expected range. All other flows, along with the MIP, are within normal limits. The MEP and the MVV are reduced.

Impression: Spirometry results are inconsistent. The FVC and FEV_1 are not reproducible. Expiratory muscle pressure and MVV are reduced. Overall, inadequate subject effort or technical errors are present.

Cause of Symptoms

This test shows poor repeatability, especially for effort-dependent measurements. The figure shows the variability for three FVC maneuvers. The tracings show incomplete end of forced exhalation (EOFE) and variability.

The low FVC seems to be consistent with a mild restrictive process. The FEV_1, however, is close to normal. If simple restriction were present, both FVC and FEV_1 should be reduced similarly. The subject's other flows are normal. Flows that depend on the FVC (e.g., the $FEF_{25\%-75\%}$) might also be in error if the FVC is incorrect. The MVV is much less than 40 times the FEV_1, so the MVV is probably not accurate and most likely reflects poor effort. Because MVV was low, respiratory pressures were measured. MIP appears to be normal but was variable. MEP was also variable. The best effort was only 24% of expected.

Examination of the volume–time spirograms reveals that the subject terminated each FVC maneuver after approximately 2 seconds. The FVC values varied by more than 150 mL, confirming poor effort. However, a lack of repeatability of the FVC maneuvers is not a sufficient reason for discarding the test results. This subject's FVC maneuvers lasted 2 seconds despite repeated coaching by the operator. The maneuvers did not meet the current defined standard of EOFE, which is a 1-second plateau, regardless of total exhalation time. Failure to exhale completely is one of the most common errors in spirometry. This error may be caused by the lack of cooperation on the part of the subject or by the inability to continue exhalation caused by cough. It may also occur if the operator does not adequately explain or demonstrate the maneuver.

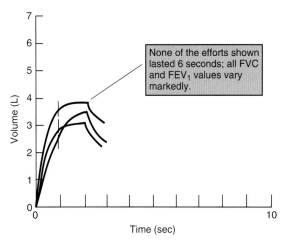

None of the efforts shown lasted 6 seconds; all FVC and FEV_1 values vary markedly.

The operator performing this test repeated the FVC maneuver eight times. Only the three best efforts were recorded. Appropriate comments were added at the end of the test data. The poor quality of the data makes it impossible to determine whether the subject's symptoms are real. The subject appears to be malingering—that is, not giving maximal effort on tests that are effort dependent. Poor reproducibility in a subject who is free of symptoms at the time of the test suggests poor effort or lack of cooperation.

Other Tests

Alternative tests for this subject should be independent of subject effort. A simple blood gas analysis was performed. The results indicated normal oxygenation and acid–base status. Testing of lung volumes and diffusing capacity was postponed because both of these depend on subject effort and cooperation. A bronchoprovocation challenge test (see Chapter 9) might have been indicated because the subject had asthma-like symptoms. However, airway resistance or FOT should be considered as alternative methods to assess the response because the subject was unable to perform acceptable spirometry (see this chapter and Chapter 4).

Treatment

Before suggesting any treatment, the referring physician contacted the subject's employer to ask about possible environmental hazards that might cause the symptoms. He learned that the subject was facing possible termination for excessive absence from work. The subject's supervisor revealed that the subject claimed to have asthma, which may have contributed to his excessive absenteeism.

CASE 10.2

HISTORY

A 39-year-old male presents for evaluation of shortness of breath and cough. He was a healthy competitive cyclist on no medications until he developed an upper respiratory infection last spring, which was treated with an antibiotic and inhaled corticosteroid. Later that fall, he developed wheezing and a productive cough, which was treated with 60 mg of prednisone. His symptoms continued to worsen, and he went to his local emergency room. He was admitted for a 7-day hospital stay that included intravenous (IV) Solu-Medrol, oxygen, moxifloxacin, and nebulizers.

He now presents to a tertiary medical center for a follow-up. His current medications include Combivent and Advair 250/50. His symptoms have stabilized, but he still has daily cough and sputum production. A PFT is ordered.

PULMONARY FUNCTION TESTING
Personal Data

Sex:	Male
Age:	39 yr
Height:	69 in. (174.5 cm)
Weight:	152 lb (68.6 kg)

	Before Drug	Predicted	LLN	% Predicted	Post Drug	% Change
TLC_{pleth} (L)	6.82	6.57	>5.20	104		
RV (L)	1.73	1.64	<2.14	105		
RV/TLC	25.0	<32.7	25.4	102		
FVC (L)	4.99	5.13	4.23	97	5.09	+2
FEV_1 (L)	3.35	4.10	3.34	83	3.41	+2
FEV_1/FVC	67	80	70.3		66.9	
D_{LCO}	24.7	32.7	24.7	76		

QUESTIONS

1. What is the interpretation of the following?
   a. Spirometry
   b. Lung volumes
   c. D_{LCO}
2. What is the cause of the subject's symptoms?
3. What other tests might be indicated?
4. What treatment might be recommended, based on these findings?

DISCUSSION
Pulmonary Function Interpretation

The FEV_1/FVC is reduced with a normal FEV_1 and is consistent with mild obstruction. There is no response to bronchodilator and no evidence of hyperinflation and/or air trapping with a normal TLC and RV/TLC ratio. The diffusing capacity is within normal limits.

Impression: Mild obstruction with no response to bronchodilator. Normal diffusing capacity.

Multiple FVC maneuvers are superimposed. All of the recorded efforts are acceptable.

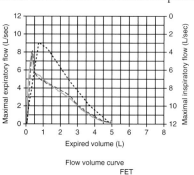

Flow volume curve

FET

····· PRED Mayo
—— Control   7.2
— — Postdilator   8.2

Cause of Symptoms

The subject has continued cough and sputum production with mild obstruction and no significant response to bronchodilator. This degree of obstruction would probably not explain the subject's level of dyspnea.

Other Tests

The clinician may want to assess the subject's exercise tolerance with a cardiopulmonary exercise test, evaluate airway hyperreactivity with a bronchoprovocation study, or assess airway inflammation with eNO. The clinician decided to order an eNO test, with the following result: eNO = 396 ppb.

According to the 2011 American Thoracic Society–European Respiratory Society (ATS-ERS) Exhaled Nitric Oxide Interpretation Guidelines, an $F_{E_{NO}}$ value > 50 ppb confirms airway inflammation.

Treatment

The clinician increased his Advair to 500/50 twice a day, with a follow-up scheduled to monitor the treatment effectiveness and titrate his ICS accordingly.

CASE 10.3

HISTORY

A 53-year-old woman sustained multiple abdominal injuries in a motor vehicle accident. After surgical repair of a perforated bowel, acute renal failure developed, followed by respiratory failure. She was placed on a mechanically supported ventilation and became increasingly dependent on the ventilator. After 13 days, a metabolic study was requested to assess the adequacy of parenteral nutrition.

METABOLIC ASSESSMENT
Personal Data

Sex: Female
Age: 53 yr
Height: 62 in. (157.5 cm)
Weight: 110 lb (50 kg)

Nutritional Information

	Total Calories	Nonprotein Calories	Protein (g)
Parenteral	1717	1393	75
Enteral	(None)		
24-hour UUN	9 g		
Resting energy expenditure	1176 kcal/24 hours (estimated)		

Ventilator Settings

F_{IO_2}	0.35
V_T	750 mL
Rate	10
Mode	Synchronized intermittent mandatory ventilation (SIMV)
Status	Awake, resting

Metabolic Measurements

$\dot{V}CO_2$ (mL/min)	205
$\dot{V}O_2$ (mL/min)	200
RER (RQ)	1.03
$\dot{V}_E$ (L/min)	10.2
REE (kcal/day)	1442
RQ_{np}	1.07

Energy Substrate Use

Carbohydrate	1480 kcal/day
Fat	–289 kcal/day
Protein	243 kcal/day

Arterial Blood Gases	
pH	7.37
Pa_{CO_2} (mm Hg)	51
Pa_{O_2} (mm Hg)	71
HCO_3^- (mEq/L)	29

QUESTIONS

1. What is the interpretation of the following?
   a. REE
   b. Substrate utilization
2. Why does the subject have an RER (RQ) greater than 1?
3. Are the data representative of the subject's caloric requirements?
4. What changes in therapy (ventilator settings, nutritional support) are indicated?

DISCUSSION

Interpretation

Exhaled gases for this study were collected over 15 minutes and appear to represent a steady state. A UUN sample was collected for 24 hours before the test. The subject was receiving 1717 kcal/day of parenteral nutrition. REE, as determined by metabolic assessment, indicates a requirement of 1442 kcal/24 hours. Substrate utilization showed carbohydrate oxidation (104%). The negative value for fat utilization is consistent with lipogenesis. Replacement of glucose with lipids and reduction of total calories to approximately 1450 kcal/day are recommended. The subject should be reassessed within 24 hours.

Cause of Elevated RER (RQ)

This study involves factors commonly encountered in the nutritional support of critically ill subjects. These elements include the subject's clinical status, estimated and actual caloric requirements, and the role of nutritional status in ventilatory support.

The subject was critically ill and required ventilatory support. Parenteral nutrition was being supplied at approximately 45% above the estimated resting caloric requirements. Estimation of caloric requirements is often performed by calculating the basal rate using the Harris–Benedict equations (see the section

Metabolic Measurements: Indirect Calorimetry). BMR is then adjusted with factors that consider the clinical status of the subject (e.g., disease state, trauma).

The metabolic study indicated that the subject required fewer calories per day than the current amount being given. In addition, carbohydrates were supplying the entire caloric need. The negative value calculated for fat utilization indicates that some of the carbohydrates were probably being stored as fat (i.e., lipogenesis). When carbohydrates are oxidized, CO_2 is produced. The RER of 1.03 supports excess CO_2 production in relation to metabolic demands.

Valid Data (Steady State)

The interpretation notes that the data were representative of a steady state. Steady-state measurements are essential to estimate caloric requirements for an entire 24-hour period. Each metabolic assessment should include adequate data so that steady-state conditions can be verified. The length of the study should be appropriate to establish that a steady state existed. Analysis of the variability of $\dot{V}O_2$ and $\dot{V}CO_2$ may be helpful. O_2 consumption and CO_2 production during measurements ideally should vary less than 5%. RER values outside of the normal range of 0.70 to 1.00 should be carefully evaluated to ensure that measurement errors did not occur. Difficulty measuring $\dot{V}O_2$ in subjects receiving supplemental O_2 is well documented. Calorimetry using open-circuit methods is usually limited to measurements when F_{IO_2} is 0.60 or less.

Changes in Therapy

The subject was switched to a 50/50 mixture of lipid and carbohydrate. The total caloric intake was also reduced to 1450 kcal/day. Her ventilation decreased, and ventilatory support was gradually reduced. An additional metabolic study indicated agreement between the prescribed nutritional support and her metabolic demands. RER on the subsequent study was 0.79 with an REE of 1395 kcal/day. This RER value compares favorably with 0.82, which is a target value for metabolism of appropriate amounts of carbohydrate, fat, and protein. She was successfully weaned from the ventilator 4 days after the initial assessment.

SELF-ASSESSMENT QUESTIONS

Entry-level

1. Which of the following would be considered indications for performing respiratory muscle strength measurements?
   1. Congestive heart failure
   2. Myasthenia gravis
   3. Amyotrophic lateral sclerosis
   4. Pulmonary fibrosis
      a. 2 and 3
      b. 1 and 3
      c. 1 and 4
      d. 2 and 4

2. What SNIP is associated with a higher mortality rate in subjects with amyotrophic lateral sclerosis?
   a. -80 cm H_2O
   b. -65 cm H_2O
   c. -55 cm H_2O
   d. -40 cm H_2O

3. Which of the following types of analyzers can measure eNO?
   1. Chemiluminescent
   2. Polarographic
   3. Wheatstone bridge
   4. Electrochemical
      a. 1 only
      b. 2 and 3
      c. 3 and 4
      d. 1 and 4

4. A 10-year-old performs an acceptable eNO test. What value would confirm airway inflammation according to the current ATS Interpretation Guidelines?
   a. >10 ppb
   b. >25 ppb
   c. >35 ppb
   d. >50 ppb

5. Which of the following would be considered indications for preoperative testing in a patient scheduled for lung resection?
   1. Age greater than 40 years
   2. Current smoker
   3. Shortness of breath on exertion
   4. BMI of 26.6
      a. 1 and 3 only
      b. 1 and 4 only
      c. 2 and 3 only
      d. 2 and 4 only

Advanced

6. A patient with a history of COPD is being evaluated for a disability. His FEV_1 is 1.44 L (43% of predicted), and his D_{LCO} is 14.5 mL CO/min/mm Hg (61% of predicted). Which of the following tests is most appropriate to perform next?
   a. Lung volumes by plethysmography
   b. Room air arterial blood gases
   c. Treadmill exercise test with pulse oximetry
   d. Postbronchodilator spirometry

7. A 50-kg patient in respiratory failure on a ventilator has a metabolic study performed at an F_{IO_2} of 0.30 (30%); the following data are reported:

Time (min)	1	2	3	4	5	6
$\dot{V}O_2$ mL/min	244	255	259	256	250	255
$\dot{V}CO_2$ mL/min	150	155	160	153	151	154
RER (RQ)	0.61	0.61	0.62	0.60	0.60	0.60
REE kcal/24	1596	1665	1695	1667	1631	1663

Which of the following statements best describes these results?
   a. A steady state was not achieved.
   b. The patient is being overfed.
   c. There is a gas analyzer malfunction.
   d. The REE was calculated incorrectly.

8. Bronchoconstriction may result in which of the following changes in respiratory system impedance, as measured by the FOT?
   1. Rise in the real part of impedance
   2. Increase in the frequency dependence of resistance
   3. Increase in resonant frequency
      a. 1 only
      b. 2 and 3 only
      c. 1 and 3 only
      d. 1, 2, and 3

9. A 39-year-old patient has her $F_{E_{NO}}$ measured at a flow of 0.05 L/sec; the average of three repeatable efforts is reported as 65 ppb. She then performs spirometry, and her FVC, FEV_1, and FEV_1/FVC are all within normal limits. Which of the following should the pulmonary function technologist conclude from these results?

    a. The patient has eosinophilic inflammation in her airways and/or alveoli.
    b. The patient is malingering.
    c. The $F_{E_{NO}}$ was measured at the incorrect flow.
    d. All results are within normal limits.
10. Which of the following results suggests that a patient may have asthma?
    1. 10% or 100-mL increase in postbronchodilator FEV_1 (whichever is greater)
    2. 20% decrease in FEV_1 after inhaling 4 mg/mL of methacholine
    3. 14% fall in FEV_1 after 8 minutes of exercise at 90% of the predicted heart rate
    4. $F_{E_{NO}}$ of 100 ppb measured at a flow of 50 mL/sec
    a. 1 and 4 only
    b. 2 and 3 only
    c. 1, 2, 3
    d. 2, 3, 4

SELECTED BIBLIOGRAPHY

Respiratory Muscle Strength Testing

Black, L. F., & Hyatt, R. E. (1971). Maximal static respiratory pressure in generalized neuromuscular disease. *American Review of Respiratory Diseases*, *103*, 641.

Bruschi, C., Cerveri, I., Zoia, M. C., et al. (1992). Reference values of maximal respiratory mouth pressures: A population-based study. *American Review of Respiratory Diseases*, *146*(Suppl. 3), 790–793.

Fauroux, B., Aubertin, G., Cohen, E., et al. (2009). Sniff nasal inspiratory pressure in children with muscle, chest wall, or lung disease. *European Respiratory Journal*, *33*, 113–117.

Morgan, R. K., McNally, S., Alexander, M., et al. (2005). Use of sniff nasal-inspiratory force to predict survival in amyotrophic lateral sclerosis. *American Journal of Respiratory and Critical Care Medicine*, *171*(Suppl. 3), 269–274.

Polkey, M. I., Lyali, R. A., Yang, K., et al. (2016). Respiratory Muscle Strength as a Predictive Biomarker for Survival in Amyotrophic Lateral Sclerosis. *American Journal of Respiratory and Critical Care Medicine*, *195*(1).

Sachs, M. C., Enright, P. E., Hinckey, K. D., et al. (2009). Performance of maximum inspiratory pressure tests and maximum inspiratory pressure reference equations for 4 race/ethnic groups. *Respiratory Care*, *54*(Suppl. 10), 1321–1328.

Exhaled Nitric Oxide

Berkman, N., Avital, A., Breuer, R., et al. (2005). Exhaled nitric oxide in the diagnosis of asthma: Comparison with bronchial provocation tests. *Thorax, 60*, 383–388.

Buchvald, F., Baraldi, E., Carraro, S., et al. (2005). Measurements of exhaled nitric oxide in healthy subjects ages 4 to 17 years. *Journal of Allergy and Clinical Immunology*, *115*, 1130–1136.

Franklin, P. J., Stick, S. M., LeSouef, P. N., et al. (2004). Measuring exhaled nitric oxide levels in adults: The importance of atopy and airway responsiveness. *Chest*, *126*, 1540–1545.

Khatri, S. B., Iaccarino, J. M., Barochia, A., et al. (2021). Use of Fractional Exhaled Nitric Oxide to Guide the Treatment of Asthma: An Official American Thoracic Society Clinical Practice Guideline. *American Journal of Respiratory and Critical Care Medicine*, *204*(10), e97–e109.

Lim, K. G., & Mottram, C. D. (2008). The use of fraction of exhaled nitric oxide in pulmonary practice. *Chest*, *133*, 1232–1242.

Petsky, H. L., Cates, C. J., Li, A. M., et al. (2008). Tailored interventions based on exhaled nitric oxide versus clinical symptoms for asthma in children and adults. *Cochrane Database of Systematic Reviews*, *2*, CD006340.

Smith, A. D., Cowan, J. O., Brassert, K. P., et al. (2005). Use of exhaled nitric oxide measurements to guide treatment in chronic asthma. *New England Journal of Medicine*, *352*, 2163–2173.

Zitt, M. (2005). Clinical applications of exhaled nitric oxide for the diagnosis and management of asthma: A consensus report. *Clinical Therapeutics*, *27*, 1238–1250.

Forced Oscillation Technique

Dencker, M., Malmberg, L. P., Valind, S., et al. (2006). Reference values for respiratory system impedance by using impulse oscillometry in children aged 2–11 years. *Clinical Physiology and Functional Imaging*, *26*, 247–250.

Komarow, H. D., Myles, I. A., Uzzaman, A., et al. (2011). Impulse oscillometry in the evaluation of diseases of the airways in children. *Annals of Allergy, Asthma, and Immunology*, *106*, 191–199.

Marotta, A., Klinnert, M. D., Price, M. R., et al. (2003). Impulse oscillometry provides an effective measure of lung dysfunction in 4-year-old children at risk for persistent asthma. *Journal of Allergy and Clinical Immunology, 112,* 317–322.

Nowowiejska, B., Tomalak, W., Radlinski, J., et al. (2008). Transient reference values for impulse oscillometry for children aged 3–18 years. *Pediatric Pulmonology, 43,* 1193–1197.

Preoperative Pulmonary Function Testing

Algar, F. J., Alvarez, A., Salvatierra, A., et al. (2003). Predicting pulmonary complications after pneumonectomy for lung cancer. *European Journal of Cardio-Thoracic Surgery, 23,* 201–208.

Beckles, M. A., Spiro, S. G., Colice, G. L., et al. (2003). The physiologic evaluation of patients with lung cancer being considered for resectional surgery. *Chest, 123*(Suppl), 105S–114S.

Behr, J. (2001). Optimizing preoperative lung function. *Current Opinion in Anaesthesiology, 14,* 65–69.

Ferguson, M. K., & Durkin, A. E. (2002). Preoperative prediction of the risk of pulmonary complications after esophagectomy for cancer. *Journal of Thoracic and Cardiovascular Surgery, 123,* 661–669.

Fisher, B. W., Majumdar, S. R., & McAlister, F. A. (2002). Predicting pulmonary complications after nonthoracic surgery: A systematic review of blinded studies. *American Journal of Medicine, 112,* 219–225.

Fuso, L., Cisternino, L., Di Napoli, A., et al. (2000). Role of spirometric and arterial gas data in predicting pulmonary complications after abdominal surgery. *Respiratory Medicine, 94,* 1171–1176.

Older, P., Smith, R., Hall, A., & French, C. (2000). Preoperative cardiopulmonary risk assessment by cardiopulmonary exercise testing. *Critical Care and Resuscitation, 2,* 198–208.

Smith, T. B., Stonell, C., Purkayastha, S., et al. (2009). Cardiopulmonary exercise testing as a risk assessment method in non-cardio-pulmonary surgery: a systematic review. *Anaesthesia, 64*(8), 883–893.

Respiratory Impairment for Disability

Sood, A., & Beckett, W. S. (1997). Determination of disability for patients with advanced lung disease. *Clinics in Chest Medicine, 18,* 471–482.

Taiwo, O. A., & Cain, H. C. (2002). Pulmonary impairment and disability. *Clinics in Chest Medicine, 23,* 841–851.

U.S. Social Security Administration. (n.d.). Disability evaluation under Social Security. https://www.ssa.gov/disability/professionals/bluebook/3.00-Respiratory-Adult.htm#3_00D4 (accessed September 2020).

Metabolic Measurements: Indirect Calorimetry

Battezzati, A., & Vigano, R. (2001). Indirect calorimetry and nutritional problems in clinical practice. *Acta Diabetologica, 38,* 1–5.

Compher, C., Frankenfield, D., Keim, N., et al. (2006). Best practice methods to apply to measurement of resting metabolic rate in adults: A systematic review. *Journal of the American Dietetic Association, 106,* 881–903.

Da Rocha, E. E., Alves, V. G., & da Fonseca, R. B. (2006). Indirect calorimetry: Methodology, instruments and clinical application. *Current Opinion in Clinical Nutrition and Metabolic Care, 9,* 247–256.

Harris, J. A., & Benedict, F. G. (1919). *Biometric studies of basal metabolism in man.* Publication No. 279 Washington, D.C: Carnegie Institution of Washington.

Miles, J. M. (2006). Energy expenditure in hospitalized patients: Implications for nutritional support. *Mayo Clinic Proceedings, 81,* 809–816.

Moreira da Rocha, E. E., Alves, V. G. F., Barcellos, V., & da Fonseca, R. (2006). Indirect calorimetry: methodology, instruments, and clinical application. *Curr Opin Clin Nutr Metab Care, 9,* 247–256.

Roffey, D. M., Byrne, N. M., & Hills, A. (2006). Day-to-day variance in measurement of resting metabolic rate using ventilated-hood and mouthpiece & nose-clip indirect calorimetry systems. *Journal of Parenteral and Enteral Nutrition, 30,* 426–432.

Stewart, C. L., Goody, C. M., & Branson, R. (2005). Comparison of two systems of measuring energy expenditure. *Journal of Parenteral and Enteral Nutrition, 29,* 212–217.

Weir, J. B. (1949). New methods for calculating metabolic rate with special reference to protein metabolism. *Journal of Physiology, 109,* 1–9.

Guidelines and Standards

ATS-ERS statement on respiratory muscle testing. (2002). *American Journal of Respiratory and Critical Care Medicine, 166,* 518–624.

American Association for Respiratory Care. (2004). Clinical practice guideline: Metabolic measurements using indirect calorimetry during mechanical ventilation–2004 Revision & Update. *Respiratory Care*, *49*, 1073–1079.

Beydon, N., Davis, S. D., Lombardi, E., et al. (2007). An official American Thoracic Society/European Respiratory Society (ATS/ERS) statement. Pulmonary function testing in preschool children. *American Journal of Respiratory and Critical Care Medicine*, *175*, 1304–1345.

Dweik, R. A., Boggs, P. B., Erzurum, S. C., et al. (2011). An official ATS clinical practice guideline: Interpretation of exhaled nitric oxide levels ($F_{E_{NO}}$) for clinical applications. (2011). *American Journal of Respiratory and Critical Care Medicine*, *184*, 602–615.

King, G. G., Bates, J., Berger, K. I., Calverley, P., de Melo, P. L., Dellacà, R. L., et al. (2020). Technical Standards for Respiratory Oscillometry. European Respiratory Society Statement. *Eur Respir J 2020*, 55.

Chapter 11

Pulmonary Function Testing Equipment

CHAPTER OUTLINE

LEARNING OBJECTIVES

After studying the chapter and reviewing the figures and tables, you should be able to do the following:

Entry-level
1. Describe two types of volume-displacement spirometers.
2. List at least two principles used by flow-sensing spirometers to measure volume.
3. Select a directional breathing valve for a specific testing situation.
4. Identify the types of gas analyzers used for diffusing capacity and dilutional lung volume tests.
5. Describe the function of commonly used gas-conditioning devices.

Advanced

1. Select and set up the basic components of a body plethysmograph.
2. Contrast and compare the measurement of oxygen saturation by multiwavelength and pulse oximeters.
3. Identify the measurement principles of pH, P_{CO_2}, and P_{O_2} blood gas devices.
4. Describe the important characteristics of an "office or screening" spirometer.

KEY TERMS

ambient temperature, pressure, and saturation (ATPS)
amperometric
chemiluminescence analyzers
CO-oximeter
dry rolling seal spirometer
electrochemical
emission spectroscopy
Fleisch-type pneumotachometer
flow-sensing spirometer
fluorescence quenching

free breathing valves
gas chromatography
heated-wire flow sensors
hemoximeter
light-emitting diode (LED)
office/home spirometer
peak flowmeter
pitot tube flow sensor
polarographic electrode
potentiometer
pressure-differential flow sensor

pressure plethysmograph
pulse oximeter
reflective spectrophotometry
resistive element
screening spirometer
Silverman/Lilly pneumotachometer
spectrophotometric oximeter
thermal conductivity analyzers
turbine
ultrasonic flow sensor
wedge bellows spirometer

The chapter describes pulmonary function equipment used for common testing applications, including spirometers (volume and flow), body plethysmographs, and blood gas analyzers.

Hutchinson introduced the precursor of the modern spirometer around 1844. This spirometer was a water-sealed, volume-displacement device. Although the water-seal spirometer has its place in history, it is no longer used in modern testing, so the discussion of it has been removed from this chapter. Regardless, some aspects of this original device are still evident in today's spirometers. Flow-sensing spirometers have become the most common with the advent of sophisticated electronics and software that can integrate flow signals to measure volume by a variety of methods. Microprocessor-based spirometers are now small enough to be handheld.

Haldane pioneered the analysis of respiratory gases by volumetric methods in the early part of the 20th century. However, modern gas analyzers use indirect means (e.g., electrodes or sensors) to measure partial pressures of gases or physical separation of gases to measure fractional concentrations (gas chromatography). Almost every instrument in the pulmonary function laboratory today combines signal transducers, analog-to-digital converters, and computer software to process and record physiologic data. Some devices, such as the pulse oximeter, are based almost entirely on electronic components. Computers eliminate many tedious calculations, allowing the technologist to concentrate on obtaining high-quality, repeatable data.

VOLUME-DISPLACEMENT SPIROMETERS

Dry-Seal Spirometers

The Stead-Wells *dry-seal spirometer* is a type of volume-displacement spirometer that is still used, although not commonly. The Stead-Wells spirometer uses a lightweight plastic bell (Fig. 11.1). A rubberized seal is used to connect the bell to the internal wall of the spirometer wall. The rubber seal then rolls over itself, much the same as the vertical dry rolling seal spirometer described in the next section. The Stead-Wells bell is usually attached to a linear potentiometer that provides analog signals proportional to volume and flow. These signals are passed to a computer through an A/D converter. The **potentiometer** is a device that produces an analog DC voltage signal proportional to its position

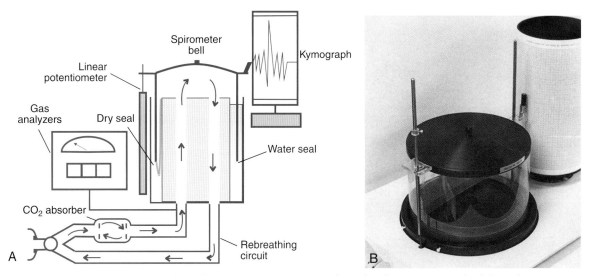

FIG. 11.1 Stead-Wells dry-seal spirometer. The conventional Stead-Wells spirometer used a lightweight plastic bell that floated in water. This version uses a silicon seal similar to that found in the dry rolling seal spirometer. The spirometer bell carries a pen that traces directly on a rotating kymograph (rarely used today). With appropriate circuitry and gas analyzers, helium (He) dilution FRC determinations and DLCO measurements are easily performed.

or displacement. The Stead-Wells design is capable of meeting the minimum requirements for flow and volume accuracy recommended by the American Thoracic Society and European Respiratory Society (ATS-ERS) (see Chapter 12).

Problems associated with a dry-seal spirometer usually involve leaks in the bell or in the breathing circuit. Gravity causes the spirometer to lose volume in the presence of leaks. Raising the bell and plugging the patient connection can detect leaks in the spirometer, tubing, or valves. Any change in volume can be detected easily by recording the spirometer volume over several minutes. Weights can be added to the top of the bell to enhance the detection of small leaks. During patient testing, improper positioning of the spirometer can cause inaccurate measurements. If positioned too high, the bell reaches the top of its travel range. This causes the volume–time tracing to appear abruptly flattened. The pattern observed may be mistaken for a normal end of expiration. If a Stead-Wells spirometer is positioned too low, it may empty completely, not allowing a subject to inhale completely.

Because lung volumes and flows are corrected to body temperature, pressure, and saturation (BTPS)

conditions, careful attention to the ambient conditions of volume-displacement spirometers is required. Although the temperature of gas in the spirometer can be easily measured, the temperature may change significantly during maneuvers such as a forced vital capacity (FVC). These changes can be difficult to monitor, resulting in volumes and flows that are not representative of lung physiology.

PF TIP 11.1

The use of volume-displacement spirometers accounts for some of the display conventions used in spirometry today. Plotting expiratory volume in the upward direction mimics the graph originally made by the pen of a Stead-Wells–type spirometer on a rotating kymograph (see Fig. 11.1).

Dry Rolling Seal Spirometers

Another type of volume-displacement spirometer is the **dry rolling seal spirometer.** A typical unit consists of a lightweight piston mounted horizontally in a cylinder. A rod that rests on frictionless bearings supports the piston (Fig. 11.2A and B). The piston is

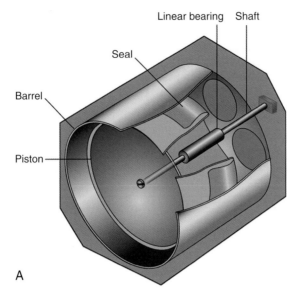

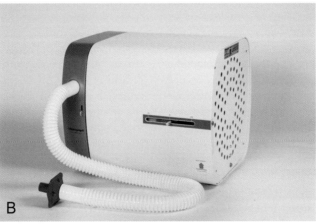

FIG. 11.2 (A) Cutaway view of a dry rolling seal spirometer and (B) a dry rolling seal spirometer integrated with a pulmonary function system. A flexible seal attaches the piston to the wall of the cylinder and rolls on itself. The piston has a large surface area, so horizontal movement is minimized. This allows for the recording of normal breaths and maximal respiratory excursions with little resistance. The piston is supported by a shaft that rides on a linear bearing. The shaft activates a rotary potentiometer (not shown). Rotation of the potentiometer generates analog signals for flow and volume. (A, Illustration by Jennifer Pryll, courtesy Vitalograph LTD, Buckinghamshire, UK.)

coupled to the cylinder wall by a flexible plastic seal. The seal rolls on itself rather than sliding as the piston moves. A similar type of rolling seal may also be used with a vertically mounted, lightweight piston that rises and falls with breathing (as in the dry-seal Stead-Wells described in the preceding section). The maximum volume of the cylinder with the piston fully displaced is usually 10 to 12 L. The piston has a large diameter, so excursions of just a few inches are all that is necessary to record large volume changes. The piston is normally constructed of lightweight aluminum to reduce inertia. Mechanical resistance is kept to a minimum by the bearings supporting the piston rod and by the rolling seal itself.

Although they can be used with a mechanical recorder, most dry rolling seal spirometers use linear or rotary potentiometers. As described previously, the potentiometer responds to piston movement to produce DC voltage outputs for volume and flow. For example, a 10-volt (V) potentiometer attached to a 10-L spirometer may produce an output of 1 V/L. On a separate channel, a flow of 1 L/sec may produce an output of 1 V. Flow in this case is proportional to the speed of the moving piston. These analog outputs for volume and flow are digitized so that a computer can store and manipulate the data.

The piston of the standard dry rolling seal spirometer (Fig. 11.2B) travels horizontally, eliminating the need for counterbalancing. The vertically mounted version (see Fig. 11.1) depends on a lightweight piston and the rolling seal to reduce resistance to breathing. Volumes measured in this way reflect the gas in the spirometer that is at **ambient temperature, pressure, and saturation (ATPS)**. These volumes, such as vital capacity (VC), had to be corrected to BTPS. These temperature corrections (from ATPS to BTPS) are made by applying a correction factor to the digital value stored in the computer. A one-way breathing circuit and CO_2 scrubber may be added so that dry rolling seal spirometers can be used for rebreathing tests, such as helium dilution.

To perform studies such as the open-circuit nitrogen-washout test, a "dumping" mechanism is attached to the spirometer. The dumping device empties the spirometer after each breath or after a predetermined volume has been reached. The addition of an automated valve and alveolar sampling device allows the dry rolling seal spirometer to be used for single-breath diffusion studies. Dry rolling seal spirometers are capable of meeting the minimum standards recommended by the ATS-ERS (see Chapter 12).

Common problems encountered with dry rolling seal spirometers are sticking of the rolling seal and increased mechanical resistance in the piston-cylinder assembly. These difficulties can usually be avoided by adequate maintenance of the spirometer. As for other types of volume-displacement spirometers, simple correction of volumes from ATPS to BTPS may not completely reflect physiologic flow or volume changes. Infection control of the dry rolling seal involves disassembling the piston-cylinder. The interior of the cylinder and the face of the piston are usually wiped with a mild antibacterial solution. The rolling seal itself is also wiped with disinfectant. Alcohol or similar drying agents may cause deterioration of the seal and should not be used. The seal should be routinely checked for leaks or tears. After reassembly, the piston should be positioned at the maximum-volume position. When the rolling seal is extended completely, the material of the seal is less likely to develop creases that can result in uneven movement of the piston. With the previously described reservations, bacteria filters may be used to avoid contamination of the spirometer.

Bellows-Type Spirometers

A third type of volume-displacement spirometer is the bellows or **wedge bellows spirometer.** Both devices consist of a collapsible bellows that folds or unfolds in response to breathing excursions. The conventional bellows design is a flexible accordion-type container. One end is stationary, and the other end is displaced in proportion to the volume inspired or expired. The wedge bellows operates similarly except that it expands and contracts like a fan (Fig. 11.3A-B). One side of the bellows remains stationary; the other side moves with a pivotal motion around an axis through the fixed side. Displacement of the bellows by a volume of gas is translated either to movement of a pen on chart paper or to a potentiometer. For mechanical recording, chart paper moves at a fixed speed under the pen while a spirogram is traced. For computerized testing, displacement of the bellows is transformed into a DC voltage by a linear or rotary potentiometer. The analog signal is routed to an A/D converter and then to a computer.

The conventional and wedge bellows may be mounted either horizontally or vertically. The horizontal bellows is mounted so that the primary direction of travel is on a horizontal plane. This design minimizes the effects of gravity on bellows movement. The horizontal bellows (either conventional or wedge) with a large surface area offers little mechanical resistance. This type is normally used in

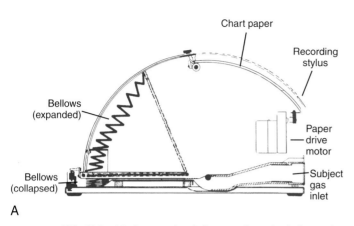

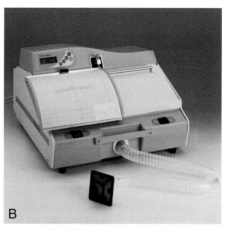

A

B

FIG. 11.3   (A) Cross-sectional diagram of a wedge bellows spirometer. (B) Wedge bellows spirometer with direct writing recorder. Fanlike movements of the wedge bellows carry the recording stylus across moving graph paper. Some manufacturers suspend the bellows so that the primary movement is in a horizontal rather than vertical plane. Large wedge bellows offer little resistance and are comparable to dry-seal or water-seal spirometers in accuracy and linearity. (A and B, Modified from Vitalograph LTD, Buckinghamshire, UK.)

conjunction with a potentiometer to produce analog volume and flow signals. Small (approximately 7–8 L) vertically mounted bellows are available and may be used for portable spirometry and bedside testing. Most of these types offer simple mechanical recording, digital data reduction, or both by means of a small, dedicated microprocessor.

Both bellows-type spirometers (see Fig. 11.3A-B) can be used to measure VC and its subdivisions, as well as FVC, forced expiratory volume in the first second (FEV$_1$), expiratory flows, and maximal voluntary ventilation (MVV). Some bellows-type spirometers, especially those that are mounted vertically, are designed to measure expiratory flows only. These types expand upward when gas is injected and then empty spontaneously under their own weight. Horizontally mounted bellows can usually be set in a midrange to record both inspiratory and expiratory maneuvers. This allows F-V loops to be recorded. With appropriate gas analyzers and breathing circuitry, bellows systems may be used for gas dilution functional residual capacity (FRC) determinations and D$_{LCO}$ measurements. Most bellows-type spirometers meet ATS-ERS recommendations for flow and volume accuracy.

One problem that may occur with bellows-type spirometers is inaccuracy resulting from sticking

of the bellows. The folds of the bellows may adhere because of dirt, moisture, or aging of the bellows material. Some bellows-type spirometers require the bellows to be partially distended when not in use. This technique allows moisture from exhaled gas to evaporate and prevents deterioration of the bellows. Leaks may also develop in the bellows material or at the point where the bellows is mounted. Leaks can usually be detected by filling the bellows with air, plugging the breathing port, and attaching a weight or spring to pressurize the contained gas.

Infection control of bellows-type spirometers depends on the method of construction. In some instruments, the bellows can be entirely removed; in others, the interior of the bellows must be wiped clean. Many bellows are made from rubberized or plastic-based material that can be cleaned with a mild detergent and dried thoroughly before reassembly. Bacteria filters may be used to avoid contamination of the bellows, with the reservations described previously.

Volume-displacement spirometers were once the main devices used for pulmonary function testing. Many such devices are still in use, and some manufacturers continue to produce sophisticated spirometers based on the volume-displacement principle. Volume-displacement spirometers in general are sometimes referred to as the "gold standard" in lung function testing because they physically measure the volume expired and are sometimes used as verification devices for flow-based systems.

FLOW-SENSING SPIROMETERS

In contrast to the volume-displacement spirometer is the flow-sensing spirometer or pneumotachometer. The term *pneumotachometer* describes a device that measures gas flow (i.e., *pnuemo* = air; *tacho* = speed; *meter* = measure). Flow-sensing spirometers use various physical principles to produce a signal proportional to gas flow. This signal is then integrated to measure volume in addition to flow. *Integration* is a process in which flow (volume per unit of time) is divided into a large number of small intervals (time). The volume from each interval is summed (Fig. 11.4). Integration can be performed easily by an electronic circuit or by computer software. Accurate volume measurement by flow integration requires an accurate flow signal, accurate timing, and sensitive detection of low flow.

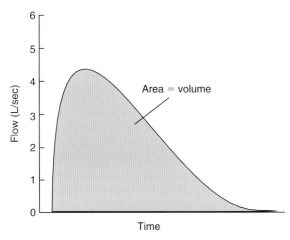

FIG. 11.4 Volume measurement by flow integration. The flow signal from many types of flow-sensing spirometers is integrated to compute volume. Flow is measured against time. The area under the flow–time curve is subdivided into a large number of small sections. Each section represents a small interval of time. Volume is equal to the sum of the areas of all sections. By dividing the curve into a large number of sections, even irregular flow curves can be accurately integrated. Integration is usually performed by a dedicated electronic circuit or by software.

1. One type of device that responds to the bulk flow of gas is the turbine or impeller. Integration may be unnecessary because the turbine directly measures gas volumes. Some turbine spirometers produce volume pulses in which each pulse equals a fixed volume. These spirometers count pulses very accurately. Most flow-sensing spirometers use tubes through which laminar airflow is possible (see the Evolve website, http://evolve.elsevier.com/Mottram/Ruppel/). Five basic types of flow sensors are commonly used:
   1. Turbines
   2. Pressure-differential flow sensors
   3. Heated-wire flow sensors
   4. Pitot tube flow sensors
   5. Ultrasonic flow sensors

> **PF TIP 11.2**
>
> Most spirometers use flow sensors. **Flow-sensing spirometers** have several advantages over volume-displacement devices. They are smaller, easier to maintain, and easier to clean and can even use disposable sensors. Their small size makes them ideal for portable systems, making simple spirometry a powerful diagnostic tool that can be used in settings such as the primary care practitioner's office.

Turbines

The simplest type of flow-sensing device is the **turbine,** or respirometer. This instrument consists of a vane connected to a series of precision gears. Gas flowing through the body of the instrument causes the vane to rotate, registering a volume (Fig. 11.5). The respirometer can be used to measure slow VC. It can also be used for ventilation tests such as V_T and $\dot{V}_E$. One such device is the *Wright respirometer*. This respirometer can measure volumes accurately at flows between 3 and 300 L/min. At flows greater than 300 L/min (5 L/sec), the vane is subject to distortion. Because of this limitation, it should not be used to measure FVC when the patient is capable of flows greater than 300 L/min. At low flows (<3 L/min), inertia of the vane-gear system may underestimate volume.

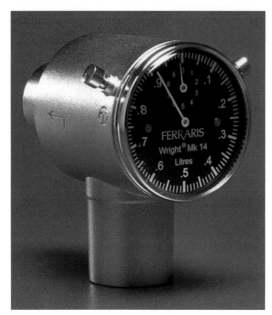

FIG. 11.5 Turbine-type flow sensor. The Wright Mk14 respirometer is shown. A rotating vane mounted on jeweled bearings drives reduction gears connected to the main dial.

A special advantage of this type of respirometer is its compact size and usefulness at the bedside. Most respirometers can register a wide range of volumes using multiple scales. The standard Wright respirometer measures 0.1 to 1 L on one scale and up to 100 L on another scale. Turbine devices are also widely used for measurements of bulk flow in various dry gas meters.

An adaptation of the turbine flow device includes a photocell and light source that is interrupted by the movement of the vane or impeller (Fig. 11.6D). Rotation of the vane interrupts a light beam between its source and the photocell. This produces a pulse, with each pulse equivalent to a fixed gas volume. The pulse count is summed to obtain the volume of gas flowing through the device. The signal produced may not be linear across a wide range of flows because of inertia or distortion of the rotating vane. However, these variables can be corrected through software when integrated into a computerized system.

Simple stand-alone turbine devices may be used for monitoring or screening. Because of their simplicity and small size, several such devices are

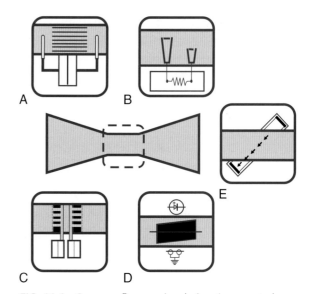

FIG. 11.6 Common flow-sensing devices (pneumotachometers). Each flow-sensing device is mounted in a tube that promotes laminar flow *(center)*. (A) Pressure-differential pneumotachometer in which a resistive element causes a pressure drop proportional to the flow of gas through the tube. A sensitive pressure transducer monitors the pressure drop across the resistive element and converts the differential to an analog signal. The resistive element may be a mesh screen or capillary tube; it is usually heated to 37°C or higher to prevent condensation of water from expired gas. (B) A heated-wire pneumotachometer contains heated elements of small mass that respond to gas flow by heat loss. An electric current heats the elements (thin wires). Gas flow past the elements causes cooling. In one element, current is increased to maintain a constant temperature; the other element acts as a reference (see also Fig. 11.9). The current change is proportional to gas flow, and a continuous signal is supplied to an integrating circuit as for the pressure-differential flow sensor. (C) A pitot tube flow sensor uses a series of small tubes that are placed at right angles to the direction of gas flow. Sensitive pressure transducers detect changes in gas velocity. The pitot tubes are mounted in struts in the flow tube; separate devices face either way so that bidirectional flow can be measured (see also Fig. 11.10). (D) Electronic rotating-vane flow sensor. A vane or impeller is mounted in the flow tube. A light-emitting diode (LED) is mounted on one side of the vane and a photodetector on the other side. Each time the vane rotates, it interrupts the light from the LED reaching the detector. These pulses are counted and summed to calculate gas volume. (E) Ultrasonic flow sensor. High-frequency sound waves pass through membranes on either side of a flow tube at an angle to the stream of gas. The sound waves speed up or slow down depending on which direction the gas is flowing. By measuring the transit time of the sound waves, gas flow can be measured very accurately and integrated to compute volume. (See also Fig. 11.11.)

marketed for home use. This type of spirometer allows FVC, FEV_1, and peak expiratory flow (PEF) to be monitored outside of the usual clinical setting.

Infection control of turbine-type respirometers depends on their construction and intended use. Devices such as the Wright respirometer usually must be gas sterilized. Water condensation from exhaled gas can damage the vane-gear mechanisms. Some turbine spirometers use disposable impellers. This avoids cross-contamination, but accuracy may be limited by the quality of the disposable sensor.

Pressure-Differential Flow Sensors

Pressure-differential flow sensors are among the most common implementations of flow sensing. They consist of a tube containing a **resistive element**. The resistive element allows gas to flow through it but causes a pressure drop (see Fig. 11.6A). The pressure difference across the resistive element is measured by means of a sensitive pressure transducer. The transducer usually has pressure taps on either side of the element (Fig. 11.7A). The pressure differential across the

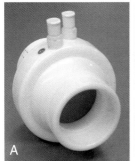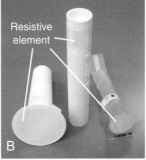

FIG. 11.7   Pressure-differential flow sensors (pneumotachometers). (A) Small, reusable pressure-differential flow sensor is shown. This pneumotachometer consists of an unheated screen that acts as a resistive element. Two Luer-type fittings provide for connection to a pressure transducer so that the pressure drop across the resistive element can be measured. (B) Three types of disposable pressure-differential flow sensors are shown. Each device uses a porous paper or plastic screen-like material to act as a resistive element. A single pressure tap upstream of the resistive element allows pressure to be measured and compared with ambient pressure. Disposable flow sensors are calibrated at the time of manufacture. Some manufacturers print a calibration code or calibration bar code on the disposable sensor that can be used by the spirometer software to achieve accurate measurement of flow and volume.

resistive element is proportional to gas flow as long as flow is laminar. This flow signal is integrated to measure volume (see Fig. 11.4). Turbulent gas flow upstream or downstream of the resistive element may interfere with the development of true laminar flow. Most pneumotachometers attempt to reduce turbulent flow by tapering the tubes in which the resistive elements are mounted.

Although there are many designs for resistive elements, two types are commonly used. The **Fleisch-type pneumotachometer** uses a bundle of capillary tubes (or similar material) as the resistive element. Laminar flow is ensured by the size and arrangement of the capillary tubes. The cross-sectional area and length of the capillary tubes determine the actual resistance to flow through the Fleisch pneumotachometer. The dynamic range of the Fleisch device must be matched to the range of flows to be measured. Different sizes (i.e., resistances) of pneumotachometers may be used to accurately measure high or low flows.

The other common type of pressure-differential flow sensor is the Silverman or Lilly type. The **Silverman/Lilly pneumotachometer** uses one or more screens to act as a resistive element. A typical arrangement has three screens mounted parallel to one another. The middle screen acts as the resistive element with the pressure taps on either side, whereas the outer screens protect the middle screen and help ensure laminar flow. The Silverman/Lilly pneumotachometer usually has a wider dynamic flow range than the Fleisch type. As a result, it is better suited for measuring widely varying flows.

Most Fleisch and Silverman/Lilly pneumotachometers use a heating mechanism to warm the resistive element to 37°C or higher. Heating the resistive element prevents condensation of water vapor from exhaled gas on the element. Condensation or other debris lodging in the resistive element changes the resistance across it, thus changing its calibration. A change in the resistive element, such as condensation or a hole, causes a change in the pressure–flow relationship. Pneumotachometers need to be recalibrated after cleaning or similar maintenance.

Some flow-sensing spirometers use resistive elements such as porous paper, rendering the flow sensor disposable (see Fig. 11.7B). These devices usually have a single pressure tap upstream of the resistive element. Pressure measured in front of the resistive element is referenced against ambient pressure. This design requires that the flow sensor be carefully zeroed before making any flow measurements. These types of flow sensors may be more susceptible to moisture or debris on the resistive element, causing volumes and flows to increase with each successive blow. The flow sensor will need to be replaced or cleaned if the technologist notices this occurring. The accuracy of spirometers using this type of flow sensor often depends on how carefully the disposable resistive elements are manufactured. If the resistance varies widely from sensor to sensor, each unit may need to be calibrated before use to ensure accuracy. Some manufacturers calibrate their disposable sensors and provide a calibration code with each sensor. This code is used to identify a particular sensor by the software in the spirometer. One method of identifying the correct calibration factor for individual flow sensors is to imprint the sensor with a bar code (see Fig. 11.7B). The spirometer then includes a simple bar code reader to identify the appropriate calibration factors. Some portable spirometer systems that use precalibrated flow sensors do not provide for user calibration. However, verification of accuracy (using a 3-L syringe) is usually possible, even if the manufacturer has not provided for this in the software accompanying the spirometer.

Systems that use permanent pressure-differential flow sensors usually meet or exceed the ATS-ERS minimal recommendations for spirometers. Spirometers that use disposable sensors can meet or exceed the minimal requirements, depending on the quality of the sensor and the application software responsible for signal processing. Gas composition affects the accuracy of flow measurements in pressure-differential pneumotachometers. Correction factors for gases other than air can be applied by software so that these types of flow sensors can be used for most types of pulmonary function tests.

Infection control of pressure-differential flow sensors depends on their placement in the spirometer. In open-circuit systems in which only exhaled

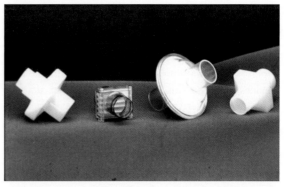

FIG. 11.8 Barrier filters are often used to prevent droplet moisture/debris from affecting a pneumotachograph and may be an effective and less expensive method of preventing equipment contamination.

gas is measured, only the mouthpiece needs to be changed between patients. If inspiratory and expiratory flows are measured, the flow sensor itself may need to be disinfected between patients. Disassembly and cleaning of flow sensors usually require that the spirometer be recalibrated. Disposable or single-use sensors avoid this problem. In-line bacteria filters may be used to isolate the pneumotachometer from potential contamination. The spirometer should meet all ATS-ERS requirements for range, accuracy, and flow resistance with the filter in place (see Chapter 12 and Fig. 11.8). If a filter is used, calibration with the filter in-line is usually required. The effect of bacteria filters on spirometric measurements has been reported to cause small errors in measured flows and volumes (30–50 mL). The use of in-line filters can be an efficient and effective component of the pulmonary function laboratory's infection control program.

Heated-Wire Flow Sensors

Heated-wire flow sensors are a third type of flow-sensing spirometer. They are based on the cooling effect of gas flow. A heated element, usually a thin platinum wire, is situated in a laminar flow tube (see Fig. 11.6B). Gas flow past the wire causes a temperature decrease, so more current must be supplied to maintain a preset temperature. The current needed to maintain the temperature is proportional to gas flow. The heated element usually has a small

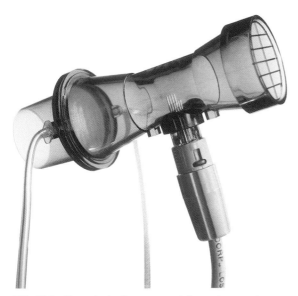

FIG. 11.9 Heated-wire flow sensor. A flow tube contains very thin, paired stainless steel wires. The wires are maintained at two temperatures exceeding body temperature and are connected by a Wheatstone bridge. The tube streamlines gas flow into laminar flow. The temperature of the wires decreases in proportion to the mass of the gas and its flow. Two wires are used; one measures expiratory flow, and the other serves as a reference. (Courtesy Vyaire, Mettawa, IL.)

mass so that slight changes in gas flow can be detected. The flow signal is integrated electronically or by software to obtain volume measurements. The heated wire is usually protected behind a screen to prevent impaction of debris on the element. Debris or moisture droplets on the element can change its thermal characteristics. Some systems use two wires (Fig. 11.9). One measures gas flow, and the second serves as a reference. Most heated-wire flow sensors maintain a temperature higher than 37°C. Heating prevents condensation from expired air that might interfere with the sensitivity of the element.

Most heated-wire flow sensors meet or exceed ATS-ERS recommendations for accuracy and precision. Gas composition may affect the accuracy of flow measurements. Correction factors for gases other than room air can be applied via software. This allows heated-wire devices to accurately measure gases for pulmonary function tests using helium (He), oxygen (O_2), and other gases. Heated-wire sensors can be used for routine pulmonary function

tests, exercise testing, and metabolic studies. Infection control for heated-wire sensors is similar to that for pressure-differential devices. Disposable or single-use devices avoid cross-contamination even when the sensor is located proximal to the patient's airway.

Pitot Tube Flow Sensors

Pitot tube flow sensors are a fourth type of flow sensor. They use the pitot tube principle. The pressure of gas flowing against a small tube is related to the gas's density and velocity. Flow can be measured by placing a series of small tubes in a flow sensor and connecting them to a sensitive pressure transducer (see Fig. 11.6C). The pressure signal must be linearized and integrated as described for other flow-sensing devices. In practice, two sets of pitot tubes are mounted in the same sensor so that bidirectional flow can be measured (Fig. 11.10). Using two or more pressure transducers with different sensitivities can accommodate a wide range of flows. Because this type of flow-sensing device is affected by gas density, software correction for different gas compositions is necessary. This is accomplished by sampling the gas, analyzing O_2 and CO_2, and applying the necessary correction factors. Software corrections for test gases used for various pulmonary function tests (e.g., D_{LCO}) can be easily applied.

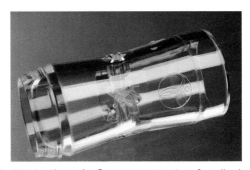

FIG. 11.10 Pitot tube flow sensor. A series of small tubes is mounted on struts in the flow tube. The tubes are connected to very sensitive pressure transducers (not shown). Using a series of transducers allows a wide range of flows to be accurately measured. Pitot tubes are mounted with struts facing both directions so that inspiratory and expiratory flow can be detected. (Courtesy MGC Diagnostics, St. Paul, MN.)

Pitot tube flow sensors meet or exceed ATS recommendations for accuracy and precision. Their practical applications include routine pulmonary function tests, metabolic measurements, and exercise testing. Infection control for this type of device includes single-use or disposable flowmeters. If pitot tube flow sensors are cleaned, care must be taken that disinfectant solution or rinse water is completely removed from the small tubes used to sense flow.

Ultrasonic Flow Sensors

Gas flow can be detected and measured by passing high-frequency sound waves across the stream of gas. Ultrasonic transducers on either side of the flow tube transmit sound waves alternately across the tube. By passing the sound waves at an angle to the flow of gas in two different directions, bidirectional flow can be measured (see Fig. 11.6E). The sound waves are sped up by gas flowing in one direction and slowed down by gas flowing in the opposite direction. By measuring the transit time of the pulses with a very accurate digital clock, flow can be integrated to measure volume. Analyzing the change in frequency of the sound waves passing through the flowing gas has the advantage of not being affected by the gas composition, temperatures, or humidity. In addition, there are no moving parts or elements to become occluded when measuring exhaled gas.

A distinct advantage of measuring gas flow by means of ultrasonic pulses is that a disposable flow tube can be inserted between the transducers, thus eliminating problems with cross-contamination between subjects. A further advantage of this design is that the disposable flow tube does not require calibration because it simply acts as a transparent barrier separating exhaled gas from the sensing transducers (Fig. 11.11). A filter can be used with the ultrasonic flow tube in Fig. 11.11, which has been shown to be an effective infection barrier.

Flow Sensor Summary

Flow-sensing spirometers have some advantages over volume-displacement systems. When combined with appropriate gas analyzers and breathing circuits, flow-sensing spirometers can be used to perform lung volume determinations by the open-circuit method. Diffusing capacity can be measured with flow-sensing spirometers as well. Pressure-differential, heated-wire, turbine, and pitot tube pneumotachometers are used to measure flow and volume in body plethysmographs, exercise testing systems, and metabolic carts. Because flow sensors require electronic circuitry to integrate flow or sum volume pulses, flow-based spirometers are integrated into a spirometer system where

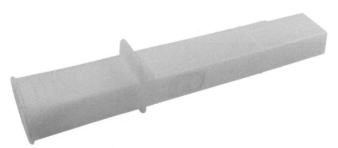

FIG. 11.11 Ultrasonic flow sensor tube. A tube with membranous ports on either side permits high-frequency sound waves to be passed through the stream of gas. The ports are angled so that the sound waves speed up or slow down, depending on the direction of gas flow. By measuring the transit time of the sound pulses compared with conditions of no flow, flow can be accurately measured. This method allows an inexpensive disposable tube to be used and prevents contamination of the ultrasonic transducers themselves. (Courtesy ndd Medical Technologies, Inc., Andover, MA.)

computer-generated graphics are used to produce volume-time or flow-volume (F-V) tracings.

Most flow-based spirometers can be easily cleaned and disinfected. Some flow sensors can be immersed in a disinfectant without disassembly. As noted, many systems use inexpensive disposable sensors that can be discarded after one use. The use of in-line bacteria filters to prevent contamination of flow-based spirometers may result in changes in the operating characteristics of the spirometer. Any resistance to airflow through the filter will be added to the resistance of the spirometer. For this reason, the spirometer may need to be calibrated with the filter in place. Although the resistance offered by most filters is low, it may change with use. This may occur if water vapor from expired gas condenses on the filter media. The use of barrier filters does not eliminate the need for routine cleaning of spirometers.

Flow sensors may produce a signal that is not linear across a wide range of flows. Better accuracy can be obtained for flow and volume by matching the flow range of the sensor to the physiologic signal. Most flow-based spirometers "linearize" the flow signal electronically or by means of software corrections. In many systems, a simple "look-up table" is stored in the computer. The flow signal is continuously checked against the table and corrected. By combining a calibration factor (see Chapter 12) with the look-up table corrections, very accurate flow and integrated volume measurements are possible. Flows and volumes are corrected before variables such as FEV_1 are measured.

Turbine, pressure-differential, heated-wire, and pitot tube flow-sensing spirometers are affected by the composition of the gas being measured. Changes in gas density or viscosity require correction of the transducer signal to obtain accurate flows and volumes. In most systems, these corrections are performed by computer software with a stored table. A flow-sensing spirometer may be calibrated with air but then used to measure mixtures containing He, neon, O_2, or other test gases. Some gases cause a linear shift in flow proportional to their concentrations. Corrections are usually made by applying a simple multiplier to the signal.

The accuracy of flow-based spirometers depends on the electronics and software that process the flow signal. Pulmonary function variables measured on a time basis (e.g., FEV_1 or FEV_6) require precise timing and accurate flow measurement. Detection of the start or end of the test is critical in flow-based spirometers. Timing is usually triggered by a minimum flow or pressure change. Signal integration begins when flow reaches a threshold limit, usually 0.1 to 0.2 L/sec. Spirometers that initiate timing in response to volume pulses usually have a similar threshold that must be achieved to begin recording. Contamination of resistive elements, thermistors, or pitot tubes by moisture or other debris can alter the flow-sensing characteristics of the transducer and interfere with the spirometer's ability to detect the start or end of the test. Similar problems can occur when flow drops to very low levels near the end of a forced expiration, causing measurement of flow (and volume) to be terminated prematurely. As a result, the volume (e.g., FVC or VC) may be underestimated.

Problems related to electronic drift require flow sensors to be zeroed frequently (see Chapter 2). Zeroing is simply a one-point calibration in which the output of the transducer is set to zero under a condition of no flow. Many systems zero the flow signal immediately before a measurement. Zeroing corrects for much of the electronic drift that occurs. A true zero requires no flow through the flow sensor. Thus the flow sensor must be held still or occluded during the zero maneuvers. Most flow-based systems use a 3-L syringe for calibration. By calibrating with a known volume signal, the accuracy of the flow sensor and the integrator can be checked with one input. Calibration and quality control (QC) techniques for volume-displacement and flow-sensing spirometers are included in Chapter 12.

Portable (Office or Home) Spirometers

The widespread availability of microprocessors has resulted in a large number of small, portable spirometers based on various flow-sensing principles.

These spirometers can be separated into two general categories: (1) those that interface with a laptop or desktop computer and (2) stand-alone devices that incorporate a dedicated microprocessor. In both cases, these devices may be referred to as **screening spirometers** or **office/home spirometers.**

Many flow-sensing spirometers interface directly with personal computers (Fig. 11.12A–C), typically a laptop computer. Other spirometers use an interface card that plugs directly into a personal computer (PC). With the appropriate software installed on the PC, spirometry can be

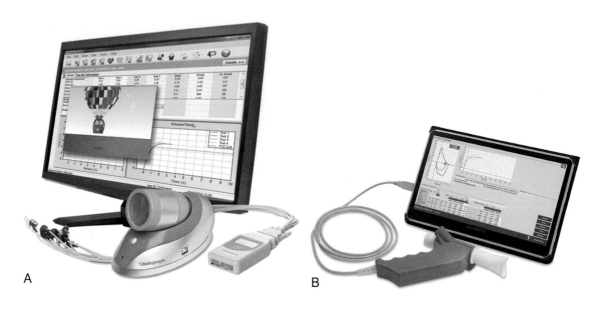

A

B

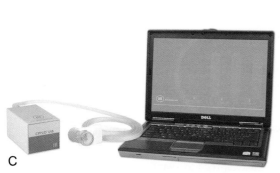

C

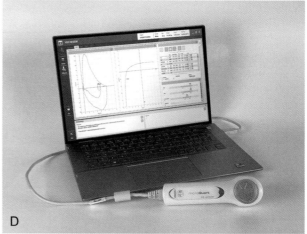

D

FIG. 11.12 Examples of pneumotachograph systems interfaced with a personal computer (PC). The laptop computer runs software that provides calculations, data storage, and printing of results. (A, Vitalograph Pneumotrac PC, courtesy Vitalograph LTD Buckinhamshire UK. B, ndd PC, courtesy ndd Medical Technologies, Andover, MA. C, CPSF-D, courtesy MGC Diagnostics, Saint Paul, MN. D, MicroQuark, courtesy Cosmed, Concord, CA.)

performed. Other spirometers place the necessary electronic components in the flow sensor head or in an external adapter. This implementation allows the flow sensor to be connected to a serial port or universal serial bus (USB) port, both of which are standard on most computers. The pressure transducer and electronics for flow-based spirometry can also be mounted on a removable card. These cards allow spirometry to be performed with handheld computers, laptop computers, or personal digital assistants (PDAs). Many flow-based spirometers use dedicated microprocessors (Fig. 11.13). Some of these are very compact so that the entire device is not much larger than a calculator. These designs allow the units to be handheld and portable.

Many portable spirometers use disposable flow sensors. Disposable sensors can provide accurate measurements if they are manufactured according to rigid specifications. Disposable flow sensors are usually precalibrated at the time of manufacture. Some manufacturers include calibration codes (or bar codes) on the sensor to be used in conjunction with the spirometer software. Ideally, each spirometer should provide a means for calibration using a 3-L syringe. At a minimum, the software in portable spirometers should allow verification of volumes even if precalibrated flow sensors are used.

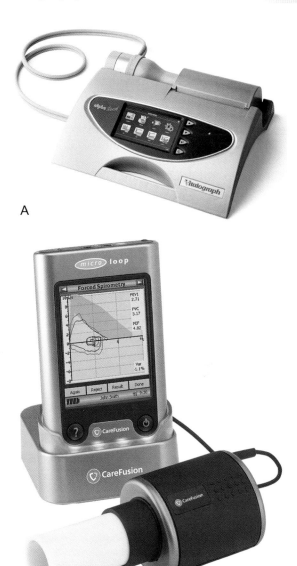

A

B

FIG. 11.13 Examples of flow-based spirometers integrated with a dedicated microprocessor. This system includes a display and a printer for hard-copy results. (A, Alpha Spirometer, courtesy Vitalograph, Buckinghamshire, UK. B, Micro Loop, courtesy Vyaire, Chicago, IL.)

PF TIP 11.3

Most office spirometers include software features to help the user obtain high-quality data. These features include prompts to direct the patient's efforts, along with messages regarding the quality of the data obtained. These quality indicators are usually based on ATS-ERS recommendations for spirometry. Many spirometers also include a grading system to assess the overall acceptability and repeatability of the patient's efforts.

Interfacing a flow sensor to a PC or laptop computer makes spirometry available in a variety of clinical settings. Handheld or PC-based systems provide a relatively inexpensive way to perform spirometry, before-and-after bronchodilator studies, and even bronchial challenges. Increasingly sophisticated software allows spirometric data to be stored, manipulated, and displayed graphically. In spite of the availability of small, accurate spirometers, spirometry is still not widely used in primary care. Because spirometry is effort dependent, poorly performed maneuvers can result in misclassification (i.e., obstruction versus restriction versus normal). The choice of inappropriate reference equations and incorrect interpretation of results further limit the usefulness of spirometry.

The National Lung Health Education Program (NLHEP) provides recommendations for office spirometers to be used in primary care settings (Box 11.1). The goal of these recommendations is to standardize spirometry to promote the early detection of chronic obstructive pulmonary disease (Fig. 11.14). Office spirometers should be simple and designed to measure the major parameters: FEV_1, FEV_6, FVC, and the FEV_1/FEV_6 or FEV_1/FVC ratio. To provide accurate measurements, office spirometers should display automated messages describing the acceptability and repeatability of efforts. Automated interpretation of simple spirometry can be performed if test quality is acceptable

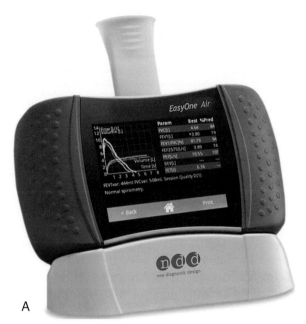

A

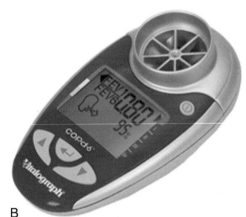

B

FIG. 11.14 (A) EasyOne. (B) COPD-6. (A, Courtesy ndd Medical Technologies Inc., Andover, MA. B, Courtesy Vitalograph, Lenexa, KS.)

and appropriate reference values are used. Display or printouts of spirograms are optional. Office spirometers should meet the accuracy recommendations of the ATS-ERS (see Chapter 12).

BOX 11.1   NLHEP SPIROMETER RECOMMENDATIONS

- Office spirometers must meet or exceed current ATS-ERS minimum standards.
- Office spirometers should report FEV_1, FEV_6, and FEV_1/FEV_6 ratios only.
- Measurement end of test should be terminated at 6 seconds (FEV_6).
- NHANES III reference set should be used for determining lower limits of normal (LLNs).
- Automated maneuver acceptability/repeatability messages should be displayed and reported.
- Airway obstruction is determined when FEV_1/FEV_6 and FEV_1 are below respective LLNs.
- Display/printout of spirograms and F-V curves is optional.
- Office spirometers should include easy-to-understand educational materials.
- A simple means of checking calibration should be included.

ATS-ERS, American Thoracic Society–European Respiratory Society; *FEV*, forced expiratory volume; *F-V*, flow–volume; *NHANES III*, Third National Health and Nutrition Examination Survey; *NLHEP*, National Lung Health Education Program. Adapted from Ferguson, G. T., Enright, P. L., Buist, A. S., et al. (2000). Office spirometry for lung health assessment in adults: a consensus statement from the National Lung Health Education Program. *Chest 117*, 1146–1161.

PEAK FLOWMETERS

Peak expiratory flow (PEF) can be measured easily with most spirometers, particularly the flow-sensing types. Many devices are available that measure PEF exclusively. PEF has become a recognized means of monitoring patients who have asthma. By incorporating a simple measurement into an inexpensive package, portable peak flowmeters allow monitoring of airway status in a variety of settings.

Most **peak flowmeters** use similar designs. The patient expires forcefully through a resistor or flow tube that has a movable indicator attached (Fig. 11.15). An orifice provides the resistance in most devices. The movable indicator is deflected in

TABLE 11.1		
Peak Flowmeter Recommended Ranges		
	Children	**Adults**
National Asthma Education Program	100–400 L/min ± 10%	100–700 L/min ± 10%
American Thoracic Society (1994)	60–400 L/min ± 10% or 20 L/min, whichever is greater	100–850 L/min ± 10% or 20 L/min, whichever is greater

proportion to the velocity of air flowing through the device. PEF is then read directly from a calibrated scale. Because these devices are nonlinear, different flow ranges are usually available. High-range peak flowmeters typically measure flows as high as 850 L/min. Low-range meters measure up to 400 L/min (Table 11.1). Low-range peak flowmeters are useful for small children or for patients who have marked obstruction.

The absolute accuracy of portable peak flowmeters is less important than their precision (i.e., repeatability of measurements). Within-instrument variability should be less than 5% or 0.15 L/sec (10 L/min), whichever is greater. Between-instrument variability should be less than 10% or 0.3 L/sec (20 L/min), whichever is greater. These devices are intended to provide serial measurements of peak flow as a guide to treatment. Patients who are carefully instructed should be able to reproduce their peak flow measurements within 0.67 L/sec (40 L/min). However, patients with asthma may have difficulty repeating their PEF, particularly during exacerbations. PEF meters must be easy to use and easy to read. Scale divisions of 5 L/min for low-range devices and 10 L/min for high-range devices allow small changes in PEF to be detected. The scale should be calibrated to read flow in BTPS units. Corrections for altitude should be included because PEF meters tend to underestimate flow as altitude increases (i.e., approximately 7% per 100 mm Hg change in barometric pressure).

Although the simple design of portable peak flowmeters allows them to be used repeatedly, moisture or other debris can cause sticking of the movable parts. This can be problematic because it

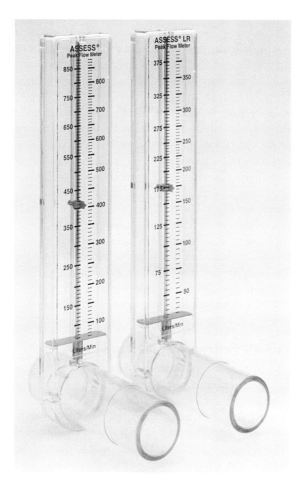

FIG. 11.15 Portable peak flowmeters. Portable peak flowmeters for measuring peak expiratory flow (PEF) outside of the pulmonary function laboratory. The patient exhales forcefully through the mouthpiece at the bottom. Pressure generated by the flow of gas deflects the movable indicator up the scale. Two flow ranges are available, for normal and reduced peak flows. (Courtesy Respironics, Inc., Murrysville, PA.)

may suggest that the patient's asthma has worsened. Some instruments can be cleaned but may need to be replaced periodically. Because portable peak flowmeters may have a limited life span, variability between same-model instruments should be 10% or 20 L/min, as noted. This allows the patient to continue monitoring with a new device. Clear instructions on how to use and maintain the peak flowmeter should come with each device. Most peak flowmeters comply with the National Asthma Education Program's "color zone" scheme for identifying clinically significant changes (see Chapter 2).

BODY PLETHYSMOGRAPHS

Body plethysmographs (Fig. 11.16A–C) are used in many pulmonary function laboratories. Body plethysmographs are also called *body boxes.* Two types of plethysmographs are available: the constant-volume, variable-pressure plethysmograph and the flow or variable-volume plethysmograph. These are sometimes called the **pressure plethysmograph** and *flow plethysmograph,* respectively. Pressure-type plethysmographs are more commonly used than flow types. Both designs are used to measure thoracic gas volume (V_{TG}) and/or FRC_{pleth} and airway resistance (Raw) and its derivatives (see Chapter 4). Both types of boxes use some type of pneumotachometer to measure flow and a mouth pressure transducer with a shutter to measure alveolar pressure. They differ in the method used to measure volume change in the box and therefore in the lungs.

Pressure Plethysmographs

The pressure plethysmograph is based on an adaptation of Boyle's law (see the Evolve website, http://evolve.elsevier.com/Mottram/Ruppel/). Volume changes in a sealed box are inversely related to pressure changes if temperature is constant. A sensitive pressure transducer monitors changes in box pressure. Pressure change is related to volume change by calibration (see Chapter 12 for calibration techniques). Pressure changes result from compression and decompression of gas within both the patient's chest and the box. If box

temperature remains constant, each unit of pressure change equals a specific volume change. For example, a volume change of 15 mL may result in a pressure change of 1 cm H_2O. After the box has been calibrated empty, the calibration factor changes slightly when a patient enters the plethysmograph. This change is easily corrected using an estimate of the volume displaced by the patient (based on the patient's weight).

The pressure plethysmograph must be essentially leak-free. Most pressure boxes use a solenoid to vent the box and maintain thermal equilibrium. In some implementations, the vent remains open until the pressure measurement begins, so that the box is continually being vented. Making V_{TG} and Raw measurements with the patient panting reduces unwanted pressure changes caused by thermal drift, leaks, or background noise. Some pressure plethysmograph systems use a controlled leak to facilitate thermal equilibrium. The leak allows gas to escape as the interior of the box warms but does not interfere with high-frequency changes such as those that occur with panting. Similarly, connecting the atmospheric side of the box pressure transducer to a container within the box dampens the effects of thermal drift. Both methods reduce the effect of temperature changes within the box and maintain a good frequency response. Pressure plethysmographs are best suited to maneuvers that measure small volume changes (i.e., 100 mL or less). Measurements of VC or FVC can usually be made only with the door open or the box adequately vented to the atmosphere.

Flow Plethysmographs

The flow plethysmograph uses a flow transducer in the box wall to measure volume changes in the box. Gas in the box is compressed or decompressed, causing flow through the opening in the box wall. Flow through the wall is integrated, corrections are applied, and volume change is recorded as the sum of the volume passing through the wall and the volume compressed. In one implementation, the patient breathes through a pneumotachometer connected to the room (*transmural breathing*). The transmural pneumotachometer allows larger gas volumes (i.e., the VC or F-V curves) to be measured while the patient is enclosed in the plethysmograph.

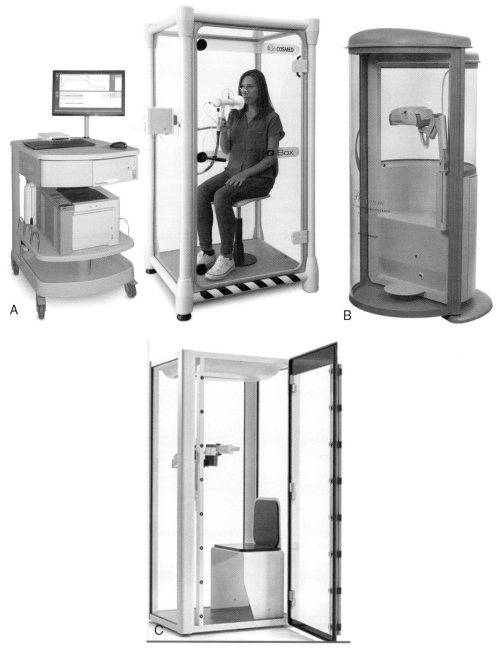

FIG. 11.16 Body plethysmograph. Examples of modern plethysmographs, with a highly transparent box, self-contained calibration equipment, and computerized data reduction and display. (A) Cosmed Q-Box. (B) MGC Platinum Elite. (C) Vyaire Wheelchair box. (A, Q-Box, courtesy Cosmed, Concord, CA. B, Platinum Elite, courtesy MGC Diagnostics, St. Paul, MN. C, Vyntus Body, with permission from Vyaire, Mettawa, IL.)

The transmural flow is redirected to the plethysmograph for Raw measurements so that the ratio of flow to box volume can be plotted. For V_{TG} measurements, the flow transducer in the plethysmograph wall is occluded so that the device works like a pressure box. The flow-type plethysmograph requires that the pressure, volume, and flow signals be measured in phase. Although thermal changes must be accounted for, the flow plethysmograph does not need to be rigorously airtight. The flow box's primary advantage is the ability to measure flows at absolute lung volumes (i.e., corrected for gas compression).

In both types of plethysmographs, a flow sensor (i.e., pneumotachometer) is needed to measure airflow at the mouth (Fig. 11.17). Flow measurement is required to compute Raw. The flow signal is also used to determine end expiration for shutter closure in V_{TG} measurements. The pneumotachometer must be linear across the range of flows encountered in spontaneous breathing and panting (± 2 L/sec) and should meet all ATS-ERS requirements for spirometers (e.g., range, accuracy, frequency response) for measurement of VC and/or FVC. Heated Fleisch or Silverman/Lilly types of pressure-differential pneumotachometers are often used in the plethysmograph. Pitot tube or heated-wire flow transducers can also be used.

A mouth pressure transducer is normally coupled to a shutter mechanism. The shutter can be an

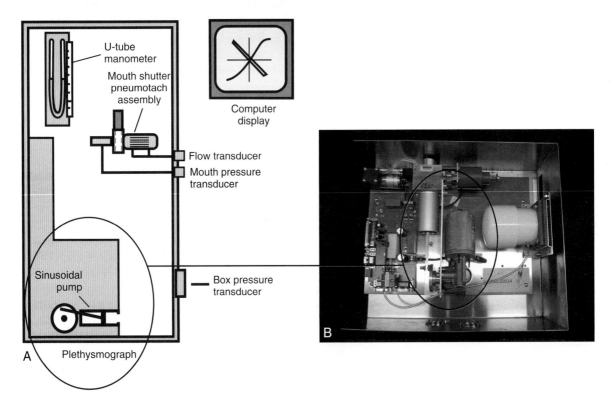

FIG. 11.17 Diagram of a pressure plethysmograph. (A) A pneumotachometer (flow sensor) with an automatic shutter mechanism is mounted at a height that is comfortable for a patient sitting in the plethysmograph. Pressure transducers for flow, mouth pressure, and box pressure provide signals that are digitized and processed by a computer. A sinusoidal pump allows calibration of the box pressure signal; a small, known volume change can be repeatedly generated. A pressure manometer (U-tube) or similar device is used to calibrate the mouth pressure transducer. A 3-L syringe is used to calibrate the pneumotachometer. Flow plethysmographs are arranged similarly, with an additional pneumotachometer in the wall of the box so that volume changes in the box are measured as gas flows through the wall. (B) Actual panel with a mechanical 50-mL pump for pressure–volume calibration of a body plethysmograph.

electric solenoid, a scissors-type valve, or a balloon valve. The mouth pressure transducer records pressures in the range of -20 to $+20$ cm H_2O when the airway is occluded but should be able to measure pressures of more than ± 50 cm H_2O with a flat frequency response greater than 8 Hz. Some systems require the technologist to close the shutter by remote control at end expiration. This may be accomplished by observing the tidal breathing maneuver on a display and actuating the shutter at end expiration. However, most systems automatically close the shutter at a preselected point in the breathing cycle. The technologist initiates a sequence in which the computer monitors flow and closes the shutter when expiratory flow becomes zero. Automated shutters allow the airway to be occluded for a fixed length of time or for a specified number of panting breaths.

Plethysmograph or box pressure is recorded by a sensitive pressure transducer connected to the box chamber. This transducer needs to be able to accurately measure pressure changes as small as ± 0.2 cm H_2O with a flat frequency response that accommodates the panting rates that are commonly encountered (e.g., > 8 Hz). The box pressure transducer should have a range that can accommodate the pressures typically encountered because of thermal drift, tidal breathing, and so forth. If a slow leak is incorporated into the box to promote thermal stability, it should have a time constant of approximately 10 seconds.

Recording of plethysmographic maneuvers is usually performed by a computer. Breathing efforts are displayed in real time, allowing the technologist to elicit proper maneuvers from the patient. The real-time display assists in ensuring that panting maneuvers are performed correctly; some systems display prompts or flags so that the patient can be coached to pant at the correct frequency. The computer then stores the data and performs the necessary calculations to compute thoracic gas volume and airway resistance. Because the computer can track volume changes in the body box, V_{TG} and airway resistance are sometimes measured from the same maneuver. The patient breathes normally to establish the end-expiratory level, the shutter is closed, and the patient pants. When the preset number of seconds has elapsed, the shutter opens (see Chapter 4). The volume change between the established end-expiratory level and the point at which the shutter was closed is then used to correct the measured V_{TG} so that it equals the patient's FRC. If V_{TG} is measured at lung volumes other than FRC, the alveolar pressure should also be corrected for any difference from ambient pressure (i.e., P_B).

Computerized plethysmographs compute a best-fit line to determine the slope (i.e., tangent) for both the open-shutter (flow versus box pressure) and closed-shutter (mouth pressure versus box pressure) panting maneuvers. The technologist can also manipulate the tangent by means of the computer keyboard or mouse. This allows some degree of correction for efforts in which the patient panted incorrectly or noise was introduced into the recorded signal. Plethysmography software provides data on lung volume and airway resistance immediately after completion of the maneuver. This aids in selecting acceptable maneuvers to report. The test can also be repeated as required when questionable values are obtained. With the use of the computer-displayed panting frequency, the technologist can coach the patient to maintain a desired rate.

Most plethysmographs include the necessary signal-generating devices to perform physical calibration (see Chapter 12). A pressure manometer (or fluid-filled U-tube) may be mounted on the box for calibration of the mouth pressure transducer. Some systems provide a fixed pressure signal for mouth pressure calibration. A small syringe (50 mL) driven by an electric motor allows calibration of the box pressure transducer (Fig. 11.17B). The motorized syringe usually produces a sine-wave flow with a frequency that can be varied. This allows checking of box pressure calibration at various frequencies. Most computerized plethysmographs use a standard 3-L syringe to calibrate the pneumotachometer or flow sensor. However, a flow generator and rotameter (i.e., a flowmeter) may be included for flow calibration. Computerized plethysmograph systems provide automated calibration of transducers. The output of the transducer (i.e., its amplified signal) is measured, and the computer generates a software correction factor. This correction is then applied to every measurement made with the transducer. Some manufacturers also supply quality control (QC) devices such as an isothermal lung analog (see Chapter 12). These devices provide QC to verify calibration of transducers and appropriateness of software correction factors.

PF TIP 11.4

Most patients can perform plethysmographic measurements acceptably, even if they experience some claustrophobia. Modern body plethysmographs use Plexiglas or similar transparent material so that the subject feels less confined. Plethysmographic measurements can usually be made quickly, reducing the length of time spent with the door closed. Plethysmography may not be practical for some patients, such as those who have orthopedic impairments.

The ease with which a patient can enter the plethysmograph and perform the required maneuvers is an important feature. Some patients may experience claustrophobia when inside the plethysmograph. Older boxes used a plywood cabinet to provide the necessary rigidity so that pressure changes were not attenuated. Boxes made of durable plastics are largely transparent and less confining for the patient (see Fig. 11.16) while maintaining the necessary rigidity. Most plethysmographs contain 500 to 700 L of volume and can accommodate even large patients. Careful design allows the patient to easily enter the box. Some plethysmographs are large enough to accommodate patients in wheelchairs. Others use a clamshell design so that the patient may be seated and the box closed around him or her. Most plethysmographs provide an internal switch or mechanism that allows patients to open the box from inside if they become uncomfortable.

Equally important is a communication system that allows both voice and visual contact with the patient. Panting against a closed shutter may be difficult for some individuals, and continuous coaching is often necessary to elicit valid maneuvers. An intercom system that provides continuous two-way communication is essential.

Adjuncts that do not affect the operation of the box yet aid in reducing anxiety or improve safety have been found to be of benefit. Plastic decals, such as fish, can be very effective in reducing anxiety, in particular for the younger subject (Fig. 11.18A). Likewise, a suction cup safety handle may aid the subject in entering or exiting the box (see Fig. 11.18B).

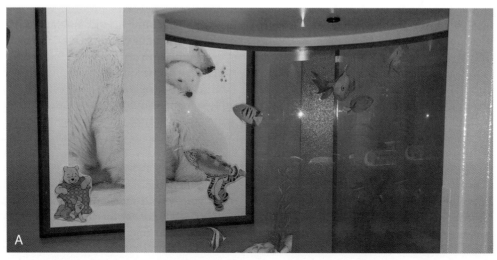

FIG. 11.18 Body box adjuncts. (A) Plastic decals that make the box appear as a fish tank.

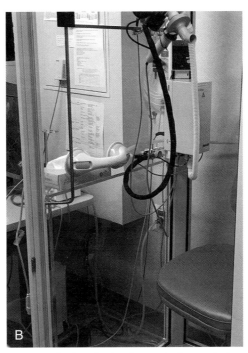

FIG. 11.18, CONT'D   (B) Suction safety handle placed strategically to assist in entering and exiting the box.

BREATHING VALVES

Various types of valves are commonly used for pulmonary function tests, particularly for dilutional lung volume, DLCO, and exercise tests. These valves direct inspired or expired gas through the spirometer or provide a means of sampling for gas analysis.

Free Breathing and Demand Valves

The simplest type of valve allows the patient to be switched from breathing room air to breathing gas contained in a spirometer or special breathing circuit. **Free breathing valves** are often used in both open-circuit and closed-circuit FRC determinations. The free breathing valve is designed so that the patient can be switched into the system either manually or by computer controls at a specific point in the breathing cycle.

The typical free breathing valve consists of a body with two or more ports. A drum in the valve body rotates to connect different combinations of ports. Because these valves are used mainly for tidal breathing or slow vital capacity (SVC) maneuvers, resistance to flow is usually not critical. Most have ports with diameters of 1.5 to 3 cm. For studies involving gas analysis, such as FRC determination, the valve must be free of leaks. The dead space of valves used in measurements of FRC should be less than 100 mL.

Some systems use a breathing manifold that consists of multiple ports and valves, all connected to the patient mouthpiece. The different ports allow inspired or expired gas to be directed to the spirometer or gas-sampling devices. The valves may be electric or gas-powered solenoids, balloon valves that inflate with compressed air, or scissors-type valves that pinch flexible tubing to control flow. Under computer control, different combinations of valves and ports are opened and closed. This type of manifold permits spirometry, dilutional lung volumes, and DLCO tests to be performed with the same breathing circuit. A similar manifold is used in many body plethysmograph systems to permit measurement of V_{TG} (FRC_{pleth}) and Raw along with DLCO.

Infection control of free breathing valves and multiple-port manifolds involves disassembly, cleaning, and disinfection or sterilization. Because cleaning between patients may not be practical, in-line filters may be used to prevent contamination of these devices.

PF TIP 11.5

The most common problem encountered in breathing circuits that use valves is a failure of the valves to operate correctly. Balloon-type valves often develop leaks. Demand valves sometimes stick or require excessive inspiratory pressure to open. Solenoid-type valves have O-rings that must be properly lubricated to prevent leaks. Directional valves (one-way and two-way) may have leaflets that stick or have been assembled incorrectly.

Demand valves (also sometimes referred to as *demand-flow regulators*) are used in many circuits in which the patient inspires a test gas (e.g., D_{LCO}, FRC_{N2}). The primary considerations for demand valves are the pressure required to trigger gas flow and the adequacy of flow once the valve opens. Most demand valves consist of a valve body that contains a sensitive diaphragm. The diaphragm moves in response to the patient's inspiratory effort, opening the valve and allowing gas to flow from a high-pressure source. Maximal flow is controlled by the valve and usually depends on the driving pressure (typically 20–50 psi). Demand valves are often adjustable, allowing the sensitivity to be set so that minimal pressure is needed to trigger gas flow. Problems typically encountered with demand valves include inadequate source pressure (turned off or not connected) and sticking or incorrectly adjusted diaphragms. Demand valves used in D_{LCO} circuits should be able to deliver 6 L/sec flow with less than 10 cm H_2O pressure.

Directional Valves

Directional (one-way and two-way) valves are used in many types of breathing circuits. The simplest type consists of a flap or diaphragm that opens in only one direction. The valve is then mounted in a rigid tube that can be inserted into a breathing circuit. Because gas is permitted to flow in one direction only, these valves are called *one-way valves*.

Another common valve design is that used to separate inspired from expired gas, often called a *two-way nonrebreathing valve*. This type of directional valve consists of a T-shaped body with three ports and two separate diaphragms (Fig. 11.19A). The diaphragms allow gas to flow in one direction only. The patient connection is between the diaphragms, effectively separating inspired from expired gas. Two-way nonrebreathing valves are used in exercise testing; metabolic studies; or any procedure requiring collection, measurement, or analysis of exhaled gas. The valve body may contain a tap for the connection of gas sample tubing. This tap is typically placed between the diaphragms so that both inspired and expired gas can be sampled.

Two factors must be considered in the selection of appropriate directional valves: dead-space volume and flow resistance. For one-way valves, only flow resistance is a concern. In two-way nonrebreathing valves, dead space is the volume contained between the two diaphragms along with the volume of any connectors (e.g., a mouthpiece). Most manufacturers supply information about the dead space of individual valves. Sometimes, the dead-space value is printed on the valve body. Unknown dead space can be determined by blocking two of the three ports and measuring the water volume required to fill the dead-space portion of the valve.

Low dead-space valves (<50 mL) may be required for children or if the patient already has increased dead space, particularly if only tidal breathing is being assessed. Valves with large-bore ports and low-resistance diaphragms usually have larger dead-space volumes. For exercise testing, large-bore nonrebreathing valves are used to minimize resistance at high flows. These valves may have a dead-space volume of 100 to 200 mL. The selection of an appropriate-sized nonrebreathing valve should be based on the maximal flow anticipated during the test. For example, a maximal exercise test for a healthy adult patient may include flows greater than 100 L/min. A large-bore valve would be selected to accommodate the high flow. Valve dead space would be less of a concern because large tidal

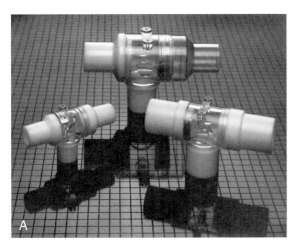

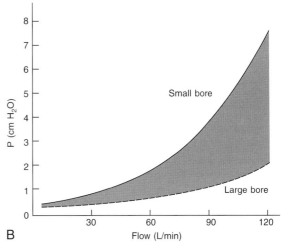

FIG. 11.19 (A) Two-way nonrebreathing valves. Three different-sized valves used for the measurement of expired gas are shown. Each valve consists of a T-shaped body containing two diaphragms that separate inspired and expired gas. The smaller valves have less dead space but higher resistance to flow; the large valve has low flow resistance but more dead space. The small and medium valves are used for studies in which low flows are encountered, such as metabolic measurements. The large valve is appropriate for high flow rates such as those occurring during maximal exercise testing. (B) Breathing valve resistance. Graph plots the pressure developed across two different-sized valves in relation to gas flow through the valves. For small-bore valves, pressures of less than 1 cm H_2O are generated up to approximately 60 L/min (1 L/sec). Large-bore valves have less resistance (pressure per unit of flow) and are typically used for studies in which the patient has high flow rates. Other factors affecting resistance include the design and material used for the diaphragms in the valve and whether the diaphragms move freely. Resistance increases nonlinearly in all types of valves; high resistance can occur even in large-bore valves at very high flows. (A, Courtesy Hans Rudolph, Inc., Kansas City, MO.)

volumes are necessary to generate the increased flow. Mechanical (i.e., valve) dead space must be accurately determined for use in calculations involving gas analysis, such as physiologic dead-space measurements.

Low resistance to flow is also a critical characteristic of one-way and two-way valves. Resistance to flow through most valves is nonlinear and depends on the cross-sectional area of valve leaflets or diaphragms (see Fig. 11.19B). Resistance is usually not critical for tests in which flows of less than 1 L/sec occur. Small-bore (15- to 22-mm) directional valves can be selected based on an appropriate dead-space volume. Most small-bore nonrebreathing valves have a resistance in the range of 1 to 2 cm H_2O/L/sec at flows of up to 1 L/sec (60 L/min). However, if the patient breathes through the valve for long intervals, even a small resistance may result in respiratory muscle fatigue and changes in the ventilatory pattern. Applications such as exercise testing typically involve increased flows. Large-bore,

two-way valves are indicated when flows greater than 1 L/sec (60 L/min) can be expected to develop. Pressures less than 3 cm H_2O can be maintained even at flows of 5 L/sec (300 L/min) with large-bore valves. Saliva and moisture may collect in valves during prolonged tests (e.g., exercise or eucapnic hyperventilation). Valves with saliva traps may be needed for these procedures. If a valve is used in a spirometry circuit, it must have very low resistance to meet the ATS-ERS recommendation of less than 1.5 cm H_2O/L/sec at flows of 12 L/sec. Valves used in a DLCO circuit should produce a total resistance of less than 1.5 cm H_2O/L/sec at flows of 6 L/sec.

Any valve can cause increased resistance if not properly maintained. Rubber, plastic, or silicon leaflets and diaphragms can stick or become rigid with age. Valves should be disassembled and cleaned after each use, according to the manufacturer's directions, and allowed to dry thoroughly before reassembly. Care must be taken when reassembling valves to ensure that all diaphragms are oriented properly. Valves should be visually inspected to make sure that diaphragms are mounted correctly and that they open and close properly before being used.

Gas-Sampling Valves

Specialized valves (valve manifolds) may be used to sample gas during tests such as the single-breath D_{LCO}. These valves open and close during the breathing maneuver to allow the patient to inspire test gas and expire to a gas collection device. The same mechanisms are often used to occlude the airway near the patient's mouth for breath-holding maneuvers or to measure mouth pressure. Many of these valves use electrically or pneumatically powered solenoids to direct flow to a spirometer or sample collection device. Other systems use scissors-type valves to pinch compressible tubing. The primary concern with gas-sampling valves is smooth operation with appropriate direction of the gas to be sampled. Electrically activated solenoids may deteriorate with age, particularly if exposed to high-humidity conditions (e.g., expired air). Replacement of O-rings or similar types of seals may be necessary to ensure uncontaminated gas samples. Some sampling valves use balloons that inflate to block or direct the flow of gas. These balloons require periodic replacement because small leaks can prevent the balloon from occluding flow. When this occurs, gas may not be directed to the appropriate device, or the gas itself may be contaminated. Scissors-type valves offer an advantage in that the compressible tubing can be changed easily between patients.

Infection control for sampling valves usually requires disassembly and cleaning. Some complex valve manifolds may be difficult or impossible to disassemble. In such devices, an in-line filter may be needed to avoid cross-contamination.

PULMONARY GAS ANALYZERS

Various types of gas analyzers are used in pulmonary function testing. O_2 and CO_2 analyzers are used for metabolic studies and exercise testing. Helium (He) analysis is used for closed-circuit FRC determinations and for several types of D_{LCO} tests.

N_2 analysis is used in the open-circuit FRC method. CO measurements are integral to all of the diffusion capacity methods currently used. Analyses of neon, argon, methane, and acetylene are used in specialized tests for diffusion, lung volume measurements, and cardiac output determination. NO (nitric oxide) analyzers are used to assess airway inflammation in the diagnosis and treatment of asthma.

How rapidly a gas analyzer can detect and display a change in gas concentration is termed *response time*. Response time is commonly measured in seconds or milliseconds (thousandths of a second). Manufacturers of gas analyzers list response time as the interval required for an analyzer to measure some fraction of a given step change in gas concentration. For example, an O_2 analyzer might require 2 seconds to respond to an increase in O_2 concentration from 21% to 100%. The response time may be listed as the time required for 90% of the total change to be detected. The response time of an analyzer often depends on the size of the step change in gas concentration. A related factor in gas analysis is transport time. *Transport time* is how long it takes to move the gas from the sample site to the analyzer itself. How rapidly a gas (e.g., O_2) can be analyzed depends on both the response time and the transport time of the instrument. A third consideration is *phase delay* (or phase shift) in the gas analyzer signal. When the gas analyzer signal is integrated with a flow signal, the two signals may be out of phase; that is, the flow signal may be considered instantaneous while the gas analyzer signal lags slightly behind (because of transport and response time). The two signals can be aligned by measuring the phase delay (or shift) and offsetting one of the signals; this is usually done with software. In breath-by-breath gas analysis, response time, transport time, and phase delay are critical, and rapidly responding analyzers are required. Tests such as the D_{LCO} or FRC measurement by He dilution require very accurate gas analysis, but a rapid response is not necessary.

Oxygen Analyzers

O_2 analysis can be performed by several different methods. Table 11.2 lists some types of O_2 analyzers available. Two types are used for rapid analysis

TABLE 11.2

Oxygen Analyzers

Type	Applications	Advantages/ Disadvantages
Paramagnetic	Monitoring	Discrete sampling only
Polarographic electrode	Monitoring, exercise testing, metabolic studies	Discrete or continuous sampling; requires special electronic circuitry for fast response (200 ms)
Galvanic cell (fuel cell)	Monitoring	Continuous sampling; similar to polarographic but does not require polarizing voltage
Zirconium cell	Breath-by-breath exercise and metabolic studies	Heated (650°C–800°C) electrochemical sensor; fast response useful for continuous sampling; thermal stabilization required
Gas chromatograph	Exercise testing, monitoring, metabolic measurements	Discrete sampling; response time approx. 30 sec; very accurate; multiple gas analysis

of O_2, such as breath-by-breath exercise tests: the polarographic electrode and zirconium fuel cell. The other O_2 analyzers listed are used for specialized applications, including patient monitoring.

Polarographic Electrodes

The **polarographic electrode** is similar to the blood gas O_2 electrode (see the section on blood gas analyzers, oximeters, and related devices). For gas analysis, a platinum cathode is used without a membrane covering the tip. A gas pump draws the sample past the polarized electrode at a constant flow. O_2 is reduced in proportion to its partial pressure. The electrode is calibrated by exposing it to known fractional concentrations of O_2 at a known barometric pressure. Response times of approximately 200 ms can be attained by using special electronic circuitry. Rapid response allows continuous analysis for breath-by-breath

measurements. Contamination of the electrode can degrade its response time and cause difficulty with calibration.

Zirconium Fuel Cells

An electrode is formed by coating a zirconium element with platinum. The zirconium, when heated to 700°C to 800°C, acts as a solid electrolyte between the platinum coating on either side. When the two sides of the electrode are exposed to different partial pressures of O_2, gas traverses the electrode, creating a voltage proportional to the difference in concentrations. Sample gas is drawn past the element at a constant low flow. This allows rapid, continuous analysis without altering the temperature of the electrode. The electrode temperature must be held constant, so the electrode requires adequate insulation. A warm-up period of 10 to 30 minutes is typically required to reach thermal equilibrium at the elevated temperature. Response times of less than 200 ms are possible with the zirconium fuel cell, making it useful for breath-by-breath measurements.

The zirconium fuel cell and the polarographic electrode each measure the partial pressure of O_2. Pressure changes in the sampling circuit can affect the concentration measurement. Such pressure changes can be caused by gas flow in a breathing circuit or by positive pressure in a mechanical ventilator circuit. The presence of water vapor in the sample affects both electrodes similarly. O_2 concentration is measured accurately but is diluted in proportion to the water vapor pressure present in the sample. Zirconium fuel cells eventually degrade in relation to the volume of O_2 analyzed. The cell may be refreshed by passing a current through it, thus reversing the O_2 uptake process.

Infrared Absorption (CO_2, CO) Analyzers

Several types of respiratory gas analyzers are based on the absorption of infrared radiation to measure gas concentrations. Infrared absorption is used in CO analyzers for D_{LCO} tests. Infrared CO_2 analyzers are used for exercise testing, metabolic studies, and bedside monitoring (capnography) in critical care (Fig. 11.20A–C).

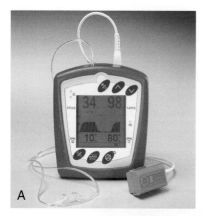

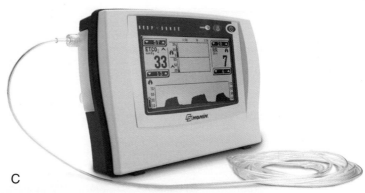

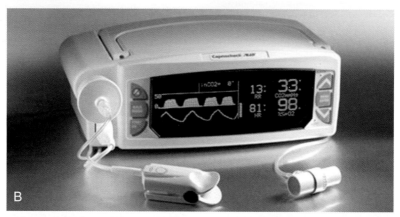

FIG. 11.20 Examples of portable capnographs. These portable capnographs include a pulse oximeter. It measures and displays end-tidal CO_2, SpO_2, heart rate, respiratory rate, and the CO_2 waveform. (A) Capnocheck II. (B) BCI Capnograph. (C) Infrared CO_2 monitor. (A and B, courtesy Smiths Medical, Dublin, OH. C, Courtesy Nonin Medical Inc., Plymouth, MN.)

Certain gases (e.g., CO_2 and CO) absorb infrared radiation. A common type of infrared analyzer uses two beams of infrared radiation directed through parallel cells. One cell contains sample gas, and the other contains a reference gas. The two beams converge on a single infrared detector (Fig. 11.21). A small motor rotates an interrupter, or "chopper," between the infrared source and the cells. The chopper blades alternately interrupt the infrared radiation passing through the sample and reference cells. If the sample and reference gases have the same concentration, the radiation reaching the detector is constant. However, when a sample with a different gas concentration is introduced, the radiation reaching the detector varies in a rhythmic fashion. This causes a vibration in the detector that

PF TIP 11.6

For accurate gas analysis, most analyzers require that measurements be made under the same conditions in which calibration was performed. Analyzers that pump the gas from a sample port to the measuring chamber should not have flow adjustments made after calibration. Sample lines should remain the same lengths as those used in calibration. Carrier gas flow (gas chromatographs) should not be changed after calibration. Gas-conditioning devices, such as water absorbers, should be inspected and changed before calibration, as necessary. Chemiluminescence analyzers are susceptible to changes in ambient temperature and need to be maintained in a stable environment.

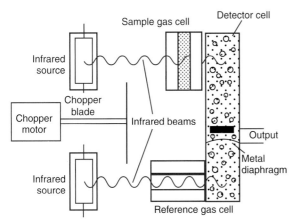

FIG. 11.21 Infrared absorption gas analyzer. Components of an infrared analyzer used to measure CO_2 are depicted. Infrared sources emit beams that pass through parallel cells. One cell contains a reference gas; the other contains a gas sample to be analyzed. A rotating blade "chops" the infrared beams in a rhythmic fashion. When both reference and sample cells contain the same gas, the radiation reaching each half of the detector cell is the same. When a gas sample is introduced, it absorbs some infrared radiation. Different amounts of radiation reach the two halves of the detector cell, causing the diaphragm separating the compartments of the detector to oscillate. This oscillation is transformed into a signal proportional to the difference in gas concentrations. The infrared analyzer is ideal for determining small changes in concentration in gas samples. (From Beckman Instruments, Inc., Medical Gas Analyzer LB-2: operating instructions, FM-149997-301, Schiller Park, IL.)

is translated into a pulsatile signal proportional to the difference between the two beams.

Infrared analyzers can measure small changes in gas concentrations, such as the difference between inspired and expired CO in DLCO tests. Infrared analyzers respond rapidly once the gas has been transported to the measuring chamber. Gas can be sampled either continuously or discretely with infrared analyzers. For continuous sampling, the gas flow must be constant. The analyzer must be calibrated using the same flow at which measurements are made. Pump settings and the sample line should not be altered after calibration. Water condensation or other debris in the sample line can significantly alter the flow and affect the accuracy of the measurement. Water vapor in the sample will dilute the gas being analyzed. Water vapor can be removed if the response time is not critical. For rapid response times, as required for breath-by-breath analysis, the

effects of water vapor can be corrected mathematically by assuming that expired gas is fully saturated or by using semipermeable tubing that equilibrates the sample with ambient saturation (see the section on gas-conditioning devices).

Infrared analyzers used to measure CO (and in some cases, tracer gas) during the DLCO test need to have a linear output because the calculation of DLCO commonly uses the ratio of CO to tracer gas (see Chapter 3). The analyzer should display nonlinearity of 0.5% or less of full scale across the range of gas concentrations typically used (approximately 0.3% for CO). Although the output of the infrared detector may be nonlinear, it can be easily corrected electronically or by means of a look-up table in software. For measuring CO and tracer gases during DLCO tests, the analyzer needs to be stable (i.e., no drift) for at least as long as the test may last (typically 30 seconds). Because water vapor and CO_2 affect the measurement of CO, these gases need to be removed (scrubbed) before reaching the infrared detector.

Common problems occurring with infrared analyzers involve the chopper motor, sample cell, and infrared detector. Motors turning the chopper blades may wear out or work intermittently. Some analyzers use a nonmechanical means of alternating the infrared beams, thus eliminating the problem. The sample cell can easily become contaminated. Water or other debris can be aspirated into the analyzer and contaminate the cell window, interfering with thr transmission of the infrared beam. Infrared detector cells degrade over time and become less sensitive. Both contamination of the sample cell and detector aging can alter the response time or make the analyzer impossible to calibrate.

Emission Spectroscopy Analyzers

The single-breath and multiple-breath N_2-washout tests (open-circuit FRC determination) use N_2 analysis. The *Geissler tube ionizer* is an N_2 analyzer based on the principle of **emission spectroscopy** (Fig. 11.22). This instrument consists of an enclosed ionization chamber that contains two electrodes and a photocell. A vacuum pump creates a constant low pressure in the ionization chamber by bleeding gas through a needle valve. The needle valve draws

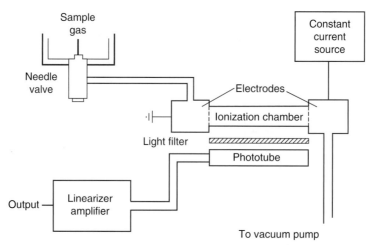

FIG. 11.22 Emission spectroscopy gas analyzer. The optical emission analyzer (Geissler tube) is commonly used for N_2 analysis. A vacuum pump draws a small gas sample through a needle valve (usually in the breathing circuit). The gas sample passes through an ionization chamber, where the ionized gas emits light. All light except that from the desired gas is filtered out, and the remaining light is monitored by a phototube or similar detector. The detector transmits a signal proportional to the intensity of the light, allowing rapid gas analysis. (From Hewlett-Packard, Application Note AN 729, San Diego, CA.)

gas to be sampled from the breathing circuit. When current is supplied to the electrodes, the N_2 between them is ionized and emits light. After being filtered, this light is monitored by a photodetector. The intensity of the light is directly proportional to the concentration of N_2 in the sample. The current, distance between electrodes, and gas pressure must remain constant. The photodetector converts the light signal into a DC voltage. This analog signal is then amplified, linearized, and directed to an appropriate meter or A/D converter. The Geissler tube ionizer allows continuous and rapid analysis of N_2, with response times typically less than 100 ms.

Emission spectroscopy analyzers used for measuring FRC by N_2 washout should have a range of 0% to 80% and should be linear ($\leq 0.2\%$ error) across this range. N_2 analyzers need to have a resolution of 0.01% or less with a 95% response time of 60 ms or less. Because these analyzers measure rapidly changing concentrations of N_2, correction for phase delay in the N_2 signal may be required.

Analyzers using emission spectroscopy usually require a vacuum pump. Vacuum pressure must be maintained at a stable level to ensure accuracy and linearity. Leaks in the seals around the needle valve or in the pump itself may occur. Inability to zero or

span the analyzer (i.e., adjust the gain) often indicates a leak or faulty vacuum source. The photodetector, ionizing electrodes, and light filter may all degrade over time. Periodic linearity checks allow adjustment for small changes in these components.

Thermal Conductivity Analyzers

Measurement of FRC by the closed-circuit method requires He analysis. Some DLCO systems also analyze He as the tracer gas. **Thermal conductivity analyzers** measure gas concentrations in a sample by detecting the rate at which different gases conduct heat. Heated wires or beads (thermistors) are exposed to the gas sample. The concentration of a specific gas can be detected by measuring the change in electrical resistance of the thermistors. Two glass-coated thermistors serve as sensing elements connected by a *Wheatstone bridge circuit* (Fig. 11.23). Thermistors change temperature and electrical resistance as a function of the molecular weight of the gases surrounding them. One thermistor serves as a reference. A difference in the concentration of gases between two thermistors can be detected because differences in heat conducted away alter the electrical resistance in the circuit. He analyzers use a reference cell containing no He. Other gases can

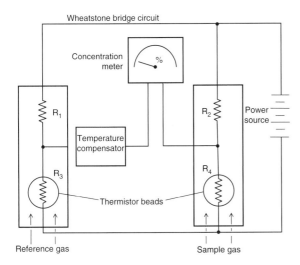

Wheatstone bridge circuit

Concentration meter

%

R₁

Temperature compensator

R₃

Thermistor beads

Reference gas

R₂

Power source

R₄

Sample gas

FIG. 11.23 Thermal conductivity analyzer. A thermal conductivity gas analyzer, as used for helium (He) analysis or gas chromatography, is shown. Two thermistor beads (temperature-sensitive electrical resistors) are connected in a Wheatstone bridge circuit. When the thermistors are subjected to the same gas concentrations, their electrical resistances are equal, and the meter registers zero (by calibration). When a gas is applied to the sample thermistor (R_4) and the reference thermistor is submitted to a reference gas, an electrical potential occurs. This deflects the meter (i.e., a voltmeter) by an amount proportional to the difference in gas concentrations.

be analyzed by means of thermal conductivity if no interfering gases are present. Thermal conductivity analyzers are used in conjunction with gas chromatography (see the section on gas chromatography). Water vapor and CO_2 must be removed before He analysis. Thermal conductivity analyzers can be used for continuous or discrete measurements but have response times in the range of 10 to 20 seconds. Thermal conductivity analyzers cannot be used to detect rapid changes in gas concentration.

When a thermal conductivity analyzer is used for FRC_{He} measurements, a range of 0% to 10% of full scale is required with a resolution of 0.01% or less over this range. The 95% response time should be 15 seconds or less for step changes in He concentration of 2%. The analyzer should show minimal drift ($\leq 0.02\%$) for as long as the test may last (up to 10 minutes).

Thermal conductivity analyzers are very stable. Other than the pump used to draw gas into the analyzer, there are no moving parts. Unless the

thermistor in the sampling chamber is contaminated or physically damaged, the analyzer remains accurate for an extended period. Gas pressure and temperature should be maintained at levels similar to those used during calibration in order for the analyzer to produce accurate results. Water vapor or CO_2 in the sample circuit (caused by malfunctioning absorbers) is a common cause of errors with this type of analyzer. Some He analyzers also use a water absorber in line with the reference thermistor. This allows dry room air to be used to zero the analyzer. Exhaustion of this absorber can result in calibration errors.

Gas Chromatography

Gas chromatography combines a means of separating a sample into component gases and a detector for measuring concentrations of the components. The detector is usually a thermal conductivity analyzer as previously described. Most chromatographs use the principle of column separation to segregate the component gases of the sample (Fig. 11.24). The chromatograph column contains a packing material that impedes the movement of gas molecules depending on their size. The material is usually a high-surface-area inorganic or polymer packing. Some columns also use materials that combine chemically with specific gases. A combination of columns allows a wide range of gases to be analyzed with a single detector. He is used as a carrier gas because of its high thermal conductivity. The sample gas, along with the He carrier gas, is injected into the column. Component gases exit the column at varying rates and are detected by a thermal conductivity analyzer. The concentrations of each gas can be determined by comparing the output of the thermal conductivity analyzer with a known calibration gas. When He is used as the carrier gas, it cannot be used as an inert indicator for lung volume determinations or diffusing capacity measurements. Neon, which is relatively insoluble, may be substituted for He in these tests. Water vapor and CO_2 are usually removed from the sample to prevent contamination of the separator column.

Gas chromatographs are well suited to applications requiring analysis of multiple gases, such as D_{LCO} determinations. If gas chromatography

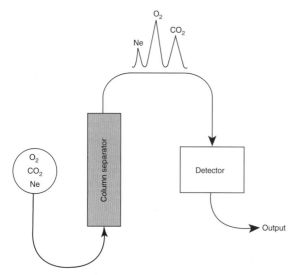

FIG. 11.24 Gas chromatograph. Diagram of the components of a gas chromatograph for analyzing respiratory gases. The gas sample moves through a separator column via a carrier gas, usually helium (He). Gases of different molecular sizes pass through the column at different rates and are monitored sequentially by a thermal conductivity detector. The output of the detector is proportional to the concentration of the gases in the sample. Gases can be analyzed accurately by using appropriate separator columns.

is used for DLCO measurements, the linearity of the device should be 0.5% of full scale for both CO and the tracer gas. As for infrared analyzers, gas chromatographs in DLCO systems need to be stable (i.e., no drift) for the interval between calibration and test gas analysis. Gas chromatograph response times are typically from 15 to 90 seconds, depending on the gas to be detected and the flow of carrier gas.

Chromatography is very accurate and is widely used for the analysis of certified reference gases. Column material must be replaced when exhausted to maintain accuracy. Some chromatographs heat the column to enhance separation. Failure of the heating mechanism can lead to inaccurate analyses. Exhaustion of water or CO_2 absorbers can also cause the column to become contaminated.

Chemiluminescence Analyzers

Chemiluminescence analyzers are based on the principle that when two reactants are mixed to form an excited intermediate state, the intermediate may emit light as it decays back to a lower energy level. Chemiluminescence is routinely used to measure nitric oxide (see FE_{NO} in Chapter 10) to assess airway inflammation. Ozone may be combined with NO to form NO_2 (nitrogen dioxide) in an excited state:

$$NO + O_3 \rightarrow NO_2[\lozenge] + O_2$$

where:

NO = nitric oxide
O_3 = ozone
NO_2 = nitrogen dioxide
$[\lozenge]$ = decay to a lower-energy state
O_2 = oxygen

The activated NO_2 luminesces (i.e., emits light) in visible and infrared wavelengths as it decays to a lower-energy state. A photomultiplier or charge-coupled device (CCD) counts photons emitted at a specific wavelength, which are proportional to the amount of NO in the sample. Fig. 11.25 shows an example of one commercially available chemiluminescence analyzer for the measurement of NO.

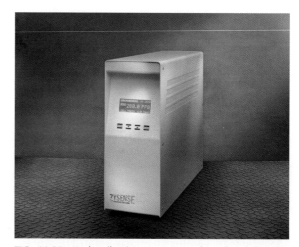

FIG. 11.25 A chemiluminescent gas analyzer for nitric oxide (NO). A commercially available analyzer designed to measure trace amounts of NO in the exhaled breath. The monitor includes an NO scrubbing device so that the subject can inhale NO-free gas and immediately exhale into the sampler. The analyzer uses the chemiluminescence effect to measure NO (see text). (Courtesy Dr. Rengarajan Ramesh, Zysense LLC, Waxhaw, NC.)

Specific recommendations for chemilumines-cence NO analyzers have been published by the ATS-ERS. Calibration of NO analyzers is critical be-cause of the small gas concentrations typically in-volved (parts per billion [ppb]). Chemiluminescence analyzers used to measure F_{ENO} should be cali-brated with gases that span the range of values en-countered in clinical practice. These ranges differ depending on whether airway or nasal NO is be-ing measured. In addition to appropriate calibra-tion gases, a zero gas free of NO is also required. Ambient air can be drawn through an NO scrubber to provide the zero gas. Chemiluminescence analyz-ers are sensitive to changes in ambient conditions, especially temperature, and may require recalibra-tion if conditions change. Sample inlet flow also af-fects the temperature of the reaction chamber and must be carefully controlled.

An **electrochemical** sensor has been devel-oped, based on the amperometric technique that can measure exhaled nitric oxide. The technique uses the production of a current when a voltage potential is applied between two electrodes (basic principle used in the P_{O_2} electrode). The utiliza-tion of this analyzer allowed for the development of a handheld (portable) exhaled nitric oxide de-vice (Fig. 11.26).

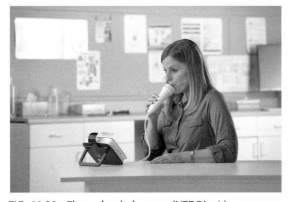

FIG. 11.26 **Electrochemical sensor (VERO)** with a computer incentive that gives the patient feedback so that he or she exhales at the correct flow rate into the analyzer. (Courtesy Aerocrine with Circassia Pharmaceuticals Inc., Chicago, IL.)

Gas-Conditioning Devices

Interference from water vapor or CO_2 in expired gas is common to many types of gas analyzers. These two gases are usually removed by chemical scrubbers.

CO_2 may be absorbed by passing the sample through granules containing either barium hy-droxide ($Ba[OH]_2$) or sodium hydroxide (NaOH). Granules containing NaOH usually have a light-brown appearance that changes to white when saturated with CO_2. $Ba(OH)_2$ (Baralyme) is usually supplied with an indicator (ethyl violet), which changes from white to purple when saturated with CO_2. Both NaOH and $Ba(OH)_2$ are mildly corrosive and may generate heat if exposed to high concen-trations of CO_2. Both generate water as a product of combination with CO_2. Therefore they should be placed upstream of any water vapor absorber used in the same circuit.

Water vapor is absorbed by passing the humidi-fied gas over granules of anhydrous calcium sulfate ($CaSO_4$ [Drierite]) or silica gel. These substances are termed *desiccants*. $CaSO_4$ usually contains an indica-tor that changes from blue to pink when saturated with water vapor. Some analyzers use silica gel to remove water vapor.

Conditioning of gas that contains water va-por may also be accomplished with special sam-ple tubing (Nafion). This tubing is permeable to water vapor. Sample gas passing through the tub-ing equilibrates its water vapor pressure with that of the surrounding atmosphere. Water vapor is not removed; it remains constant at a known level. If wet gas (e.g., expired air) is passed through the tubing, the sample falls to ambient humidity. If dry gas (e.g., calibration gas) is passed through the tubing, the sample rises to ambient humidity. This allows corrections for water vapor pressure to be ac-curately applied, as long as the ambient humidity level is known.

Failure to adequately remove water vapor or CO_2 from a gas sample usually results in dilution of the remaining gases. Dilution lowers the fractional concentration of the gas being analyzed. In some types of analyzers (e.g., thermal conductivity), CO_2 or water vapor may also directly alter the output of the analyzer. Chemical scrubbers or permeable tubing should always be replaced according to the manufacturer's recommendations.

BLOOD GAS ANALYZERS, OXIMETERS, AND RELATED DEVICES

Measurements of arterial or mixed venous blood gases include the determination of Po_2, Pco_2, and pH. Calculation of arterial oxygen concentration (Sao_2), bicarbonate (HCO_3^-), total CO_2, base excess, and other variables depends on measurements derived from one or more of the three primary electrodes. Oxyhemoglobin saturation, as well as other forms of Hb, is measured with a multiwavelength oximeter. Oxyhemoglobin saturation may also be estimated with a pulse oximeter. Other methods of assessing blood gases and oxygen saturation rely on transcutaneous electrodes and reflective spectrophotometry.

pH Electrodes

The traditional glass pH electrode contains a solution of constant pH on one side of a glass membrane. The sample to be analyzed is brought into contact with the other side of the pH-sensitive glass (Fig. 11.27). The difference in pH on either side of the glass causes a potential difference or voltage. To measure this potential, two half-cells are used: one for the constant solution and one for the sample. The constant solution half-cell (i.e., the measuring electrode) is usually a silver–silver chloride wire. The external half-cell is usually a saturated calomel (i.e., approximately 20% KCl) electrode called the *reference electrode.* The reference electrode makes contact with the unknown solution by means of a permeable membrane or a liquid junction. These half-cells are connected to a voltmeter calibrated in pH units. The voltage difference between the two electrodes is proportional to the pH difference of the solutions. Because the pH of one solution is constant, the developed potential is a measure of the pH of the sample. This type of analysis is thus referred to as *potentiometric* because a potential is measured. Potentiometric

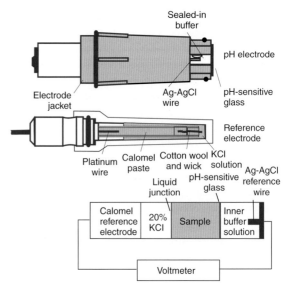

FIG. 11.27 pH and reference electrodes. The pH electrode is a microelectrode, shown here with its plastic jacket *(top).* At the tip is a silver–silver chloride wire in a sealed-in buffer behind pH-sensitive quartz glass. The reference electrode *(center)* contains a platinum wire in calomel paste that rests in a 20% KCl solution. The blood sample is introduced in such a way that it contacts the measuring electrode tip and the KCl. A voltmeter measures the potential difference across the sample, which is proportional to the pH.

electrodes are widely used in instruments with permanent electrodes and in some disposable cartridge-based systems.

pH can also be measured by an optical pH indicator. The indicator is an azo-dye substance in a cellulose membrane; the indicator exists in an acidic and basic form. Each of the two forms absorbs light in different regions of the spectrum (i.e., blue and red). The acidic form absorbs blue light, whereas the basic form absorbs red light. Light is passed through the blood sample and analyzed at different wavelengths. Increased absorbance in the blue wavelength indicates a lower pH, whereas increased absorbance in the red portion of the spectrum indicates a higher pH. By analyzing the absorptions at multiple wavelengths, the actual pH can be determined. This method is used in some cartridge-based blood gas analyzers.

A third method used for measuring pH in blood gas analysis uses a fluorescent chemosensor or optode. The optode has a pH-sensitive fluorescent indicator dye that exists in two forms (protonated and deprotonated). The deprotonated form fluoresces (emits light), but the protonated form (higher H^+ concentration) does not. By measuring the fluorescence, the pH can be measured.

Protein contamination of the pH-sensitive glass is a common problem that increases with the number of specimens analyzed. Routine cleaning with a proteolytic agent (e.g., bleach) reduces the buildup of protein on the electrode tip. KCl depletion or blockage of the reference junction can also cause pH electrode malfunction. Contamination of reagents used for pH electrode calibration may also result in measurement errors. Daily (or more frequent) use of suitable QC materials can detect these and other problems (see Chapter 12). pH measurements made with optical methods are dependent on how well the sample is mixed. Poorly mixed specimens may result in absorbances that do not accurately reflect the acid–base status of the patient. Fluorescent optodes are designed to separate the blood specimen from the sensor itself using an isolation layer to prevent contaminants from affecting the sensor.

Pco₂ Electrodes

Traditional Pco_2 electrodes (Severinghaus electrodes) measure Pco_2 potentiometrically using an adaptation of the pH electrode (Fig. 11.28). A combined pH-reference electrode is placed inside of a membrane-tipped plastic jacket. The jacket is filled with a bicarbonate electrolyte. The membrane is usually Teflon or a similar material permeable to CO_2 molecules. A spacer or wick made of nylon is sometimes placed between the pH-sensitive glass and the membrane. The spacer ensures that a thin layer of bicarbonate electrolyte is in contact with the electrode. When the blood sample is introduced at the tip of the electrode, CO_2 diffuses across the membrane. CO_2 is hydrated in the electrolyte according to the following equation:

$$CO_2 + H_2O \leftrightarrow H_2CO_3 \leftrightarrow H^+ + HCO_3^-$$

The higher the Pco_2, the more the equation is driven to the right. The change in H^+ concentration is proportional to the change in Pco_2. The electrode detects the change in Pco_2 as a change in pH of the electrolyte (i.e., a potentiometric measurement). The voltage developed is exponentially related to Pco_2. A tenfold increase in Pco_2 is approximately equal to a decrease of 1 pH unit. The partial pressure of CO_2 can be determined by calibrating the pH change when the electrode is exposed to gases with known Pco_2 values.

PF TIP 11.7

Computerized blood gas analyzers do an excellent job of monitoring analyzer function and detecting problems. Automated calibration allows tracking of electrode or sensor performance. The function of traditional electrodes is monitored by evaluating drift or trends during calibration. Optical sensors can be checked before and during measurements to detect abnormal responses. If either electrode or sensor errors are discovered, an alert is displayed.

Another method of measuring Pco_2 uses infrared absorption of dissolved CO_2 at three different wavelengths. By modulating the length of the light path through the specimen, absorption caused by factors other than the blood itself can be factored out. Once the concentration of CO_2 has been determined (solving for three different wavelengths), the Pco_2 can be calculated by dividing the concentration by the solubility factor for CO_2.

Pco_2 can also be measured with optical fluorescence. An optode similar to that used for pH measurements (see the preceding section) is covered by a membrane that is permeable to CO_2. CO_2 diffuses into the optode, where it forms carbonic acid and lowers the pH. As the pH decreases (more H^+), there is less fluorescence, and Pco_2 can be measured indirectly in much the same way as in the traditional electrode.

The most common problem with traditional Pco_2 electrodes is degradation or contamination

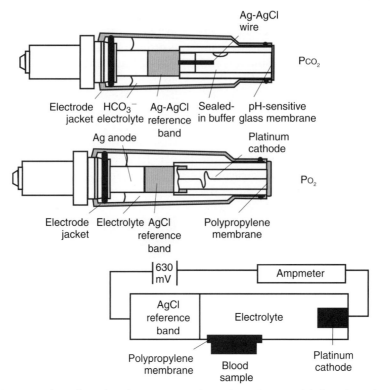

FIG. 11.28 P_{CO_2} and P_{O_2} electrodes. The P_{CO_2} (Severinghaus) electrode is a modified pH electrode. The electrode has a sealed-in buffer; an Ag-AgCl reference band is the other half-cell. The entire electrode is encased in a Lucite jacket filled with a bicarbonate electrolyte. The jacket is capped with a Teflon membrane that is permeable to CO_2. A nylon mesh (not shown) covers the pH-sensitive glass, acting as a spacer to maintain contact with the electrolyte. CO_2 diffuses through the Teflon membrane, combines with the electrolyte, and alters the pH (see text). The change in pH is displayed as the partial pressure of CO_2. The P_{O_2} (polarographic or Clark) electrode contains a platinum cathode and a silver anode. The electrode is polarized by applying a slightly negative voltage of approximately 630 mV. The tip is protected by a polypropylene membrane that allows O_2 molecules to diffuse but prevents contamination of the platinum wire. O_2 migrates to the cathode and is reduced, picking up free electrons that have come from the anode through a phosphate–potassium chloride electrolyte. Changes in the current flowing between the anode and cathode result from the amount of O_2 reduced in the electrolyte and are proportional to the partial pressure of O_2.

of the permeable membrane. Protein or debris deposited on the membrane slows the diffusion of CO_2. Equilibrium between the sample and electrode may not be achieved. Electrolyte depletion or exhaustion in the jacket around the electrode may also occur with extended use. Careful attention to shifts in electrode performance, during either calibration or control runs, can detect these common problems. Routine maintenance includes replacing the membrane and refilling the electrode with fresh electrolyte. Most manufacturers provide a kit

that contains a disposable jacket with a membrane and fresh electrolyte. Analyzers that use single-use electrodes eliminate most of the listed problems related to the membrane and electrolyte in the electrode.

Analyzers that use the infrared photometric methodology typically have single-use measurement cuvettes, eliminating problems of contamination of the measuring chamber. However, photometric absorption measurements require that the specimen be well mixed. Fluorescent optode analyzers use an optical isolation layer to prevent contaminants and stray light from entering the optode. Guidelines for QC of blood gas electrodes are included in Chapter 12.

Po₂ Electrodes

The standard Po₂ electrode (Clark electrode) consists of a platinum cathode that is usually a thin wire encased in plastic or glass, together with a silver–silver chloride (Ag-AgCl) anode (see Fig. 11.28). Both anode and cathode are placed inside a plastic jacket tipped with a polypropylene or polyethylene membrane. This membrane is semipermeable and allows the diffusion of oxygen molecules. The jacket is filled with phosphate–potassium chloride buffer. A polarizing voltage of approximately 630 mV is applied to the electrode. The cathode is slightly negative with respect to the anode. Because the electrode is polarized, it is referred to as a *polarographic* electrode. Oxygen is reduced (i.e., takes up electrons) at the cathode according to the following equation:

$$O_2 + 2H_2O + 4e^- \rightarrow 4OH^-$$

Electrons (e in the preceding equation) are supplied by the Ag-AgCl anode. Electrons flow from the anode to the cathode with a current proportional to the number of molecules of O_2 reduced. Each O_2 molecule can take up four electrons, and the greater the number of O_2 molecules present, the greater the current. The membrane causes a diffusion limitation to the number of molecules reaching the electrode. The greater the partial pressure on the sample side of the membrane, the higher the rate of diffusion. The measurement of the current **(amperometric)** developed within the electrode is therefore proportional to Po₂.

Optical methods of measuring Po₂ include phosphorescence and **fluorescence quenching.** In each of these methods, a dye that emits light and is sensitive to the presence of O_2 is used (Fig. 11.29). The higher the Po₂ is in the sensor or optode, the lower the phosphorescence or fluorescence (i.e., increased quenching of emitted light).

As with the Pco₂ electrode, contamination or degradation of the membrane alters diffusion of O_2 and can result in erratic measurements.

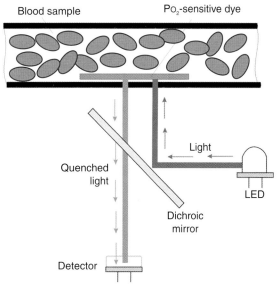

FIG. 11.29 Phosphorescence and luminescence quenching. Quenching of light emitted either by phosphorescence or luminescence can be used to measure the concentration of an analyte, such as the partial pressure of oxygen in blood. Light from a light-emitting diode (LED) bounces off a dichroic mirror and is directed toward an indicator (e.g., dye) that fluoresces. In the case of oxygen, the higher the Po₂, the more the emitted light is quenched. The emitted light then passes through the dichroic mirror and strikes a detector (e.g., a photocell or coupled charge device) that provides a measure of the Po₂.

Depletion of the phosphate buffer can also cause a change in electrode sensitivity. Most polarographic electrodes use a platinum wire of a small diameter to reduce the actual consumption of O_2 at the tip of the electrode. The exposed surface of the platinum cathode gradually becomes plated with metal ions and must be periodically polished to maintain its sensitivity. Alternatively, the entire electrode can be replaced.

Because the membrane causes a diffusion limit to O_2 molecules reaching the cathode, the electrode performs differently when exposed to liquid versus gas samples. Many blood gas systems use gas to calibrate the Po₂ electrode. Noticeable differences may result when the electrode is then used to analyze the tension of O_2 dissolved in a liquid (e.g., blood). These differences are usually compensated for by correcting the Po₂ with an empirically determined gas-to-liquid factor.

Laboratory Analyzers

Although the gas-measuring (Po_2 and Pco_2) electrodes and the pH electrode system can each be used separately, all three are usually implemented together in a blood gas analyzer (Fig. 11.30). The three electrodes are mounted in a single measuring chamber. This allows a small blood sample (≤ 200 μL) to be analyzed. Most blood gas analyzers are microprocessor controlled. Sample aspiration, rinsing, and calibration can all be done automatically with program control. Standardization of these functions, especially calibration, reduces measurement error and improves precision. The microprocessor can calculate other blood gas values derived from pH, Pco_2, and Po_2, including HCO_3^-, total CO_2, and base excess (BE). In addition to pH, Pco_2, and Po_2, most modern laboratory analyzers incorporate a hemoximeter to provide total Hb and its derivatives (e.g., O_2Hb, COHb). Computerized analyzers can monitor automated calibrations and electrode performance to alert the technologist of existing or impending problems. The computer can monitor the level of reagents and calibrating solutions/gases as well. Some analyzers automatically perform QC runs (i.e., auto QC) and monitor the results.

Point-of-Care Analyzers

To provide rapid results of critical analytes (e.g., blood gases and electrolytes), portable or bedside analyzers (i.e., point-of-care [POC]) have become widely available (Fig. 11.31). These devices are typically designed for use in the emergency department, critical care unit, or outpatient clinic. Most can be battery operated, but some POC instruments require standard power. Techniques for blood gas measurement differ slightly among models. Some

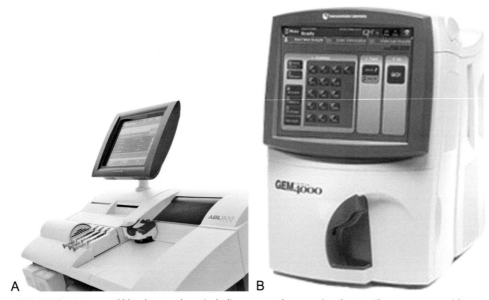

FIG. 11.30 Automated blood gas analyzer, including spectrophotometric oximeter. These systems provide automatic sample handling, flushing, and calibration. Results of sample analysis and calibrations are displayed using an integrated computer and display terminal. pH, Pco_2, and Po_2 are measured; HCO_3^-, total CO_2, standard bicarbonate, and other variables are calculated. This system also incorporates a spectrophotometric oximeter for analysis of Hb, O_2Hb, COHb, and MetHb. Base excess is calculated with HCO_3^-, calculated from the blood gas analysis and Hb measured by the oximeter. Additional parameters can include bilirubin, electrolytes, glucose, and lactate. (A, ABL800, courtesy Radiometer America, Westlake, OH. B, GEM, courtesy Instrumentation Laboratories, Bedford, MA. C, Siemens Rapid Lab, courtesy Siemens Healthcare, Tarrytown, NY.)

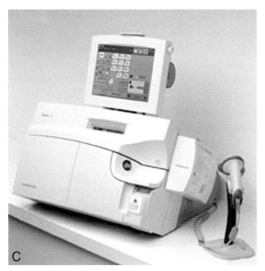

FIG. 11.30, CONT'D

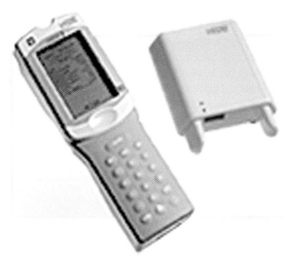

FIG. 11.31 Point-of-care (POC) blood gas analyzer. This handheld POC blood gas analyzer uses microelectrodes. It is battery powered, so it can be used in a variety of clinical settings. (Courtesy i-Stat Corp., East Windsor, NJ.)

POC blood gas analyzers use microelectrodes similar to those described previously, whereas others use spectrophotometry, infrared spectroscopy, or fluorescence quenching methods. Reagents, calibration materials, and waste containers are usually contained in disposable cartridges. Some POC systems use cartridges that allow a fixed number of analyses, whereas others use a single-patient sample chamber. Calibrations for POC systems that use multiple-specimen cartridges are usually performed in the traditional manner (see Chapter 12). These POC instruments use aqueous buffers in the single-patient chamber to perform calibration immediately before sample analysis. Single-use devices often have the sample chamber precalibrated by the manufacturer. Many POC instruments include ion-specific electrodes for analysis of electrolytes (e.g., K^+, Na^+, and Ca^+) along with other metabolites and hematocrit. A few POC analyzers also incorporate hemoximetry in addition to pH, P_{CO_2}, and P_{O_2}.

The accuracy and precision of most POC blood gas analyzers appear comparable to those obtained with standard laboratory instruments. Routine analysis of multiple levels of QC material is required to assess precision. However, because of the design of the sensors and the fact that reagents and reference electrodes may not be required, some cartridge-based systems require QC only when the cartridge is changed. Analysis of unknown specimens and comparison with other instruments or laboratories (proficiency testing) are required to determine accuracy.

Transcutaneous P_{O_2} and P_{CO_2} Electrodes

The transcutaneous O_2 electrode (tcP_{O_2}) operates on a principle similar to that of the polarographic electrode. The tcP_{O_2} electrode typically consists of a ring-shaped silver anode heated by a coil to increase blood flow at the skin placement site. Inside the circular anode is a platinum cathode (Fig. 11.32). All elements are enclosed in a plastic case. The face of the sensor is covered by a Teflon membrane. Electrolyte (KCl) is placed between the membrane and the sensor. A second layer of electrolyte and a cellophane membrane are added to form a double membrane. The current between the silver anode and platinum cathode is proportional to the P_{O_2} diffusing through the skin and membrane. A feedback controller keeps the temperature constant at the skin site. This also compensates for changes in capillary blood flow and stabilizes the measurement.

The gradient between tcP_{O_2} and Pa_{O_2} is relatively constant in patients with normal cardiac output. In neonates, there is a close correlation between transcutaneous and Pa_{O_2}. In hemodynamically stable adults, tcP_{O_2} is approximately 80% of Pa_{O_2}.

Measurement of tcP_{O_2} can trend oxygenation when this gradient has been established. In patients with reduced cardiac output, the gradient between tcP_{O_2} and Pa_{O_2} widens. Conditions that affect perfusion to the skin may also alter the gradient between arterial and tcP_{O_2}.

Transcutaneous measurements of P_{CO_2} are possible with a sensor that uses a CO_2-permeable membrane like that in the traditional blood gas electrode. CO_2 diffuses through the skin and into the sensor. tcP_{CO_2} and tcP_{O_2} sensors typically require calibration. This is usually accomplished by attaching the sensor to a port that exposes it to a calibration gas. Several types of transcutaneous monitors combine tcP_{CO_2} with tcP_{O_2} or pulse oximetry (Sp_{O_2}).

Most transcutaneous monitors heat the skin site from 40°C to 45°C. The increased temperature "arterializes" capillary blood flow. The fastest response times are usually attained at the highest temperature setting. However, this necessitates moving the electrode every 3 to 4 hours to prevent burns. Changing sensor sites is particularly important in neonates because of the reduced thickness of their epidermis. Periodic recalibration of the electrode is necessary even if the sensor site has not been changed. After placement of the sensor, an interval of 5 to 30 minutes may be required for equilibration to be reached.

Spectrophotometric Oximeters

The **spectrophotometric oximeter** uses light absorption to analyze the saturation of hemoglobin (Hb) with O_2. The concentration of carboxyhemoglobin (COHb) or other forms of Hb (e.g., methemoglobin, sulfhemoglobin) can also be determined. This type of spectrophotometer is sometimes called a **CO-oximeter** or **hemoximeter.** In addition to various forms of Hb, spectrophotometric measurement principles (absorption of light) can be used to measure pH and P_{CO_2}, as described previously.

The hemoximeter analyzes the absorption of light in a blood sample at multiple wavelengths. At certain wavelengths, two or more forms of Hb have similar absorbances (Fig. 11.33). These common wavelengths are termed *isobestic points.* An isobestic point for oxyhemoglobin (O_2Hb), reduced Hb

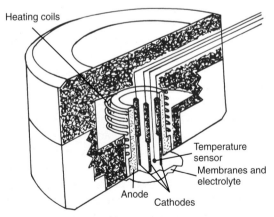

Heating coils

Temperature sensor

Membranes and electrolyte

Anode

Cathodes

FIG. 11.32 Transcutaneous P_{O_2} (tcP_{O_2}) electrode. Cross-sectional diagram of a tcP_{O_2} electrode showing a circular anode around a series of cathodes and a temperature sensor. A heating coil causes local hyperemia so that skin P_{O_2} closely resembles Pa_{O_2}. A double membrane separates the electrode proper from the skin. Because the electrode warms the skin, it must be moved periodically. A similar design uses a modified P_{CO_2} electrode to provide tcP_{CO_2}.

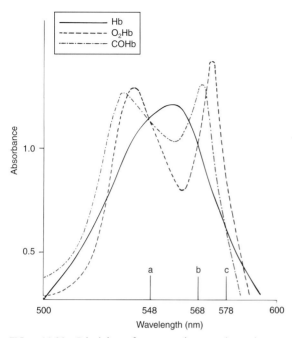

FIG. **11.33** Principle of spectrophotometric oximetry. Absorbance measurements are made at three or more distinct wavelengths (548, 568, 578 nm) as light passes through a sample of hemolyzed blood. At 548 nm, all three forms of Hb (Hb, O_2Hb, and COHb) have identical absorbances. At 568 nm, only Hb and HbO_2 coincide, whereas at 578 nm, Hb and COHb coincide. The solution of simultaneous equations provides the relative proportions of each species, as well as total Hb (see text).

(RHb), and COHb is 548 nm. At this wavelength, the absorbance of a mixture of the three pigments is directly proportional to the total concentration of Hb. An isobestic point for O_2Hb and RHb is 568 nm. The absorbance of COHb at this point is considerably higher. A change in absorbance at 568 nm compared with 548 nm indicates a change in the concentration of COHb relative to the sum of the concentrations of the other two species. The isobestic point for RHb and COHb is 578 nm, with O_2Hb absorbance being considerably greater. The difference in absorbance at 578 nm indicates the concentration of O_2Hb relative to the other two pigments. The total Hb concentration, O_2Hb, COHb, and methemoglobin (MetHb) saturation can be determined by analyzing absorbances and solving simultaneous equations.

The hemoximeter provides the true O_2Hb saturation (see the section on oxygen saturation in Chapter 6). This is particularly important if increased concentrations of COHb, MetHb, or other abnormal hemoglobins are present. Some automated blood gas analyzers calculate O_2Hb saturation. Calculated saturation is based on the measured P_{O_2} and pH at 37°C. This calculation assumes that the Hb has a normal P_{50} (see Chapter 6). Calculated O_2Hb may significantly overestimate true saturation in the presence of increased levels of COHb or methemoglobin. The hemoximeter provides the most accurate estimate of the actual O_2 saturation. Most laboratory blood gas analyzers and some POC analyzers combine blood gases and hemoximetry. These instruments provide pH, P_{CO_2}, P_{O_2}, and spectrophotometric measurements of Hb saturation, all performed with the same blood sample.

Hemoximeters may give erroneous Hb, O_2Hb, or COHb readings if forms of hemoglobin are present that the instrument does not recognize. For example, blood from a newborn (e.g., containing fetal Hb) will give erroneous values if analyzed by an oximeter set up for adult blood. Substances that cause light scattering in the specimen (e.g., lipids resulting from lipid therapy) may also cause false readings. To function properly, the hemoximeter must hemolyze the sample so that Hb molecules are suspended in solution rather than contained within the red cells. Hemolysis is accomplished by chemical or mechanical disruption of red cell membranes. Incomplete hemolysis results in light scattering within the sample rather than simple absorption. Sickle cells are not easily disrupted, particularly by chemical lysis, and may result in false readings for O_2Hb and COHb. Incomplete hemolysis may be difficult to detect unless whole-blood QC or proficiency testing is performed (see Chapter 12). Blood specimens used for hemoximetry must be well mixed, or the concentration of Hb (i.e., total Hb) may be incorrect. Most hemoximeters report errors such as incomplete hemolysis or light scattering.

In addition to measurements of O_2Hb, COHb, and MetHb saturations, the hemoximeter can calculate oxygen content and P_{50}. P_{50} can be estimated by measuring the actual saturation of a specimen (usually a venous sample with a saturation of less than 90%) and comparing this value with the calculated saturation based on Po_2 and pH of the same blood. This simplified method compares favorably with tonometering of the blood sample with various low-oxygen concentrations and constructing a dissociation curve.

Pulse Oximeters

Pulse oximeters (Fig. 11.34) are commonly used to assess oxygenation noninvasively. Pulse oximeters treat Hb as a filter that allows only red and near-infrared light to pass. The *Lambert–Beer law* relates

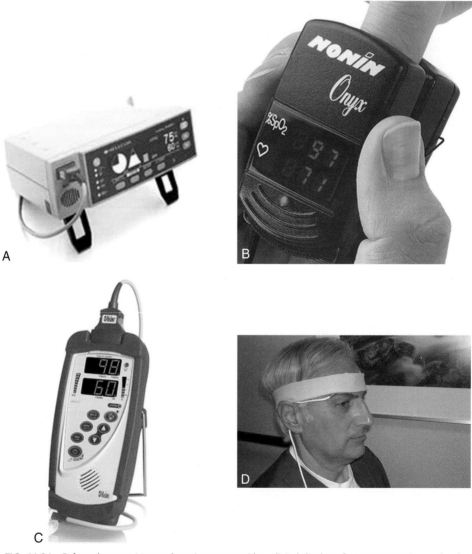

FIG. 11.34 Pulse oximeters. Most pulse oximeters provide a digital display of oxygen saturation and pulse rate. (A) Desktop unit. (B) A small, portable pulse oximeter that fits over the patient's finger. Miniaturized components allow a device of this size to be easily transported. (C) A sophisticated multiwavelength pulse oximeter that is capable of measuring Hgb, COHb, and MetHb, in addition to O_2Hb and pulse rate. (D) Reflectance pulse oximetry probe placed on a subject's forehead. (A and D, courtesy Nellcor, a Covidien brand, Mansfield, MA. B, Courtesy Nonin Medical, Inc., Plymouth, MN. C, Courtesy Masimo Corporation, Irvine, CA.)

total absorption in a system of absorbers to the sum of their individual absorptions.

In principle, the standard pulse oximeter measures the absorption of a mixture of just two substances, O_2Hb and RHb. The concentration of either one can be determined whether their extinction is measured while the path length stays constant. The wavelengths of light used in standard pulse oximetry are near 660 nm in the red region of the spectrum and near 940 nm in the near-infrared region. Extinction curves for O_2Hb and RHb show that reduced Hb has absorption 10 times higher than oxyhemoglobin at 660 nm, whereas O_2Hb has a higher absorbance (two to three times) at 940 nm. Calculating all possible combinations of the two forms of Hb (i.e., varying the saturation from 0% to 100%) allows the ratio of absorbances at the two wavelengths to be determined. As a result, a calibration curve can be constructed. The capillary bed does not follow the optical principles exactly as described by the Lambert–Beer law, so the calibration curve is derived empirically. The ratio of absorbances at the two distinct wavelengths is expressed as follows:

$$R = A_{660nm} / A_{940nm}$$

A series of R values (e.g., the calibration curve) is determined by relating this ratio to actual saturation measurements. Unlike the hemoximeter, which measures absorption in a hemolyzed blood sample, the pulse oximeter measures light passing through living tissue. The transmitted light is not only absorbed but also refracted and scattered. This causes the absolute accuracy of the pulse oximeter to be less than the accuracy of a hemoximeter.

The transmitted light at each wavelength consists of two components, the AC and DC components (Fig. 11.35). The AC component varies with the pulsation of blood. The DC component represents light absorbed by tissue and venous blood. The DC component is larger than the AC and is relatively constant. The amplitude of both AC and DC levels depends on the intensity of the incident light. The AC component represents the arterial blood because the arterioles pulsate in the light path. By dividing the AC level by the DC level at each of the

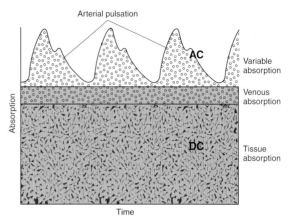

FIG. 11.35 Measurement principle of standard pulse oximetry. Transmitted light (at wavelengths of 660 and 940 nm) consists of two components. A large, fixed component, the DC component, represents light passing through tissue and venous blood without being absorbed. A smaller portion is pulsatile in nature and changes absorption as blood pulses through the arterioles; this is represented as the AC component. The pulse oximeter divides the AC signal by the DC signal at each wavelength, effectively canceling the DC component. The ratio of the AC signals at the two wavelengths is then a function of the relative absorptions of O_2Hb and RHb (see text). Modern pulse oximeters include sophisticated digital filters to better distinguish the AC and DC components of the signal. Some oximeters operate with additional wavelengths and can detect other forms of Hb (e.g., COHb and MetHb).

two wavelengths, the AC component is effectively corrected. The AC component then becomes a function of the extinction of O_2Hb and RHb. The ratio just described then becomes:

$$R = \frac{AC_1 / DC_1}{AC_2 / DC_2}$$

where:

1 = red wavelength (660 nm)
2 = near-infrared wavelength (940 nm)

Correcting the pulsatile component (AC) in this manner allows the pulse oximeter to ignore absorbances caused by venous blood, tissue, and skin pigmentation.

The light source used in pulse oximetry is the **light-emitting diode (LED).** LEDs are capable of emitting a very bright light near the 660- and 940-nm wavelengths required for analysis of Hb saturation. Light intensity is controlled by a feedback circuit that regulates the driving current to the LED. The greater the DC component resulting from pigmentation or venous blood, the greater the current supplied to the LED. One problem with LEDs is that the exact wavelength of light emitted varies with individual diodes. Each LED has its own center wavelength that may differ from 660 nm or 940 nm by as much as 15 nm. To overcome this variation, each oximeter must have a series of calibration curves programmed into it so that it can accommodate a range of LEDs. The extinction curves for RHb and O_2Hb are steep and different at 660 nm, so 10 or more calibration curves are typically required for the red-light range. Slight variations in center wavelength are less critical in the 940-nm region because the extinction characteristics of O_2Hb and RHb are the same from 800 to 1000 nm.

A photodiode detects transmitted light in the pulse oximeter. A single photodiode senses both red and near-infrared light. The microprocessor that controls the oximeter cycles the LEDs on and off separately 400 to 500 times per second. The oximeter also turns both LEDs off during each cycle. This allows the photodiode to detect ambient light caused by scattering and to offset the LED signals.

Pulse oximeter accuracy tends to decrease at low saturations. Low saturations occur as the concentration of RHb increases. RHb has a much higher absorbance at 660 nm than does O_2Hb. Therefore slight variations in the center wavelength of the red LED (as described) exaggerate the error in measured saturation. This is one reason pulse oximeters exhibit decreasing accuracy at lower saturations.

PF TIP 11.8

The standard pulse oximeter measures the saturation of available hemoglobin at two wavelengths. In these devices, the presence of COHb causes absorption at wavelengths similar to O_2Hb, and the pulse oximeter tends to read higher than the true saturation. MetHb causes increased absorption at both red and infrared wavelengths. This causes the ratio of the absorptions to be close to unity, and the pulse oximeter tends to read 85%. However, some pulse oximeters are capable of multiwavelength analysis and can detect COHb and MetHb, as well as O_2Hb (see text).

Because the AC, or pulsatile component, is usually much smaller than the DC component, detecting it can sometimes cause problems. Low perfusion or poor vascularity can cause the oximeter to be unable to measure the pulsatile component. Most oximeters display a warning message if the photodetector senses inadequate light levels. Motion artifact can also cause inaccuracy with pulse oximeters. Movement, especially shivering, often occurs in the same frequency range as the signal to be detected (i.e., arterial pulsations). If the motion is consistent and lasts long enough, it introduces a signal of approximately the same amplitude into both red and infrared channels. The pulse oximeter senses motion artifact as part of the DC component. This adds a large value to both the numerator and denominator of the ratio (R). The motion signal forces R toward a value of 1, which is equal to a saturation of 85% on the typical oximeter calibration curve. Some oximeters use multiple digital filters to discriminate motion artifact and produce a more reliable signal.

Most pulse oximeters use the AC signal from one channel (660 or 940 nm) to calculate pulse rate. An algorithm implemented by the microprocessor locates peaks in the waveform of the AC signal and counts them (see Fig. 11.35). Some oximeters use this signal to display graphic representations of pulse waveforms. Pulse oximeters that measure absorption at multiple wavelengths (see Fig. 11.34) can detect Hgb (SpHb), COHb (SpCO), and MetHb (SpMet), in addition to the standard SpO_2.

Reflective Spectrophotometers

Reflective spectrophotometry is based on the variable reflection of light by O_2Hb and RHb at different wavelengths. Just as the light absorbed by O_2Hb and RHb is a function of wavelength, so is the intensity of reflected or back-scattered light. Carefully spaced optical fibers can be used as transmitting and receiving paths for light. Reflective spectrophotometry can be used to monitor arterial saturation in a manner similar to that of pulse oximetry. Reflective spectrophotometry can also be incorporated into a pulmonary artery catheter to measure mixed venous oxygen saturation ($S\bar{v}_{O_2}$).

A reflective sensor can be placed at a site where a thin layer of tissue covers bone, such as the forehead. The oximeter then measures O_2Hb in a manner similar to that used for pulse oximetry but uses reflected rather than absorbed light. Pulse oximeters are available that can use either the regular sensor (i.e., absorption) or a reflective sensor.

A specially designed pulmonary artery (Swan-Ganz) catheter contains fiberoptic bundles (Fig. 11.36). This catheter has regular pressure-sensing ports, a balloon tip for flotation through the right side of the heart, and the capability for cardiac output determinations. Three LEDs similar to those used in pulse oximeters illuminate blood flowing past the tip of the catheter via one of the optical fibers. A photodetector senses the reflected light and converts its intensity into a signal. A microprocessor calculates two independent ratios of reflected light intensities from the three wavelengths. Combining two reflected light-intensity ratios reduces the instrument's sensitivity to pulsatile blood flow or changing hematocrit. This design also minimizes changes caused by light scattering from red cell surfaces and the walls of the blood vessel. $S\bar{v}o_2$ is calculated from the light ratios using programmed calibration curves, similar to those used for a pulse oximeter. As in a pulse oximeter, saturation measured is the saturation of functional Hb (see Chapter 6). $S\bar{v}o_2$ determination by this method tends to be higher than that measured by a hemoximeter, especially if large amounts of COHb or MetHb are present. $S\bar{v}o_2$ is then displayed and may be printed using a trend recorder (Fig. 11.37).

The reflective spectrophotometer must be routinely calibrated to ensure that observed changes in $S\bar{v}o_2$ are the result of physiologic phenomena rather than instrument drift. The catheter is usually standardized by calibrating it against an absolute color reference before insertion. After the catheter is in place, calibration is accomplished by adjusting the output to match saturation measured by a CO-oximeter. This type of calibration is accurate at the time it is performed but may change if there are shifts in pH or hematocrit. Because reflective spectrophotometers measure reflected light in whole blood that is flowing rather than transmitted light in a hemolyzed blood sample, their absolute accuracy is less than that of a hemoximeter.

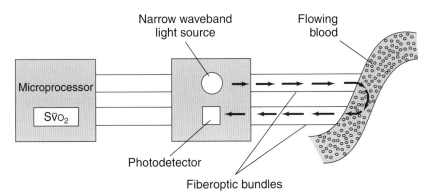

FIG. 11.36 Principle of reflective spectrophotometry. A diagrammatic representation of the components of an optical pulmonary artery catheter. This type of catheter (Swan-Ganz) is used for continuous monitoring of $S\bar{v}o_2$. Light-emitting diodes (LEDs) provide a narrow-waveband light source. Light is transmitted along one fiberoptic filament to blood flowing past the tip of the catheter. Light reflected from the blood is transmitted back to a photodiode by the second fiberoptic bundle. The light-intensity signals are then evaluated by a microprocessor to calculate light-intensity ratios. These ratios (usually two ratios are determined from three wavelengths) determine the $S\bar{v}o_2$. The principle of reflective absorption can also be used for pulse oximetry.

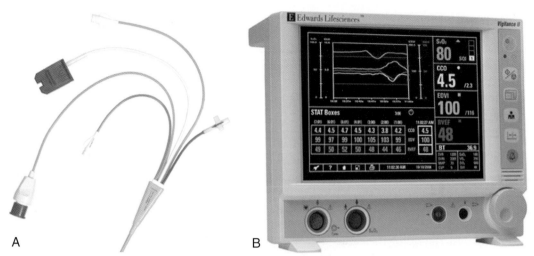

A   B

FIG. 11.37 (A) Pulmonary artery catheter. (B) Reflective spectrophotometer. A microprocessor-controlled reflective spectrophotometer. The pulmonary artery catheter contains fiberoptic bundles for continuous measurement of $S\overline{v}O_2$, as well as the usual pressure-measuring ports and sensors for both continuous cardiac output determinations and thermodilution cardiac output. The instrument displays mixed venous saturation digitally and as a trend graph that can be printed. High- and low-saturation alarms are included, along with a light-intensity alarm to detect artifact caused by catheter motion or problems with the fiberoptics. (Courtesy Edwards Lifesciences Corp., Irvine, CA.)

COMPUTERS FOR PULMONARY FUNCTION TESTING

All modern pulmonary function equipment uses computers in one form or another. Many spirometers use either a dedicated microprocessor (see Fig. 11.13) or are interfaced to a desktop or laptop (Fig. 11.38; see also Fig. 11.12). Computerized pulmonary function systems allow sophisticated data handling and storage, accurate calculations, graphic display of maneuvers, and enhanced reporting capabilities. Some laboratories use networked computers in which each pulmonary function system has a dedicated workstation. Networked systems allow rapid exchange of information and centralized data storage and retrieval.

Data Acquisition and Instrument Control

Computerized pulmonary function systems process analog signals from spirometers, plethysmographs, and gas analyzers. Equally important is the computer's capacity to control instrument functions, such as switching valves or recording signals. Computer control allows the technologist to manage complex test maneuvers. Data-acquisition software can be helpful in other ways too. Interactive incentives, such as candles that extinguish with flow and volume criteria, or other animations, can facilitate acceptable testing behaviors through visual feedback. These can be especially helpful with young subjects (Fig. 11.39A and B). Data-acquisition testing software may display the testing maneuvers in real time or once the maneuver is completed. Regardless, the software can provide feedback to the operator. This feedback may be related to a specific maneuver or on the overall test session (Fig. 11.39C and D). These visual prompts are helpful to the technologist in assessing the quality of the maneuver and test sessions, and they may also include the grading schemes provided by the ATS-ERS technical standard criteria.

Pulmonary Function Data Storage and Programs

Computerized pulmonary function systems, even small, portable spirometers, generate large volumes of patient data. Managing these large amounts of data is relatively easy via computer networks. Almost all PC-based systems support networking to some extent. Networked computers allow multiple

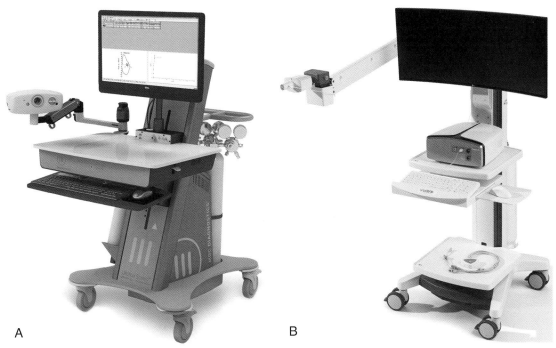

FIG. 11.38 **Computerized pulmonary function system.** Modern laboratory systems use personal computers (PCs) interfaced to spirometers, gas analyzers, body plethysmographs, and associated breathing circuitry. These automated systems (A and B) include a flow-sensing spirometer, gas analyzers, and a computer-controlled breathing circuit. The PC allows rapid and accurate processing of data, including calculation of test variables; calibration; body temperature, pressure, and saturation (BTPS) and standard temperature, pressure, dry (STPD) corrections; and graphic display. Data can be stored locally on a high-capacity hard disk or on a networked server. (A, courtesy MGC Diagnostics, St. Paul, MN. B, courtesy Vyaire, Mettawa, IL. B, The images of Vyntus One are © 2021 Vyaire Medical, Inc.; Used with permission.)

users to share data, as well as peripheral devices such as printers. The network typically consists of a primary computer or server. Other computers are then linked by one of several types of networks. Data can be transferred between any two computers linked by the system. The server usually maintains programs and data that all of the networked users need.

The format in which test data is stored is determined by (1) the complexity of the data, (2) the volume of data (i.e., number of tests done per month or year), and (3) how the data will be accessed. Three methods for data management are used with computerized pulmonary function systems.

Permanent Individual Patient Data Files

Patient data records are stored by creating individual files, usually on the PC's hard drive or the network. The volume of data stored in files of this type is limited only by the computer's operating system and the physical capacity of the storage device. Tabular and graphic data (e.g., F-V curves) may be stored in a single file or in separate files. Graphic data often requires more storage space than tabular data, depending on the format in which it is stored.

Database Storage

Many pulmonary function systems use a relational database format. Tests from different patients are stored as individual records in a file. Files (sometimes called *tables*) are then linked to form a database. One table may contain all spirometry records, a second all lung volume records, a third table D_{LCO} measurements, and so on. Complete tests are linked across files by an index using patient number or test date. A database structure allows for sorting, selecting, searching, and editing of patient data. Some applications of a database system for pulmonary function data include the following:

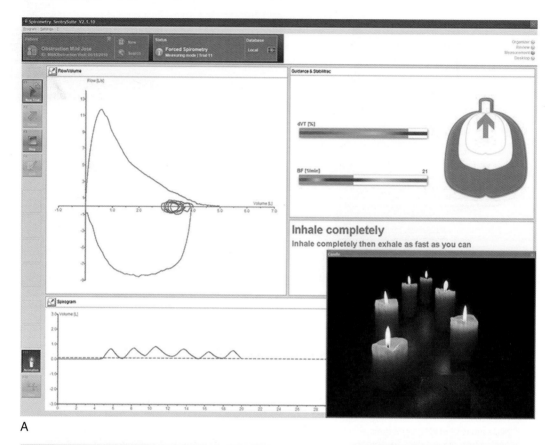

A

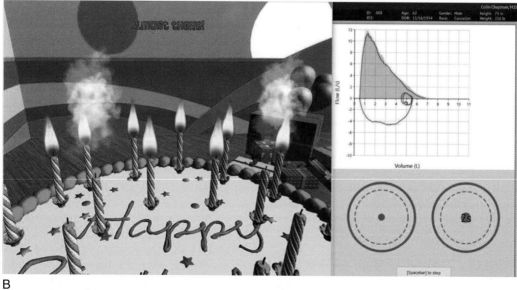

B

FIG. 11.39 Data-acquisition software. (A) Data-acquisition software can be helpful in testing subjects via visual incentives such as blowing out candles as in these examples. (B) These interactive programs may help in achieving acceptable spirometry results, especially in the younger population. (A, © 2021 Vyaire Medical, Inc.; Used with permission; D, Courtesy of Morgan Scientific Inc, Haverhill, MA.)

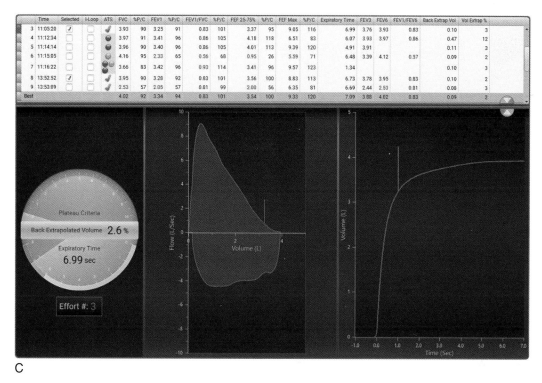

	Time	Selected	I-Loop	ATS	FVC	%P/C	FEV1	%P/C	FEV1/FVC	%P/C	FEF 25-75%	%P/C	FEF Max	%P/C	Expiratory Time	FEV3	FEV6	FEV1/FEV6	Back Extrap Vol	Vol Extrap %
3	11:05:20	✓		✓	3.93	90	3.25	91	0.83	101	3.37	95	9.05	116	6.99	3.76	3.93	0.83	0.10	3
4	11:12:34				3.97	91	3.41	96	0.86	105	4.18	118	6.51	83	6.07	3.93	3.97	0.86	0.47	12
5	11:14:14				3.96	90	3.40	96	0.86	105	4.01	113	9.39	120	4.91	3.91			0.11	3
6	11:15:05				4.16	95	2.33	65	0.56	68	0.95	26	5.59	71	6.48	3.39	4.12	0.57	0.09	2
7	11:16:22				3.66	83	3.42	96	0.93	114	3.41	96	9.57	123	1.34				0.10	3
8	13:52:52	✓		✓	3.95	90	3.28	92	0.83	101	3.56	100	8.83	113	6.73	3.78	3.95	0.83	0.10	2
9	13:53:09			✓	2.53	57	2.05	57	0.81	99	2.00	56	6.35	81	6.69	2.44	2.53	0.81	0.08	3
Best					4.02	92	3.34	94	0.83	101	3.54	100	9.33	120	7.09	3.88	4.02	0.83	0.09	2

C

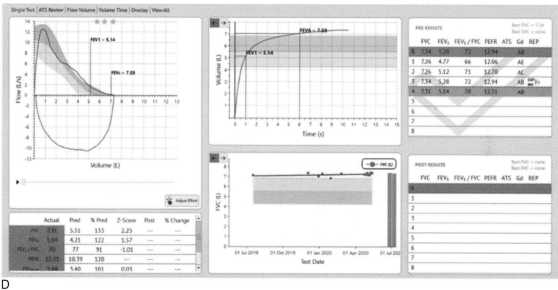

D

FIG. 11.39, CONT'D   (C and D) Data-acquisition software can also assist the operator in assessing the quality of the test by assigning grades and visual color feedback to the testing personnel. (A, courtesy Vyaire, Mettawa, IL. B and C, courtesy Morgan Scientific Inc, Haverhill, MA. D, courtesy MGC Diagnostics, St. Paul, MN.)

Serial comparisons of multiple tests on a single patient may be extracted to plot a trend:

- Data from longitudinal studies on groups of patients may be extracted for statistical analysis or exported to an external program.
- Queries may be performed to extract data that match selected criteria.
- An unlimited number of report formats may be generated.
- Reference equations may be stored in a database format. This structure allows input of user-defined equations for predicting normal values.
- Data may be retrieved and posted to an electronic medical record (EMR)

Relational database systems support a special command language called *Structured Query Language* (SQL). SQL databases (or similar) provide a standardized means for the user to enter and retrieve data, generate reports, and perform functions such as importing or exporting records. SQL databases can be easily restructured so that additional information can be added to existing databases.

Pulmonary function software often includes interpretation programs. Various interpretation algorithms may be available for the laboratory management team to select in the software as either a preliminary or final interpretation. Interpretation programs use algorithms for identifying obstructive, restrictive, combined, or normal patterns of pulmonary function. Spirometers designed for detecting obstruction in the primary care setting (i.e., office spirometers) typically include a computerized interpretation. More sophisticated algorithms can evaluate spirometry, lung volumes, and D_{LCO}, comparing measured and reference values. Although algorithms use logic similar to that of a clinician, they are usually not able to consider the patient's clinical history or other laboratory findings. Some programs are very sophisticated and can diagnose obstruction or restriction reasonably well. An incorrect computer interpretation may occur if test data are not acceptable or repeatable because of poor patient effort or technical problems. However, most spirometers include software functions that assess the acceptability and repeatability

of efforts. If the computerized interpretation considers data quality, an accurate interpretation is possible. Even if computerized interpretation is not implemented, computer-generated statements regarding test quality can be useful for traditional interpretation. Computer interpretation in no way substitutes for evaluation by a qualified clinician. It may be helpful when an immediate report of abnormalities is necessary, such as for screening purposes. If a computerized interpretation is included in the final report, it should be clearly labeled as such.

SUMMARY

- Spirometers that use either volume-displacement or flow-sensing principles are used for many different pulmonary function tests.
- Small, computerized spirometers (office spirometers) are often used for testing in many areas outside of the traditional pulmonary function laboratory.
- Small, portable peak flow devices have been developed and are widely used in clinical and home settings.
- Body plethysmography, using either a pressure box or flow box, is commonly used for measuring lung volumes and airway resistance. Its design and ease of use have benefited from advances in electronics and computerization.
- Various types of pulmonary gas analyzers and their principles of operation are discussed, along with how they are used for pulmonary function testing.
- Breathing valves and gas-conditioning devices are described, with particular attention to selection and maintenance.
- Blood gas electrodes, along with other technologies used for blood gas analysis, are reviewed. Spectrophotometric oximeters, pulse oximeters, and related monitors are illustrated.
- Information on the components of computer systems, data acquisition and storage, and specific interfaces to pulmonary function equipment are presented.

SELF-ASSESSMENT QUESTIONS

Entry-Level

1. Which of the following are true in regard to a dry rolling seal spirometer?
   1. It cannot be used to measure D_{LCO} by the single-breath method.
   2. Measured volumes need to be corrected to BTPS.
   3. Inspiratory and expiratory flows can be measured.
   4. Leaks do not affect spirometric measurements.
      a. 1, 3
      b. 2, 4
      c. 2, 3
      d. 1, 4

2. A 3-L syringe is used to check a wedge bellows spirometer, and the following results are observed:

Trial	Volume
1	2.78
2	2.55
3	2.92

   Which of the following best explains these findings?
   a. Automatic BTPS correction was turned off.
   b. The calibration syringe has a leak.
   c. The spirometer has a leak.
   d. The 3-L volume was injected too rapidly.

3. Flow integration is used to measure volume in which of the following?
   a. Dry-seal spirometer
   b. Pressure-differential pneumotachometer
   c. Turbine respirometer
   d. Dry rolling seal spirometer

4. Which of the following principles are used in flow sensing spirometers?
   1. Paired heated wires to detect temperature change
   2. Ultrasonic sound waves passing through a gas stream
   3. Molecular impaction on a gel membrane
   4. Pressure drop across a resistive element
      a. 1 and 4 only
      b. 2 and 3 only
      c. 1, 2, 4
      d. 2, 3, 4

5. A demand flow valve used to supply test gas for single breath D_{LCO} testing should provide
   a. a dead space of less than 10 mL.
   b. 6-L/sec flow at less than 10 cm H_2O.
   c. less than 5 cm H_2O flow resistance at 1 L/sec.
   d. a built-in, high-efficiency bacteria filter.

6. Which of the following are commonly used to measure carbon monoxide concentration for the $D_{LCO}sb$?
   1. Emission spectroscopy-type analyzer
   2. Gas chromatograph
   3. Fuel cell analyzer
   4. Infrared analyzer
      a. 1, 2
      b. 3, 4
      c. 1, 3
      d. 2, 4

7. Which of the following is commonly used to measure the He concentration in dilutional lung volume determinations?
   a. Thermal conductivity analyzer
   b. Emission spectroscopy analyzer
   c. Infrared absorption analyzer
   d. Chemiluminescence analyzer

8. A gas analyzer circuit uses chemical absorbers to remove water vapor and CO_2 from exhaled gases. Which of the following describes how these should be used?
   a. Both chemical absorbers should contain granules of the same color.
   b. The water vapor absorber should be placed before the CO_2 absorber.
   c. The CO_2 absorber should be placed before the water vapor absorber.
   d. The order of the absorbers is not important.

Advanced

9. Some plethysmographs have a built-in slow leak; the purpose of this leak is to
   a. allow oxygen to slowly enter the box while the door is closed.
   b. compensate for differences in the size of patients.
   c. prevent excessive pressure that may cause ear discomfort.
   d. help maintain thermal equilibrium when a patient is in the box.

10. Which of the following principles can be used to measure the pH in a blood gas analyzer?
    1. Molecular resonance spectroscopy
    2. Potential difference across pH-sensitive glass
    3. Optical absorption in a dye indicator at multiple wavelengths
    4. Chemiluminescent optodes sensitive to pH
       a. 1 and 3 only
       b. 2 and 4 only
       c. 1, 2, 3
       d. 2, 3, 4

11. A patient in the emergency department has his O_2 saturation measured by standard pulse oximetry, and an SpO_2 of 85% is recorded. Blood gases are drawn immediately, and the Sao_2 (by hemoximetry) is reported as 98%. A possible explanation of these findings is that the patient
    a. had polycythemia (increased hemoglobin).
    b. was shivering.
    c. was hyperventilating.
    d. had an elevated level of COHb.

12. Some pulse oximeters use sensors that can be placed on the forehead rather than on a finger or earlobe; these types of sensors
    a. are based on the principle of reflective spectrophotometry.
    b. measure absorption at five to eight distinct wavelengths.
    c. use the chemiluminescent quenching principle.
    d. can measure the total Hb concentration in addition to SpO_2.

13. Office spirometers used to screen for chronic obstructive lung disease should do which of the following?
    1. Incorporate automated interpretation of acceptable spirometry
    2. Measure the FEV_1, FEV_6, and FEV_1/FEV_6 ratio
    3. Provide feedback concerning test acceptability and repeatability
    4. Calculate the forced expiratory flow (FEF) 25% to 75% based on the largest FVC
       a. 1 and 3 only
       b. 2 and 4 only
       c. 1, 2, 3
       d. 1, 3, 4

14. When selecting a body plethysmograph, the box pressure transducer should be
    a. able to measure pressures of ± 50 cm H_2O at 8 Hz.
    b. calibrated with a 3-L volume injected at 1 to 2 Hz.
    c. connected to a slow leak with a time constant of 30 to 60 seconds.
    d. capable of measuring pressure changes as small as ± 0.2 cm H_2O at 8 Hz.

15. A pulmonary function laboratory wants to screen a large number of healthy subjects at multiple locations to establish reference values for spirometry. Which of the following methods would be the most appropriate?
    a. Office spirometers capable of producing printed reports
    b. Several volume-based spirometers interfaced to laptop computers
    c. Different types of flow-based spirometers to provide comparative values
    d. Portable spirometers communicating with an SQL database

SELECTED BIBLIOGRAPHY

Spirometers

Ferguson, G. T., Enright, P. L., Buist, A. S., et al. (2000). Office spirometry for lung health assessment in adults: a consensus statement from the National Lung Health Education Program. *Chest, 117*, 1146–1161.

Fuso, L., Accardo, D., Bevignani, E., et al. (1995). Effects of a filter at the mouth on pulmonary function tests. *European Respiratory Journal, 8*(2), 314–317.

Hiebert, T., Miles, J., & Okeson, G. (1999). Contaminated aerosol recovery from pulmonary function equipment. *American Journal of Respiratory and Critical Care Medicine, 159*, 610–612.

Johns, D. P., Ingram, C., Booth, H., et al. (1995). Effect of a microaerosol barrier filter on the measurement of lung function. *Chest, 107*, 1045–1048.

Kendrick, A. H., Johns, D. P., & Leeming, J. P. (2003). Infection control of lung function equipment: a practical approach. *Respiratory Medicine, 97*, 1163–1179.

Pulmonary function standards for cotton dust, 29 Code of Federal Regulations; 1910.1043 Cotton Dust, Appendix D, Occupational Safety and Health Administration; 1980.

Townsend, M. C., Hankinson, J. L., Lindesmith, L. A., et al. (2004). Is my lung function really that good? Flow-type spirometer problems that elevate test results. *Chest, 125,* 1902–1909.

Peak Flowmeters

Bongers, T., & O'Driscoll, B. R. (2006). Effects of equipment and technique on peak flow measurements. *BMC Pulmonary Medicine, 6,* 14.

Fonseca, J. A., Costa-Pereira, A., Delgado, L., et al. (2005). Pulmonary function electronic monitoring devices: a randomized agreement study. *Chest, 128,* 1258–1265.

Irvin, C. G., Martin, R. J., Chinchilli, V. M., et al. (1997). Quality control of peak flow meters for multicenter clinical trials. The Asthma Clinical Research Network (ACRN). *American Journal of Respiratory and Critical Care Medicine, 156,* 396–402.

Jensen, R. L., Crapo, R. O., & Berlin, S. L. (1996). Effect of altitude on hand-held peak flowmeters. *Chest, 109,* 475–479.

Plethysmographs

American Association for Respiratory Care. (2001). Clinical practice guideline: body plethysmography—2001 update. *Respiratory Care, 46,* 506–513.

DuBois, A. B., Bothello, S. Y., Bedell, G. N., et al. (1956). A rapid plethysmographic method for measuring thoracic gas volume: a comparison with nitrogen-washout method for measuring functional residual capacity in normal subjects. *Journal of Clinical Investigation, 35,* 322–326.

Wanger, J., Clausen, J. L., Coates, A., Pedersen, O. F., et al. (2005). Standardisation of the measurement of lung volumes. *European Respiratory Journal, 26,* 511–522.

Gas Analyzers

Alving, K., Jansson, C., & Nordvall, L. (2006). Performance of a new hand-held device for exhaled nitric oxide measurement in adults and children. *Respiratory Research, 7,* 67.

Hemmingsson, T., Linnarsson, D., & Gambert, R. (2004). Novel hand-held device for exhaled nitric oxide analysis in research and clinical applications. *Journal of Clinical Monitoring and Computing, 18,* 379–387.

Norton, A. C. (1979). Accuracy in pulmonary measurements. *Respiratory Care, 24,* 131–147.

Zar, H. A., Noe, F. E., Szalados, J. E., et al. (2002). Monitoring pulmonary function with superimposed pulmonary gas exchange curves from standard analyzers. *Journal of Clinical Monitoring and Computing, 17,* 241–247.

Blood Gas Electrodes, Oximeters, and Related Devices

Barker, S. J., Curry, J., Redford, D., et al. (2006). Measurement of carboxyhemoglobin and methemoglobin by pulse oximetry: a human volunteer study. *Anesthesiology, 105,* 892–897.

Berkenbosch, J. W., & Tobias, J. D. (2006). Comparison of a new forehead reflectance pulse oximeter sensor with a conventional digit sensor in pediatric patients. *Respiratory Care, 51,* 726–731.

Cariou, A., Monchi, M., & Dhainaut, J. F. (1998). Continuous cardiac output and mixed venous oxygen saturation monitoring. *Journal of Critical Care, 13,* 198–213.

Franklin, M. L. (1995). Transcutaneous measurement of partial pressure of oxygen and carbon dioxide. *Respiratory Care Clinics of North America, 1,* 119–131.

Gehring, H., Hornberger, C., Matz, H., et al. (2002). The effects of motion artifact and low perfusion on the performance of a new generation of pulse oximeters in volunteers undergoing hypoxia. *Respiratory Care, 47,* 48–60.

Kozlowski-Templin, R. (1995). Blood gas analyzers. *Respiratory Care Clinics of North America, 1,* 35–46.

Nishiyama, T., Nakamura, S., & Yamashita, K. (2006). Effects of the electrode temperature of a new monitor, TCM4, on the measurement of transcutaneous oxygen and carbon dioxide tension. *Journal of Anesthesia, 20,* 331–334.

Peruzzi, W. T., & Shapiro, B. A. (1995). Blood gas measurements. *Respiratory Care Clinics of North America, 1,* 1–157.

Severinghaus, J. W. (2002). The invention and development of blood gas analysis apparatus. *Anesthesiology, 97,* 253–256.

Severinghaus, J. W., & Bradley, A. F. (1958). Electrodes for blood P_{O_2} and P_{CO_2} determination. *Journal of Applied Physiology, 13,* 515–523.

Tremper, K. K., & Waxman, K. S. (1986). Transcutaneous monitoring of respiratory gases. In M. L. Nochomovitz, & N. S. Cherniack (Eds.), *Noninvasive respiratory monitoring.* New York, NY: Churchill Livingstone.

Tusa, J. K., & He, H. (2005). Critical care analyzer with fluorescent optical chemosensors for blood analytes. *Journal of Materials Chemistry, 125,* 2640–2647.

Computers

American Thoracic Society. (1986). Committee on Proficiency Standards for Clinical Pulmonary Laboratories. Computer guidelines for pulmonary laboratories. *American Review of Respiratory Disease, 134,* 628–632.

Beardsmore, C. S., Paton, J. Y., Thompson, J. R., et al. (2007). Standardizing lung function laboratories for multicenter trials. *Pediatric Pulmonology, 42,* 51–59.

Chapter 12

Quality Systems in the Pulmonary Function Laboratory

SUSAN BLONSHINE, BS, RRT, RPFT, FAARC, AE-C

CHAPTER OUTLINE

LEARNING OBJECTIVES

After studying the chapter and reviewing the figures, tables, and case studies, you should be able to do the following:

Entry-level

1. Describe the 12 quality system essentials and the path of workflow for pulmonary function testing.
2. Describe three types of mechanical quality control devices.
3. Perform and evaluate spirometry linearity testing on a flow-based system.
4. Determine whether spirometers, single-breath diffusing equipment, a plethysmograph, or a blood gas analyzer is "in control" using a control chart.
5. Compose technologist's comments to describe acceptable and unacceptable spirometry, D_{LCO}, and lung volumes.

Advanced

1. Evaluate results from a customer satisfaction survey and apply to process improvement.
2. Apply results obtained from biologic control subjects to troubleshoot pulmonary function equipment.

3. Describe two methods for performing quality control of a D$_{LCO}$ system.
4. Apply results obtained from D$_{LCO}$ system quality control to troubleshoot pulmonary function equipment.
5. Define and describe the three components of a quality manual—policy, process, procedure—as applied to each quality system essential (QSE).
6. Describe key components of an information management QSE.
7. Identify key components of a safety and infection control QSE for arterial blood gas collection and prevention of cross-contamination of pulmonary function equipment.

KEY TERMS

accuracy	decommissioning	procedures
back-pressure	D$_{LCO}$ simulator	processes
biologic control	drift	proficiency testing (PT)
calibration factor	gas analysis certificate	quality control (QC)
coefficient of repeatability (CR)	isothermal lung analog	quality system essential (QSE)
coefficient of variation (CV)	leak check	random error
computerized syringe	lung analog	serial dilution
control	maintenance	shift
correction factor	multiple-rule method	sine-wave rotary pump
corrective action	path of workflow (POW)	validation

The chapter discusses issues related to a quality system, as introduced in Chapter 1. Although an in-depth review of the quality system is beyond the scope of this chapter, an introduction to the basics of each **quality system essential (QSE)** and the path of workflow is included to move the laboratory toward total quality management. *Total quality management* may be defined as a management system for a customized customer-focused organization that involves all employees in continual improvement. The referenced Clinical and Laboratory Standards Institute (CLSI) documents will broaden the reader's understanding of each of the concepts introduced in the chapter and may be essential for meeting accreditation and regulatory standards. The concept of developing a quality manual that addresses policies, processes, and procedures is introduced. Each of the 12 QSEs is discussed, with examples for application to the pulmonary function (PF) laboratory. The *personnel QSE* addresses personnel standards, training, and competence assessment. Personnel who perform PF tests must make decisions during the **path of workflow** (**POW**; pretesting, testing, and posttesting) that determine the quality of the data obtained. Special attention is given to methods by which the PF technologist can

assess data quality through discussion of each component of the path of workflow. Documentation of PF data quality (e.g., acceptability, repeatability, and reproducibility) is discussed. *Repeatability* is the variance within a test session, whereas *reproducibility* refers to variance across test sessions.

The *equipment QSE* includes equipment standards for spirometers, plethysmographs, gas analyzers, D$_{LCO}$ systems, blood gas analyzers, and metabolic systems. Proper instrument maintenance and calibration are bases for obtaining acceptable and repeatable data. Records are maintained to document each of these activities. The chapter also deals with the *process control QSE,* which addresses specific **quality control (QC)** methods for equipment used in PF testing and blood gas analysis. Problems commonly encountered with various types of equipment are listed to guide in troubleshooting.

The *facilities and safety QSE* discusses safety and infection control as they relate to patients and to those performing PF tests.

Using the QSEs as a foundation for quality and incorporating each component of the path of workflow for each test performed leads to a final quality output. As in previous chapters, case studies and self-assessment questions are included.

QUALITY MANUAL

The initial step in building the quality system is developing a quality manual. The quality manual addresses policies for each of the 12 QSEs. Policies are written to answer the question: What do we do in our organization? Each policy describes the organization's intent and provides direction for the specific QSE. Policies for the *personnel QSE* often include the intent and direction for job descriptions and qualifications, orientation, training, competence assessment, and continuing education. Processes are described to transform the policy into action and answer the question: How does this happen in our pulmonary laboratory? **Processes** are generally a group of activities or procedures. There is a process to obtain reliable spirometry data that may result in a need for several procedures, such as QC, test performance, test result selection and reporting, selection of reference values, and interpretation of results (Table 12.1). **Procedures** answer the question: How do I do this activity? Each QSE incorporates policies, processes, and procedures to build a platform for the path of workflow to be followed for each test procedure.

TABLE 12.1

Spirometry Operating Process

Operating Process: Spirometry Test Result Selection and Reporting

Purpose	To describe the process for spirometry test result selection and reporting.	
Process	This process is supported by the steps and documents in the table that follows.	

What Happens	Who's Responsible	Results: Documents
1. Spirometry performed meeting ATS-ERS acceptability and repeatability criteria	Therapist/technologist	Procedures for • Spirometry performance
2. Largest FVC selected from acceptable maneuvers	Therapist/technologist	Procedures for • Data selection • Selection of best curve
3. Largest FEV_1 selected from acceptable maneuvers		
4. Instantaneous flows from the "best curve" selected[a]		
5. Highest peak flow selected		
6. All acceptable curves printed	Therapist/technologist	Procedures for • Data to print and maintain hard copies
7. Patient cooperation, effort, and standards not met documented	Therapist/technologist	Procedures for • Report comments • Data-entry criteria
8. Accuracy of demographic, environmental, and anthropometric data verified		
9. Accuracy of selected data verified		
10. Data stored	Therapist/technologist	
11. Report generated	Support staff	Procedures for • Report generation and entry into interpretation process

ATS-ERS, American Thoracic Society–European Respiratory Society; *FEV₁,* forced expiratory volume in the first second; *FVC,* forced vital capacity.
Expected results: Accurate and reliable test results.
[a] The "best curve" is selected from the largest sum of FVC + FEV_1.
From Blonshine, S., Mottram, C. D., Berte, L. M., et al. (2006). *Application of a quality management system model for respiratory services: Approved guidelines* (2nd ed.). CLSI document HS4-A2. Wayne, PA: Clinical and Laboratory Standards Institute.

QUALITY SYSTEM ESSENTIALS

Organization and Leadership

The organizational commitment to quality is essential and may be a requirement to comply with governmental and accreditation standards. The organization is responsible for the development of the quality manual and integration into the system by committing time and personnel to the process. The department and PF laboratory organizational structure is available in the quality manual. A visible management commitment to the implementation of the quality policies, seeking customer feedback, and responding to quality reports is required for success. Risk assessment of the pulmonary laboratory's work operations processes is included in the *organization QSE*. The pulmonary laboratory should set quality goals and objectives integrated with the organization's quality planning.

Customer Focus

The pulmonary laboratory should identify its customers and expectations. Customers include both external and internal groups. Examples of external customers include accreditation and governmental agencies, patients, physicians, nurses, clinical support services, asthma educators, home care companies, and payers. All staff members involved in the path of workflow are considered internal customers. An initial step is to evaluate the laboratory's capability to meet the identified expectations. Physicians ordering tests likely will have an expectation of how long it should take to schedule a patient for testing and the length of time to receive an interpreted copy of the report. Surveys will identify expectations met and the potential for continual improvement (Box 12.1). Complaints are recorded and managed according to the *nonconforming event management QSE*.

Facilities and Safety

The facility should be designed to support the workflow and accommodate the equipment to meet manufacturers' and standards expectations. It should support efficient processes. The environment, processes, and safety procedures must be compliant

---

BOX 12.1 PULMONARY FUNCTION LABORATORY CUSTOMER SERVICE SUMMARY

- How close to your scheduled appointment time were you called in for your test?
  - ☐ Before appointment time
  - ☐ On time
  - ☐ 30 minutes late
  - ☐ 1 hour late
  - ☐ Longer than 1 hour
- How well did the technologist explain your test?
  - ☐ Excellent
  - ☐ Very good
  - ☐ Good
  - ☐ Fair
  - ☐ Poor
- How knowledgeable and technically skilled was the technologist performing your procedure?
  - ☐ Excellent
  - ☐ Very good
  - ☐ Good
  - ☐ Fair
  - ☐ Poor
- How courteous and professional was your technologist?
  - ☐ Excellent
  - ☐ Very good
  - ☐ Good
  - ☐ Fair
  - ☐ Poor

Test performed: PFT ABG CPET O_2 titration
Comment: _____

Courtesy Mayo Clinic PF Laboratory, Rochester, MN.

---

with organizational and accreditation standards. Environmental conditions that may affect the quality of the test results are monitored and documented. The use of accurate room temperature, humidity, and barometric pressure monitors is a standard requirement. Although some equipment uses internal sensors, it is also prudent to maintain external (certified) monitors for environmental factors.

PF tests, including blood gas analysis, often involve patients with blood-borne or respiratory pathogens. Reasonable precautions applied to testing techniques and equipment handling can prevent cross-contamination among patients. Similar techniques can prevent infection of the technologist performing the tests.

Each laboratory should have written guidelines defining safety and infection control practices. The guidelines should be part of a policy and procedure manual (Box 12.2). Procedures should include, but not be limited to, handwashing techniques, the use of protective equipment such as laboratory coats and gloves, and guidelines for equipment cleaning. The handling of contaminated materials (e.g., waste blood) should be clearly described. Policies and procedures should include education of technologists regarding proper handling of biologic hazards. Department policies and procedures should be consistent with those mandated by individual hospitals or institutions. Most accrediting agencies require written plans for safety, waste management, and chemical hygiene. In the United States the Occupational Safety and Health Administration (OSHA) has published strict guidelines regarding the handling of blood and other medical waste (see the Evolve website at http://evolve.elsevier.com/Mottram/Ruppel). Safety training should be documented, and the training records should be maintained per institutional requirements, accreditation, and regulatory requirements in the records management system. Generally, some areas will require retraining on an annual basis.

BOX 12.2   PULMONARY FUNCTION PROCEDURE MANUAL

Items to be included in a typical procedure manual for a pulmonary function laboratory. For each procedure performed, the following should be present:

1. Description of each test performed in the laboratory and its purpose
2. Indications for ordering the test and contraindications, if any
3. Description of the general method(s) and any specific equipment required, including disposable supplies
4. Calibration of equipment required before testing (manufacturer's documentation may be referenced)
5. Patient preparation for the test, if any (e.g., withholding medication) and patient assessment before beginning the test
6. Step-by-step procedure for measurement/calculation of results; how to perform the measurement or calculation manually is useful for quality monitoring
7. Quality control guidelines with acceptable limits of performance and corrective actions to be taken when control values are outside of their limits
8. Safety precautions related to the procedure (e.g., infection control, hazards) and alert values that require physician notification with read-back of critical results
9. Description of results reporting
10. References for all equations used for calculating results and for predicted normals, including a bibliography
11. Documentation of computer protocols for calculations and data storage; guidelines for computer downtime and software upgrades
12. Dated signatures of medical and technical directors (may be electronic)

Pulmonary Function Tests

Historically, PF testing has not presented a significant risk of infection for patients or technologists. Most respiratory pathogens are spread by either direct contact with contaminated equipment or by an airborne route. Airborne organisms may be contained in droplet nuclei, on epithelial cells that have been shed, or in dust particles. The following guidelines can help reduce the possibility of cross-contamination or infection:

1. Disposable mouthpieces and nose clips should be used by the patient during spirometry. Reusable mouthpieces should be disinfected or sterilized after each use. Proper handwashing should be done immediately after direct contact with mouthpieces or valves. Gloves should be worn when handling potentially contaminated equipment. Hands should always be washed between patients and after removing gloves.
2. Tubing or valves through which subjects rebreathe should be changed after each test. Any equipment that shows visual condensation from expired gas should be disinfected before reuse. This is particularly important for maneuvers, such as the forced vital capacity (FVC), where there is a potential for mucus, saliva, or droplet nuclei to contaminate the device. Breathing circuit components should be stored in sealed containers (e.g., plastic bags) after disinfection.

3. Spirometers should be cleaned according to the manufacturer's recommendations. The frequency of cleaning should be appropriate for the number of tests performed. For open-circuit systems, only that part of the circuit through which air is rebreathed needs to be decontaminated between patients. Some flow-based systems offer pneumotachometers that can be changed between patients. Pneumotachometers not located proximal to the patient are less likely to be contaminated by mucus, saliva, or droplet nuclei. Disposable flow sensors should not be reused. Volume-displacement spirometers should be flushed using their full volume at least five times between patients. Flushing with room air helps clear droplet nuclei or similar airborne particulates. Water-sealed spirometers should be drained at least weekly and allowed to dry completely. They should be refilled with distilled water only. Bellows and rolling-seal spirometers should be disinfected on a routine basis. The spirometer may require recalibration after disinfecting.

4. Systems used for spirometry, lung volumes, and diffusing capacity tests often use breathing manifolds that are susceptible to contamination. Bacteria filters may be used to prevent contamination of these devices. Filters may impose increased resistance, affecting the measurement of maximal flows as well as Raw or conductance. Some types of filters show increased resistance after continued use in expired gas. The filter specifications and filtering capabilities should match the intended use. For example, a filter used with spirometry should have the filtering capabilities known for high flow. Spirometers with bacteria filters should be calibrated with the filter in line. If filters are used for procedures such as lung volume determinations, their volumes must be included in the calculations to account for the additional dead space.

5. Small-volume nebulizers, such as those used for bronchodilator administration or bronchial challenge, offer the greatest potential for cross-contamination. These devices, if reused, should be sterilized to destroy vegetative microorganisms, fungal spores, tubercle bacilli, and some viruses. Disposable single-use nebulizers are preferable but may not be practical for routines such as inhalation challenges. Metered-dose devices may be used for bronchodilator studies by using disposable mouthpieces or "spacers" to prevent colonization of the device. Common canister protocols for metered-dose inhaler usage have been evaluated in the laboratory, but usage is dependent on institutional guidelines.

6. Gloves or other barrier devices minimize the risk of infection for the technologist who must handle mouthpieces, tubing, or valves. Special precautions should be taken whenever there is evidence of blood on mouthpieces or tubing. There is a risk of acquiring infections such as tuberculosis or pneumonia caused by *Pneumocystis carinii* from infected patients. The technologist should wear a mask when testing subjects who have active tuberculosis or other diseases that can be transmitted by coughing. A face shield may be required in some scenarios. Refer to Chapter 1 for additional infection control considerations and information on testing in a pandemic.

7. Patients with respiratory diseases such as tuberculosis may warrant specially ventilated rooms, particularly if many individuals need testing. The risk of cross-contamination or infection can be greatly reduced by filtering and increasing the exchange rate of air in the testing room. Equipment can be reserved for testing infected patients only. Examples include the use of a spirometer for *Cepacia*-positive patients in a clinic patient room. Special patient organizations such as the Cystic Fibrosis Foundation may have additional requirements for infection control. Patients with known pathogens can also be tested in their own rooms or at the end of the day (to facilitate equipment decontamination).

8. Surveillance may include cultures of reusable components such as mouthpieces, tubing, and valves after disinfection.

Blood Gases

The Centers for Disease Control and Prevention (CDC) has established standard precautions that apply to personnel handling blood or other body fluids containing blood. Standard precautions apply to blood, semen, vaginal secretions, cerebrospinal fluid, synovial fluid, pleural fluid, pericardial fluid, and amniotic fluid. Some of these fluids (i.e., blood) are commonly encountered in the blood gas or PF laboratory. These fluids present a significant risk to the health care worker. Hepatitis B, HIV, and other blood-borne pathogens must be assumed to be present in these fluids.

Body fluids to which the standard precautions do *not* apply include feces, nasal secretions, sputum, sweat, tears, urine, and vomitus, unless they contain visible blood. Some of these fluids may be encountered in the PF laboratory. These fluids present an extremely low or nonexistent risk for HIV or hepatitis B. However, they are potential sources for nosocomial infections from other non–blood-borne pathogens. Standard precautions do not apply to saliva, but infection control practices such as the use of gloves and handwashing further minimize the risk involved in contact with the mucous membranes of the mouth.

PF TIP 12.1

The two most important practices for infection control in the PF laboratory are proper use of gloves and handwashing. Gloves should be worn anytime blood is handled or drawn, including handling of blood-tinged mouthpieces. Handwashing is essential to prevent cross-contamination. Hands should be washed between patient contacts; anytime mouthpieces, tubing, or nebulizers are handled; and when gloves are removed.

---

1. These standard precautions should be applied in the PF and/or blood gas laboratory: Treat *all* blood and body fluid specimens as potentially contaminated.
2. Exercise care to prevent injuries from needles, scalpels, or other sharp instruments. Do not resheath used needles by hand. If a needle must be resheathed, use a one-handed technique or a device that holds the sheath. Do not remove used unprotected needles from disposable syringes by hand. Do not bend, break, or otherwise manipulate used needles by hand. Use a rubber block or cork to obstruct used needles after arterial punctures. Use needle safety devices (now used in almost all blood gas kits) as described by the manufacturer. Place used syringes and needles, scalpel blades, and other sharp items in puncture-resistant containers. Locate the containers as close as possible to the area of use.
3. Use protective barriers to prevent exposure to blood, body fluids containing visible blood, and other fluids to which standard precautions apply. Examples of protective barriers include gloves, gowns, laboratory coats, masks, and protective eyewear. Gloves should be worn when drawing blood samples, whether from a needle puncture or an indwelling catheter. Gloves cannot prevent penetrating injuries caused by needles or sharp objects. Gloves are also indicated if the technologist has cuts, scratches, or other breaks in the skin. Protective barriers should be used in situations where contamination with blood may occur. These situations include obtaining blood samples from an uncooperative patient, performing finger or heel sticks on infants, and receiving training in blood drawing. Examination gloves should be worn for procedures involving contact with mucous membranes. Masks, gowns, and protective goggles may be indicated for procedures that present a possibility of blood splashing. Blood splashing may occur during arterial line placement or when drawing samples from arterial catheters.
4. Wear gloves while performing blood gas analysis. Laboratory coats or aprons resistant to liquids should also be worn. Protective eyewear may be necessary if there is a risk of blood splashing during specimen handling. Maintenance of blood gas analyzers, such as repair of electrodes and emptying of waste containers, should be performed while wearing similar protective gear. Laboratory coats or aprons should be left in the specimen-handling area. Blood waste products (e.g., blood gas syringes) should be discarded in clearly marked biohazard containers.
5. Immediately and thoroughly wash hands and other skin surfaces that are contaminated with blood or other fluids to which the standard precautions apply. Hands should be washed after removing gloves. Blood spills should be cleaned up using a solution of one part 5% sodium hypochlorite (bleach) in nine parts of water. Bleach should also be used to rinse sinks used for blood disposal.

Personnel

The *personnel QSE* is one of the most important elements in the PF laboratory quality system because of the impact of the technologist on the quality of the final product. The American Thoracic Society–European Respiratory Society (ATS-ERS) technical standard for spirometry also observed that the importance of the technologist was a key message from a patient survey. Job qualifications and duties across the path of workflow are outlined and maintained in job descriptions for all personnel in the pulmonary laboratory. The American Association of Respiratory Care (AARC) Clinical Practice Guidelines (CPGs) and the ATS-ERS standards outline job requirements and qualifications for individuals employed to perform PF tests. The ATS-ERS standards also suggest training and ongoing education for individuals in the laboratory. Both the training and the experience of the technologist affect the ability to engage with the patient and achieve optimal results.

An orientation/training plan and process are required for all new employees. An orientation manual and a training guide are developed and updated as required. The training manual may include, but is not limited to, quality management, safety, computer systems, ethics, work processes, and procedures. Records documenting the orientation and training processes are maintained according to the *document and records management QSE* (Table 12.2). Training occurs, and documentation is maintained when processes or procedures are updated or added. Performance of QC procedures has been identified as a primary training need in PF laboratories globally, regardless of professional credentials. Orientation also includes a review of the quality manual and application to work duties in the laboratory.

Competence assessment is required by The Joint Commission. Competence may be established initially through formal training programs and professional credentialing. One method of evaluating ongoing competence is completing the National Board for Respiratory Care (NBRC) examinations for the certified pulmonary function technologist (CPFT) or the registered pulmonary function technologist (RPFT). Both training and maintenance of competence are required elements of all pulmonary diagnostics services.

Adequate staffing is based on performance requirements, published time standards, and the number and type of patients to be tested. For example, young patients typically require additional time for testing. Infection control requirements may also affect patient flow in the laboratory. The AARC has published time standards for the PF laboratory. Performance appraisals are developed and maintained according to organizational requirements. Records are also maintained for personnel hiring, orientation, training, competence assessment, continuing education, and performance appraisals according to the quality policies and institutional, governmental, and accreditation requirements. The CLSI document on personnel and training and competence assessment provides more guidance that can be applied to PF laboratories.

Supplier and Inventory Management

The *supplier QSE* portion requires the laboratory to establish criteria for vendor qualification, selection, and evaluation. This is typically accomplished in partnership with the materials management team and involves identifying the supplies required for the work processes. It is good practice for the laboratory to maintain a copy of all purchase agreements, particularly for major equipment purchases.

The *inventory QSE* portion requires the laboratory to develop an inventory management system that identifies and maintains supplies for the work processes in a fiscally responsible environment. To meet regulatory requirements for consumables or critical supplies such as blood gas reagents, the laboratory must have processes and procedures documented. Records should be maintained with the date received, lot number, expiration dates, a note documenting whether acceptance criteria were met, date placed in service, expiration date, and disposition date if not used.

Equipment

The *equipment QSE* incorporates a management plan for selection and acquisition (SQ), installation qualification (IQ), identification, **validation,** reverification (also referred to as *performance qualification (PQ)*), calibration, use, maintenance, service, repair, and decommissioning. The QSE also

TABLE 12.2

Components of a Complete Clinical Service Training Program

Type of Employment Training	Contents
Quality	• Organization's quality system
	• Quality manual
	• Service's path of workflow
	• Quality control program
	• Quality assurance program
	• Occurrence management program
	• Customer service program
	• Quality system responsibilities
	• [Good manufacturing practice (GMP): blood banking only]
	• [Proficiency testing: screening and diagnostic laboratory testing only]
Computer	• Main organization's system (e.g., hospital information system [HIS])
	• Department's system (e.g., laboratory information system [LIS])
	• Personal computer (PC) applications (e.g., email, scheduling, word processing, spreadsheets, database)
	• Intranet
	• Online documents
	• Other computer applications used in the job (e.g., documentation of training, continuing education, competence assessment)
Safety	• Accident reporting
	• Emergency preparedness
	• Hazardous waste disposal
	• Chemical hygiene program
	• Infection control (universal precautions, bioterrorism, etc.)
	• Radiation safety, where needed
Work processes and procedures	• Processes in the path of workflow in which the employee works
	• Procedures performed
Compliance (United States only)	• Medical necessity requirements
	• Fraud and abuse reporting
	• Health Insurance Portability and Accountability Act (HIPAA)

From Blonshine, S., Mottram, C. D., Berte, L. M., et al. (2006). *Application of a quality management system model for respiratory services: approved guidelines* (2nd ed.). CLSI document HS4-A2. Wayne, PA: Clinical and Laboratory Standards Institute.

includes a process for operational qualification (OQ). Calibration is addressed with equipment QC in the *process control QSE*. Computer system hardware, middleware, and software are also included in the *equipment QSE* but are not covered in depth in the chapter. Equipment files and records are developed and maintained for all processes and results.

The CLSI document on equipment outlines multiple areas to consider and provides examples of how to develop a comprehensive equipment management plan. The CLSI guideline addresses all of the activities required, from selection through the life of the equipment until it is decommissioned. The plan should include a master list of all equipment, with identifying information, calibration and maintenance schedules, individuals responsible, and documentation of periodic review by management and the medical director.

Equipment acquisition includes meeting the minimum equipment standards as outlined by the ATS-ERS standards for spirometers. Spirometers are required to meet the current International Organization for Standardization (ISO) 26782 requirements. Additional guidance may be found in the ATS-ERS standards for other types of equipment. The selection process may include a list of acceptable vendors, development of a product-evaluation matrix, equipment evaluation (onsite is preferred), written acceptable limits of accuracy and precision, information management options, computer standards, warranty and service agreements, and training options (Box 12.3). The initial selection may include an onsite evaluation with a comparison of old and new equipment.

Installation, Validation, and Verification

The selection of equipment locations in the pulmonary laboratory includes consideration of environmental conditions that affect acceptable function. For example, equipment specifications outline temperatures appropriate for spirometry equipment. A plethysmograph is sensitive to pressure changes in the room, vibrations close to the device, or other significant changes such as a fan blowing on the device. The installation process should include a correlation study between old and new equipment. Correlation studies are required for blood gas equipment by the Clinical Laboratory Improvement Amendments of 1988 (CLIA) and would be considered best practice when replacing PF equipment. Studies have shown bias between vendors and equipment within a specific vendor. Equipment function is validated initially to determine compliance with the manufacturer's specifications, expected accuracy and precision, and QC standards. The question to answer is: Have the requirements for the intended use or application been fulfilled? *Verification* means that the specified requirements are fulfilled, such as calibration verification. All institutional, regulatory, or governmental requirements should be considered during the installation process (Box 12.4).

Equipment Maintenance

An equipment maintenance plan should be developed and approved. If maintenance is provided by an outside contractor, it should follow the institutional plan. The type and complexity of instrumentation for a specific test determine the long-term and short-term maintenance that will be required. Daily **maintenance** includes replacing disposable

---

BOX 12.3   AREAS OF CONSIDERATION IN EQUIPMENT ACQUISITION

In addition to the policies, processes, and procedures, the respiratory service needs to maintain a history file for each piece of equipment (including replacement equipment):
- Selection
- Acquisition
- Installation qualification
- Identification
- Validation or verification
- Calibration program
- Maintenance program
- Service and repair
- Equipment files and records

From Blonshine, S., Mottram, C. D., Berte, L. M., et al. (2006). *Application of a quality management system model for respiratory services: approved guidelines* (2nd ed.). CLSI document HS4-A2. Wayne, PA: Clinical and Laboratory Standards Institute.

BOX 12.4   INSTALLATION PROCESS VERIFICATION ACTIVITIES

- Development of an installation manual
- Equipment validation performed by the manufacturer
- Equipment validation performed by the pulmonary laboratory staff
- Biomedical safety checks performed by an internal or external biomedical department (may be included in the preventive maintenance provided by the manufacturer)
- Validation of selected reference values by the laboratory under medical supervision (i.e., medical director)

From Blonshine, S., Mottram, C. D., Berte, L. M., et al. (2006). *Application of a quality management system model for respiratory services: approved guidelines* (2nd ed.). CLSI document HS4-A2. Wayne, PA: Clinical and Laboratory Standards Institute.

items such as filters and gas conditioning devices. Refer to Chapter 3 and Chapter 11 for other examples and explanations of equipment maintenance requirements or device-specific manufacturer instructions. Preventive maintenance is scheduled in anticipation of equipment malfunction to reduce the possibility of equipment failure. Corrective maintenance or repair is unscheduled service required to correct equipment failure. These types of failures are often detected by QC procedures or unusual test results. Familiarity with the operating characteristics of spirometers, gas analyzers, D_{LCO} systems, plethysmographs, metabolic systems, and application software requires manufacturer support and thorough documentation. Accurate records are essential to a comprehensive maintenance program. Documentation of procedures and repairs is required by most accrediting organizations. Upgrades to application software should be considered an essential component of equipment maintenance in the PF laboratory. Software upgrades generally require a reverification process. Reverification is often required after preventive maintenance and repairs (Table 12.3).

When equipment is removed from service **(decommissioning),** the date should be documented, along with the final disposition of the equipment. Special attention should be given to items such as equipment with biohazard material requiring decontamination or hard drives with patient information.

Process Management

The *process management QSE* includes multiple areas: analysis, design, and documentation of the pulmonary laboratory path of workflow; process validation or verification; process control or QC; and a process for making changes to established processes. Process management assists in meeting accreditation requirements, optimizes the efficient use of resources, and contributes to patient safety and positive outcomes. This should be a major component in the pulmonary laboratory quality plan, record keeping, and procedure manual because of the impact on the accuracy and precision of test results. Process changes should be controlled, validated, and verified before implementation. Members of a process team should be staff who currently work within a process or those who will be involved in a new process.

QC is essential in the operation of a PF laboratory to obtain valid and reliable data. The type of equipment used (e.g., volume-based versus flow-based spirometer) often determines the specific procedures that are required for calibration and QC. For example, both flow-based and volume-based spirometers require calibration with a 3-L syringe, but only volumetric spirometers need to be checked for leaks. The number and complexity of the tests performed may also dictate which equipment and methods are used. Methods and equipment that have been validated in the scientific literature should be used whenever possible. QC is usually easier to perform when standardized techniques are used. The final QC plan includes the schedule of activities, QC methods, procedures for performing the QC methods, tolerance limits, and corrective action. It also must meet accreditation and regulatory requirements.

Control Methods: Mechanical and Biologic

A **control** is any known test signal for an instrument that can be used to determine its accuracy and precision. Controls or control materials must be available for spirometers, gas analyzers, D_{LCO}

TABLE 12.3				
Maintenance and Problem Log				
Date	Time	Maintenance or Problem	Resolution	Technologist

Courtesy Mayo Clinic, Rochester, MN.

systems, plethysmographs, blood gas analyzers, metabolic systems, and other instruments. Because many laboratories use computerized PF or blood gas analyzers, controls are required to ensure that both software and hardware are functioning within acceptable limits. In many instances, application software is used to record and evaluate control assessments (e.g., automated blood gas analyzers). Control methods may vary from a mechanical control, such as the use of 3-L syringes for spirometers, to commercially prepared materials for blood gas analyzers. Another control method is the use of **biologic controls,** which assesses the test results from healthy human beings with their prior test results to evaluate equipment function.

Quality Control Tools and Materials

Syringes

A large-volume syringe is the most common and frequently used mechanical QC tool in PF testing. Syringes used for calibration should be accurate to within ±15 mL or ±0.5% of the stated volume (i.e., 15 mL for a 3-L syringe). The accuracy of calibration syringes should be verified annually or according to the manufacturer's recommendations. Several companies provide the service (Fig. 12.1A and B). Syringes can be checked for leaks simply by occluding the port and trying to empty the syringe. This

procedure should occur at the frequency required in current ATS-ERS standards and at several volumes up to the maximum. Some laboratories use two syringes to exclude the syringe as a source of error. One strategy is to use a 3-L syringe to calibrate and another 3-L syringe to verify volume accuracy. An alternative approach is using a 3-L and 7-L syringe as depicted in Fig. 12.1.

A syringe of at least 3-L volume (see Fig. 12.1) should be used to calibrate spirometers. A 3-L syringe can be used to verify volume-displacement device accuracy and to check the volume accuracy of flow-based spirometers. Computerized systems often have the user inject (or withdraw) a 3-L volume to calibrate the spirometer and then immediately perform additional injections to verify the calibration. Some portable flow-based spirometers (i.e., those using disposable flow sensors) do not provide for calibration but do allow checking or verification of a stored calibration. The calibration or verification should minimally be completed each day testing is completed.

Sine-Wave Rotary Pumps

Sine-wave rotary pumps produce a biphasic volume signal. A biphasic or sine-wave signal may be useful for checking volume and flow accuracy for both inspiration and expiration. A rotary-drive syringe may

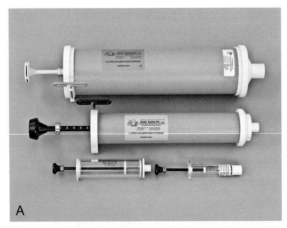
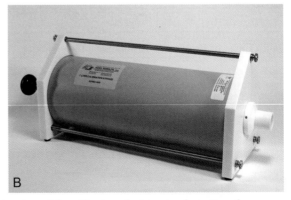

FIG. 12.1 Calibration syringes. (A) Standard 3-L syringe is used for calibration of spirometers for testing of adults and adolescents. Smaller-calibration syringes may be used for calibration and verification of pulmonary function equipment used for small children and infants. (B) A 7-L syringe. (Courtesy Hans Rudolph, Inc., Shawnee, KS.)

be useful for checking the frequency response of a spirometer or to evaluate a spirometer's ability to adequately record tests such as the maximal voluntary ventilation (MVV). Sine-wave pumps are also commonly used in the calibration of body plethysmographs (Fig. 12.2).

Computerized Syringes

Computerized syringes are also available for assessing the accuracy of commonly measured parameters such as forced expiratory volume (FEV_1) and $FEF_{25\%-75\%}$. These syringes use a built-in microprocessor to time the volume injection and calculate the flows. The microprocessor displays volume and flows for comparison with those produced by the spirometer. A computerized syringe provides a 3-L volume for calibration or volume checks and tests accuracy for commonly reported flows.

Computer-Driven Syringes

Computer-driven syringes incorporate large-volume syringes with a computer-controlled motor drive.

Computerized syringes are usually used only by equipment manufacturers or for research applications. The ATS has developed a series of standard waveforms that may be used to drive a computer-controlled syringe. These waveforms are used to validate spirometers and peak flowmeters.

Explosive Decompression Devices

Explosive decompression devices simulate the exponential flow pattern of a forced expiratory maneuver. Such devices use compressed gas, such as carbon dioxide (CO_2), released through an orifice. The gas from the device is injected into a spirometer to generate a simulated forced exhalation. The primary advantage of these devices is that they allow flow and volume signals to be reproduced. When the control signal can be reproduced, both accuracy and precision can be assessed. Using a gas other than air may not work properly with certain types of flow-sensing spirometers.

Dlco Simulator

A **Dlco simulator** is a commercially available device, as depicted in Fig. 12.3. This simulator uses precision gas mixtures to allow repeatable Dlco measurements at different levels (e.g., high Dlco, low Dlco) to simulate Dlco results over the range of expected results for patient testing. Two large-volume syringes are included; an adjustable 5-L syringe provides measured inspiratory volumes. A smaller second syringe is loaded with one of the precision gases; this gas is "exhaled" at the end of the breath-hold interval and sampled by the gas analyzers. Application software calculates the expected Dlco with the known gas concentrations (inspired and expired), along with the inspired volume, breath-hold time, and environmental conditions. The measured Dlco is then compared with the expected value, and the percent error is reported. By using different precision gases and varying the inspired volume, a range of expected Dlco values can be generated. This type of simulator is useful for all laboratories to identify the source of error in Dlco measurements and may also be used for performance qualification when installing new equipment. Use of the device is standard practice by manufacturers developing Dlco systems and in the evaluation of systems before shipment. It is

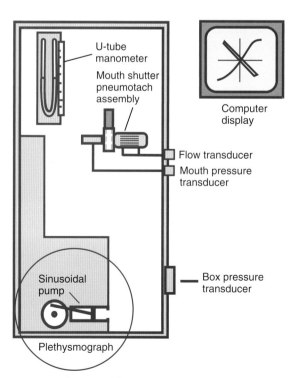

FIG. 12.2   The sinusoidal pump of the pressure plethysmograph.

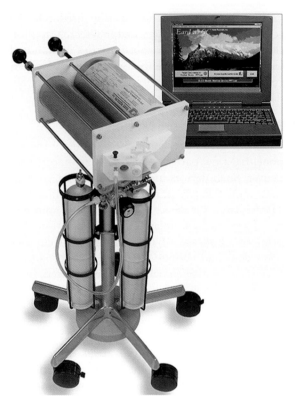

FIG. 12.3   Dʟᴄᴏ simulator. A Dʟᴄᴏ simulator that incorporates two large-volume syringes and multiple precision gas mixtures provides quality control for Dʟᴄᴏ systems. The simulator attaches to the patient port of the Dʟᴄᴏ system. (Courtesy Hans Rudolph, Inc., Kansas City, MO.)

also very useful for large laboratories with multiple Dʟᴄᴏ systems, multicenter research applications in which accurate Dʟᴄᴏ measurements are critical, and accreditation or regulatory programs. Studies have shown that the Dʟᴄᴏ simulator data correlates with biologic data but may be more sensitive in identifying the source of the problem or error. In a recent large multicenter study, the use of a Dʟᴄᴏ simulator allowed identification of the source of and correction of errors prior to testing in 114 laboratories. Initial Dʟᴄᴏ device failures occurred in 13 (11.4%) of the 114 devices. The failure sources were inaccurate medical gas (46%), CO analyzers (46%), and software (8%). Posttraining, Dʟᴄᴏ simulations failed at a rate of 12.7%. Over approximately 3 years, 51.9% of devices had zero failures, and 28.7% had more than one failure.

Plethysmograph volumes can be verified with an isothermal bottle. This device is available commercially (Fig. 12.4) or can be constructed. An isothermal device can be constructed from a glass bottle or jar of 4 to 5 L (for adult-size plethysmographs). The jar is filled with metal wool, usually copper or steel. The metal wool acts as a heat sink (see Fig. 12.4) so that small pressure changes within the jar can be measured with minimal temperature change. The mouth of the bottle is fitted with two connectors. One connector attaches to the mouth shutter (or the patient connection). The other is attached to a rubber bulb with a volume of 50 to 100 mL (e.g., the bulb from a blood pressure cuff). The actual volume of the lung analog can be determined by subtracting the volume of the metal wool from the volume of the bottle. The volume occupied by metal wool is calculated from its weight times its density. The gas volume of the empty bottle may be measured by filling it with water from a volumetric source. The volume of the connectors and rubber bulb should be added to the total volume.

Quality Control Concepts

Two concepts central to QC are accuracy and precision. **Accuracy** may be defined as the extent to

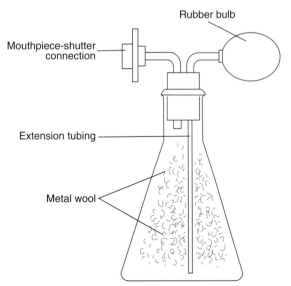

FIG. 12.4   Isothermal lung analog. A schematic of an isothermal lung analog for quality control of the body plethysmograph.

which the measurement of a known quantity results in a value approximating that quantity. For most laboratory tests, repeated measurements of a control are made and the mean, or average, is calculated. If the mean value approximates the known value of the control, the instrument is considered accurate.

Precision may be defined as the extent to which repeated measurements of the same quantity can be reproduced. If a control is measured repeatedly and the results are similar, the instrument may be considered precise. Precision is often defined in terms of variability based on the standard deviation (SD) of a series of measurements (Box 12.5).

Accuracy and precision are desirable but may not always be present together in the same instrument. For example, a spirometer that consistently measures a 3-L test volume as 2.5 L is precise but not very accurate. A spirometer that evaluates a 3-L test volume as 2.5, 3.0, and 3.5 L on repeated maneuvers produces an accurate mean of 3.0 L, but the measurements are not precise. Determining both the accuracy and precision of instruments such as spirometers is critical because many PF variables are effort dependent. The largest observed value, rather than the mean, is often reported as the best test (see Chapter 2). Reporting the largest result observed is

---

BOX 12.5   THE MEAN AND THE STANDARD DEVIATION

Calculation of the Mean and the Standard Deviation

The mean ($\bar{X}$) and standard deviation (SD) are computed to determine the variability of a series of values. Performing multiple measurements of the same quantity (i.e., the "control") allows the mean to be determined and precision to be expressed by the SD of the measurements. Assuming that all of the values sampled are normally distributed, 68.3% of them will be within ±1 SD of the mean, 95.5% will be within ±2 SD, and 99.7% within ±3 SD. When the mean and standard deviation have been determined for a series of measurements, subsequent values may be checked to see whether they are "in control." Values between ±2 and ±3 SD from the mean should occur 5% of the time only (i.e., random error), and values more than ±3 SD from the mean should occur less than 1% of the time.

The mean ($\bar{x}$) may be calculated as:

$$\bar{x} = \frac{\Sigma(x)}{N}$$

where:

Σ = a symbol meaning "the sum of"
x = individual data values
N = number of items sampled
    The SD is calculated as follows:

$$SD = \sqrt{\frac{\Sigma(x)^2}{N}}$$

where:

X^2 = deviations from the mean $(X - \bar{X})$ squared
N = number of items sampled

If the SD is computed from a sample of 30 data points or less, N − 1 is usually substituted for N.

Example Calculation of the Mean and SD for a Series of P_{CO_2} Values

Sample	P_{CO_2} (mm Hg)	Deviation from the Mean (X)	Deviation Squared (X^2)
1	39	−0.9	0.81
2	40	0.1	0.01
3	43	3.1	9.61
4	42	2.1 s	4.41
5	39	−0.9	0.81
6	38	−1.9	3.61
7	40	0.1	0.01
8	41	1.1	1.21
9	38	−1.9	3.61
10	39	−0.9	0.81
Total	399		24.90
Mean	39.9		

$$SD = \sqrt{\frac{24.9}{10 - 1}}$$
$$= \sqrt{2.77}$$
$$= 1.66$$

The range of P_{CO_2} values (in this example) within 2 SD of the mean is 39.9 ± (2 × 1.66), or from 36.6 to 43.2 mm Hg.

based on the rationale that the subject cannot over-shoot on a test that is effort dependent. Other PF tests, such as the DLCO, are reported as an average of two or more acceptable maneuvers; in these instances, the precision of the measuring devices (e.g., gas analyzers) needs to exceed the normal physiologic variability of the parameter being measured.

For instruments such as blood gas analyzers, accuracy is determined by measuring an unknown control and comparing the results with a large number of laboratories using similar equipment and methods. This is commonly referred to as **proficiency testing (PT).** Precision for blood gas analyzers is determined by checking the day-to-day variability of controls and expressing the variability in terms of the standard deviation. These general principles for assessing accuracy and precision can be applied to most types of PF equipment.

Calibration is the process in which the output signal from an instrument is adjusted to match a known input. This may be accomplished by one of several methods:

1. Adjustment of the analog output signal or a continuous signal from the primary transducer (e.g., flow sensor, gas analyzer)
2. Adjustment of the sensitivity of the recording device (specifically mechanical recorders)
3. Software correction or compensation

Calibration involves adjustment of the instrument (or its signal). It should not be confused with calibration verification or QC. Calibration verification confirms the device is within the expected calibration range, and QC assesses the function of the instrument after it has been calibrated. Most PF systems use software-based calibration but allow for adjustment of analog outputs as well.

Spirometry Calibration and Mechanical Quality Control

Spirometers that produce a voltage signal by means of a potentiometer (see Chapter 2) normally allow some form of "gain" adjustment so that the analog output can be matched to a known input of either volume or flow. For example, a 10-L volume-displacement spirometer may be equipped with a 10-V potentiometer. The potentiometer amplifier would be adjusted so that 0 V equals 0 L (zero), and 10 V equals 10 L (gain). The calibration could be verified by setting the

spirometer at a specific volume and noting the analog signal (e.g., 5 L should equal 5 V).

Most spirometer systems are computerized. In computerized systems, the signal produced by the spirometer is often corrected by applying a software **correction factor.** A known volume or flow is injected into the spirometer with a large-volume (usually 3-L) syringe. A correction (i.e., calibration) factor is calculated based on the measured versus expected values:

$$\text{Correction factor} = \frac{\text{Expected volume}}{\text{Measured volume}}$$

The correction factor derived by this method is then stored in memory and applied to all subsequent volume measurements. For example, if a syringe with a volume of 3.00 L were injected into a spirometer and a volume of 2.97 L recorded, the correction factor would be as follows:

$$1.010 = \frac{3.00\,\text{L}}{2.97\,\text{L}}$$

The correction factor 1.010 would then be used to adjust subsequent measured volumes. This method assumes that the spirometer's output is linear and that the same factor would be correct for any volume, large or small. Most automated spirometers allow the correction factor to be verified by reinjecting a known volume, usually 3 L. Taking into account the accuracy of the syringe (0.5%), after calibration, the spirometer should display a volume of 3.0 L ± 3.0%. Three percent of a standard 3-L volume means that the spirometer should read 3.00 ± 0.09 L (range, 2.91–3.09 L). Manufacturers are required to alert the technologist if the new correction factor varies more than ±2 SDs from the mean **calibration factor** or more than 6% from the previous calibration factor.

Care should be taken that the gas in the syringe, which is at ambient temperature (ambient temperature, ambient pressure, and saturated with water vapor [ATPS]), is not "temperature corrected" by the software. Many computerized spirometers provide software functions specifically for calibration and verification. This allows the use of a 3-L syringe without applying corrections that are necessary when patients are tested. Inaccurate temperature corrections produce an erroneous correction factor. Ambient temperature should be available from an accurate thermometer, both for calibration and for testing. If the ambient temperature changes significantly, the temperature used by the software should be updated, or recalibration may be needed. Many spirometers automatically measure ambient temperature. These devices should be checked regularly to verify that appropriate temperature corrections are being applied. The calibration syringe should be maintained at the same environmental conditions as the spirometer.

PF TIP 12.2

Most spirometers provide a means of verifying the volume calibration. This step typically uses the 3-L calibration syringe. After calibration, additional injections and withdrawals of a known volume (usually 3 L, but other volumes may be used) can be used to verify that the spirometer produces a known output. The verification step should include a range of flows to demonstrate volume accuracy that is independent of flow. For example, the range should include a low flow of less than 2 L/s, mid flows (3–7 L/s, and a high flow > 8 L/s).

Other factors that may influence establishment of the spirometer calibration include the accuracy of the large-volume syringe and the speed with which injections are performed. An inaccurate syringe or leaks in the connection to the spirometer may produce erroneous software corrections.

Some spirometers, particularly those that are flow based, may require that the calibration volume be injected within certain flow limits. The ATS-ERS guidelines recommend a range from 0.5 to 12 L/s with injection times of about 6 seconds and less than 0.5 seconds. Flow-based spirometers that measure both inspiratory and expiratory volumes require the syringe volume to be injected and withdrawn. This allows separate correction factors for inspired and expired gas to be generated. Many flow-sensing spirometers also require a "zero" before measuring exhaled volume. This means that the flow sensor must be held motionless (so that

there is no flow through it) while the software adjusts the output of the sensor to equal zero. Lack of a zero-flow baseline is a potential cause of a falsely increased or decreased FVC caused by a **drift** in the zero. When an in-line bacteria filter is used for testing, calibration should be performed with the device in place.

Spirometers that use disposable flow sensors may or may not allow calibration. Many disposable sensors are calibrated during manufacture and are coded so that the spirometer software applies appropriate correction factors (see Chapter 11). If these types of spirometers provide for user calibration, they should be calibrated at least daily. At a minimum, a daily calibration check (see the following paragraphs) should be performed with a sensor from the lot used for patient testing.

QC of spirometers is closely related to calibration, and the two are sometimes confused. An important distinction is that calibration (i.e., adjustment) may or may not be needed, but QC should be performed on a routine basis. Calibration, whether it includes the output of the spirometer or generation of a software correction factor, involves adjustment of the device to perform within certain limits. QC is a test performed to determine the accuracy, precision, or both of the device based on a known standard. Various control methods (e.g., signal generators) are available for spirometers.

Calibration for spirometer volume measurements should be performed at least once each day that the device is to be used. For field studies, accuracy may need to be checked more often. Frequent checks are recommended for industrial applications or epidemiologic research, especially if the spirometer is moved or used for a large number of tests or if the ambient temperature and humidity change rapidly. The accuracy of any spirometer can be calculated as follows:

$$\%Error = \frac{Expected\ volume - Measured\ volume}{Expected\ volume} \times 100$$

where:

Expected volume = known syringe volume (usually 3 L)
Measured volume = volume recorded for the test

The maximum acceptable error for spirometers, according to ATS-ERS recommendations, is ± 3.0% or ± 90 mL, whichever is larger. If the error exceeds these limits, careful examination of the spirometer, software, most recent calibration, and testing technique should be performed (Box 12.6).

Flow-based spirometers should have their accuracy checked (calibration performed) using at least three different flows ranging from 0.5 to 12.0 L/sec. This can be accomplished easily by injecting the 3-L volume over intervals of less than or equal to 0.5 seconds up to about 6 seconds. At each flow, the volume accuracy of ± 3.0% should be maintained.

The linearity of volume-based spirometers should be verified at least quarterly. Volume-displacement spirometers should be checked in 1-L increments across their volume range (i.e., 0–8 L). A 3-L syringe injection performed when the spirometer is nearly empty or nearly full should yield accurate results. The linearity of flow-sensing spirometers should be tested weekly by injecting a series of 3-L volumes at low, moderate, and high flows. Different flows can be generated by varying the speed at which the syringe is emptied. Applying different flows and measuring the resulting volumes may indicate if the spirometer (and its software) is accurate across the range of flows. For example, three different injection times, 0.5 to 1.0 seconds, 1.0 to 1.5 seconds, and 5.0 to 6.0 seconds, may be used with a 3-L syringe to simulate a wide range of flows. The variance between volumes at low and high should not exceed 90 mL or 3.0%.

In addition to checking the volume and flow accuracy of spirometers, several other important aspects of QC require routine evaluation. **Leak checks** should also be performed on volume-based spirometers daily before assessing volume accuracy. The spirometer should be filled with air to approximately half of its capacity, and pressure of 3 cm H_2O should be applied with the breathing port occluded. The pressure may be generated by a weight or spring. Any volume loss greater than 30 mL/min is a significant leak and should be corrected before calibration or patient testing.

To assess flow resistance, the **back-pressure** from a spirometer should be less than 1.5 cm H_2O up to flows of 14 L/sec. Resistance to flow is measured by placing an accurate manometer or pressure transducer at the patient connection and applying a known flow. This is easily accomplished with flow-sensing devices but somewhat difficult with volume-displacement devices. Measurement of flow resistance is normally performed only when there is some reason to suspect that the spirometer is causing undue resistance. The total resistance requirement must be met with all tubing, valves, and filters in place.

Frequency response refers to the spirometer's ability to produce accurate volume and flow measurements across a wide range of frequencies. Frequency response is most critical for peak expiratory flow (PEF) and MVV maneuvers. Frequency response is usually evaluated by means of a sine-wave pump or computer-driven syringe. It should be measured as part of the manufacturer's validation and rechecked if the spirometer's function is questioned.

Flow-sensing spirometers directly measure flow and indirectly calculate volume by integration or by counting volume pulses. It may be necessary to assess the flow accuracy of such devices. Inaccurate measurement of flow usually results in inaccurate volume determinations. A rotameter (a large calibrated flow-metering device) may be used in conjunction with an adjustable compressed gas source to supply a gas at a known flow to the device.

BOX 12.6   COMMON SPIROMETER PROBLEMS

Some problems detected by routine quality control of spirometers include the following:
- Inappropriate signal correction (body temperature, pressure, and saturation [BTPS])
- Improper software calibration (corrections)
- Defective software or computer interface
- Obstructed or dirty flow sensors
- Excessive drift in flow sensors
- Sticking or worn bellows
- Inaccurate or erratic potentiometers
- Mechanical resistance (in volume-displacement spirometers)
- Leaks in tubes and connectors
- Faulty computer or mechanical recorder timing

A weighted volume-displacement spirometer, such as a water-seal type, can also be used to generate a known flow. Most commercial flow-sensing spirometers use a volume signal (e.g., a 3-L syringe) to perform software calibration/verification as previously described. It may be useful to check the flow signal from the spirometer at different known flows if the volume accuracy is observed to vary with flow.

Printed records or computer-generated displays of spirometry signals are required for diagnostic functions or validation or when waveforms are to be measured manually. Printed copies of volume–time or flow-volume (F-V) graphs should be available for diagnostic spirometry. Flow-volume curves should be plotted with expired flow in the positive direction on the vertical (y) axis and expired volume from left to right on the horizontal (x) axis. A flow-to-volume aspect ratio of 2:1 should be maintained (i.e., 2 L/sec flow for each 1 L of volume). Most PF systems are computerized, and printed tracings are generated by ink-jet, thermal, or laser printers. The output of these devices should adhere to the recommended scale factors but often does not. In effect, it may be difficult or impossible to check the timing during forced spirometry using computer-generated tracings.

QC for spirometers should be performed as if a patient were being tested. The 3-L syringe should be connected to the patient port with the circuitry used for the actual test. Spirometer temperature correction may need to be set to 37°C (i.e., no correction applied). Most computerized spirometers provide a specific routine for volume checks or calibration that disables temperature corrections. In some systems, temperature correction cannot be disabled. In these spirometers, injection of 3 L at ATPS results in a reading greater than 3 L because the system attempts to "correct" the volume to body temperature, pressure, and saturation (BTPS). Some flow-sensing spirometers require a length of tubing between the flow sensor and syringe to reduce artifact caused by turbulent flow in the syringe. When an in-line bacteria filter is used, volume verification should be performed with it in place. The action to be taken if controls exceed specified limits should be documented in the procedure manual.

Gas Analyzers and D$_{LCO}$ Systems

Accurate analysis of inspired and expired gases is required to measure lung volumes by dilution methods, D$_{LCO}$, and gas exchange during exercise or metabolic testing. The validity of these tests depends on the accuracy of both the spirometer and the gas analyzers used. Various types of gas analyzers are commonly used in PF testing (see Chapter 11). *Calibration* refers to the process of adjusting analyzer output to match the input of a known concentration of gas. *QC* refers to a method for routinely checking the accuracy and/or precision of the gas analyzer. Important factors related to calibration techniques for gas analyzers include those discussed in the following subsections.

Physiologic Range

Many gas analyzers are not linear or exhibit poor accuracy over a wide range of gas concentrations. Analyzers should be calibrated to match the physiologic range over which measurements will be made. For example, an oxygen (O_2) analyzer may be used to measure fractional concentrations from 0.00 to 1.00, representing a wide physiologic range. If the O_2 analyzer is to be used for exercise tests in subjects who are breathing air, an appropriate calibration range might be from 0.12 to 0.21. This narrow interval represents the physiologic range of expired O_2 likely to be encountered during an exercise test in a patient breathing air. Reducing the physiologic range of an analyzer generally allows better accuracy and precision. Some types of analyzers provide range adjustments for this purpose. Calibration gases should represent the extremes of the physiologic range. In the example of the O_2 analyzer described, air and a gas containing 16% O_2 would be appropriate.

Sampling Conditions

Gas analyzers should be calibrated under the same conditions that will be encountered during the test. Analyzers that are sensitive to the partial pressure of gas may be affected by the sample flow rate. For some tests, gas is sampled continuously from the breathing circuit using a pump (e.g., breath-by-breath gas analysis during exercise). Sample flow through the pump must be adjusted before calibration and then left unchanged during sampling. If gas flow stops before analysis is actually performed (e.g., some types of DLCO systems), sample flow is usually not critical. A gas analyzer in this type of system should be calibrated under conditions of zero flow. Measurement errors may occur if an analyzer is calibrated and then the configuration of the sampling circuit is changed. This may happen if tubing, valves, or stopcocks are added or changed. Any gas conditioning devices, such as those used for CO_2, H_2O vapor, or dust, should be in place during calibration as well. If a CO_2 or H_2O absorber is changed, calibration should be repeated. The gas conditioning devices described in Chapter 11 should be changed at the frequency recommended by the manufacturer.

Two-Point Calibration

The most common technique for analyzer calibration, two-point calibration, involves introducing two known gases. One gas is typically used to "zero" or adjust the low end of the range, whereas the second gas is used to "span" or adjust the high end of the range. Adjusting the span is actually setting the gain of the analyzer so that a known input produces a known output. For some PF tests, the gas to be analyzed is not normally present in expired air (e.g., helium [He], CO, CH_4 [methane], or neon [Ne]). For such tests, air may be used to zero the analyzer. Calibration gas (Cal gas) representing the other end of the physiologic range may be used to adjust the gain of the analyzer. He dilution, functional residual capacity (FRC), and DLCOsb are examples of such tests. He and CO analyzers are zeroed by drawing ambient air into the measuring chambers. He and CO are assumed to be absent from the atmosphere. Compressed air from a cylinder or other source may instead be used if there is concern about trace amounts of other gases (e.g., CO_2, CO, argon) in the ambient air. Then calibration gas containing a known concentration of the gas to be analyzed is introduced. The analyzer gain is adjusted to match the known concentration. The calibration gas approximates the concentration to be analyzed during the test.

The analyzer may then be rezeroed, and the entire process repeated, to verify the calibration. A similar technique may be used with two gases of known concentration if the exhaled sample normally contains varying concentrations of the gas. For example, air and 16% O_2 may be used to perform a two-point calibration of an O_2 analyzer for exercise testing. Depending on the stability of the analyzer, calibration may need to be repeated before (and after) each test or measurement. Gas analyzers should be calibrated before each patient for gas dilution lung volumes, DLCO, exercise tests, and metabolic studies. Gas analyzers used for monitoring (e.g., capnographs) should be calibrated on a schedule appropriate for the extent of use. Calibration should be performed according to the manufacturer's recommendations. The accuracy of the calibration gas should reflect the necessary accuracy of the measurements involved. For DLCO, exercise, or metabolic studies, calibration gases should be accurate to at least two decimal places (i.e., hundredth of a percent). Calibration gases may require verification by an independent method. Patient test gases should also meet the manufacturer's recommendations and be verified with a **gas analysis certificate.** The relative accuracy of all gases used in calibration or patient testing should be known.

Multiple-Point (Linearity) Calibration

An assumption made by a two-point calibration is that analyzer output is linear between the points used. To verify linearity or to determine the pattern of nonlinearity, three or more calibration points must be determined (Fig. 12.5). A multiple-point calibration is performed in a manner similar to the two-point calibration, except that concentrations of known gases across the range to be analyzed are checked and plotted. If multiple points are determined, regression analysis may be used to determine the slope (or type of curve) relating the measured gas concentrations to the expected gas concentrations. A spreadsheet or graphing calculator can be used to analyze the data points. If the analyzer is linear, the points plotted will approximate a straight line. A minimum of three points

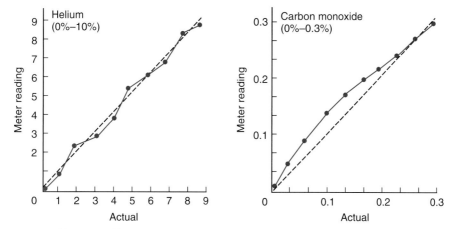

FIG. 12.5 Calibration and linearity check of gas analyzers. Two plots of varying gas concentrations (for helium [He] and carbon monoxide [CO]) are shown. Each graph plots the meter reading of the analyzers against the actual concentration of the gas. Different dilutions of each gas are prepared and then analyzed. The He analyzer shows good linearity in the comparison of measured versus expected concentrations. The CO analyzer shows a nonlinear pattern, typical of an infrared analyzer.

(i.e., gases) is required to demonstrate linearity. If the analyzer is nonlinear, a calibration curve must be constructed to correct the results. In most instances, an equation describing a nonlinear curve can be generated. This equation can then be used either manually or by software to correct analyzer readings. Computerized systems often use an equation or a table of points representing a calibration curve. This allows an analyzer to be calibrated using two points only. Most nonlinear analyzers incorporate electronics that linearize their output. Per the ATS-ERS technical standard, the linearity of analyzers used for D_{LCO} should be assessed monthly. Lung volumes, exercise, and metabolic studies should be assessed at least quarterly.

D_{LCO} **Systems**

Gas analyzer accuracy and linearity are particularly important in PF systems that measure D_{LCO}. For the measurement of D_{LCO} by the single-breath method, analyzer linearity is more critical than the absolute measurement of gas concentrations. Small errors in which the analyzer outputs for CO and tracer gas are not linear with respect to one another

Can result in significant errors in the calculation of D_{LCO}. The nonlinearity of each of the analyzers should be 1.0% or less of the full scale. Analyzers used for D_{LCO} tests also need to be stable, with minimal drift (less than ±0.5% of full scale over 30 seconds) between calibration and testing. To detect drift or similar problems during testing, the actual readings of the analyzers should be displayed. Limited systems use discrete analysis and the majority of systems use rapid gas analyzers (RGAs). Additional specifications apply to the RGAs because of the lag time (travel of the sampled gas through the sampling tube to the analyzer) and the analyzer response time (time required to reach 90% of the actual measurement from the time the gas sample reaches the analyzer). The gas concentration signal must align with the flow signal. The RGA response time should be ≤ 150 ms. Removal of water vapor and CO_2 is usually accomplished by chemical absorbers or related devices (see Chapter 11). Some analyzers use software corrections for the effects of water vapor and CO_2 rather than physically removing or altering the interfering gases.

QC of gas analyzers can be performed by submitting known concentrations of gases to the analyzer, by testing a lung analog, or by using biologic controls. Several gases with concentrations that span the range of the analyzer can be maintained. This can be a costly means of QC for PF laboratories. A simpler technique is to prepare **serial dilutions** of a known gas using a large-volume syringe. The syringe may be the type used for volume calibration. For example, 100 mL of He and 900 mL of air may be mixed in a syringe to produce a 10% He mixture that is then injected into the analyzer. Subsequently, 100 mL of He may be diluted in 1000 mL, then 1100 mL, and so on, with the expected concentrations calculated as follows:

$$\text{Expected test gas} = \frac{\text{Volume of test gas}}{\text{Total volume of gas}}$$

where:

$$\text{Total volume of gas} = \text{Test gas} + \text{Added air} + \text{Syringe dead space}$$

As each dilution is analyzed, the meter reading is recorded and plotted against the expected percentage (see Fig. 12.5). This method is simple and available in most laboratories. Care must be taken when preparing samples so that air does not leak into the syringe, further diluting the test gas. The volume of air in the syringe connectors (i.e., dead space) must be included when calculating the dilution of the test gas. Some calibrated syringes include their dead-space volume.

A second method of verifying analyzer performance involves simulating either lung volume or DLCO tests. This may be accomplished using a lung analog. A **lung analog** is simply an airtight container of known volume. The lung volume simulator is attached at the patient connection with the system set up for a lung volume or DLCO test. A large-volume syringe is used to "ventilate" the lung analog, mimicking the patient's breathing. The resulting lung volume (e.g., FRC) is compared with the known volume of the analog system. A calibration syringe may also be used by itself as the lung analog. Many calibration syringes feature a locking collar that can be adjusted so that only a portion of the syringe's volume can be emptied. With a known volume of air in the syringe, the test is performed by filling and emptying the syringe to the starting volume.

PF TIP 12.3

The 3-L calibration syringe can often be used as a lung model to evaluate the accuracy of gas analyzers used for lung volumes or DLCO tests. For example, a DLCO test can be simulated by setting the calibration syringe to a volume of 1 L and then connecting it to the patient port of the PF system. The syringe is then withdrawn to "inspire" 2 L of test gas. After a 10-second breath hold, the syringe is emptied. This simulates a lung with a total volume (total lung capacity [TLC]) of 3 L and an inspired volume (VC) of 2 L. With this technique, the DLCO should be close to zero (target ≤ 0.5) because no diffusion occurred in the syringe.

Simulation of the DLCOsb maneuver with a calibration syringe can be used to check analyzer linearity and should be completed weekly (How To ... 12.1). Both the tracer gas (He, Ne, CH_4) and CO are diluted equally in the syringe, and their relative concentrations should be identical if the two analyzers used are linear with respect to one another. This causes the calculated DLCOsb to be near zero (approximately ± 0.5 mL CO/min/mm Hg with a 3-L syringe). If the two analyzers are not linear in relation to one another, the ratio of tracer gas to CO will not equal 1. Calculated DLCOsb may be either slightly above or below zero. This method tests not only the gas analyzers but also the volume transducer, breathing circuit, and software. Temperature or gas corrections should be disabled. A linearity check at different dilutions can be performed by varying the volume of the calibration syringe. For each different syringe volume, however, the calculated DLCOsb should be close to zero (≤ 0.5).

A DLCO simulator is commercially available (see Fig. 12.3). This simulator uses precision gas mixtures to allow repeatable DLCO measurements at different levels (e.g., high DLCO, low DLCO). Two large-volume syringes are included; an adjustable 5-L syringe provides measured inspiratory volumes. A smaller second syringe is loaded with one of the precision gases; this gas is "exhaled" at the end of the breath-hold interval and sampled by the gas analyzers. Application software calculates the expected DLCO with the known gas concentrations (inspired and expired), along with the inspired volume, breath-hold time, and environmental

12.1   How To ...

Perform a Syringe D_{LCO}

Steps to performing a weekly syringe D_{LCO} test:
1. Turn the body temperature, pressure, and saturation (BTPS) correction off if possible or set the temperature to 37°C and barometric pressure to 760 mm Hg.
2. Set up a patient file labeled "Syringe D_{LCO}."
3. Enter a standard height and weight.
4. Use a 3-L syringe to perform a D_{LCO} exactly the same as testing a patient. (Some manufacturers also provide instructions and software to perform the maneuver.)
   a. Tidal volume—emulate tidal breathing with the syringe.
   b. Exhale to residual volume or empty the syringe completely.
   c. Inhale the test gas to total lung capacity or fill the syringe completely.
   d. Hold the breath for 10 seconds.
   e. Completely empty the syringe after the breath hold.
5. Complete at least two separate D_{LCO} maneuvers.
6. Evaluate the inspiratory vital capacity (IVC), V_A, and target D_{LCO}. The IVC and V_A measured results should not exceed 5% of the expected result or manufacturer specifications. The target D_{LCO} is < 0.5 mL/min/mm Hg or < .166 mmol/min/kPa. Some newer systems will not display the D_{LCO} when zero or a negative result is obtained.

BOX 12.7   COMMON GAS ANALYZER PROBLEMS

Some problems detected by routine calibration or quality control of gas analyzers include the following:
- Leaks in sample lines or connector
- Blockage of sample lines
- Exhausted water vapor or CO_2 absorbers
- Exhausted water vapor permeable tubing (Nafion)
- Contamination of photocells or electrodes
- Inadequate warm-up time
- Unstable ambient conditions (chemiluminescence analyzers)
- Deterioration or contamination of column packing material (gas chromatographs)
- Poor vacuum pump performance (emission spectroscopy analyzers)
- Chopper motor malfunction (infrared analyzers)
- Electrolyte or fuel cell exhaustion (O_2 analyzers)
- Aging of detector cells (infrared analyzers)
- Poor optical balance (infrared analyzers)
- Medical gas inaccuracies

conditions. The measured D_{LCO} is then compared with the expected value, and the percent error is reported. By using different precision gases and varying the inspired volume, a range of expected D_{LCO} values can be generated. This type of simulator is useful for large laboratories with multiple D_{LCO} systems or for multicenter research applications in which accurate D_{LCO} measurements are critical.

Some computerized PF systems may make lung simulators more challenging to use, although it has become common practice for manufacturers to develop D_{LCO} systems with a lung simulator. The device may also be used to verify the function of new systems before shipment and in the laboratory during installation. When using a D_{LCO} simulation device, the laboratory staff must understand how calculations are completed, both in the testing software of the PF equipment and in the D_{LCO} simulation calculation software, to avoid errors. The

software may be designed to make all necessary corrections for human subjects, giving erroneous results when a simulator is used. However, if the software reports gas analyzer values, the accuracy and linearity of various dilutions can usually be checked (Box 12.7). In a current study of 114 PF laboratories, the initial D_{LCO} simulations failed in 13 systems. Of the 13 failures, 46% were inaccurate medical gas, 46% for CO analyzers, and 8% were software errors. Over the next 4 years, the D_{LCO} systems were evaluated every 12 weeks. Two percent of the failures were attributed to a CO analyzer error.

Body Plethysmographs

The calibration techniques described here apply primarily to variable-pressure, constant-volume plethysmographs. Flow-based plethysmographs may require slightly different calibration procedures for the box transducer. Mouth pressure and pneumotachometer calibrations are similar for both types of plethysmographs.

Mouth Pressure Transducer

Calibration is done by connecting the pressure transducer to a water manometer or a similar device that can generate an accurate pressure. The manometer is a fluid-filled, U-shaped tube with a calibration scale that allows very accurate pressures

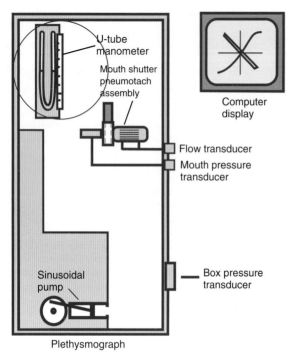

FIG. 12.6 U-tube manometer highlighted in the pressure plethysmograph.

to be generated (Fig. 12.6). Some plethysmographs use a weighted piston to produce a calibration pressure signal. The mouth pressure transducer should be able to accurately record pressures greater than ± 50 cm H_2O at frequencies of 8 Hz or more. The actual mouth pressures encountered are often less than this level. Air is injected into one port of the U-tube manometer. For example, a small volume of air may be introduced to cause a deflection of 5 cm. In effect, this creates a difference of 10 cm between the two columns of the manometer. The gain of the mouth pressure amplifier is then adjusted so that its signal display deflects by an amount equivalent to 10 cm H_2O/cm. The display device is most commonly a computer screen. The deflection then equals the calibration factor for the mouth pressure transducer. In the previous example, if a pressure change of 10 cm H_2O resulted in a 1-cm deflection on the display, the calibration "factor" would be 10 cm H_2O/cm. Because almost all plethysmograph systems are computerized, the analog output of the transducers is measured, and a software correction factor is determined. The correction (or calibration) factor is calculated in a manner similar to that used for spirometer output (see section on spirometers). The correction factor is then applied by the software as the mouth pressure signals are acquired.

Box Pressure Transducer

Calibration of the box pressure transducer is accomplished by closing the door of the plethysmograph and applying a volume signal comparable to what occurs during patient testing. In a plethysmograph of 500 to 700 L, a volume signal of 25 to 50 mL is typical. The box pressure transducer should be capable of accurately measuring pressures as small as ± 0.2 cm H_2O. The box pressure transducer typically requires a range of up to 5 to 10 cm H_2O to accommodate large changes in box pressure (e.g., thermal drift). An adjustable sine-wave pump connected to a small syringe is ideal for box calibration. A small volume is pumped into and out of the box (see Fig. 12.6). With the pump operating, the gain of the box pressure transducer is adjusted so that volume change in the box causes a specific pressure change. For example, if the pressure signal generated by a 30-mL volume change is adjusted to cause a 2-cm deflection on the display, the box pressure calibration factor would be 15 mL/cm. For computerized systems (most plethysmographs), a software calibration factor is derived rather than an actual adjustment of the displayed signal. In other words, no actual adjustment of the output of the box pressure transducer is necessary; the software correction is simply applied to all signals generated during measurements. The calibration procedure may be repeated by adjusting the pump speed from 0.5 to 8.0 cycles/sec (Hz). Varying the frequency allows the frequency response of the box and transducer to be checked. The volume deflection or calibration factor should not change at frequencies up to 8.0 Hz. Flow-based plethysmographs may be calibrated similarly. The output of the box flow transducer is adjusted (instead of a pressure transducer) to correspond to a known volume change within the plethysmograph chamber. Flow boxes can be used as pressure boxes simply by occluding the flow sensor in the box wall. For plethysmographs that use this method, a box pressure transducer may need calibration as well.

Plethysmographs are normally calibrated empty. A volume correction for the displacement of gas by the patient can be calculated from the patient's weight. This correction is then applied in the calculation of results (see Evolve website, http://evolve.elsevier.com/Mottram/Ruppel/).

Flow Transducer

The pneumotachometer (flow sensor) may be calibrated by applying either a known flow or a known volume. A precise flow may be generated with a rotameter or similar calibrated flow meter. Most systems, however, calibrate the pneumotachometer with a 3-L syringe. The flow is integrated, and the gain of the flow signal is then adjusted until the output of the integrator matches the 3-L volume, just as is done for most flow-based spirometers. The flow sensor used in the plethysmograph should meet the volume range and accuracy requirements for spirometers. Just as for the box and mouth pressure transducers, a software calibration factor may be computed rather than physically adjusting the output of the flow sensor. Pressure-differential, heated-wire, or Pitot tube flow sensors may be used (see Chapter 11). Once the flow sensor is calibrated, both volumes and flows (as needed for measurement of airway resistance [Raw]) can be measured.

QC of body plethysmographs may be accomplished with one or more of the following: an **isothermal lung analog,** fixed resistors, biologic controls, or comparison with gas dilution or radiologic lung volumes.

The accuracy check is performed with an assistant seated in the sealed plethysmograph. The isothermal volume device is connected to the mouthpiece. The mouth shutter is then closed. While the assistant holds his or her breath, the bulb is squeezed at a rate of 1 to 2 times per second. A P_{MOUTH}/P_{BOX} tangent is recorded just as would be done when testing a patient. Thoracic gas volume (V_{TG}) is calculated as usual, except that P_{H_2O} is not subtracted. The V_{TG} calculated should equal the volume of the isothermal lung analog (as determined previously) within 50 mL or ± 3%, whichever is greater. Correction should be made for the assistant's volume (based on body weight) plus the known volume of the isothermal lung analog.

The procedure may be repeated by squeezing the bulb at 0.5 to 5.0 cycles/sec to check the frequency response of the box. If the box's frequency response is "flat," tangents should not change when the bulb is squeezed at different rates. The lung analog must contain a sufficient mass of metal wool to act as a heat sink (i.e., isothermal). The metal wool "absorbs" changes in temperature that would result from the compression and decompression of gas in the bottle. If there is not enough metal wool, small temperature changes may affect the volume determination. Some manufacturers provide an automated isothermal lung analog that can be placed in the plethysmograph and operated under software control to provide measurements across the range of expected results for both pediatrics and adults (see Fig. 12.4).

The accuracy of the box for measuring Raw can be assessed with known resistances. A resistor can be made using a plug with a small-diameter orifice. Alternatively, a resistor can be constructed from capillary tubes arranged lengthwise in a flow tube. In either case, the pressure drop across the resistor must be measured at a known flow rate. Some manufacturers supply resistors with known resistances. The resistor is then inserted between the pneumotachometer/mouth shutter assembly and a test subject. The subject, whose Raw has been previously measured, then has Raw measured with the resistor in place. The increase in measured Raw should approximate that of the resistor (Box 12.8).

BOX 12.8   COMMON PLETHYSMOGRAPH PROBLEMS

Some problems detected by routine quality control of body plethysmographs include the following:
- Leaks in door seals or connectors (pressure boxes)
- Improperly calibrated mouth or box pressure transducers
- Damaged flow sensors (pneumotachometers) or mouth shutter mechanisms
- Excessive thermal drift
- Poor frequency response
- Inappropriate software calibration factors
- Procedural errors (e.g., testing before thermal equilibrium is reached)

A third method of checking plethysmograph accuracy is to compare the V_{TG} with FRC determined by gas dilution. Correlations greater than 0.90 have been demonstrated between gas dilution and plethysmograph lung volumes in healthy individuals. Differences greater than 10% (in healthy individuals) for volumes measured by plethysmograph and gas dilution are not specific but may indicate equipment malfunction. This method, as well as the use of biologic controls, is based on measurements of healthy individuals with normal day-to-day variability. It is important that control subjects perform the breathing maneuvers correctly (see Chapter 4).

Biologic Controls

Biologic controls are healthy subjects who are available for repeated tests. These controls can be laboratory personnel or other individuals who can be tested repeatedly. The use of biologic controls does not eliminate other control devices, such as large-volume syringes. Although a 3-L syringe can verify the volume and flow accuracy of a spirometer, biologic controls can evaluate an entire system, including spirometers, gas analyzers, plethysmographs, and software. A disadvantage of using biologic controls is that PF varies from day to day. However, by establishing means and measures of variability from repeated tests, real problems with most PF equipment can be identified (How To . . . 12.2).

12.2 How To ...

Use Biologic Controls

1. *Performance of a single instrument.* Test *healthy* biologic controls on a regular basis. Compare variables (e.g., forced expiratory volume in the first second [FEV_1], DL_{CO}) to the established mean. Control values should fall within a range of ± 2 standard deviations (SD) of the mean (at least 95% of the time). If the value is outside of this range, the cause of the change should be identified. Is the biologic control healthy on the day of testing? Was the last calibration performed correctly? Have any modifications been made to the spirometer hardware? Have any software upgrades or modifications been made? If the source of the problem is found and corrected, the control should be retested to confirm that the instrument performs as expected.
2. *Establish precision of the system.* Include data in the control database that falls within the 2-SD limit. Data outside of 2 SD may be included if they are clearly caused by variability and not an equipment problem. This may be verified by repeating the test. If the second test produces another result that is more than 2 SD from the mean, there is likely an equipment or procedural error. Alternatively, a second biologic QC could be tested to verify if the result more than 2 SD from the mean is related to the subject and not the equipment. By calculating SD from repeated measures, the precision of a particular instrument or system can be established.
3. *Use the coefficient of variation (CV) to reduce variability.* The CV for most spirometry and lung volume pulmonary function variables should be approximately 5% or less. Some parameters, such as $FEF_{25\%-75\%}$, are more variable in healthy subjects and may show CV values closer to 10%. If the CV is greater than 10%, calibration and testing procedures should be reviewed to see whether sources of error can be eliminated. The DL_{CO} CV will approximate 6% to 8%, based on current published studies.
4. *Compare instruments or laboratories.* Biologic controls can be used to perform interinstrument or interlaboratory evaluation. Similar devices should produce similar control results. However, if different instruments (e.g., a flow-based and a volume-based spirometer) are compared, slightly different values for the same control may be obtained. This difference is the bias between the two systems. The true value for a particular variable (e.g., forced vital capacity [FVC], DL_{CO}) may be considered the average of the means for the two instruments or laboratories. Alternatively, one instrument may be considered the "gold standard"; the other instrument can be described as having a negative or positive bias, depending on whether its measurement is less than or greater than the gold standard.
5. *Compare methods.* Biologic controls may also be used to compare different methods within the same laboratory. For example, functional reserve capacity (FRC) might be measured with a gas-dilution technique and by plethysmography. The mean, SD, and CV of each method can then be compared.
6. *Troubleshooting.* Biologic controls can be used to troubleshoot a problem instrument. For example, if a system produces low DL_{CO} values in several otherwise healthy patients, a problem might exist. Test a biologic control; if the control value is within expected limits, the low DL_{CO} values may be valid.

Control subjects should have normal lung function (i.e., no asthma or other respiratory symptoms) and, ideally, span a range of values. For example, a 64-inch-tall female and a 72-inch-tall male will provide a wide range of values for most PF parameters. PF studies on controls should be performed on a regular basis (weekly or monthly). All tests should use the same protocols applied to the patient population. Control measurements should meet all criteria for acceptability and repeatability. Tests should be performed at the same time of the day to minimize the effects of diurnal variation. If the laboratory has multiple PF systems, controls may be tested on each instrument on the same day to provide a check of interinstrument bias.

To provide useful statistics, 20 sets of measurements should be recorded. Ten measurements may be adequate to develop an initial range. PF variables that are not derived from other measurements should be recorded. These include FVC, FEV_1, FRC, and D_{LCO}. Calculated values such as TLC or DL/V_A can also be used; however, if subsequent control tests show significant differences, it may be unclear which component test is at fault. Typical values selected from metabolic studies may include $\dot{V}O_2$, CO_2, tidal volume, $\dot{V}_E$, and respiratory rate at different work rates. See Chapter 7 for specifics on metabolic QC performance. A calculator or a computer spreadsheet may be used to perform the simple statistics required (Table 12.4). Most spreadsheets have built-in functions to calculate the mean and standard deviation (SD) and to allow data to be graphed. An increasing number of manufacturers provide these functions as a part of the PF software. The **coefficient of variation (CV)** may be calculated by dividing the SD by the mean. The **coefficient of repeatability (CR)** may also be calculated. Separate statistics should be calculated for each biologic control and for separate instruments. Data more than 1 or 2 years old should be evaluated with more recent measurements to account for small normal changes in PF that occur over time (Fig. 12.7).

Testing biologic controls is also a means of evaluating gas analyzers. This method may not detect small changes in analyzer performance because of day-to-day variability of lung volumes, D_{LCO}, or resting energy expenditure. Despite variability

TABLE 12.4

Example Spreadsheet for a Biologic Control[a]

Control Subject: J.S.

Date	FVC	FEV_1	FRC	D_{LCO}
2/1/12	4.51	3.93	3.51	25.1
2/15/12	4.61	3.99	3.55	26.2
3/14/12	4.49	3.95	3.65	27.2
3/19/12	4.40	3.90	3.50	25.5
4/21/12	4.57	3.89	3.60	26.0
5/1/12	4.50	3.94	3.66	27.2
5/15/12	4.55	3.95	3.65	27.0
Mean	4.52	3.94	3.59	26.31
SD	0.07	0.03	0.07	0.85
CV	1.49%	0.85%	1.91%	3.21%

CV, Coefficient of variation; FEV_1, forced expiratory volume in the first second; *FRC*, functional residual capacity; *FVC*, forced vital capacity; *SD*, standard deviation.
[a]Most spreadsheet programs have built-in functions to calculate means and standard deviations; additional calculations, such as coefficient of variation, can be entered by the user. Quality control charts may be constructed with mean and standard deviation data for each variable.

as high as 10% for D_{LCO} or exercise parameters in healthy patients, gas analyzer malfunctions may be detected. Current research has shown that the variability in biologic controls for D_{LCO} may be as low as 5% if the equipment is well maintained. Biologic controls may be the simplest means of checking automated exercise/metabolic systems that depend on accurate gas analysis. Abnormal results from biologic controls can suggest which component of the gas analyzer may be faulty (see Chapter 7 for a complete explanation of biologic QC with metabolic systems). For D_{LCO} systems, studies suggest that changes in the weekly biologic controls trend well with the mechanical simulation device; the simulation devices may be more sensitive to identification of the source of the error.

A simple but effective means of checking plethysmograph function is to measure TLC, V_{TG}, and Raw from biologic control subjects. A series of 20 box measurements when QC is in control (usually done over a period of days or weeks) provides an appropriate mean value for comparison with subsequent results. Day-to-day variability in trained subjects is usually less than 10% for FRC_{pleth}, so changes

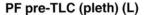

PF pre-TLC (pleth) (L)

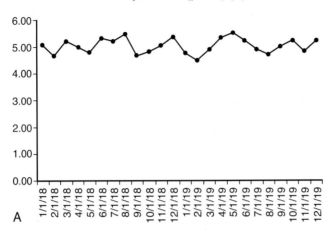

A

PF pre-TGV (L)

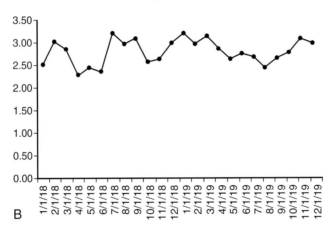

B

PF pre-SVC (L)

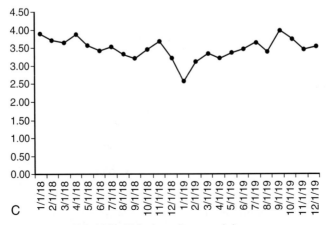

C

FIG. 12.7   Biologic quality control charts.

in FRC_{pleth} of greater than 10% suggest a problem with the box. TLC variability is generally less than 5% with linked maneuvers. This method allows for checking of the box, the transducers, the recording devices (if any), and the software. A discrepancy between the established mean and an individual QC measurement will detect a problem but may not indicate which component is causing the problem. For example, a control with an established FRC_{pleth} of 3 L is measured again, and the FRC_{pleth} is calculated to be 2 L. The biologic control establishes that there is a problem, but the cause of the discrepancy requires further investigation. In this example, either incorrect calibration of box or mouth pressure transducers or a leaky door seal may be the cause. Biologic control data from other methods for lung volume determinations is also helpful in troubleshooting the cause of the discrepancy. If multiple methods are used for lung volume determinations, the methods must be compared with biologic QC.

Table 12.5 defines expected CVs for several biologic QC parameters. The CVs displayed in column 2 are representative of a recent large global study consisting of five separate vendor equipment types. The data were monitored by an external group and met all current test standards for the recorded results. The CVs in column 3 are *target values* for a

TABLE 12.5

Biologic QC Ranges

Biologic Quality Control Recommended Ranges

Parameter	Coefficient of Variation in Large Multisystem Global Studies	Coefficient of Variation in Multisystem Single-Country Studies—Target Values
FVC	≤4%	≤3%
FEV_1	≤4%	≤3%
SVC	≤4%	≤3%
D_{LCO}	≤8%	≤5%
IVC	≤5%	≤3%
FRC_{pleth}	≤7.5%	≤5%
TLC	≤5%	≤5%

FEV₁, Forced expiratory volume in the first second; *FRC,* functional residual capacity; *FVC,* forced vital capacity; *IVC,* inspiratory vital capacity; *SVC,* slow vital capacity; *TLC,* total lung capacity.

well-controlled system derived from an accreditation program in one Canadian province with quality oversight.

Calibration and Quality Control of Blood Gas Analyzers

Modern blood gas analyzers rely on a microprocessor or computer to control functions such as calibration. The user selects a "calibration schedule" appropriate for the complexity and number of tests performed. For example, in a laboratory that performs many blood gas analyses, automated one-point calibration may be performed every 30 minutes, with two-point calibration every 2 hours. Government agencies and some voluntary credentialing organizations have specific schedules for the frequency and types of calibrations that must be performed. Different calibration schedules may be required for different types of blood gas analyzers (e.g., point-of-care devices versus laboratory instruments).

For traditional blood gas electrodes, calibration involves exposing the gas electrodes (i.e., Po_2, Pco_2) to one or two gases (or liquids) with known partial pressures of O_2 and CO_2. If only one gas is used, the calibration is termed a *one-point calibration;* if two gases are used, it is called a *two-point calibration.* Similarly, one or two known buffers may be used to calibrate the pH electrode. Calibration gases spanning the physiologic ranges of the Po_2 and Pco_2 electrodes are used, just as for gas analyzers. Typical combinations include one calibration gas with a fractional O_2 concentration of 0.20 (20%) and a fractional CO_2 concentration of 0.05 (5%). A second calibration gas may have a CO_2 concentration of 0.10 (10%) with an O_2 concentration close to zero.

As for gas analyzers, a "low" gas (or buffer solution) is used to zero or balance each electrode. A "high" gas (or buffer) is used to adjust the gain (also called the *slope*) of the electrode's amplifier. "Electronic" zeroing may be done without exposing the electrode to a gas with a partial pressure of zero. Some blood gas analyzers use this method to zero the Po_2 electrode. Computerized systems allow the user to select how frequently and what type of calibration is performed on the gas and pH electrodes. The Po_2 electrode is usually calibrated over a range of 0 to 150 mm Hg. The P_{CO_2} electrode is typically calibrated for the range of 40 to 80 mm Hg. The pH electrode is usually calibrated using buffers with pH values of 6.840 (low) and 7.384 (high).

Most blood gas analyzers use precision gases to calibrate the gas electrodes, even though gas tensions are measured in liquid (i.e., blood). Some differences may exist when the partial pressure of gas is analyzed in a gaseous versus liquid medium, especially for O_2. The reduction of O_2 at the tip of the polarographic electrode occurs more rapidly in a gaseous medium than in a liquid. If the electrode is calibrated with a gas, its response when measuring a liquid will be to read slightly lower. This difference is termed the *gas–liquid factor*. Gas–liquid corrections may be clinically important when measuring high partial pressures of O_2, particularly above 400 mm Hg.

Computerized calibration brings calibration gases or buffers into contact with the electrodes. Electrode responses to the calibration gas or buffer are then stored. The microprocessor compares the measured responses to expected calibration values. The computer then "corrects" the zero and gain (for a two-point calibration) so that measured and expected values match. Most computerized blood gas analyzers compare the current calibration results with the previous calibration. The difference between calibrations is termed **drift** and indicates an electrode's stability.

Automatic calibrations can be programmed to occur at predetermined intervals. Adjustments are performed automatically based on the response of the electrodes. Because of this, all conditions for an acceptable calibration must be met before the procedure actually begins. Automated blood gas analyzers check most conditions that may affect accurate results, such as the temperature of the measuring chamber. During automatic calibration, inadequate buffer or the wrong calibration gas may cause the microprocessor to correct inappropriately for a properly functioning electrode. A similar problem arises if protein contaminates the electrode tip, altering its sensitivity. The microprocessor adjusts the electrode's output in an attempt to bring it into range. This process works well for minor changes in electrode sensitivity. However, electrodes cannot be properly calibrated if they are contaminated with protein, if membranes are damaged, or if the electrolyte is depleted. The user must maintain reagents, calibration gases, and electrodes so that automatic calibration can occur successfully. Systematic errors can sometimes be masked by automatic calibration. Contamination of the calibration gases or buffers is a common example. If the microprocessor adjusts electrodes to match a contaminated calibration standard, the calibrations appear normal, but analysis of control samples will show differences. Detection of these errors usually requires appropriate QC and PT (described later in this section). Automated blood gas analyzers reduce variability by controlling calibration and sample analysis but require careful attention to function appropriately.

Many blood gas analyzers (such as point-of-care devices) use electronic checks of the function of the various sensors (e.g., P_{O_2}, P_{CO_2}). Some analyzers use a combination of electronic checks and traditional calibration methods. Electronic checks are typically performed immediately before sample processing, and some checks are performed during analysis to detect bubbles, clots, and so forth. Electronic checks are sufficient for ensuring proper functioning of sensors such as optodes, spectrophotometers, or fluorescence quenching devices. The adequacy of electronic sensor checks and traditional calibration methods must be demonstrated by appropriate QCs and calibration verification.

The primary method of QC for blood gas analysis is the use of commercially prepared controls. Although tonometry is no longer commonly used in blood gas laboratories, the method is the basis for commercially prepared controls. Interpretation of blood gas QC is the same for either method.

Commercially Prepared Controls

There are two types of commercially prepared controls: aqueous and fluorocarbon-based emulsions. The aqueous material is usually a bicarbonate buffer. The fluorocarbon-based control material is a perfluorinated compound that has enhanced O_2-dissolving characteristics. Multiple levels (e.g., acidosis, alkalosis, normal) of these materials provide control over the range of blood gases seen clinically. Aqueous and fluorocarbon-based controls usually contain dyes that generate known absorptions when injected into hemoximeters designed for blood. These dyes allow the materials to be used for QC of blood gases and hemoximetry at the same time.

Both types of controls are packaged in sealed glass ampoules of 2- to 3-mL volume. They require minimum preparation for use. Aqueous and fluorocarbon-based controls can be stored under refrigeration for long periods or at room temperature for day-to-day use. Most aqueous and fluorocarbon-based controls have shelf lives of 1 year or longer. Each requires agitation for 10 to 15 seconds before use to ensure equilibration with the gas sealed in the ampoule. Care must be taken when handling the glass ampoules because temperature changes (from the hands) can affect the amount of gas dissolved in the liquid, particularly for O_2. If the ampoules are stored at a temperature significantly different from 25°C, the control values for Po_2 may need to be adjusted.

PF TIP 12.4

Most laboratories use commercially prepared controls. These controls should be prepared according to the manufacturer's instructions. This usually involves shaking the contents to mix the liquid and gaseous contents of the ampoule. Once opened, the contents should be immediately aspirated into the analyzer. Delay in aspirating blood gas controls results in Po_2 values drifting toward 150 mm Hg and Pco_2 values drifting toward zero. The temperature at which the ampoule is stored may be needed to correct for small differences in the Po_2 of the control.

One problem with aqueous controls (and to a lesser extent with fluorocarbon solutions) is poor precision of Po_2. The O_2 carrying capacity of these materials is much lower than that of whole blood. Consequently, the Po_2 in the control material changes rapidly on exposure to air. Controls with low Po_2 values (50–60 mm Hg) become quickly contaminated after opening. Aqueous or fluorocarbon controls may produce a wide range of "expected"

Po_2 values, limiting their usefulness in detecting an out-of-control device. Some of these difficulties may be overcome by careful statistical evaluation of Po_2 control data as described in this section.

Some analyzers provide automatic measurement of QC materials. In these devices, control materials are contained in cartridges, similar to cartridge-based reagents. Controls are then run on a predetermined schedule with little operator intervention. In most instruments, the auto-QC software can be set to "lock out" the analyzer for those analyses (e.g., pH, Po_2) that fail QC. This prevents the analyzer from being used to report values that might be inaccurate.

A sound statistical method of interpreting "control runs" is necessary to detect blood gas analyzer malfunctions (Box 12.9). The most commonly used method for detecting out-of-control situations is calculating the control mean $\pm 2\,SD$. A series of runs of the same control material is performed. Twenty to 30 runs will provide an adequate base for calculation of the mean and SD (see Evolve website, http://evolve.elsevier.com/Mottram/Ruppel/). One SD on either side of the mean in a normal distribution includes approximately 67% of the data points. Two SD include 95% of the data points in a normal distribution. Three SD include 99% of the data points in a normal series. A QC value that falls within $\pm 2\,SD$ of the mean is usually considered to be "in control." If the control value falls between 2 and 3 SD from the mean, there is only a 5% chance that the run is in control. The normal variability that occurs when multiple measurements are performed is called **random error.** One of 20 control runs (i.e., 5%) can be expected to produce a result in the 2- to 3-SD range and still be acceptable. In practice, if a control run shows a value more than 2 SD above or below the mean, the control is usually repeated. If the second run shows a value within 2 SD of the mean, the first value was probably a random error. Conversely, if the second run produces a result similar to the first run (> 2 SD on the same side of the mean), the instrument is probably "out of control." This simple approach works very well for detecting most types of errors that occur in analytic instruments like blood gas analyzers. The same method has also been applied to PF equipment.

BOX 12.9   COMMON BLOOD GAS ANALYZER PROBLEMS

Some problems detected by routine quality control or proficiency testing of blood gas analyzers include the following:

- *Electrode or sensor malfunction.* Protein deposited on membranes or sensors is common and can usually be remedied by cleaning. Leaks in membranes, electrolyte depletion, or sensor failure can cause drift or shifts in performance.
- *Temperature control.* Failure to maintain 37°C in the measuring compartment or thermometer inaccuracy causes quality control (QC) results to be out of control.
- *Improper calibration.* Problems during calibration are almost always related to inadequate or contaminated buffer or calibration gas. QC data that is consistently high or low may indicate a problem with reagents.
- *Mechanical problems.* Leaks in pump tubing or poorly functioning pumps allow calibrating solutions, controls, and patient samples to be contaminated. Air bubbles introduced during analysis may cause gas tensions to be in error. Inadequate rinsing may also occur with pump problems or improperly functioning valves. This usually results in blood clotting in the transport tubing or measuring chamber.
- *Improper sampling technique.* Failure to anaerobically collect arterial specimens or improperly storing samples (e.g., plastic syringes in ice water), excessive or incorrect anticoagulant, or bubbles in the specimen all may result in questionable results. Another common problem related to sampling is inadvertently obtaining a venous specimen. Adequately functioning electrodes or sensors, as demonstrated by good QC, can distinguish poor sampling from actual clinical abnormalities.

More complex sets of rules have been developed to distinguish true out-of-control situations from random errors. A widely used set of rules is that proposed by Westgard (see Selected Bibliography). The rules are selected to provide the greatest probability of detecting real errors and rejecting false errors. This approach to QC is termed the **multiple-rule method.** An example of the multiple-rule method may be applied as follows:

1. When one control observation exceeds the mean ± 2 SD, a "warning" condition exists.
2. When one control observation exceeds the mean ± 3 SD, an out-of-control condition exists.
3. When two consecutive control observations exceed the mean $+2$ SD or the mean -2 SD, an out-of-control condition exists.
4. When the range of differences between consecutive control runs exceeds 4 SD, an out-of-control condition exists.
5. When four consecutive control observations exceed the mean $+1$ SD or the mean -1 SD, an out-of-control condition exists.
6. When 10 consecutive control observations fall on the same side of the mean ($\pm$), an out-of-control condition exists.

These are just some of the rules that may be applied; not all rules have to be used at all times. Rules 1 and 2 detect marked changes in electrode performance, sometimes called a **shift,** by examining how far from the mean a single control value falls. Rule 3 looks for a shift by comparing two consecutive control runs. Rule 4 looks for shifts in electrode performance by noting excessive variability between consecutive runs. Rules 5 and 6 look for "trends" in instrument response by evaluating an unexpected pattern (i.e., multiple consecutive values on the same side of the mean) in the recent history of control runs.

The multiple-rule method can also be applied when two or more levels of controls are evaluated on the same measurement device (electrode). The rules may be applied by linking multiple levels (e.g., high, normal, low) of control material. For example, if three levels of controls all show values greater than 2 SD above their respective means, it is likely that the electrode (sensor) is out of control.

One problem with a strict statistical approach is that if outliers (i.e., values more than 2 SD from the mean) are sometimes excluded, the SD becomes smaller with repeated calculations. Eventually, valid control data may be rejected. This situation can be managed by including data in the calculations that are clinically acceptable, although they may be more than 2 SD above or below the mean.

When using the multiple-rule method, it is necessary not only to evaluate the mean and SD of the current control run but also to keep a control history. This is often accomplished by means of a control chart (Fig. 12.8), also called a *Levey–Jennings plot.* A graph for each control is created with the

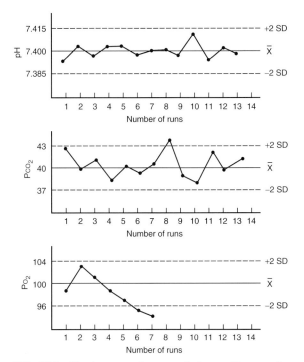

FIG. 12.8 Blood gas quality control charts. (See text for explanation.)

mean ±2 SD on the *y*-axis and control run number (or time) on the *x*-axis. Individual controls are then plotted as they are run to track electrode performance.

To provide adequate QC for a blood gas analyzer, three levels of control materials are normally used. Three levels of controls for each of the three electrodes (i.e., pH, PCO_2, and PO_2) require that 9 means and 9 SD must be calculated for each instrument. Controls may also be used for blood oximeters, and this adds more control histories to be managed. When controls are run several times daily, tracking multiple runs can become complex. To simplify this task, computerized QC programs are often used. Such programs are usually included in the software for automated blood gas analyzers. Many laboratory computer systems also support statistical databases for control data. The chief advantages of computerized QC are simplified data storage and maintenance of necessary statistics. Multiple rules can be applied easily to each new control run to detect problems. Computerized records and control charts can be printed. These types of routine QC records are required by many accrediting agencies. (See the Evolve website, http://evolve.elsevier.com/Mottram/Ruppel/ for a list of regulatory agencies.)

QC of blood gas analyzers should be performed on a schedule appropriate for the number of specimens analyzed. In most laboratories, controls must be performed daily or more often. In busy laboratories, multiple levels of controls may be required on each shift. QC is also usually required after any significant maintenance is performed to verify proper function of the instrument.

QC charts, or Levey–Jennings plots, are used to assess the QC. Fig. 12.8 illustrates three examples of Levey–Jennings charts for pH, PCO_2, and PO_2. The mean for each control material is plotted as a solid line, and the ±2 SD lines are dashed. The left *y*-axis on each graph is labeled with the actual mean and ±2 SD values. Consecutive control runs are plotted on the *x*-axis. On the pH control chart *(top)*, all values vary about the mean in a regular fashion; the electrode appears in control (all values within ±2 SD) for the 13 measurements plotted. The PCO_2 chart *(middle)* shows somewhat more variability. Control run 8 shows a value outside of the ±2 SD range. This may be considered a random error because subsequent controls show normal variability about the mean. The PO_2 chart *(bottom)* shows a trend of decreasing control values. Runs 6 and 7 both produce values of more than 2 SD below the mean. This pattern suggests that the electrode or sensor is malfunctioning and needs to be serviced. By applying multiple rules to the interpretation of consecutive control runs, with or without charts, most out-of-control situations can be detected.

In addition to providing regular checks of acceptable instrument performance, routine QC establishes the precision (variability) of each measurement. Instrument precision must be determined so that blood gas interpretation can be related to a range of values. For example, the variability of the PO_2 measurement for a specific analyzer may be determined to be ±6 mm Hg (i.e., 2 SD) around a mean of 50 mm Hg. Each PO_2 result (near 50 mm Hg) can then be interpreted with some certainty that it is within 6 mm Hg of the reported value.

Several other techniques related to QC of blood gas analyzers are commonly used. Interlaboratory comparison of control results can compare the performance of similar instruments for measuring the same lot of control materials. Manufacturers of control materials and some voluntary credentialing agencies provide such interlaboratory databases. Each laboratory submits its control values for a specific period, usually once per month. The laboratory then receives a report showing its performance related to all participating laboratories. This type of comparison is useful for detecting systematic errors that may go unnoticed when running daily controls. Accreditation standards may also require interlaboratory comparison for specific analyses.

Documents and Records

The *documents and records QSE* is central to a quality system. Accreditation and/or regulatory bodies require document management systems. It encompasses a management system for document and record creation, control, retention, and retirement. Records are generated based on the documents and activities that are performed in the PF laboratory. Forms are created to record data or results from all procedures in the path of workflow and each QSE. Specific recommended documents and records are addressed with each QSE. They may be electronic or paper.

The system for creating, reviewing, and approving documents is an example of a process document (see Table 12.1). The document for maintaining a record of procedures, effective dates, and location is an example of a form and could be created in an electronic database, a paper form, or as a spreadsheet. A procedure manual that outlines the steps for each test performed is a required document. The ATS has published the *Pulmonary Function Laboratory Management and Procedure Manual.* Templates are recommended for documentation creation and are available in this manual. Multiple forms may also be required to document other processes and procedures, such as QC procedures and results, equipment maintenance, quality improvement activities, equipment validation procedures, ordering forms, and pretest instructions. Box 12.2 outlines a typical technical procedure manual for the PF laboratory.

Process maps and flow charts are effective methods to clearly define the work processes. The key components of activities required across the path of workflow are included. This also supports training activities for new staff or when a change in process is implemented for current staff.

Reference documents received from outside agencies may serve as resource materials for the development of processes and procedures. These documents should also be referenced and maintained. Examples include operator manuals, examination inserts, notices from manufacturers (e.g., software updates), ATS-ERS standards and guidelines, accreditation requirements, and manufacturer instructions.

Information Management

The *information management QSE* provides the guidance for managing information generated in the pulmonary laboratory in either paper or electronic format and dissemination of the information with adherence to organizational, accreditation, and regulatory requirements. An example of a required procedure is instructions that define the flow of information. The process for meeting confidentiality requirements such as those outlined in the Health Insurance Portability and Accountability Act (HIPAA) should be available to staff members. Security for data access, both paper and electronic, along with levels of access, is determined. This may include assigning one individual with authority to change predicted author sets or primary-user configurable files that affect data integrity. Record-keeping processes should also be identified. *A process for verifying data integrity during equipment installation, after repairs, and after software changes is a critical component in the laboratory.* Software upgrades can cause unanticipated changes in formulas or how data are obtained and processed. Repeating all QC is recommended as a part of the process to ensure data integrity after any change in hardware of software. Data integrity may also be affected when transferring data between electronic systems, such as from the pulmonary laboratory system to the electronic medical record. This includes agreement of the terms and/or abbreviations used in each system. When electronic systems are used to collect and disseminate data, a downtime procedure is required. Systems used for interpretation of the results also require specific processes and procedures for managing the data, maintaining standards, and tracking availability of the data for clinical use within specified timeframes. Planning for information management may involve both staff and users of the data to increase satisfaction. Billing processes related to tests performed and interpretations should be outlined to avoid errors and maintain compliance with regulations.

Nonconforming Event Management

The *nonconforming event management QSE* provides guidance to detect, document, and monitor nonconforming events (NCEs). This may also be known as *occurrence management*. According to the CLSI guideline, an NCE is an occurrence that does not conform to the laboratory's policies, processes, and/or procedures; does not conform to applicable regulatory or accreditation requirements; or has the potential to affect patient and/or employee safety. This is a central document for patient safety and a quality management system. This QSE provides the framework for managing equipment or events that do not meet specified requirements, classifying events, and analyzing the data to correct problems. This allows the laboratory to identify and correct system problems. Analysis and intervention are key elements for this QSE. For example, QC results that are unacceptable are documented and investigated, and the root cause is evaluated to prevent further problems. This improves troubleshooting efficiency and often aids in the prevention of further events. Root causes are often associated with a limited number of recurring events, such as equipment problems; software errors; a lack of effective training; a lack of effective communication; and/or a lack of a well-defined policy, process, or procedure. The NCE process creates a nonthreatening culture of continual improvement. Unacceptable blood gas PT results must be investigated, and the probable cause and resolution must be documented. The nonconforming QSE is also linked to the organization's risk management and serves as a supplement.

The PF laboratory should review the NCEs at regular intervals so that trends and patterns can be assessed. The NCE process can also be linked to laboratory costs. The quality costs are categorized as prevention costs, appraisal costs, and failure costs. For example, a process failure may result in additional work and potential work to correct the failure.

Assessments

The *assessment QSE* addresses the use of external and internal monitoring (Box 12.10). The purpose is to determine whether the defined process meets the requirements and evaluate how well the process is functioning. It is a building block for quality to support all activities within the path of workflow. The assessment QSE provides guidance for meeting regulatory and accreditation requirements for external assessments. It also offers guidance, suggestions, and examples for fulfilling the requirements. Several countries are using specific external assessment criteria for the accreditation of pulmonary diagnostic services. An external assessment may be an inspection, site visit, audit, or survey. It gives the laboratory objective feedback on how it is performing related to quality objectives, processes, and whether it is complying with expected requirements. A laboratory should always be in a state of readiness for any type of inspection. There are several activities required for external assessments that are generally outlined and required by the organization providing the assessment. Accreditation visits or an audit for a clinical study are examples of external assessments for the PF laboratory. Another example includes the PT program for the blood gas laboratory. In both scenarios there is a report with findings from the assessment. The laboratory is responsible for responding to the findings and developing corrective action plans that will sustain improvements. It is helpful to organize deficiencies and corrective action related to the specific QSE. For example, a common nonconformance for the assessment QSE is a lack of documentation for a failed PT. Nonconformance for the personnel QSE would be incomplete training and competency records or not having personnel qualifications or position descriptions available. An external assessment requires significant planning and

---

BOX 12.10   EXAMPLES OF PULMONARY FUNCTION (PF) LABORATORY QUALITY INDICATORS BY OPERATING SYSTEM

Patient Assessment

- Unstated reasons for test orders
- Inappropriate reasons for test orders

Test Request Process

- Requests missing required or critical information
- Missing patient instructions
- Incorrect scheduling

Patient Preparation

- Inaccuracies in entry of patient demographics
- Lack of adherence to pretest instructions

Equipment Preparation

- Lack of calibration data
- Incorrect reference values

Patient Training

- Ineffective or lack of test performance instructions
- Laboratory Information System
- Security violations
- Unscheduled downtimes
- Inability to retrieve archived patient results and information

Testing and Review

- Lack of trial acceptability
- Lack of reproducibility
- Inadequate number of trials

Laboratory Interpretation

- Disparities in: PF results obtained by two separate methods
- Calculated and measured parameters

Results Reporting

- Times alert values were not reported or documented
- Completeness/correctness of reports
- Delayed reports
- Corrected reports due to reporting errors
- Disparities between preliminary and final reports

Posttest Data Management

- Retained data unable to be retrieved

Clinical Interpretation and Application

- Inappropriate action taken after report of results
- Inappropriate test performed per protocols

From Blonshine, S., Mottram, C. D., Berte, L. M., et al. (2006). *Application of a quality management system model for respiratory services: approved guidelines* (2nd ed.). CLSI document HS4-A2. Wayne, PA: Clinical and Laboratory Standards Institute.

---

preparation for an optimal experience. Both CLSI and ATS provide useful documents to achieve a positive outcome that results in improved processes and quality.

Internal assessments are quality indicators such as monitoring turnaround time for PF results, from performance to release of the interpretation results. The use of comparative data among pulmonary laboratories or clinics within a health care organization is another method for completing an internal assessment. The percentage of tests meeting acceptable and repeatable criteria for spirometry for each technologist, laboratory, or clinic could be used as an internal assessment.

Interlaboratory PT consists of comparing unknown control specimens from a single source in multiple laboratories. This allows an individual laboratory to compare its results with other laboratories using similar methods. Results from laboratories that used different methods (e.g., analyzers) may also be compared. The results of PT are usually reported as means and SD for each instrument participating in the program. PT does not measure day-to-day precision, as does daily QC. However, it provides a measure of the absolute accuracy of the individual laboratory. An analyzer may have acceptable precision as determined by daily QC but be inaccurate compared with analyzers from other laboratories. PT often detects systematic errors that occur because of improper calibration, contaminated reagents, or procedural problems. Multiple levels of unknowns (for PT) are usually provided to check the range of values seen in clinical practice. PT programs are available from professional organizations, such as the College of American Pathologists, as well as from commercial vendors. Satisfactory performance on interlaboratory PT has been mandated by the U.S. Department of Health and Human Services under CLIA (see Evolve website).

Continual Improvement

The *continual improvement QSE* identifies opportunities for improvement from multiple sources, such as customer surveys, NCEs, evidence-based practice, ATS-ERS standards, PT results, internal assessments, external inspections or evaluations, and quality indicators. Improvement opportunities may be within a specific QSE or the path of workflow. A defined strategy for continual improvement should be used. A quality report is submitted at least annually to upper management (Box 12.11). One common effective strategy in pulmonary laboratories is the provision of a technologist's feedback loop.

BOX 12.11   QUALITY REPORT

Date of Report:

Medical Director or Designee Review/Date:

Table of Contents

QSE—Organization ....
QSE—Documents and Records....................
QSE—Personnel................................
QSE—Purchasing and Inventory........................
QSE—Equipment...
QSE—Process Control......................................
QSE—Event Management................................
QSE—Assessments..
QSE—Process Improvement..............................
QSE—Safety and Facilities.................................
QSE—Customer Service and Satisfaction..................

Special Pulmonary Evaluation Laboratory

Quality Report by QSE Summary

Organization

See Organization Chart

Staff Changes: Number of new allied health employees—None

- Number of new supplemental employees—2

Personnel

Orientation of New Employees: Employees who attended the human resources orientation this year—None

Training: New employee training accomplished this year—2

- Emergency Preparedness Plan (EPP) training specific to laboratory location
- Employee Right to Know Act (ERTKA) training (hazardous chemicals and infection control)
- Integrity training
- Hazard and Infection Control training

Competency Assessments: Competency assessments performed—10

Performance Appraisals: Performance appraisals completed—10

Purchasing and Inventory

Utilization of the Inventory Center (coined "PAR Stocking"). Moved some blood gas supplies to PAR Stocking.

Continued

BOX 12.11   QUALITY REPORT—cont'd

Product Recalls—None

Process Control

New Tests Implemented—None

Significant Process Changes: Noted in Standard Operating Procedure (SOP)

Validation Performed: Intralaboratory comparison data

Test Delays—None

Event Management

Summary of Reported Events

Event log reviewed by medical director

Assessments

Quality Indicator (Charts)

Appointment availability

1. Customer (patient) satisfaction

Proficiency Testing

College of American Pathologists—Blood gas and CO-oximetry surveys

Comparability Studies

Intralaboratory comparison with the hospital arterial blood gas labs (see comparison binder)

Internal Audits

Daily quality control (QC) statistical reports (see lab binder)

External Assessments/Audits

College of American Pathologists—Blood gas, CO-oximetry, and linearity surveys

Computer-Generated Patient Results Audit

Computer check audits completed.

Process Improvement

1. Process Improvement Activities: Improve ordering process for the pediatric cardiopulmonary exercise studies
   Code cart monitoring process improvement
   Arterial blood gas order verification process

Documents and Records

New or Revised Documents

Updated policy and procedure manual with medical director review and signature.

Equipment

New Equipment Installation Qualification—None

Retired Equipment

Major Repairs/Maintenance Issues

Maintenance log, but in summary, no issues arose that caused delayed analysis or reporting of patient data.

BOX 12.11	QUALITY REPORT—cont'd

Unplanned Computer Outages—None

Customer Service and Satisfaction

Customer Surveys Conducted

Customer (patient) satisfaction survey—Key indicator

Customer Complaints or Comments—None

Employee Surveys

Culture of Safety survey

Tours Conducted

Facilities and Safety

Employee/Patient Incidents

Safety Audits

None

Other Safety Issues

Facility Issues (Remodeling, Unplanned Outages, etc.)

None

Courtesy Mayo Clinic, Special Pulmonary Evaluation Laboratory, Rochester, MN.

Technologist's Feedback

A well-trained and highly motivated technologist is a key component for obtaining valid data, particularly in tests that require patient instruction and encouragement. As a component of the continual improvement QSE, a program based on established criteria for acceptability and repeatability can be used to provide feedback on test performance to the individuals conducting the tests. This may also be included in performance appraisals and as a competence tool during training.

Routine review of the tests performed by each technologist is highly recommended. If criteria for acceptability and repeatability have been recorded (as described in the path of workflow), these can be used to grade the performance of the technologist. This information forms the basis for reinforcing superior performance or correcting identified problems. Feedback should include the type and extent of unacceptable or nonrepeatable tests. Feedback should also include what **corrective action** can be taken to improve performance. Feedback needs to be ongoing to maintain a high level of proficiency.

Test quality review should be included in the orientation process and updated when standards change. For research applications or in clinical trials, review of test data and performance, along with feedback to the personnel conducting the tests, may be necessary to provide the highest-quality results. An example of "Spirometry Test Quality Review" is shown later in the chapter in Table 12.7.

PATH OF WORKFLOW

The path of workflow was briefly described in Chapter 1. This section will illustrate and describe key processes in the path of workflow for the PF laboratory from the time a patient is assessed for testing to the clinical correlation of the results. The pretest processes are shown in Fig. 12.9.

Pretest Process

Patient assessment is the entry point to a therapist-driven protocol (TDP) or ordering of PF tests. TDPs are developed with current scientific evidence in partnership and with the approval of the medical

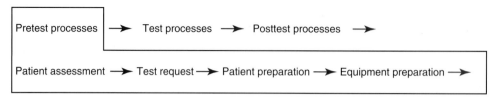

FIG. 12.9 Pulmonary diagnostics pretest key processes. (From Blonshine, S., Mottram, C. D., Berte, L. M., et al. [2006]. *Application of a quality management system model for respiratory services: approved guidelines* [2nd ed.]. CLSI Document HS4-A2. Wayne, PA: Clinical and Laboratory Standards Institute.)

director. The assessment may include, but is not limited to, the clinical history, signs and symptoms, and other abnormal tests, which will also lead to the clinical indications outlined in the ATS-ERS statements. A standardized ordering format can assist with the test request process.

The *test request* key process includes generation of the order, pretest instructions, and scheduling the tests. Test requests may be generated electronically or by paper. The request should meet all institutional, accreditation, and regulatory requirements. The requestor and location to send the final report are also required. Other important areas to consider are the patient's physical and mental status, medications that may affect test results or that need to be held before testing, special preparation instructions, and the clinical indication for testing. Ordering instructions and guidance are needed for the authorized requestor to facilitate efficiency and accurate orders and to prevent medical errors. These instructions answer questions related to tests available, patient consent requirements, how to complete the requisition, medications that need to be held for test validity, how to schedule the test with contact information, and any other special considerations. Specific preparation instructions for tests such as bronchial provocation testing may be provided both in a verbal and written format to the patient.

Patient preparation is a critical key process in obtaining valid data. The demographic information provides the data to calculate the predicated reference values. An accurate height is required to obtain reliable reference values. A stadiometer provides the most accurate height measurements. Stadiometers should be calibrated on an annual basis. All height measurements are made with shoes removed. In those cases where a standing height cannot be obtained, calculations are available in most manufacturers' software programs to use the arm span measured from fingertip to fingertip. Deviations from standard practice should be included in the technologist's comments. Calibrated scales provide an accurate weight.

The clinical indication for testing should be verified again before testing each individual because the clinical presentation can change between ordering and testing. The absence of contraindications needs to be confirmed before testing. Patient adherence to any pretest instructions, such as holding medications before a test, should be confirmed and documented. Patient preparation is the point where a final assessment of age-specific considerations that may affect test results is completed.

Equipment preparation includes the final preparation of the equipment just before testing that is required to obtain reliable results. QC is completed at the frequencies predetermined for the laboratory and typically would be completed before this step unless a probable out-of-control situation is defined after the patient has started the testing process. Equipment that is found to be out of control should not be used for patient testing. Specific instructions on how to handle out-of-control situations are included in the procedure manual. Equipment calibration is performed, and all necessary supplies are ready for testing. Reference values may be selected if there are multiple options based on specific patient populations. The reference sets selected are based on current evidence and the patient population to be tested (Chapter 13). For example, the Cystic Fibrosis Foundation currently requires PF laboratories to use defined reference authors.

Testing

Test Method Selection

The testing method is dependent on the patient population, equipment available, tests ordered, and ultimately, the patient's needs (Fig. 12.10). To decrease unwanted variations that affect test reliability, the laboratory can validate its testing processes, equipment, and software. An initial validation is completed when new equipment is installed. Reverification is completed when processes are changed, software is changed, or after repairs and preventive maintenance.

Patient training is essential to obtaining reliable results. The patient's anxiety level and understanding of why they are being tested are important considerations in obtaining maximum cooperation. Communication strategies may need to be altered based on the age of the patient. Chapter 8 addresses the training and coaching of pediatric patients. Regardless of the test performed, key steps to performing the test are explained and demonstrated to the patient. If needed, an interpreter should be available. Demonstration of the procedure should always be done to achieve a maximum understanding of the test procedure. The technologist training the patient needs to display the same effort required by the patient to achieve reliable tests.

Test Performance

A primary means of ensuring data quality is to rigidly control the procedures by which data are obtained. For many PF tests, how the data are obtained depends on the technologist's ability to train the patient adequately, to conduct the procedure, and to elicit subject cooperation in the test maneuvers. Technologist and subject performance, as well as proper equipment function, must be evaluated for each test completed. This may be accomplished by using appropriate criteria to judge the acceptability of results. Recommendations for testing procedures published by the ATS-ERS are widely recognized as standards for test performance.

Each PF laboratory should have a written technical procedure manual (documents and records QSE) that includes the following:
- Methods used for specific tests
- Specific guidelines as to how tests are to be performed
- Limitations of each procedure (if any)

Providing quality output in the PF laboratory requires not only appropriate calibration, verification, and QC but also careful attention to how the data are obtained (i.e., testing techniques). Testing technique may be compared with "sampling" technique in other laboratory sciences. In PF testing, *sampling* refers to procedures used to obtain patient data. How the data are obtained becomes extremely important because many of the tests performed are effort dependent. Eliciting maximal effort and cooperation from the patient is often just as critical as correct performance of the equipment. Applying objective criteria to determine the validity of data is one means of providing high-quality results.

Using Criteria for Acceptability/Repeatability

Criteria for assessing the validity and reliability of various tests have been described in Chapters 2 through 9. Standards for PF testing have been published by the ATS in conjunction with the ERS. Criteria for acceptability and repeatability have three primary uses:

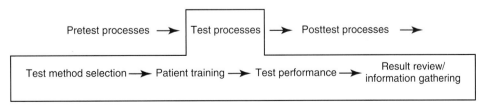

FIG. 12.10 Pulmonary diagnostics test process key activities. (From Blonshine, S., Mottram, C. D., Berte, L. M., et al. [2006]. *Application of a quality management system model for respiratory services: approved guidelines* [2nd ed.]. CLSI document HS4-A2. Wayne, PA: Clinical and Laboratory Standards Institute.)

1. To provide a basis for decision making during testing. Standards or guidelines can be used to decide whether equipment is functioning properly, whether the patient is giving maximal effort, or whether testing should be continued or repeated. Standardized criteria also help characterize the types of problems known to occur during specific tests (e.g., poor effort during spirometry).
2. To evaluate the validity of PF data from an individual patient. Criteria may be applied by the technologist performing the test, by computer software, or by the clinician responsible for interpretation. This may consist of assigning a letter grade or a code to individual efforts or tests.
3. To score or evaluate the performance of the technologist. Many PF tests, especially spirometry, depend on the interaction between the technologist and the patient. Criteria for acceptability can be used to gauge the performance of individual technologists and to provide objective feedback.

Implementation of a quality system in the PF laboratory should use acceptability and repeatability criteria during and after testing (results review process), both to evaluate individual tests and to provide feedback for technologists. For each of these, certain procedures will be similar.

Examine Printed Tracings or Displayed Graphics Whenever Available

Compare the observed tracing with the characteristics of an acceptable curve or pattern. Computer graphic displays make this particularly easy and can usually display tracings in real time. Graphics may be superimposed or displayed side by side to assess patient effort and cooperation. Similarly, expected values can be displayed graphically along with each individual effort. The user should be able to modify the graphic display (e.g., change graphing scale) to allow for extremes such as very low flows or volumes. During testing, graphs of multiple efforts should be available. Storage of graphic data (all acceptable maneuvers) may be useful for assessing data quality after testing has been completed. Some portable (office) spirometers may not display graphics of volume–time or F-V curves during testing but are able to print graphics. In these cases, the printed graphs may be used to assess test quality. Real-time displays for both F-V and volume–time displays during testing are particularly helpful in assessing test variation during the testing process rather than after testing. Current spirometry standards require real-time displays. This allows for corrective action during the testing process.

Look at Numeric Data

Are the largest values from multiple efforts within the accepted range of repeatability? The decision to perform additional maneuvers is usually based on repeatability. Most manufacturers provide software that applies current standard guidelines for repeatability. Data from multiple efforts should be maintained during testing to allow for the selection of appropriate results for the final report. Storage of all efforts may be necessary for subsequent review or editing. Data that are not repeatable may be valid (i.e., usable) but need to be identified as such.

Evaluate Key Indicators

Most PF tests have one or two features that determine whether the test was performed acceptably. For spirometry, meeting the start-of-test and end-of-forced-exhalation test criteria are key indicators. For gas dilution lung volumes, absence of leaks and test duration are key indicators. For DLCOsb, inspired volumes and breath-hold times are two of several important indicators. Key indicators vary with the method used for specific tests. In each instance, the important indicator should be assessed in relation to an accepted standard. During testing, these indicators help determine whether additional patient instruction or tests are needed. Key indicators are also useful in assessing what factors might influence the interpretation of the test (e.g., the patient was unable to achieve a 1-second plateau during spirometry).

After determining the acceptability and repeatability of maneuvers for each test, the technologist decides when an adequate number of maneuvers has been completed to ensure reliable results or the patient is unable to continue testing.

Reviewing the results against posttest results and selecting the final data for the final report follow the same standards used during the testing

---

BOX 12.12   SAMPLE CHECKLIST FOR DLCO TEST QUALITY

1. Is the breath-hold time (BHT) between 8 and 12 seconds?
2. Is the inspiratory vital capacity (IVC) at least 90% of the slow vital capacity (SVC) in the same test session, or is the IVC $\geq$ 85% of the SVC and V_A within 200 mL or 5% (whichever is greater) of the largest V_A from other acceptable maneuvers?
3. Is 85% of the inspiratory volume inhaled in less than 4 seconds?
4. Were two acceptable D_{LCO} trials completed with a maximum of five trials?
5. Is the time between trials at least 4 minutes?
6. Is sample collection completed within 4 seconds of the start of exhalation or, for rapid gas analyzer (RGA) systems, is the sample collection initiated after dead-space washout is complete?
7. Are the first two acceptable D_{LCO} trials data averaged that agree within 2 traditional D_{LCO} units (.67 SI unit) of each other?

---

process and the preestablished laboratory standards. A checklist can be helpful at each workstation to assist in the process (Box 12.12).

The results of various tests should be consistent with the clinical history and presentation of the patient. Spirometry, lung volumes, D_{LCO}, and blood gas values should all suggest a similar interpretation for a specific diagnosis. Discrepancies among tests may indicate a technical problem rather than a clinical condition. Comparing results from similar measurements is helpful, with an understanding of the expected relationships.

PF TIP 12.5

1. Slow vital capacity (SVC; lung volumes) > FVC (spirometry)
2. TLC (lung volumes) > V_A (D_{LCO})
3. FRC_{PL} > FRC_{N_2} or FRC_{He} in obstructive patterns
4. Inspiratory vital capacity (IVC; D_{LCO}) < SVC (lung volumes)

Patient assessment for further testing occurs when a TDP has been implemented or the correlation with the patient's clinical condition suggests further testing is indicated.

Scoring or grading the quality of a patient's test is an important component of quality assurance for PF testing. The technologist administering the test can accomplish this by adding notes. Spirometers should use software that grades test performance or that includes codes denoting problems with the test to assist the technologist performing the tests. Evaluation of spirometry, lung volumes, D_{LCO}, and any other tests performed should be included.

The technologist's comments or notes should be added to the test results. The commentary should be based on standardized criteria. If a particular test meets all criteria, that fact should be stated. Failure to meet any of the laboratory's criteria should be documented as well. The reason the patient was unable to perform the test acceptably should be explained whenever possible. Failure to meet the criteria for acceptability does not necessarily invalidate a test. For some patients, their best performance may fail one or more of the criteria. Table 12.6 lists examples of statements that may be used to document test quality.

The technologist's comments can be included in the final report. Many automated systems provide for "free text" comments to be included with tabular data. Current software should support "canned text" functions that allow predetermined statements (see Table 12.6) to be entered with a single keystroke. The technologist's name or initials should be included. The technologist's comments should be clearly identified to avoid confusion with the physician's interpretation.

Most current computerized spirometer systems automatically score FVC (FVC and FEV_1 independently) maneuvers. The score may be indicated by a letter or numeric code that is attached to each maneuver. For example, an FVC maneuver that meets all criteria (e.g., start of test) might be scored with an "A." Other systems allow the technologist to select a user-defined code to attach to individual maneuvers. Both techniques can be used to provide feedback that enhances quality assurance.

The evaluation of the quality of tests completed in the laboratory is a critical component of the laboratory processes in personnel orientation, competence assessment, remediation, and retraining as updates to current testing standards are

TABLE 12.6

Technologist's Comments (Examples)

Test	Comments
Spirometry	Meets all ATS-ERS recommendations.
	Poor start of test or patient effort.
	There was no obvious 1-second plateau at the end of forced exhalation.
	Back-extrapolated volume was > 5% of FVC.
	Patient was unable to continue to exhale because of _____.
	Two best acceptable FVC maneuvers were not within 150 mL
	Two best acceptable FEV_1 maneuvers were not within 150 mL
	MVV does not correlate with FEV_1.
Lung volumes (gas dilution)	Lung volumes by [method] meet ATS-ERS recommendations.
	Lung volumes reported were the average of [n] FRC determinations.
	Slow VC was [greater/less] than FVC (_____%).[a]
	Lung volumes were unacceptable because of a leak.
	Equilibration not reached within 7 minutes—He dilution.
	Alveolar N_2 > 1.5% after 7 minutes—N_2 washout.
Plethysmography	All plethysmographic measurements met ATS-ERS recommendations.
	FRC_{pleth} measurements were variable.
	Raw measurements were variable.
	Patient was unable to pant at the correct frequency.
DLcosb	Meets all ATS-ERS recommendations.
	DLco reported is average of (n) maneuvers.
	Predicted DLco corrected for an Hb of _____.
	Inspired volume < 90% of best VC (_____%).[a]
	Breath-hold time not within 8–12 seconds (_____ seconds).[a]
	DLco values not within 2 mL CO/min/mm Hg or 0.67 CO/mmol/min/kPa.
	DLco not corrected for Hb or COHb.

ATS-ERS, American Thoracic Society-European Respiratory Society; *FEV₁,* forced expiratory volume in the first second; *FRC,* functional residual capacity; *FVC,* forced vital capacity; *MVV,* maximal voluntary ventilation; *VC,* vital capacity.
[a]Values in parentheses may be filled in with appropriate values from the patient's data.

implemented. An example of a spirometry test quality report is displayed in Table 12.7.

After Testing

Results reporting occurs after the quality review is completed and the final data have been selected for the report (Fig. 12.11). A system for a secondary review of results as a routine or random evaluation leads to continual improvement. It also provides a forum to discuss methods to improve testing processes. The report format needs to provide numeric and graphic results for the interpretation process. If preliminary and final reports are used, both must be accurately labeled in the patient chart and the process defined for when a preliminary report is replaced by a final report. Turnaround times for report generation can be a quality indicator for the laboratory. If a report is

TABLE 12.7		
Spirometry Test Quality Review Example		
Acceptability/Repeatability Questions for Determining Quality Grades		
Acceptability	**Yes**	**No**
Were the ATS-ERS end-of-forced-exhalation criteria met? (1 of the 3 criteria) a. Expiratory plateau (<0.025 L in the last 1 s of expiration) b. Expiratory time > 15 s c. FVC is within the repeatability tolerance of or is greater than the largest prior observed FVC		
Was the back extrapolated volume less than 5% of the FVC or 100 mL, whichever is greater?		
Is exhalation smooth and continuous? (no cough in first second or glottic closure)		
Is there evidence of an obstructed mouthpiece?		
Is there evidence of a leak?		
Was the effort maximal based on the peak flow?		
Is the zero-setting stable with no drift?		
Repeatability	**Yes**	**No**
Are there 3 acceptable trials?		
Were repeatability criteria met for FVC and FEV_1 (150 mL)? (age 6 and older)		
Was the difference between the two largest FVC values <0.100 L or 10% of the highest value, whichever is greater, and the difference between the two largest FEV_1 values <0.100 L or 10% of the highest value, whichever is greater? (less than age 6)		
Technologist Review		
Technologist Administering Test:		
Technologist Reviewing Test:		
FVC score:		
FEV_1 score:		
Comments:		
Test Date:		
Date Review Date:		

ATS-ERS, American Thoracic Society–European Respiratory Society; *FEV_1,* forced expiratory volume in the first second; *FVC,* forced vital capacity
From Graham, B. M., Steenbruggen, I., Miller M. R., et al. (2019). Standardization of spirometry 2019 update. An official American Thoracic Society and European Respiratory Society technical statement. *American Journal of Respiratory and Critical Care Medicine, 200*(8), e70–e88..

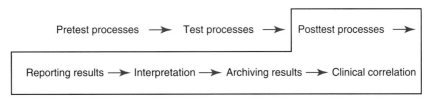

FIG. 12.11 Pulmonary diagnostics posttest process key activities.(From Blonshine, S., Mottram, C. D., Berte, L. M., et al. [2006]. *Application of a quality management system model for respiratory services: approved guidelines* [2nd ed.]. CLSI document HS4-A2. Wayne, PA: Clinical and Laboratory Standards Institute.)

found to be erroneous after release, a system for the correction and replacement of the original report is required. This includes a method to verify that the health care provider is notified. The laboratory should establish acceptable limits for each test. Notification procedures for "alert" results and a documentation process should be available in the procedure manual and immediately available for all technologists.

Interpretation of the results includes providing a process for standardization based on current standards and evidence. Some systems provide a template for interpretation and potential interpretation statements. To establish a standardized process for interpretation, objective criteria for separating normal and abnormal results are required. Additional information in the medical record or history, such as smoking, occupational exposure, recent illnesses, and medications, is useful when reviewing data. Frequently, the data also are compared with previous data, which should be easily identified or available in the medical record. The selection of reference values is a critical element in reliable interpretation systems.

The turnaround time for interpretation is an important quality indicator. As an example, in a previous ATS survey to evaluate average turnaround time for the interpretation of test results, the authors found the following results: less than 1 day (15%), 1 to 2 days (30%), 3 to 4 days (27%), 5 to 6 days (15%), more than 7 days (3%). This highlights the variability in the process among institutions. A delayed interpretation has the potential to delay the clinical consultation and important therapeutic interventions in patient care. Applying the test results to the patient is the last step in the path of workflow.

Understanding and establishing the path of workflow processes will lead to the needed procedures to develop an effective system for the delivery of patient care in the pulmonary laboratory.

SUMMARY

· The quality systems approach is outlined, with a review of the 12 QSEs and path of workflow as applied to the PF laboratory and blood gases.

· Calibration and verification of spirometers, gas analyzers, D_{LCO} systems, and body plethysmographs are discussed. Special emphasis is placed on techniques to ensure that PF equipment meets established standards of accuracy and precision. QC methods are reviewed, including the use of large-volume syringes, biologic controls, and lung simulators.

· Calibration and QC of blood gas analyzers are discussed, as well as the advantages and disadvantages of automated calibration.

· Basic statistical concepts commonly used in laboratory situations are covered, including the application of multiple control rules.

· Testing technique is a key element in ensuring the validity of PF data. Some guidelines for applying acceptability and repeatability criteria (as listed throughout the text) are given. These include decision making before the test and during testing, assessing test quality for interpretive purposes, and providing feedback on the technologist's performance.

· Infection control and safety issues are presented. Cleaning of spirometers and related equipment and techniques to avoid cross-contamination are described. Standard precautions applicable to blood gas analysis and PF testing are reviewed.

· The QSEs and path-of-workflow concepts incorporated in multiple CLSI quality management documents list five probable outcomes by implementing this approach: the ability to reduce or eliminate medical error, the likelihood of meeting customer expectations, more effective and efficient operations, the potential for successful governmental and accreditation assessments, and sustainable attainment of quality objectives.

CASE STUDIES

CASE 12.1

This case describes the use of blood gas QC to detect analytic errors.

HISTORY

A 30-year-old man who works as a firefighter is referred for PF testing and arterial blood gas analysis as part of a 5-year physical examination required by the fire district for which he works. He has no symptoms or history suggestive of pulmonary disease. He has never smoked. He performed all portions of the spirometry, lung volume, and D_{LCO} maneuvers acceptably. All results were within normal limits for his age and height. Arterial blood gases were drawn for analysis.

Blood Gases	
F_iO_2	0.21
pH	7.41
$Paco_2$ (mm Hg)	39
Pao_2 (mm Hg)	54
HCO_3^- (mEq/L)	24.1
Hb (g/dL)	15.1
Sao_2 (%)	96.0
COHb (%)	1.4
MetHb (%)	0.2

Because of the low Pao_2 in an otherwise normal subject and because Sao_2 measured independently by hemoximetry showed normal saturation, the Po_2 measurement of the automated blood gas analyzer was questioned.

A review of the two most recent automatic calibrations revealed the following:

	Calibration	Expected	Drift
9 AM			
pH	7.387	7.384	0.003
Pco_2 (mm Hg)	39.1	38.6	0.5
Po_2 (mm Hg)	132.0	140.1	− 8.1
10 AM			
pH	7.383	7.384	− 0.001
Pco_2 (mm Hg)	38.4	38.6	− 0.2
Po_2 (mm Hg)	151.2	140.1	11.1

For each automatic calibration, the instrument analyzes a calibration gas or buffer and compares the measured value with an expected value based on the local barometric pressure. Drift is the amount of adjustment applied to a particular electrode to bring it within the expected calibration limits. The drift exhibited by the Po_2 electrode prompted a review of the most recent QC runs performed on the analyzer.

Blood Gas Quality Control (Five Most Recent Po_2 Runs)							
			Runs[a]				
Control	Mean (mm Hg)	SD	1	2	3	4	5
Level A	45	±2.1	46	47	49	42	50
Level B	100	±2.0	101	99	97	96	105
Level C	150	±3.1	147	151	151	149	143

[a]Control runs performed every 8 hours.

QUESTIONS

1. What are the possible explanations for the patient's low P_{O_2}?
2. What is the significance of the 9 AM and 10 AM automated calibrations for the blood gas analyzer?
3. What do the routine QC runs show?
4. What corrective action, if any, might be necessary?

DISCUSSION

Explanation of the Low P_{O_2}

The low P_{O_2} might be caused by lung disease or might be an erroneous reading from the automated blood gas analyzer. An abnormally low Pa_{O_2} in an otherwise healthy person with normal lung function suggests that an analytic error might have occurred. The findings in this case regarding the P_{O_2} electrode function are not unusual. The P_{O_2} is the sole abnormal value; even the Sa_{O_2} measured from the same specimen (but using hemoximetry) shows a normal result. If the subject had been seen with evidence of lung disease or abnormalities in his PF test, the inaccuracy of the Pa_{O_2} might not have been questioned, resulting in inappropriate O_2 therapy.

Automatic Blood Gas Analyzer Calibrations

Excessive drift of the O_2 electrode should have prompted the immediate attention of the technologist performing the blood gas analyses. A common problem with automated analyzers is their apparent simplicity. Because calibrations are performed automatically, corrections that the analyzer makes may be overlooked. Automated analyzers adjust the zero and gain of each electrode or sensor to correct for small changes that occur in electrode performance. These small changes may be caused by a buildup of protein on the electrode, electrolyte depletion, or slight temperature alterations. If there is a large change in electrode performance, the instrument attempts to "correct" the electrode's output just as it would for small changes that occur normally. Some automated analyzers flag a large drift in electrode performance as an error, whereas others simply report the drift. In this case the reported drifts indicated that the P_{O_2} electrode seemed to be fluctuating markedly. One calibration reading was high, and the next one was lower than the expected value.

Quality Controls

The change in electrode performance should have been detected by the routine QC run before the excessive drift was observed during automatic calibration. Blood gas QC used in this laboratory consisted of multiple levels of control materials for the P_{O_2} electrode. Means and SD had been determined for each level.

Examination of control runs 1 through 4 reveals acceptable electrode performance. All values are within ±2 SD of the mean. Run 5 (the most recent run) shows values that are all 2 SD or more away from the mean. These control results may be expected to occur 5% of the time simply because of the random error associated with sampling. If run 5 is compared with the previous four runs and multiple rules are applied (see the section on calibration and quality control of blood gas analyzers), the electrode is clearly out of control. When multiple levels of controls are evaluated, more than one control value outside of the 2-SD limit suggests an out-of-control situation. For both levels A and B, there is a change of 4 SD from run 4 to run 5. Changes of this magnitude are not consistent with random error and are detected only when a control history is kept. Similarly, there are inconsistencies within run 5 across the three levels of controls. Levels A and B both show control values that are more than 2 SD above their respective means, but level C shows a value that is more than 2 SD below its mean. This pattern suggests fluctuating electrode performance as displayed during the automatic calibrations that followed.

Corrective Action

The P_{O_2} electrode was removed, inspected, and replaced. The instrument was recalibrated, and multiple levels of controls were repeated. All P_{O_2} values fell within 2 SD of the established mean. Another specimen was drawn from the subject, and a Pa_{O_2} value of 89 mm Hg was obtained.

CASE 12.2

This case addresses the use of biologic controls in the PF laboratory.

HISTORY

PF studies are performed on three consecutive patients, each of whom has a chief complaint of shortness of breath. The following data are obtained:

	Patient 1	Patient 2	Patient 3
FVC	4.04 (101%)	5.22 (97%)	3.90 (83%)
FEV$_1$	3.51 (99%)	4.10 (103%)	3.12 (82%)
FEV$_{1\%}$	87%	79%	80%
TLC	5.11 (98%)	6.96 (100%)	5.01 (81%)
D$_{LCO}$[a]	14.3 (69%)	18.2 (65%)	10.2 (50%)

[a] Percent of predicted values corrected for Hb.

The PF technologist notices that each subject has apparently normal spirometry and lung volumes but that their D$_{LCO}$ values are reduced.

QUESTIONS

1. Is the reduction in D$_{LCO}$ representative of the actual lung function of each subject, or has a technical problem occurred?
2. What can be done to evaluate the accuracy of the D$_{LCO}$ system?
3. What (if anything) needs to be done to correct the problem?

DISCUSSION
Has a Technical Problem Occurred?

This type of situation arises frequently in the PF laboratory when subjects with possible pulmonary disease are being evaluated. The technologist, in this case, noticed a pattern in which three subjects all had apparently normal results from spirometry and lung volume measurements but displayed reduced D$_{LCO}$ values. Careful attention to inconsistencies in different categories of tests can often point to technical problems with spirometers, gas analyzers, or software. In this case it is difficult to determine whether the low D$_{LCO}$ values may be caused by a physiologic abnormality or a technical problem with the D$_{LCO}$ system.

Evaluating the D$_{LCO}$ System

The first step in assessing a possible technical error would be to look for problems with the D$_{LCO}$ measurement system. In this case pretest calibrations and all other system functions appeared to be acceptable. This facility used a weekly program of testing laboratory personnel as biologic controls. Each of three technologists performed spirometry, lung volumes, and D$_{LCO}$ measurements on one another to establish representative means and standard deviations. The technologist in this case tested one of the biologic controls before performing any further tests on subjects and obtained the following values:

	Biologic Control Result	Expected Value (Control History)
D$_{LCO}$ mL CO/ min/ mm Hg	18.5	27.1 ± 1.5

The biologic control D$_{LCO}$ had been established from a series of 22 previous measurements. The measured value from the biologic control is lower than 3 SD below the expected value (i.e., 27.1 − 4.5 = 22.6). This simple comparison suggests that the D$_{LCO}$ system is malfunctioning and that the results obtained from the three patients in question were most likely erroneous.

What Needs to Be Done?

The use of a biologic control in this case demonstrated that the D$_{LCO}$ system was not functioning properly. This suggests that the low D$_{LCO}$ values obtained from three apparently normal patients do not represent real disease. Although the comparison with a biologic control subject showed that there was a problem, it did not define exactly what was causing the low values.

This laboratory was fortunate to have access to a D$_{LCO}$ simulator (see Fig. 12.3), as described previously. Simulations were performed with two different levels of precision gases. The simulator showed D$_{LCO}$ values that were similarly reduced in comparison to the expected values. Examination of the measured CO and tracer gas concentrations with the simulator revealed that the CO values were significantly higher than expected, resulting in low calculated D$_{LCO}$. The faulty gas analyzer was replaced before any further subject testing was conducted. Both biologic controls and simulations showed acceptable D$_{LCO}$ values after replacement of the analyzer.

SELF-ASSESSMENT QUESTIONS

Entry-Level

1. A PF technologist is checking a small portable spirometer that uses disposable flow sensors. Repeated injections from a 3-L syringe produce the following results: 3.24 L, 3.30 L, and 3.29 L. Which of the following best describes these results?
   a. The flow sensor is defective.
   b. Spirometer shows excessive drift.
   c. Volume is being corrected to BTPS.
   d. Volumes were injected too rapidly.

2. QC is performed on a blood gas analyzer. The P_{CO_2} electrode shows the following results when plotted on a QC chart (Levey–Jennings). Which of the following best describes the result of control run 10?
   a. An out-of-control situation
   b. A trend
   c. A random error
   d. Normal electrode performance

4. When developing a QC program, which of the following devices would the technologist select to determine the FRC_{PL}?
   a. Isothermal bottle
   b. Rotameter
   c. 3-L syringe
   d. Pressure manometer

5. After the subject performs eight FVC maneuvers, these results are recorded from the three best efforts:

	Trial 2	Trial 5	Trial 7
FVC (L)	4.90	5.41	4.79
FEV_1 (L)	1.91	2.01	1.88
PEF (L/sec)	4.90	4.41	4.67

Which of the following comments should the PF technologist use to describe the patient's spirometry?
   a. "Spirometry meets all ATS-ERS criteria."
   b. "FVC is not repeatable."
   c. "FEV_1 is not repeatable."
   d. "Peak flow is not repeatable."

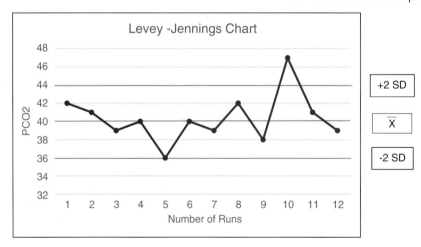

3. The PF laboratory develops and implements a training and orientation guide for new employees. This process is a requirement of which QSE?
   a. Personnel
   b. Process management
   c. Continual improvement
   d. Documents and records

Advanced

6. Daily maintenance of a body plethysmograph should include which of the following?
   1. Calibration of the box pressure transducer
   2. Calibration of the flow sensor (pneumotachometer)
   3. Checking the mouth pressure transducer against a known standard

4. Quality control using an isothermal lung analog
   a. 1 and 3 only
   b. 2 and 4 only
   c. 1 and 2 only
   d. 1, 3, and 4 only

7. A biologic control performs multiple FRC$_{pleth}$ maneuvers to check the accuracy of a variable-pressure body box. The control established FRC is 3.60 L with an SD of 0.15 L. The following FRC values are obtained from the control:
   4.55 L
   4.55 L
   4.49 L
   Based on these findings, the PF technologist should conclude which of the following?
   a. The plethysmograph is functioning within acceptable limits.
   b. The plethysmograph door seal has a small leak.
   c. The mouth pressure transducer has not been calibrated correctly.
   d. The flow sensor has not been calibrated correctly.

8. Which of the following can be used to verify the function of an automated D$_{LCO}$ system?
   1. D$_{LCO}$ simulator
   2. Biologic controls
   3. Isothermal lung analog
   4. 3-L syringe
   a. 1 and 3 only
   b. 1, 2, and 3 only
   c. 1, 2, and 4 only
   d. 2, 3, and 4 only

9. Which of the following is most likely to cause cross-contamination in the PF laboratory?
   a. Disposable mouthpieces and nose clips
   b. Volume-displacement spirometers
   c. Flow-sensing spirometers
   d. Nebulizers used for bronchial challenge

10. A PF technologist simulates D$_{LCO}$sb maneuvers using a 3-L calibration syringe. She turns the BTPS correction off, but all other settings are configured as for patient testing. Three maneuvers produce the following results:
    Trial 1: 0.13 mL CO/min/mm Hg
    Trial 2: –0.20 mL CO/min/mm Hg
    Trial 3: 0.11 mL CO/min/mm Hg
    On the basis of these results, the technologist should conclude that

    a. BTPS corrections should have been on to simulate D$_{LCO}$.
    b. the CO analyzer is malfunctioning.
    c. the signal from the tracer gas analyzer is not linear.
    d. the gas analyzers are functioning properly.

11. Which of the following should the PF technologist do when drawing an arterial blood sample?
    1. Use eye protection if there is a possibility of blood splashing.
    2. Check the patient history to see whether protective barriers are needed.
    3. Wear gloves while drawing and analyzing the specimen.
    4. Dispose of needles and syringes in red plastic bags marked "Biohazard."
    a. 1 and 3 only
    b. 2 and 4 only
    c. 1, 2, and 3 only
    d. 1, 3, and 4 only

12. Which of the following questions does a policy statement answer in the quality manual?
    a. How do we obtain reliable spirometry in our laboratory?
    b. How is quality control performed for the D$_{LCO}$ system?
    c. What is the laboratory's intent for orientation, training, and competence assessment?
    d. How do I do a spirometry linearity check?

13. The equipment software has been updated. Which of the following processes should be verified to ensure data integrity?
    a. Quality control
    b. User security codes
    c. Reference authors
    d. Abbreviations

14. The following interpretation turnaround data were included in the annual quality report:
    Clinic 1: 3 to 4 days
    Clinic 2: less than 1 day
    Clinic 3: greater than 7 days
    Which of the following external pulmonary laboratory customers need to be included in the team to identify potential sources of variability among the clinics?
    a. Patients
    b. Nurses
    c. Technologists
    d. Physicians

SELECTED BIBLIOGRAPHY

General References

American Thoracic Society. (2016). *Pulmonary function laboratory management manual* (3rd ed.). New York, NY: American Thoracic Society.

Guide for Infection Prevention for Outpatient Settings: Minimum expectations for safe care. www.cdc.gov/HAI/settings/outpatient/outpatient-settings.html. (September 2016). Accessed 03.06.20.

Guideline for Isolation Precautions: Preventing transmission of infectious agents in healthcare settings. www.cdc.gov/ncidod/dhqp/gl_isolation_standard.htm. Last updated 2007. Accessed 03.06.20.

Wanger, J. (1997). Quality assurance. *Respiratory Care Clinics of North America, 3,* 273–289.

Standards and Guidelines

CLSI. (2004). *H11-A4, Percutaneous collection of arterial blood for laboratory analysis* (4th ed.). Wayne, PA: Clinical Laboratory Standards Institute.

CLSI. (2006). *HS4-A2, Application of a quality system model for respiratory services, Approved guideline.* Wayne, PA: Clinical Laboratory Standards Institute.

CLSI. (2009). *C46-A2, Blood gas and pH analysis and related measurements.* Wayne, PA: Clinical Laboratory Standards Institute.

CLSI. (2011). *Quality management system: equipment. CLSI document QMS13-A.* Wayne, PA: Clinical Laboratory Standards Institute.

CLSI. (2013). *Assessments: laboratory internal audit program; approved guideline. CLSI document QMS15-A.* Wayne, PA: Clinical and Laboratory Standards Institute.

CLSI (Ed.). (2013). Quality management system: development and management of laboratory documents; approved guideline—6th ed. In *CLSI document QMS02-A6.* Wayne, PA: Clinical and Laboratory Standards Institute.

CLSI. (2013). *Quality management system: leadership and management roles and responsibilities; approved guideline. CLSI document QMS14-A.* Wayne, PA: Clinical and Laboratory Standards Institute.

CLSI. (2013). *The Key to Quality^{TM}. CLSI product K2Q* (2nd ed.). Wayne, PA: Clinical and Laboratory Standards Institute.

CLSI. (2013). Understanding the cost of quality in the laboratory; a report. In *CLSI document QMS20-R.* Wayne, PA: Clinical and Laboratory Standards Institute.

CLSI. (2014). *M29-A4, Protection of laboratory workers from occupationally acquired infection* (4th ed.). Wayne, PA: Clinical Laboratory Standards Institute.

CLSI. (2015). Laboratory personnel management. *CLSI guideline QMS16* (1st ed.). Wayne, PA: Clinical and Laboratory Standards Institute.

CLSI. (2015). Nonconforming event management. *CLSI guideline QMS11* (2nd ed.). Wayne, PA: Clinical and Laboratory Standards Institute.

CLSI. (2015). Process management. *CLSI guideline QMS18* (1st ed.). Wayne, PA: Clinical and Laboratory Standards Institute.

CLSI. (2016). Training and competence assessment. *CLSI document QMS03-A4.* Wayne, PA: Clinical Laboratory Standards Institute.

CLSI. (2019). External assessments, audits, and inspections of the laboratory. *CLSI guideline QMS17* (1st ed.). Wayne, PA: Clinical and Laboratory Standards Institute.

CLSI. (2019). Quality management system: a model for laboratory services, Approved guideline. *CLSI document QMS01-A5.* Wayne, PA: Clinical Laboratory Standards Institute.

Graham, B. L., Brusasco, V., Burgos, F., et al. (2017). 2017 ERS/ATS Standards for single-breath carbon monoxide uptake in the lung. *European Respiratory Journal,* 1–30.

Graham, B. M., Steenbruggen, I., Miller, M. R., et al. (2019). Standardization of Spirometry 2019 Update. An Official American Thoracic Society and European Respiratory Society Technical Statement. *Am J Respir Crit Care Med.,* 2019 Oct 15;200(8): e70–e88.

Miller, M. R., Crapo, R. O., Hankinson, J., et al. (2005). General considerations for lung function testing. *European Respiratory Journal, 26,* 153–161.

Townsend, M. (May 2011). *ACOEM Position Statement. Spirometry in the occupational health setting–2011 update, ACOEM.*

Wanger, J., Clausen, J. L., Coates, A., et al. (2005). Standardisation of the measurement of lung volumes. *European Respiratory Journal, 26,* 511–522.

Calibration and Quality Control

Becker, E., Blonshine, J. M., Bialek, K., Moran, E. M., & Blonshine, S. B. (In Press). Variations in FVC and FEV1 biologic quality control measures in a global multi-center clinical trial. *Respiratory Care.* https://doi.org/10.4187/respicare.09518.

Enright, P. L. (2003). How to make sure your spirometry tests are of good quality. *Respiratory Care, 48,* 773–776.

Ferguson, G. T., Enright, P. L., Buist, A. S., et al. (2000). Office spirometry for lung health assessment in adults:

a consensus statement from the National Lung Health Education Program. *Respiratory Care, 45,* 513–530.

Kozlowski-Templin, R. (1995). Blood gas analyzers. *Respiratory Care Clinics of North America, 1,* 35–46.

Krarup, T. (2001). New QC, process validates new blood gas technology at each measurement. *Clinica Chimica Acta, 307,* 75–85.

Leith, D. E., & Mead, J. (1974). *Principles of body plethysmography.* Bethesda, MD: National Heart, Lung, and Blood Institute, Division of Lung Diseases.

Liistro, G., Vanwelde, C., Vincken, W., et al. (2006). Technical and functional assessment of 10 office spirometers—a multicenter comparative study. *Chest, 130,* 657–665.

Olafsdottir, E., Westgard, J. O., Ehrmeyer, S. S., et al. (1996). Matrix effects and the performance and selection of quality-control procedures to monitor Po_2 measurements. *Clinical Chemistry, 42,* 392–396.

Townsend, M. C., Hankinson, J. L., Lindesmith, L. A., et al. (2004). Is my lung function really that good? Flow-type spirometer problems that elevate test results. *Chest, 125,* 1902–1909.

Westgard, J. O., Groth, T., Aronsson, T., et al. (1977). Performance characteristics of rules for internal quality control: probabilities for false rejection and error detection. *Clinical Chemistry, 23,* 1857.

Westgard rules and multi-rules. www.westgard.com/mltirule.htm. Accessed 06.03.20.

Chapter 13

Reference Values and Interpretation Strategies

DAVID A. KAMINSKY, MD

CHAPTER OUTLINE

LEARNING OBJECTIVES

After studying the chapter and reviewing the figures, tables, and case studies, you should be able to do the following:

Entry-level

1. Identify the reference set recommended for spirometry testing.
2. Determine the methodology used in defining the lower fifth percentile.
3. Understand the key parameter in determining airway obstruction.

Advanced

1. Describe a Z score in determining the lower limit of normal.
2. Define the nuances of the nonspecific pattern and simple versus complex restriction.
3. Understand grading the degree of obstruction in the mixed pattern.

KEY TERMS

all-age approach
correction factor
lower limit of normal (LLN)
mixed pattern

NHANES III
nomogram
nonspecific pattern
parallel shifts

residual standard deviation (RSD)
standard deviation (SD)
upper limit of normal (ULN)
Z score

The chapter provides an overview of selecting appropriate reference sets for the various parameters measured in pulmonary function testing. It discusses the science for the identification of normal or abnormal test results. It also describes "bringing it all together" using an algorithm for the interpretation of a pulmonary function test. The algorithm is not intended to cover all of the nuances one might encounter but is intended to provide a starting point for interpretation. It also offers suggestions for additional tests that may assist in further characterizing the abnormality. Detailed information regarding interpretation for specific test modalities is found in the preceding chapters. Many excellent reviews of interpreting pulmonary function tests are also available in the medical literature.

SELECTING AND USING REFERENCE VALUES

Reference values are important in the interpretation of lung function tests. The technologist and laboratory can ensure their testing equipment and techniques are performed according to international recommendations; however, if they do not select an appropriate reference equation for their specific patient population, the results of the test and the clinical implications for the patient may be compromised. After all, a clinician does not always review specific "numbered" data but whether the results are deemed normal or abnormal. The European Respiratory Society - American Thoracic Society - European Respiratory Society (ERS-ATS) 2021 Interpretation Technical Standard recommends the use of the three (spirometry, DLCO, and lung volumes) GLI reference equations. The laboratory should also ensure that the reference equations used are consistent throughout its organization to reduce intralaboratory variability. An example is a 2011 survey conducted in the greater Cleveland area that noted three different reference sets were used for spirometry alone. Another issue associated with commonly used reference sets is they may be 30 to 40 years old, and the instrumentation and testing techniques have changed significantly (e.g., volume versus flow spirometry, DLCO analyzer

technology). In response to these issues, the ERS, with the involvement of the ATS, assembled the Global Lung Function Initiative (GLI) task force and charged it with establishing improved lung function reference values for populations around the world by merging available data sets obtained using standardized methods.

Reference values for pulmonary function tests are derived by statistical analysis of a population of healthy subjects. These subjects are classified as healthy because they have no history of lung disease. Minimal exposure to risk factors, such as smoking or environmental pollution, is usually considered in selecting these individuals.

All lung function measurements vary in healthy individuals. Some tests vary much more than others. Arterial pH and Pa_{CO_2} have a very narrow range in healthy individuals. However, $FEF_{25\%-75\%}$ may vary by as much as ± 2 L/sec. This variability becomes important when measured values are compared with reference values. Most measurements vary in a predictable way in relation to one or more physical factors.

The physical characteristics that most influence pulmonary function include the following:
- Age
- Sex
- Height (standing/sitting)

By analyzing each pulmonary function variable with regard to the individual's physical characteristics, regression equations can be generated to predict the expected value.

Although age, sex, and height clearly influence pulmonary function, the influence of race or ethnicity is less clear. For example, differences in lung volumes have been described between Caucasians and African Americans, but how much these differences relate to innate biologic differences versus how much they relate to socioeconomic, nutritional, and environmental factors is a matter of debate. Older pulmonary function systems would apply a **"correction factor"** or "adjustment" to reference values for Caucasians to adjust for different races, but no single adjustment is applicable to all measurements. Instead, separate regression equations derived from healthy individuals of each race or ethnic background tested are preferred, and this is the aim of the GLI task force. Race-specific reference values should be used if they are representative of the population the laboratory tests. Self-identification is the accepted standard for defining racial or ethnic background, with no adjustments for mixed percentages. In the case of using the GLI reference standards, patients of mixed heritage should use the "Other" category, which develops a numerical average from values predicted for Caucasians, African Americans, and North- and Southeast Asians.

Spirometry

The GLI 2012 reference set is recommended by the ATS for use in North America, Europe, Australia and New Zealand, Asia, and other areas included in the reference set. The GLI 2012 reference set includes data for individuals in the 3- to 95-year age range using an **all-age approach** and a smooth transition from childhood to adulthood and so is preferred in children and adolescents. The GLI reference set, which included data on more than 74,000 individuals, also derived specific equations for three ethnic groups: African American, Northeast Asian, and Southeast Asian. However, many labs in North America have been using the third National Health and Nutrition Examination Survey (**NHANES III**) reference set for many years. A recent study has shown that there is approximately 89% agreement between the two data sets when they are used to diagnose and grade the severity of obstruction, with most of the differences occurring in older individuals, particularly African American men > 65 years old. The NHANES III reference set may still be used if a laboratory wishes to maintain continuity.

Lung Volumes

Identification of normal lung volume values, specifically functional residual capacity (FRC), residual volume (RV), and total lung capacity (TLC), is more challenging because the amount of published data is limited. Lung volumes are related to body size, with height being the most important variable. An additional factor that should be considered when selecting lung volume reference sets is the testing methodology used in deriving the values (e.g., plethysmography versus dilutional methods).

TABLE 13.1

Common Reference Authors for Lung Volumes

Author	Year	Journal
Adult		
Crapo	1982	*Bulletin Européen de Physiopathologie Respiratoire* 1982; 18:419–427
Goldman	1969	*American Review of Respiratory Diseases* 1969; 79:457–467
Hall (GLI)	2021	*European Respiratory Journal, 57* (3):2000289
Quanjer	1993	*European Respiratory Journal* 1993; 6(Suppl 16):5–40
Stocks	1995	*European Respiratory Journal* 1995; 8:492–506
Pediatric		
Quanjer	1989	*European Respiratory Journal* 1989; 1(Suppl 4): 184S–261S
Hsu	1979	*Journal of Pediatrics* 1979; 5:14–23

The ATS-ERS does not recommend a specific reference set, but a few popular authors are listed in Table 13.1. The GLI task force has just published a technical standard on reference values for static lung volumes. The values are derived from over 7000 measurements in healthy people between 5 and 80 years old. Sufficient data were available only from people of European ancestry. The lung volume values are similar between the methods of gas dilution and body plethysmography in healthy people and tend to be on par with many previously published reference values.

Diffusing Capacity

Although the ATS-ERS did not recommend a specific set of reference equations for diffusing capacity, the GLI task force has published a reference set for DLCO, albeit with the majority of data derived from Caucasians only. These reference values derive from over 9000 measurements in healthy people age 5 to 85 years. In general, the GLI DLCO reference values tend to be lower than many commonly used reference sets. A major problem with DLCO is the large interlaboratory variability seen. Published data have shown that even in a well-controlled clinical trial, intersession variability can range from 10% to 25%. The ATS-ERS statement did recommend that predicted values for alveolar volume (V_A), inspired volume (V_I), and DLco should come from the same source. Fig. 13.1A and B demonstrate the difference in a subject between various DLco predicted equations. A 60-year-old female of average height can have a predicted value ranging from approximately 21 to 27 mL/min/mm Hg, depending on the

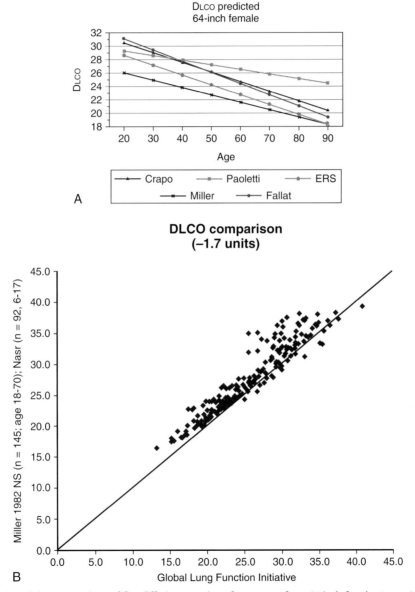

FIG. 13.1 (A) A comparison of five diffusing capacity reference sets for a 64-inch female. Depending on the author selected, the predicted value for a 20-year-old would range from a low of 26 to 31 units or, for a 70-year-old, 20 to 26 units. (B) A comparison between the Miller (adult) and Nasr (pediatric) reference equations against the Global Lung Function Initiative (GLI) predicted equations, ages 11 to 80, male and female. The mean difference was 1.7 units.

reference set selected. Thompson and others published a reference set in middle-aged to older subjects (ages 45–71) that complied entirely with the 2005 ATS-ERS recommendations for testing technique and quality assurance. Their equations compared favorably with those previously published by Miller. Several common reference authors are listed in Table 13.2, but the new GLI reference values are recommended for Caucasians.

Several methods for applying reference values are used:

- Tables of reference values
- Nomograms
- Graphs
- Regression equations used in calculators or software

Tables, nomograms, and graphs are rarely used because of the widespread availability of computerized systems, although the GLI reference set uses a so-called "look-up" table, which is done automatically

TABLE 13.2

Common Reference Authors for Diffusing Capacity

Author	Year	Journal
Adult		
Crapo	1986	*American Review of Respiratory Diseases 1986; 134:856*
Cotes	1993	*European Respiratory Journal* 1993; *6*(Suppl 16):41–52
Stanojevic[a]	2017	*Eur Respir J* 2017; 50:
Knutson	1987	*American Review of Respiratory Diseases 1987; 135:805–811*
Miller	1983	*American Review of Respiratory Diseases 1983; 127:270–277*
Paoletti	1985	*American Review of Respiratory Diseases 1985; 132:806–813*
Thompson	2008	*Thorax* 2008; *63*:889–893
Pediatric		
Hsu	1979	*Journal of Pediatrics* 1979; *95*:14–23
Nasr	1991	*Pediatric Pulmonology* 1991; *10*:267–272

[a] Preferred reference set.

by the software. Peak flowmeters and other simple devices designed for use outside of the clinic or laboratory sometimes use a **nomogram** or printed graph to allow the user to look up a predicted value. The use of computers (or calculators) allows regression equations to be available in software programs. In most automated systems, the user selects sets of prediction equations best suited to the tested population. Some software allows users to enter their own equations or modify published equations. This provides a means of adding new reference equations as they become available.

ESTABLISHING WHAT IS ABNORMAL

Determining the **lower limit of normal (LLN)** should be done by analyzing some measure (e.g., forced vital capacity [FVC], forced expiratory volume in the first second [FEV_1]) in healthy subjects and determining the variability of that measurement. In clinical medicine, the fifth percentile is often defined as the LLN because it represents the segment of healthy subjects farthest below the average. Even though subjects in the fifth percentile are healthy, they are arbitrarily defined as "abnormal" for clinical purposes. Fig. 13.2 depicts the predicted and the LLN for white females from ages 8 to 80 years (NHANES III).

Some clinicians use a fixed percentage (measured value divided by the reference value × 100) of the reference value to determine the degree of abnormality. Eighty percent (80%) is often used as the limit of normal. Unfortunately, this method leads to errors because the variability around the predicted value is relatively constant in adults with different-sized predicted values. In other words, the scatter of normal values does not vary with the size of the predicted value. Fig. 13.3 illustrates why using fixed percentages, such as 80% of the predicted, can lead to misclassification. In tall young subjects, 80% of the predicted is often less than the fifth percentile, so using 80% as the limit can allow a patient who really does have decreased lung function (in the fifth percentile or lower) to be misclassified as normal. This situation is a false-negative result; the patient has disease, but the test does not indicate

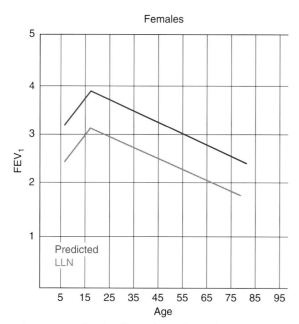

Females

FIG. 13.2 Predicted and lower limit of normal (LLN). The predicted forced expiratory volume in the first second (FEV$_1$) for females ages 8 to 80 years is shown by the upper line (blue) based on the third National Health and Nutrition Evaluation Survey (NHANES III) regression equations for Caucasian adults. The lower line (gray) represents the statistical LLN for the same group. FEV$_1$ increases from ages 8 to 18 years, with the LLN showing a similar pattern. The LLN line represents the 5th percentile.

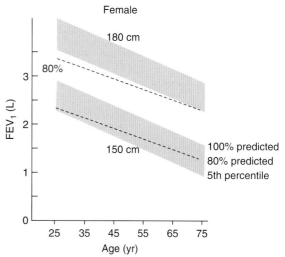

Female

FIG. 13.3 Bias introduced by using percentages of predicted. The graph illustrates the fall in predicted forced expiratory volume in the first second (FEV$_1$) for tall (180 cm) and short (150 cm) females with age. The shaded areas represent the "normal" range from 100% of the predicted value down to the fifth percentile. The *dashed line* shows a fixed percentage of the predicted, in this case 80%, as is sometimes used to represent the lower limit of normal (LLN). For a young, tall female, 80% is less than the statistical lower limit. A subject with a low FEV$_1$ (below the fifth percentile) might still be above 80% of predicted; this would result in a false-negative finding on spirometry. Similarly, a short older female might have an FEV$_1$ below 80% of predicted and be considered to have disease when her FEV$_1$ is actually above the fifth percentile. In this instance the result is a false positive. Similar bias occurs when percentages of predicted are used from adult males because the variability of FEV$_1$ (and other pulmonary function parameters) does not tend to vary with the size of the predicted value. Clinical decisions should be based on well-defined LLNs rather than fixed percentages of predicted (in adults).

abnormality. Similarly, an elderly patient who is short may have a lung function parameter of less than 80% of predicted but well within the statistically normal range (above the fifth percentile). This short, elderly subject would be misclassified as having lung disease when in fact, she is within the "normal" range (i.e., a false-positive result). The use of percentages of predicted introduces both age and height biases. The situation is slightly different in children because the variability of lung function measures tends to change proportionately with the size of the predicted value. For this reason, percentages of predicted values may be reasonable for classifying lung function in children, although the use of the LLN is still recommended.

A more statistically sound approach for classifying abnormality is to compute the **Z score** or standard deviation score (SDS). If lung function varies in a normal fashion (a Gaussian, or bell-shaped, distribution curve; Fig. 13.4), the mean ± 1.96

standard deviation (SD) defines the 95% confidence interval. In other words, statistically, 95% of the healthy population falls within approximately 2 SD of the mean. The remaining subjects fall into either the highest or lowest 2.5% of the distribution. The Z score or SDS can be calculated easily if the variability (**residual standard deviation [RSD]**) of the reference population is known:

$$Z \text{ score} = \frac{(\text{measured} - \text{predicted})}{\text{RSD}}$$

where:

RSD = residual standard deviation

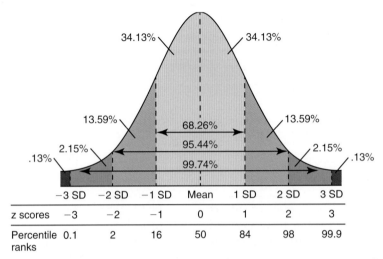

FIG. 13.4 Gaussian distribution curve with Z scores and percentile ranks. Lowest 5% of the reference population is defined as "abnormal."

The RSD is the normal variability that remains when all other sources of variability have been accounted for in the regression. Mathematically, the Z score is the number of SDs the measured value is away from the mean predicted value. If an individual's Z score is less than -1.65, there is only a 5% chance that the test result is normal. If the Z score is less than -1.96, the measured value is found in only 2.5% of healthy subjects.

For example, consider a male subject who is 70 years old and 69 inches (175 cm) tall. His FEV_1 is measured as 2.40 L; his predicted FEV_1 is 3.12 L. His FEV_1 is 77% of predicted; is this abnormal? Using 80% as the cutoff suggests that this patient has mild lung disease. However, if the patient's Z score is calculated as follows:

$$Z \text{ score} = \frac{(2.40 - 3.12)}{0.468}$$
$$= \frac{-0.72}{0.468}$$
$$= -1.53$$

where 0.468 is the residual standard deviation from the reference population, the Z score of -1.53 suggests that this subject is above the fifth percentile and likely has normal lung function. The advantage of Z scores is that they can be used for any index that is normally distributed. Because the Z score accounts for the variability occurring in healthy subjects, it tells how common, or uncommon, the finding may be in the patient being studied.

For many pulmonary function variables, only the LLN (i.e., below the mean) is significant. For example, it is not usually clinically significant if FVC is higher than predicted, only if it is lower. For normally distributed variables, $-1.645 \times$ RSD can be considered the LLN. Variables that can be abnormally high or low (e.g., RV, TLC, $PaCO_2$) must consider the **upper limit of normal (ULN)** in a similar manner ($+1.64 \times$ RSD).

The LLN can be easily calculated when the variable of interest (e.g., FEV_1, FVC) is normally distributed in the population. Using the fifth percentile to define the LLN, however, does not *require* the pulmonary function variable to be normally distributed in the population. Simple counts can determine the level for a specific variable that separates the lowest 5% of the subjects from the remainder. LLNs using the fifth percentile are sometimes defined for specific groupings of age or gender.

There are several areas in which the definition of lung function abnormality may have important clinical consequences. One such area is the use of a fixed ratio to define airway obstruction, as is frequently done with the FEV_1/FVC. The World Health Organization's Global Initiative for Obstructive Lung Disease (GOLD) recommends the use of 0.7 as a cutoff, with ratios less than this value defining the presence of airway obstruction. However, because the FEV₁/FVC ratio falls with age (sex, height, and ethnicity also may play a role), the use of a fixed ratio may misclassify younger subjects as normal *(false negative)* and older subjects as obstructed *(false positive;* Fig. 13.5). Similarly, the use of fixed percentages of predicted (e.g., 80%, 50%) to categorize the severity of obstruction may misclassify subjects who are young and tall or old and short (as discussed in a preceding paragraph). These misapplications of fixed ratios and fixed percentages of predicted can have serious consequences for individual patients and for large groups of subjects when research is involved. Misclassifying an elderly subject as having chronic obstructive pulmonary disease (COPD) based on FEV₁/FVC < 0.7 but > LLN may mean the inappropriate prescription of drugs that can have serious side effects. Similarly, classifying a young person as healthy based on

FEV₁/FVC > 0.7 but < LLN may result in missing an appropriate diagnosis of obstruction based on using the LLN. Note, however, that this issue is controversial, and the use of the fixed ratio of 0.7 may have practical use in determining risk for clinically significant COPD.

Pulmonary function laboratories should try to choose reference studies from a population similar to the patients they test. The following factors may be considerations in selecting reference values:

1. *Type of equipment used for the reference study:* Does equipment comply with the most recent recommendations of the ATS-ERS? (See Chapter 11.)
2. *Methodology:* Were standardized procedures used in the reference study similar to those to be used, particularly for spirometry, lung volumes, and DLCO?
3. *Reference population:* What were the ranges of ages of the individuals in the reference population?

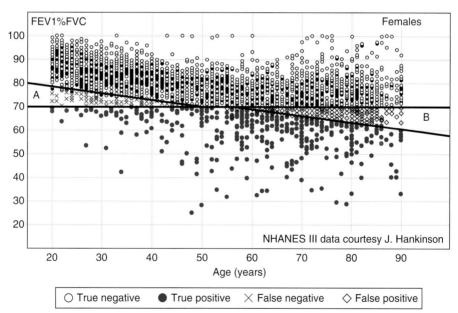

FIG. 13.5 Theoretic sample population of females for the third National Health and Nutrition Evaluation Survey (NHANES III) data set. The figure shows a theoretic sample population of females whose data fit the NHANES III equation for FEV₁/FVC ratio. All subjects plotted as black dots are truly within the normal range. Those plotted in light gray are below the lower limit of normal (LLN) and represent true positives. The subjects less than 40 years of age and plotted in blue x's are false negatives (the Global Initiative for Chronic Obstructive Lung Disease [GOLD] recommendations falsely state they are normal [> 70%] but they are in fact below the LLN), and the black ◊'s in the older population group are those where GOLD recommendations state they are abnormal when in fact they are above the LLN (false positives).

Were both males and females tested? Did the study generate different regressions for different ethnic origins? Did the study include smokers or other at-risk individuals as well as healthy individuals? If a specific group of subjects was studied, are the results applicable to the population in general?

4. *Statistical analysis:* Are LLNs specifically defined (e.g., fifth percentile, –1.645 × RSD)? Are adequate measures of variability available (RSD, standard error of estimate [SEE]) so that upper or lower limits of normal can be calculated along with the predicted values?

5. *Conditions of the study:* Was the study performed at a different altitude or under significantly different environmental conditions?

6. *Published reference equations:* Do reference values generated using the study's regressions differ markedly from other published references?

Individual laboratories may wish to perform measurements on subjects who represent a healthy cross section of the population that the laboratory usually tests. Doing this in a statistically meaningful way may require testing a large number of subjects. However, measured values from these individuals can then be compared with expected values using various reference equations. Equations that produce the smallest average differences (measured − predicted) may be preferable. Evaluation of a small number of individuals may not show much difference between equations for FVC and FEV_1. However, there may be noticeable discrepancies for D_{LCO} or maximal flows. Equations for spirometry, lung volumes, and D_{LCO} should be taken from a single reference if possible. If healthy individuals fall outside of the limits of normal, the laboratory should examine its test methods, how the individuals were selected, and the prediction equations being used.

PULMONARY FUNCTION TESTING INTERPRETATION— "BRINGING IT ALL TOGETHER"

Pulmonary function test interpretation should be structured to facilitate an understanding of the test

> ### BOX 13.1   EXAMPLE PULMONARY FUNCTION TEST INTERPRETATION
>
> Abnormal study. Severe airway obstruction with hyperinflation and air trapping. A significant response to bronchodilator. Diffusing capacity is reduced, which is consistent with a pulmonary parenchymal or vascular process. Oxygen saturation at rest is normal.
> Signature, MD

results by the attending clinician and not to further confuse the clinician. Simply reiterating numbers will not accomplish this goal. Clear, succinct terminology, such as "normal study" or "abnormal study," followed by a brief organized review of the data will be more useful to the ordering physician in caring for the patient (Box 13.1). The reported data should be structured in an organized manner to facilitate the interpretation and understanding of the clinician. Spirometers can calculate a multitude of parameters, and even though they may have benefit in specific circumstances, they serve only to confuse the novice user.

The ATS has recently published a statement recommending a standardized reporting format that will hopefully make the style of reporting more uniform (Fig. 13.6). The most important features of this reporting format are (1) reporting the measured value followed by predicted values, the latter to include the LLN, ULN, or Z score, as appropriate; (2) reporting minimal data from spirometry but to include at least FEV_1, FVC, and FEV_1/FVC (reported as decimal, not percentage), along with flow-volume (F-V) and volume–time tracings for spirometry; (3) displaying plots of inert gas washout or body plethysmography for lung volumes, and rapid gas analysis (when available) for D_{LCO}; (4) reporting the transfer coefficient as KCO rather than D_{LCO}/VA, which can be misleading in interpretation, and adjusting D_{LCO} for barometric pressure and hemoglobin and Co-Hb, as appropriate; and (5) reporting a quality grade to assist the interpreter in judging the validity of the test results as determined by the pulmonary function technologist.

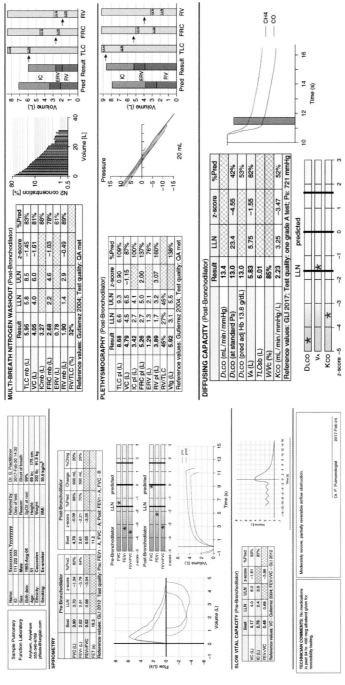

FIG. 13.6 Example of pulmonary function test (PFT) report intended to meet the suggested recommendations according to the American Thoracic Society (ATS) PFT Report Guideline.

INTERPRETATION ALGORITHM

The application of an algorithm to define the major characteristics of lung function allows for a systematic approach to interpretation (Fig. 13.7), although it does not fully describe all of the clinical nuances an interpreter may encounter. Nevertheless, machine learning incorporating such algorithms may achieve a high level of diagnostic accuracy.

Quality Review and "The Graph"

A review of the quality of the data for each testing module (see Chapter 12) and any comments documented by the testing staff are essential in the interpretation process. The interpretation of data that do not meet the ATS-ERS recommendations for acceptability and repeatability or include technologist comments related to poor effort should be conducted with caution. Data that are not repeatable but still "usable" should be noted by the interpreter in the comments (e.g., "subject could not perform repeatable FVCs"). Review of the F-V and volume–time curves can also help the interpreter in assessing quality. A slow start (e.g., back-extrapolation error), cough in the first second, sharp peak flow (e.g., effort), and end-of-forced-expiration (EOFE; formally called the "end-of-test") criteria can all be evaluated visually from the graphic data. The F-V curve can

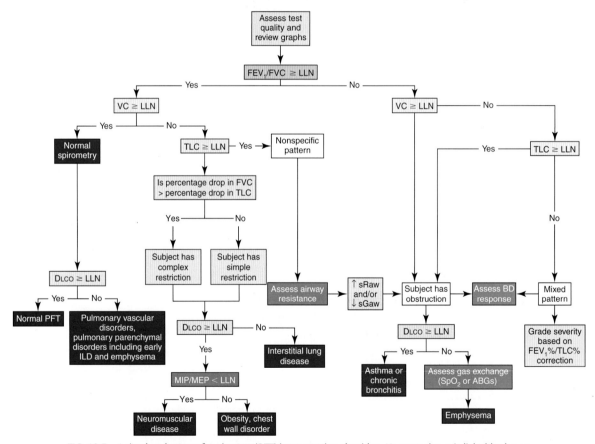

FIG. 13.7   A simple pulmonary function test (PFT) interpretation algorithm. Key steps shown in light-blue boxes. Step 1: Assess quality and review graphs. Step 2: Evaluate "the ratio." Step 3: Assess the vital capacity. Step 4: Assess total lung capacity (TLC). Step 5: Assess D$_{LCO}$. Step 6: Consider the addition of airway resistance, bronchodilator response, respiratory muscle strength, and arterial blood gases (ABGs)/pulse oximetry (medium-blue boxes). Typical diagnostic categories shown in dark-blue boxes. The 2021 ERS-ATS Interpretation Technical Standard emphasizes physiological abnormalities based on PFTs and not clinical diagnoses as shown here.

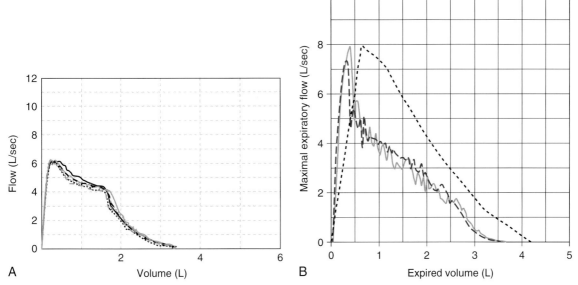

FIG. 13.8 Variants of the flow-volume curve. (A) Normal variant termed a *knee*. (B) Airway noise (not coughing) secondary to "floppy airways" or "redundant tissue" of the upper airway, which is neither specific nor sensitive for obstructive sleep apnea (OSA) but is often seen in patients with OSA.

help define obstructive and restrictive patterns, aid in the assessment of upper airway obstruction (see Chapter 2), and possibly identify normal variants or other abnormalities that may not affect the numbers but may be relevant to the patient's condition (Fig. 13.8A and B). Any spirometry data without the presence of the F-V curve graph, in particular, are just numbers and subject to question.

"The Ratio"

After reviewing the test quality, the first step of the interpretation process is to assess the FEV_1/FVC ratio. If the ratio is less than the LLN, the subject has obstruction. Other parameters such as $FEF_{75\%}$ or $FEF_{25\%-75\%}$ and/or the shape of the F-V curve (concave) may be affected earlier in the obstructive disease process and lead the interpreter to make a statement suggesting that obstruction may be present; however, no parameter has proven better at diagnosing obstruction than FEV_1/FVC.

Next is the assessment of the FVC. If the FVC is greater than the LLN in the presence of a low FEV_1/FVC, the subject has obstruction. If the ratio and the FVC are reduced, the measurement of lung volumes (e.g., TLC) is required to further define the abnormality. If the TLC is normal or elevated with a reduced FEV_1/FVC, this pattern is consistent with obstruction with air trapping or hyperinflation. Assessment of the subject's bronchodilator response may be useful in determining hyperreactive airway disease. If the TLC is reduced along with FEV_1/FVC, the subject has a **mixed pattern** of obstruction and restriction.

The subject has normal spirometry if the ratio is greater than or equal to the LLN and the FVC is also greater than or equal to LLN. However, if the FVC is less than LLN, TLC is required to further evaluate the abnormality. If the TLC is greater than or equal to the LLN when FVC is low and FEV_1/FVC is normal, it is defined as the **nonspecific pattern.** In a study published by Hyatt and others, approximately 70% of their subjects with this pattern had obstruction and/or developed obstruction on follow-up, and the other 30% were morbidly obese. The term **parallel shift** is also used to describe the pattern when both FVC and FEV_1 are reduced with a normal TLC. Airway resistance and bronchodilator response can be used to further assess the nonspecific pattern.

If the FEV_1/FVC ratio is greater than or equal to LLN and the FVC is reduced, spirometry suggests restriction; however, restriction needs to be defined by some measurement of TLC (lung volumes, chest radiograph [CXR], or computerized tomography [CT] scan). If the measured TLC is less than LLN, the subject has restriction. If the TLC and FVC are reduced in approximately the same proportion, this is known as "simple restriction." Sometimes the TLC is reduced proportionally less than the FVC, and this has been called "complex restriction." Complex restriction is most commonly seen whenever a process interferes with lung emptying, such as chest wall limitation (e.g., obesity, kyphoscoliosis), neuromuscular disease, or occult obstruction (e.g., bronchiolitis).

Gas Exchange

Gas exchange can be evaluated by several parameters. Diffusing capacity (D_{LCO}) is used to evaluate the integrity of the alveolar-capillary membrane interface (transfer factor; see Chapter 3), and arterial blood gases (ABGs) or pulse oximetry is used to assess the physiologic effect of a gas exchange abnormality (see Chapter 6). In our algorithmic scheme, we will use the former to determine the effect of the disease process on gas exchange.

If the patient has *obstruction,* mixed pattern, or nonspecific pattern included (see Fig. 13.7B) and the D_{LCO} is greater than or equal to LLN, the data would be consistent with asthma or chronic bronchitis. If the D_{LCO} is less than LLN in this setting, the data would be consistent with emphysema. According to Hadeli and others, when the D_{LCO} is less than 60%, there is a high probability of exercise desaturation and further assessment (i.e., ABGs or pulse oximetry) may be warranted.

If the patient has normal spirometry (see Fig. 13.7A) and the D_{LCO} is greater than or equal to LLN, the subject has a *normal pulmonary function test (PFT).* If the D_{LCO} is less than LLN in this setting, the data would be consistent with a pulmonary vascular disorder (e.g., pulmonary emboli, atrioventricular [A-V] malformation) and/or early pulmonary parenchymal disorders (e.g., interstitial lung disease, emphysema).

If the patient has *restriction* (see Fig. 13.7) and the D_{LCO} is greater than or equal to LLN, consider neuromuscular disease, obesity, and/or chest wall deformities. Further evaluation with respiratory muscular strength measurements (see Chapter 10) may be helpful in differentiating the abnormality. If the D_{LCO} is less than LLN in this setting, the data would be consistent with interstitial lung disease (e.g., pulmonary fibrosis).

Bronchodilator Response (BDR)

Assessing bronchodilator response may be indicated in patients complaining of chest tightness, wheeze, and/or shortness of breath. Furthermore, patients who fall into the categories of obstruction, mixed pattern, and/or nonspecific pattern may specifically warrant bronchodilator testing to further differentiate their underlying abnormality. A complete description of the test methodology and assessment of the response is provided in Chapter 2. The 2021 ERS-ATS Interpretation Technical Standard defines a significant bronchodilator response (BDR) >10% of the predicted value for either FEV1 or FVC. This new criteria being free from bias related to sex or lung size. A decrease in airway resistance of 30% to 40% occurs ($\downarrow$ sRaw or $\uparrow$ sGaw) may also be considered significant. Other methods of defining a significant bronchodilator response based on different thresholds of change in absolute FEV_1 or FVC, or change in percent predicted values or Z scores, have been proposed.

Grading Severity and Assessing Change in Lung Function

The 2021 ERS-ATS Interpretation Technical Standard dramatically simplified the grading scheme by defining the cut-points based in the Z score Table 13.3 a crossed all tests. Gardner and others recently published recommendations for grading the severity of obstruction in a patient with mixed obstruction-restriction if the TLC

TABLE 13.3

2021 ERS-ATS Interpretation 3-Tier system to assess the severity of lung function impairment using z-score values

Z score	
> −1.645	Normal
between −1.65 and −2.5	Mild
between −2.5 and −4	Moderate
< −4	Severe

is known. In their study, they applied an adjustment to FEV_1 percent predicted by dividing the FEV_1 percent predicted by the TLC percent predicted.

Example:

TLC	2.82 L	61% pred
FVC	1.11 L	44% pred
FEV_1	0.68 L	34% pred = very severe obstruction
FEV_1/FVC		61.6%

FEV_1 %predicted/TLC %predicted = 34/61 = 56% = moderately severe obstruction.

In evaluating a patient's change in lung function over time, one needs to take into account the test-to-test variability. The normal rate of decline in FEV_1 is approximately 20 to 30 mL per year in subjects greater than 30 years of age. The 2021 ERS/ATS technical standard has suggested using the FEV_1Q, which is defined as the absolute FEV_1 divided by 0.4L for women or 0.5L for men and indicates how much lung is left relative to a minimum survivable amount of lung. If the FEV_1Q falls more rapidly than 1 unit over 18 years in healthy people or more than 1 unit over 10 years in smokers, this suggests an abnormal, accelerated loss of lung function. A laboratory can also establish its own variability by analyzing its biometric quality control (BioQC;

TABLE 13.4			
Significant Change Over Time			
	FVC	**FEV_1**	**D$_{LCO}$**
Week-to-week			
Normal subjects	≥ 11%	≥ 12%	> 6 units
COPD	≥ 20%	≥ 20%	> 4 units
Year to year	≥ 15%	≥ 15%	10%
Year to year		FEV_1Q*	

COPD, Chronic obstructive pulmonary disease; *FEV_1,* forced expiratory volume in the first second; *FVC,* forced vital capacity.
* See discussion below.
Adapted from American Thoracic Society–European Respiratory Society interpretation guideline. Pellegrino, R., Viegi, G., Brusasco, V., et al. (2005). Interpretive strategies for lung function tests. *European Respiratory Journal, 26,* 948–968.

see Chapter 12) data. The Mayo Clinic Pulmonary Laboratory variability is as follows:

FVC 250 mL; FEV_1 220 mL; TLC 320 mL; DLCO 3.2 units

Table 13.4 summarizes the ATS-ERS recommendations for a clinically significant change over time.

SUMMARY

- The chapter describes the selection of reference values for spirometry, lung volumes, and diffusing capacity.
- It is important to identify the LLN and list some of the more commonly used reference sets, such as for spirometry, lung volumes, and diffusing capacity.
- An algorithm for the interpretation of PFTs can be used and will help establish the cut points used to grade severity.
- More detailed information related to test interpretation is found in specifically labeled chapters.

CASE STUDIES

CASE 13.1

51-year-old male
Weight (Wt): 83.0 kg
Body mass index (BMI): 25.5
Height (Ht): 180.3 cm

	Predicted		Control		Post-Dilator[a]	
	Normal	Range	Found	% Predicted	Found	% Change
Lung Volumes						
TLC (Pleth)	7.01	>5.64	10.75	153%		
VC	5.12	>4.29	5.69	111%		
RV	1.89	<2.46	5.06[b]	268%		
RV/TLC	26.9	<35.3	47.1	175%		
FRC			7.5			
Spirometry						
FVC	5.12	>4.29	5.91[b]	115%	6.39	+9%
FEV$_1$	4.04	>3.36	1.42[b]	35%	1.69[b]	+7%
FEV$_1$/FVC	78.9	>69.7	23.9[b]		26.4[b]	
FEFmax	9.2	>5.8	4.5[b]	49%	4.9[b]	
MVV	157	>124	51[b]	33%		
Diffusing Capacity					Found	% Predicted
D$_{LCO}$	30.9	>22.9			16.9[b]	55%
V$_A$	6.83	>5.64			7.43	109%

FEF, Forced expiratory flow; *MVV,* maximal voluntary ventilation.
[a] Bronchodilator was albuterol.
[b] Outside normal range.

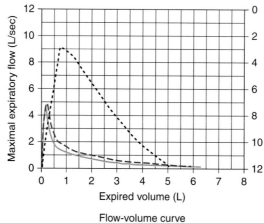

Flow-volume curve

FET

----- Predicted   —— Control   26.9   --- Post dilator   24.9

For Case Studies 13.1 to 13.3, use the interpretation flow chart to characterize the abnormality.

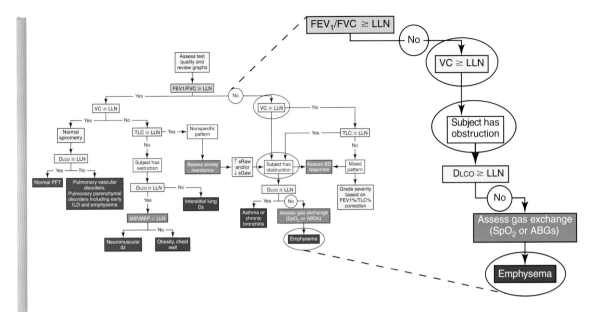

Step 1: Assess quality and review graphs. Good quality—no hesitation, good peak, no cough, expiratory time 26 seconds.
- Concave curve would suggest obstruction.

Step 2: Evaluate "the ratio." Less than LLN = obstruction.

Step 3: Assess the vital capacity. Normal.

Step 4: Assess TLC. Elevated TLC (and RV, not shown in algorithm) suggest hyperinflation and air trapping.

Step 5: Assess D_{LCO}. Less than LLN.

Step 6: Consider the addition of airway resistance, bronchodilator response, respiratory muscle strength, and ABGs/pulse oximetry. Greater than 10% predicted; no bronchodilator response.

INTERPRETATION

Abnormal study. Very severe obstruction with hyperinflation and air trapping. There is not a significant response to bronchodilator. Diffusing capacity is moderately reduced, which is consistent with a pulmonary parenchymal or vascular abnormality.

The subject had alpha-1 antitrypsin deficiency.

CASE 13.2

57-year old male
Wt: 99.1 kg
BMI: 31.8 (exceeds 95th percentile)
Ht: 176.6 cm

	Predicted		Control		Post-Dilator[a]	
	Normal	Range	Found	% Predicted	Found	% Change
Lung Volumes						
TLC (Pleth)	6.73	>5.36	3.86[b]	57%		
VC	4.71	>3.87	2.48[b]	53%		
RV	2.02	<2.63	1.38	68%		
RV/TLC	30.0	<39.3	35.8	119%		
FRC			2.4			
Spirometry						
FVC	4.71	>3.87	2.42[b]	51%	2.47[b]	+1%
FEV$_1$	3.70	>3.02	1.98[b]	53%	2.09[b]	+3%
FEV$_1$/FVC	78.5	>69.3	81.7		84.4	
FEFmax	8.6	>5.2	7.3	85%	8.3	+13%
MVV	145	>112	93[b]	65%		
Diffusing Capacity					Found	% Predicted
D$_{LCO}$	28.9	>20.9			9.5[b]	33%
D$_{LCO}$ (adjusted for Hgb = 13.9 gm/dL)					9.7[b]	34%
V$_A$	6.51	>5.36			3.31[b]	51%

[a] Bronchodilator was albuterol.
[b] Outside normal range.

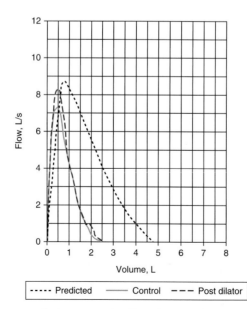

For Case Studies 13.1 to 13.3, use the interpretation flow chart to characterize the abnormality.

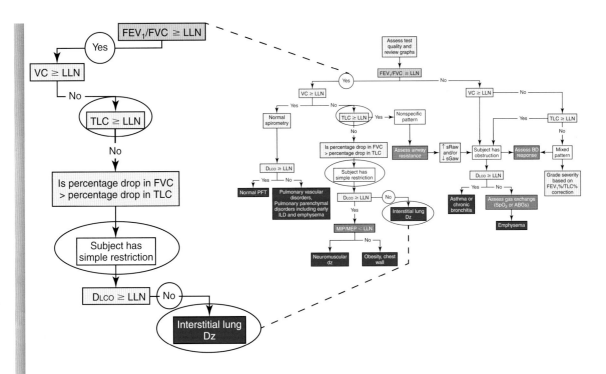

Step 1: Assess quality and review graphs. Good quality—no hesitation, good peak, no cough, expiratory time 7 seconds.
- Peaked "witch's hat" curve would suggest restriction.

Step 2: Evaluate "the ratio." Greater than LLN = normal or restriction.

Step 3: Assess the vital capacity. Reduced vital capacity suggests restriction by spirometry.

Step 4: Assess TLC. Reduced TLC is consistent with restriction.

Step 5: Assess D_{LCO}. Less than LLN.

Step 6: Consider the addition of airway resistance, bronchodilator response, respiratory muscle strength, and ABGs/pulse oximetry. No bronchodilator response.
- High probability of exercise-induced desaturation.

INTERPRETATION

Abnormal study. Moderately severe restriction with no response to bronchodilator. Diffusing capacity is moderately reduced, which is consistent with a pulmonary parenchymal or vascular abnormality.

Subject has pulmonary fibrosis.

CASE 13.3

62-year-old male
Wt: 91.1 kg
BMI: 25.4
Ht: 189.4 cm

	Predicted		Control	
	Normal	Range	Found	% Predicted
Lung Volumes				
TLC (Pleth)	7.70	>6.33	5.71[a]	74%
VC	5.60	>4.76	3.20[a]	57%
RV	2.11	<2.74	2.51	119%
RV/TLC	27.4	<35.9	44.0	161%
FRC			3.5	
Spirometry				
FVC	5.60	>4.76	3.16[a]	56%
FEV$_1$	4.26	>5.58	2.15[a]	51%
FEV$_1$/FVC	76.1	>66.9	68.1	
FEFmax	9.6	>6.2	5.6	58%
MVV	153	>120	86	56%
Diffusing Capacity				
D$_{LCO}$	29.9	>21.9	26	87%
V$_A$	7.50	>6.33	5.20[a]	69%

[a] Outside normal range.

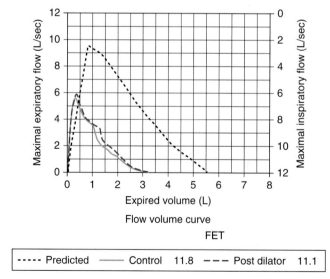

Flow volume curve

FET

····· Predicted ——— Control 11.8 – – – Post dilator 11.1

For Case Studies 13.1 to 13.3, use the interpretation flow chart to characterize the abnormality.

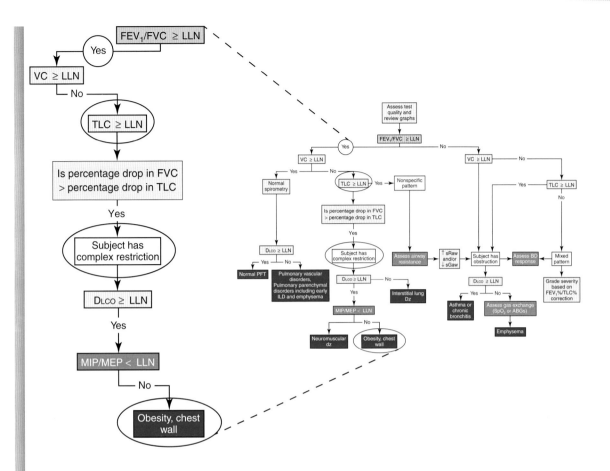

Step 1: Assess quality and review graphs. Good quality—no hesitation, good peak, no cough, expiratory time 11.8 seconds.
- F-V curve has a "knee," which is a normal variant.

Step 2: Evaluate "the ratio." Greater than LLN = normal or restriction.

Step 3: Assess the vital capacity. Reduced vital capacity suggests restriction by spirometry.

Step 4: Assess TLC. Reduced TLC, with reduction in FVC greater than reduction in TLC, is consistent with restriction, and specifically complex restriction.

Step 5: Assess DLCO. Greater than LLN.

Step 6: Consider the addition of airway resistance, bronchodilator response, respiratory muscle strength, and ABGs/pulse oximetry. No other tests ordered. Respiratory muscle strength would have been indicated, but he had an obvious chest wall abnormality, so it was not needed.

INTERPRETATION

Abnormal study. Mild restriction based on TLC. Diffusing capacity is within normal limits.

Subject has scoliosis.

SELF-ASSESSMENT QUESTIONS

Entry-level

1. What parameter is used to identify airway obstruction?
   a. FEV_1
   b. FVC
   c. FEV_1/FVC ratio
   d. TLC

2. The following data are obtained during a PFT:

TLC	4.52 L	88% pred
FVC	2.02 L	55% pred
FEV_1	1.51 L	52% pred

   With which pattern are these data most consistent?
   a. Obstruction
   b. Restriction
   c. Mixed
   d. Nonspecific

3. In a patient with a nonspecific pattern, which testing adjunct may be the most helpful in further evaluating the patient?
   a. Airway resistance
   b. Respiratory muscle strength
   c. Arterial blood gases
   d. Exhaled nitric oxide

4. The following data are obtained during a PFT:

TLC	6.56 L	99% pred
FVC	3.50 L	76% pred
FEV_1	2.09 L	57% pred

   With which pattern are these data most consistent?
   a. Obstruction
   b. Restriction
   c. Mixed
   d. Nonspecific

5. A patient with a neuromuscular disease process will most likely have which of the following PFT patterns?
   a. Obstruction
   b. Restriction
   c. Mixed
   d. Nonspecific

Advanced

6. What is another term for the Z score?
   a. Lower limit of normal
   b. Coefficient of variation
   c. Residual standard
   d. Standard deviation score

7. The following data are obtained during a PFT:

TLC	4.69 L	68% pred
FVC	3.04 L	63% pred
FEV_1	2.37 L	63% pred
D_{LCO}	16.1	56% pred

   With which of the following are these data most consistent?
   a. Neuromuscular disease
   b. Chest wall abnormality
   c. Interstitial lung disease
   d. Emphysema

8. A patient with COPD returns 6 months after the initial PFT for follow-up testing. What is the criterion for a significant change in FEV_1?
   a. 12% or 200 mL
   b. 15%
   c. 20% or 250 mL
   d. 10%

9. The following data are obtained during a PFT:

TLC	4.45 L	93% pred
FVC	2.30 L	81% pred
FEV_1	1.76 L	78% pred
D_{LCO}	10.1	50% pred

   With which of the following are these data most consistent?
   a. Neuromuscular disease
   b. Interstitial lung disease
   c. Pulmonary vascular disease
   d. Emphysema

10. What is the criterion for a significant change following bronchodilator when using airway resistance to assess response?
   a. 35%
   b. 12%
   c. 15%
   d. 25%

SELECTED BIBLIOGRAPHY

General

Bhatt, S., et al. (2019). Discriminative accuracy of FEV1:FVC thresholds for COPD-related hospitalization and mortality. *JAMA, 321*, 2438–2447.

Braun, L. (2015). Race, ethnicity and lung function: a brief history. *Can J Respir, 51*, 99–101.

Clay, R. D., et al. (2017). The "Complex Restrictive" Pulmonary Function Pattern. Clinical and radiologic analysis of a common but previously undescribed restrictive pattern. *Chest, 152*, 1258–1265.

Culver, B. H., et al. (2017). Recommendations for a Standardized Pulmonary Function Report. An Official American Thoracic Society Technical Statement. *Am J Respir Crit Care Med, 196*, 1463–1472.

Dempsey, T. M., & Scanlon, P. D. (2018). Pulmonary function tests for the generalist: A brief review. *Mayo Clin Proc, 93*, 763–771.

European Respiratory Society Global Lung Initiative (GLI). (2012). Task Force published the multi-ethnic reference values for spirometry for the 3–95-year age range: The Global Lung Function 2012 Equations. *European Respiratory Journal, 40*, 1324–1343.

Gardner, Z., Ruppel, G., & Kaminsky, D. A. (2011). Grading the severity of obstruction in mixed obstructive–restrictive lung disease. *Chest, 140*, 598–603.

Hadeli, K. O., Siegel, E. M., Sherrill, D. L., et al. (2001). Predictors of oxygen desaturation during submaximal exercise in 8,000 patients. *Chest, 120*, 88–92.

Huprikar, N. A., et al. (2019). A comparison of Global Lung Initiative 2012 with Third National Health and Nutrition Examination Survey Spirometry Reference Values. *Implications in Defining Obstruction. Ann Am Thoracic Soc, 16*, 225–230.

Hyatt, R. E., Cowl, C. T., Bjoraker, J. A., & Scanlon, P. D. (2009). Conditions associated with an abnormal nonspecific pattern of pulmonary function tests. *Chest, 135*, 419–424.

Kaminsky, D. A. (2019). What is a significant bronchodilator response? *Annals Am Thoracic Soc, 16*, 1495–1497.

Pelegrino, R., Viegi, G., Brusasco, V., et al. (2005). Interpretative strategies for lung function tests. *European Respiratory Journal, 26*, 948–968.

Quanjer, P. H.http://www.spirxpert.com/refvalues.htm and http://www.spirxpert.com/refvalueschild.htm. Accessed 12.11.16.

Quanjer, P. H., Pretto, J. J., Brazzale, D. J., & Boros, P. W. (2014). Grading the severity of airways obstruction: new wine in new bottles. *Eur Respir J., 43*, 505–512.

Stanojevic, S., Kaminsky, D. A., Miller, M., et al. (2021). ERS/ATS technical standard on interpretive strategies for routine lung function tests. *European Respiratory Journal* (in press).

Topalovic, M., et al. (2019). Artificial intelligence outperforms pulmonologists in the interpretation of pulmonary function tests. *Eur Respir J, 53*.

Vestbo, J., Edwards, L. D., Scanlon, P. D., et al. (2011). Changes in forced expiratory volume in 1 second over time in COPD. *New England Journal of Medicine, 365*(Suppl. 13), 1184–1192.

Spirometry

Crapo, R. O., Morris, A. H., & Gardner, R. M. (1981). Reference spirometric values using techniques and equipment that meet ATS recommendations. *American Review of Respiratory Diseases, 123*, 659–664.

Enright, P. L., Kronmal, R. A., Higgins, M., et al. (1993). Spirometry reference values for women and men 65 to 85 years of age. *American Review of Respiratory Diseases, 147*, 125–133.

Falaschetti, E., Laiho, J., Primatesta, P., et al. (2004). Prediction equations for normal and low lung function from the Health Survey for England. *European Respiratory Journal, 23*, 456–463.

Graham, B. L., Steenbruggen, I., & Miller, M. R. (2019). Standardization of Spirometry 2019 Update. *American Journal of Respiratory and Critical Care Medicine, 200*(8), e70–e88.

Hankinson, J. L., Odencrantz, J. R., & Fedan, K. B. (1999). Spirometric reference values from a sample of the general U.S. population. *American Journal of Respiratory and Critical Care Medicine, 159*, 179–187.

Knudson, R. J., Lebowitz, M. D., Holberg, C. J., et al. (1983). Changes in the normal maximal expiratory flow-volume curve with growth and aging. *American Review of Respiratory Diseases, 127*, 725–734.

Quanjer, P. H., et al. (2012). Multi-ethnic reference values for spirometry for the 3-95 year age range: the global lung function 2012 equations. *Eur Respir J, 40*, 1324–1343.

Quanjer, P. H., Tammeling, G. J., Cotes, J. E., et al. (1993a). Lung volume and forced ventilatory flows. Report Working Party Standardization of lung function tests. Official Statement European Respiratory Society. *European Respiratory Journal, 6*(Suppl. 16), 5–40.

Stanojevic, S., Wade, A., Stocks, J., et al. (2008). Reference ranges for spirometry across all ages. *American Journal of Respiratory and Critical Care Medicine, 177*, 253–260.

Wang, X., Dockery, D. W., Wypij, D., et al. (1993). Pulmonary function between 6 and 18 years of age. *Pediatric Pulmonology, 15*, 75–88.

Lung Volumes

Crapo, R. O., Morris, A. H., Clayton, P. D., et al. (1982). Lung volumes in healthy nonsmoking adults. *Bulletin Européen de Physiopathologie Respiratoire, 18*, 419–427.

Goldman, H. I., & Becklake, M. R. (1969). Respiratory function tests: normal values at medium altitudes and the prediction of normal results. *American Review of Respiratory Diseases, 79*, 457–467.

Hall, G. L., Filipow, N., Ruppel, G., et al. (2021). Official ERS technical standard: Global Lung Function Initiative reference values for static lung volumes in individuals of European ancestry. *European Respiratory Journal, 57*(3), 2000289.

Quanjer, P. H., Stocks, J., Polgar, G., et al. (1989). Compilation of reference values for lung function measurements in children. *European Respiratory Journal, 1*(Suppl. 4), 184S–261S.

Quanjer, P. H., Tammeling, G. J., Cotes, J. E., et al. (1993b). Lung volumes and forced ventilatory flows. Report Working Party Standardization of Lung Function Tests, European Community for Steel and Coal. Official Statement of the European Respiratory Society. *European Respiratory Journal, 6*(Suppl. 16), 5–40.

Stocks, J., & Quanjer, P. H. (1995). Reference values for residual volume, functional residual capacity and total lung capacity. *European Respiratory Journal, 8*, 492–506.

Diffusing Capacity

Bates, D. V., Macklem, P. T., & Christie, R. V. (1971). *Respiratory function in disease* (2nd ed.). Philadelphia, PA: WB Saunders.

Crapo, R. O., & Morris, A. H. (1981). Standardized single-breath normal values for carbon monoxide diffusing capacity. *American Review of Respiratory Diseases, 123*, 185–189.

Graham, B. L., Brusasco, V., Burgos, F., et al. (2017). ERS/ATS standards for single-breath carbon monoxide uptake in the lung. *European Respiratory Journal*.

Hsu, K. H. K., Bartholomew, P. H., Thompson, V., et al. (1979). Ventilatory functions of normal children and young adults—Mexican-American, white, and black. I. Spirometry. *Journal of Pediatrics, 95*, 14–31.

Knudson, R. J., Kaltenborn, W. T., Knudson, D. E., et al. (1987). The single-breath carbon monoxide diffusing capacity: reference equations derived from a healthy nonsmoking population and effects of hematocrit. *American Review of Respiratory Diseases, 135*, 805–811.

Miller, A., Thornton, J. C., Warshaw, R., et al. (1983). Single breath diffusing capacity in a representative sample of the population of Michigan, a large industrial state. *American Review of Respiratory Diseases, 127*, 270–277.

Nasr, S. Z., Amato, P., & Wilmott, R. W. (1991). Predicted values for lung diffusing capacity in healthy children. *Pediatric Pulmonology, 10*, 267–272.

Paoletti, P., Viegi, G., Pistelli, G., et al. (1985). Reference equations for the single-breath diffusing capacity: a cross-sectional analysis and effect of body size and age. *American Review of Respiratory Diseases, 132*, 806–813.

Polgar, G., & Promadhat, V. (1971). *Pulmonary function testing in children: techniques and standards*. Philadelphia, PA: WB Saunders.

Roca, J., Rodriguez-Roisin, R., Cobo, E., et al. (1990). Single-breath carbon monoxide diffusing capacity prediction equations from a Mediterranean population. *American Review of Respiratory Diseases, 141*, 1026–1032.

Stanojevic, S., et al. (2017). Official ERS technical standards: Global Lung Function Initiative reference values for the carbon monoxide transfer factor for Caucasians. *Eur Respir J, 50*, 1700010.

Thompson, B. R., Johns, D. P., Bailey, M., et al. (2008). Prediction equations for single-breath diffusing capacity in a middle aged Caucasian population. *Thorax, 63*, 889–893.

Answers to Self-Assessment Questions

CHAPTER 1, INDICATIONS FOR PULMONARY FUNCTION TESTING

1. c   2. b   3. c   4. b   5. b   6. a   7. c
8. c   9. b   10. d   11. d   12. b   13. a   14. b

CHAPTER 2, SPIROMETRY

1. b   2. c   3. c   4. b   5. b   6. d   7. b   8. b   9. c   10. a   11. c   12. b

CHAPTER 3, DIFFUSING CAPACITY TESTS

1. b   2. d   3. d   4. b   5. c   6. c   7. d   8. b   9. a   10. c

CHAPTER 4, LUNG VOLUMES, AIRWAY RESISTANCE, AND GAS DISTRIBUTION TESTS

1. a   2. c   3. b   4. c   5. c   6. c   7. c
8. c   9. c   10. c   11. b   12. d   13. d   14. a

CHAPTER 5, VENTILATION AND VENTILATORY CONTROL TESTS

1. b   2. c   3. c   4. b   5. a   6. d   7. d   8. a   9. c   10. a   11. a

CHAPTER 6, BLOOD GASES AND RELATED TESTS

1. a   2. c   3. c   4. c   5. b   6. c   7. b   8. d   9. c   10. a

CHAPTER 7, CARDIOPULMONARY EXERCISE TESTING AND FIELD TESTS

1. c   2. b   3. c   4. b   5. c   6. d   7. a   8. c   9. c   10. d   11. c   12. a

CHAPTER 8, PEDIATRIC PULMONARY FUNCTION TESTING

1. b   2. a   3. a   4. a   5. c   6. d   7. b   8. d   9. b   10. a
11. b   12. b   13. d   14. d   15. c   16. b   17. d   18. c   19. d   20. d

CHAPTER 9, BRONCHOPROVOCATION CHALLENGE TESTING

1. a   2. c   3. d   4. c   5. c   6. d   7. a   8. b   9. a   10. c

CHAPTER 10, SPECIALIZED TESTS AND EVALUATIONS

1. a   2. b   3. d   4. c   5. c   6. d   7. c   8. b   9. a   10. d

CHAPTER 11, PULMONARY FUNCTION TESTING EQUIPMENT

1. c   2. c   3. b   4. c   5. b   6. d   7. a   8. c   9. d   10. d
11. b   12. a   13. c   14. d   15. d

CHAPTER 12, QUALITY SYSTEMS IN THE PULMONARY FUNCTION LABORATORY

1. c   2. a   3. a   4. a   5. b   6. c   7. c   8. c   9. d   10. d
11. a   12. c   13. a   14. d

CHAPTER 13, REFERENCE VALUES AND INTERPRETATION STRATEGIES

1. c   2. d   3. a   4. a   5. b   6. d   7. c   8. b   9. c   10. a

Index

Note: Page numbers followed by *f* indicate figures, *t* indicate tables, and *b* indicate boxes.